OXFORD MEDICAL PUBLICATIONS

Molecular Biology and Pathology of Paediatric Cancer

Oxford University Press makes no representation, express or implied, that the drug dosages in this book are correct. Readers must therefore always check the product information and clinical procedures with the most up to date published product information and data sheets provided by the manufacturers and the most recent codes of conduct and safety regulations. The authors and the publishers do not accept responsibility or legal liability for any errors in the text or for the misuse or misapplication of material in this work.

Molecular Biology and Pathology of Paediatric Cancer

Edited by

CATHERINE J. CULLINANE
Department of Pathology
St James's University Hospital
Leeds, UK

SUSAN A. BURCHILL
Candlelighter's Children's Cancer Research Laboratory
Cancer Research UK Clinical Centre
St James's University Hospital
Leeds, UK

JEREMY A. SQUIRE
Ontario Cancer Institute
Division of Cellular and Molecular Biology
University of Toronto, Canada

JOHN J. O'LEARY
Department of Pathology
Coombe Women's Hospital,
St. James's Hospital, and Trinity College
Dublin, Ireland

IAN J. LEWIS
Yorkshire Regional Centre for Paediatric Oncology and Haematology
St James's University Hospital
Leeds, UK

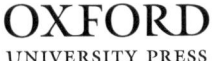

OXFORD
UNIVERSITY PRESS

Great Clarendon Street, Oxford OX2 6DP
Oxford University Press is a department of the University of Oxford.
It furthers the University's objective of excellence in research, scholarship,
and education by publishing worldwide in
Oxford New York
Auckland Bangkok Buenos Aires Cape Town Chennai
Dar es Salaam Delhi Hong Kong Istanbul Karachi Kolkata
Kuala Lumpur Madrid Melbourne Mexico City Mumbai Nairobi
São Paulo Shanghai Taipei Tokyo Toronto

Oxford is a registered trade mark of Oxford University Press
in the UK and in certain other countries

Published in the United States
by Oxford University Press Inc., New York

© Oxford University Press, 2003

The moral rights of the authors have been asserted
Database right Oxford University Press (maker)

First published 2003

All rights reserved. No part of this publication may be reproduced,
stored in a retrieval system, or transmitted, in any form or by any means,
without the prior permission in writing of Oxford University Press,
or as expressly permitted by law, or under terms agreed with the appropriate
reprographics rights organization. Enquiries concerning reproduction
outside the scope of the above should be sent to the Rights Department,
Oxford University Press, at the address above

You must not circulate this book in any other binding or cover
and you must impose this same condition on any acquirer

A catalogue record for this title is available from the British Library
Library of Congress Cataloging in Publication Data
(Data available)

ISBN 0 19 263079 2 (Hbk)

10 9 8 7 6 5 4 3 2 1

Typeset by Newgen Imaging Systems (P) Ltd., Chennai, India
Printed in Great Britain
on acid-free paper by
CPI Bath, Bath

For children everywhere with cancer

Foreword

The management of children with cancer has become a paradigm of cancer care for patients of all ages. The multidisciplinary team approach involving oncologists, surgeons, radiologists, clinical scientists, nurses, and other specialists operates on a basis of mutual respect and understanding for the roles of all disciplines. Such understanding develops through close clinical liaison but is much facilitated by the availability of readily accessible information sources which educate and guide practitioners.

This excellent book fulfils that purpose to the fullest extent. In this age of electronic media and the Internet one can be deluged with information, much of it unhelpful or misleading. In order to see the big picture, publications such as this are vital. The care of a child with cancer requires a comprehensive understanding of the biology of the disease, the diagnostic methodologies, and the way in which these impact on treatment decisions. The editors and authors of this book are to be highly commended for the quality and clarity of the text. This book is relevant not only to clinical scientists and pathologists but also to oncologists and other clinicians. It represents a one stop, comprehensive source of information and can only broaden the horizons of all those who read it. The true beneficiaries of this book will be children with cancer, for with accessible information sources such as this the quality of care can only be improved.

Allan G. Howatson
Consultant Paediatric Pathologist
Royal Hospital for Sick Children
Glasgow

Preface

Are you a clinician or scientist working in paediatric oncology who wishes to understand current developments in molecular pathology as applied to your field? Then this is the book for you! It is a broad ranging review focusing on the impact of molecular and cytogenetic techniques on understanding of the aetiology, clinical behaviour, diagnosis, and management of paediatric cancer. The first section outlines the laboratory handling of tissue samples, theory, and methodology of cytogenetic and molecular techniques and discusses predisposition syndromes. The second section highlights the application of cytogenetic and molecular methods in diagnosis and treatment of the major paediatric cancers.

C.J. Cullinane
S.A. Burchill
J.A. Squire
J.J. O'Leary
I.J. Lewis

Contents

List of contributors	xi
List of abbreviations	xiii
An introduction to children's cancer and the patient pathway *Ian J. Lewis*	1

Section 1 Methods and Clinical Application

1	Cells, tissues, and the diagnostic laboratory *Catherine J. Cullinane, Susan A. Burchill, John J. O'Leary*	15
2	Methods of genetic analysis applied to pediatric cancer *Jane Bayani, Maria Zielenska, Jeremy A. Squire*	37
3	Blots, dots, amplification, and sequencing *John J. O'Leary, Cara Martin, Orla Sheils*	56
4	Familial and predisposition syndromes *Eamonn G. Sheridan, C. Geoffrey Woods*	74

Section 2 Childhood Cancers

5	Leukemia *Sheila Weitzman, Jeremy A. Squire*	95
6	Lymphoma *Mary V. Gresik*	115
7	Tumors of the central nervous system and eye *Venita Jay, Jeremy A. Squire, Maria Zielenska*	136
8	Neuroblastoma *Sadick Variend, Susan A. Burchill*	155
9	Primitive neuroectodermal tumours *Catherine J. Cullinane, Susan A. Burchill*	171
10	Rhabdomyosarcoma *Ivo Leuschner*	186
11	Malignant soft tissue tumors of childhood *J. Robert Thomas, David M. Parham*	199
12	Pediatric renal neoplasms *Pedram Argani, Elizabeth J. Perlman*	217
13	Bone tumors (excluding Ewing's sarcoma) *Walter C. Bell, Gene P. Siegal*	238

14	Germ cell tumours *Elizabeth S. Gray*	247
15	Liver tumors *Milton J. Finegold*	264
16	Carcinoma *Catherine J. Cullinane, John J. O'Leary*	299

Glossary of molecular terms — 319

Index — 323

Contributors

Argani, Pedram, MD
Paediatric Pathologist, The National Wilms Tumor Study Group Pathology Center, Department of Pathology, The Johns Hopkins Medical Institutions, 600 North Wolfe Street, Baltimore, Maryland USA 21287

Bayani, Jane, BSc
University Health Network, Ontario Cancer Institute and the Departments of Laboratory Medicine and Pathobiology, and Medical Biophysics University of Toronto, Ontario, Canada

Bell, Walter C., MD
Division of Anatomic Pathology, Department of Pathology, The University of Alabama at Birmingham, 506 Kracke Building, 619 south 19th Street, Birmingham, Alabama 35233-6823, USA

Burchill, Susan A., PhD
Senior Scientist, Candlelighter's Children's Cancer Research Laboratory, Cancer Research UK Clinical Centre, St James's University Hospital, Leeds LS9 7TF, United Kingdom

Cullinane, Catherine J., MB, FRCPath
Paediatric Pathologist, Department of Pathology, St James's University Hospital, Leeds LS9 7TF, United Kingdom

Finegold, Milton J., MD
Professor of Pathology and Paediatrics, Department of Pathology, Texas Children's Hospital, 6621 Fannin Street, MC 1-2261, Houston, Texas 77030-2399, USA

Gresik, Mary V. MD
Associate Professor of Pathology, Baylor College of Medicine, Houston, Texas
Department of Pathology, Texas Children's Hospital, 6621 Fannin Street, MC 1-2261, Houston, Texas 77030-2399, USA

Gray, Elizabeth S. MB, FRCPath
Paediatric Pathologist, Department of Pathology, University Medical Buildings, University of Aberdeen, Foresterhill, Aberdeen AB25, 2ZD, Scotland

Jay, Venita, MD, FRCPC
Associate Professor, Departments of Laboratory Medicine and Pathobiology and Ophthalmololgy, The University of Toronto Neuropathologist and ophthalmic pathologist, Department of Pathology, The Hospital for Sick Children and Women's College Hospital, 555 University Avenue, Toronto M5G 1X8, Ontario, Canada

Leuschner, Ivo, MD, PhD
Pathologist, Institut für Paidopathologie, Universitätsklinikum Kiel, Michaelisstrasse 11, 24105 Kiel, Germany

Lewis, Ian J., MD
Paediatric Oncologist, Yorkshire Regional Centre for Paediatric Oncology and Haematology, St James's University Hospital, Beckett Street, Leeds LS9 7TF, United Kingdom

Martin, Cara, MSc
Pathology Department, Coombe Women's Hospital and Trinity College, Dublin, Ireland

O'Leary John J., MD, PhD, MSc, FRCPath
Professor of Pathology, Trinity College Dublin, and Pathologist, Coombe Women's Hospital and St James's Hospital, Dolphins Barn, Dublin, Ireland

Parham, David M., MD
Pediatric Pathologist, Departments of Pathology, University of Arkansas for Medical Sciences and Arkansas Children's Hospital, Little Rock, AR, USA

Perlman, Elizabeth J., MD
Pediatric Pathologist, The National Wilms' Tumor Study Group Pathology Center, Department of Pathology, The Johns Hopkins Medical Institutions, 600 North Wolfe Street, Baltimore, Maryland USA 21287

Shiels, Orla, PhD
Pathology Department, Trinity College, Dublin, Ireland

Sheridan, Eamonn G., MB
Clinical Geneticist, Yorkshire Regional Genetics Service, St James's University Hospital, Beckett Street, Leeds LS9 7TF, United Kingdom

Siegal, Gene P., MD, PhD
Professor of Pathology, Cell Biology and Surgery, Division of Anatomic Pathology, Department of Pathology, The University of Alabama at Birmingham, 506 Kracke Building, 619 south 19th Street, Birmingham, Alabama 35233-6823, USA

Squire, Jeremy A., PhD
Professor and Senior Scientist, Division of Cellular and Molecular Biology, Ontario Cancer Institute, University of Toronto, 610 University Avenue, Toronto, Ontario, Canada

Thomas, J. Robert, MD, PhD
Pathologist, Departments of Pathology, University of Arkansas for Medical Sciences and Arkansas Children's Hospital, Little Rock, AR, USA

Variend, Sadick, MD, FRCPath
Paediatric Pathologist, Department of Pathology, Sheffield Children's Hospital, Western Bank, Sheffield S10 2TH, United Kingdom

Weitzman, Sheila, MB
Professor of Paediatrics, University of Toronto, and Staff Oncologist, The Hospital for Sick Children, 555 University Avenue, Toronto M5G 1X8, Ontario, Canada

Woods, C. Geoffrey, MB
Clinical Geneticist, Yorkshire Regional Genetics Service, St James's University Hospital, Beckett Street, Leeds LS9 7TF, United Kingdom

Zielenska, Maria, PhD
Associate Professor, Department of Laboratory Medicine and Pathobiology, The University of Toronto and Molecular Diagnostics, Hospital for Sick Children, 555 University Avenue, Toronto M5G 1X8, Ontario, Canada

Abbreviations

AFP	alpha-fetoprotein
AI	allelic imbalance
ALCL	anaplastic large cell lymphoma
ALL	acute lymphoblastic leukaemia
AMCA	7-amino-4-methylcoumarin-3-acetic acid
AML	acute myeloid leukaemia
APAAP	alkaline phosphatase–anti-alkaline phosphatase
AT	ataxia telangiectasia
ATRA	all *trans* retinoic acid
BHCG	beta human chorionic gonadotrophin
bHLH	basic helix–loop–helix
BNLI	British National Lymphoma Investigation
BSA	bovine serum albumin
BWS	Beckwith–Wiedemann syndrome
CALLA	common ALL antigen
CCG	Children's Cancer Group
CCSG	Children's Cancer Study Group
CCSK	clear cell sarcoma of the kidney
CGH	comparative genomic hybridization
CLL	chronic lymphocytic leukaemia
CML	chronic myelocytic leukaemia
CMML	chronic monomyelocytic leukaemia
CMN	congenital mesoblastic nephroma
CNS	central nervous system
CPDN	cystic partially differentiated nephroblastoma
CPNET	central PNET
CSF	cerebrospinal fluid
CT	computerized tomography
CVS	chorionic villus sampling
DCC	deleted in colon cancer
ddNTP	dideoxy nucleotide triphosphate
DFCI	Dana Farber Cancer Institute
DIG	desmoplastic infantile ganglioglioma
DNET	disembryoplastic neuroepithelial tumor
DOP	degenerate oligonucleotide-primed
DS	Down's syndrome
DSRCT	desmoplastic small round cell tumor
EB	Epstein–Barr
EBV	Epstein–Barr Virus
EDTA	ethylene diamine tetraacetic acid
EFS	event-free survival
EGFR	epidermal growth factor receptor
ELISA	enzyme-linked immunosorbent assay
EM	electron microscopy

EMA	epithelial membrane antigen
ES	Ewing's sarcoma
ES	embryonal stem cell
ESFT	Ewing's sarcoma family of tumours
ESR	erythrocyte sedimentation rate
FAB	French/American/British
FISH	fluorescence *in situ* hybridization
FL	fluorescein
FMTC	familial medullary thyroid cancer
FNA	fine needle aspiration
GCT	germ cell tumours
GDB	genome database
GF	growth fraction
GFAP	glial fibrillary acidic protein
H&E	haematoxylin and eosin
HBV	hepatitis B virus
HCG	human chorionic gonadotropin
HL	Hodgkin lymphoma
HNPCC	hereditary non-polyposis colorectal cancer
HSR	homogenously staining regions
HTA	Health and Technology Assessment
HVA	homovanillic acid
IC	immunocytology
Ig	immunoglobulin
IGF-2	Insulin-like growth factor-2
IHC	Immunohistochemistry
ILNR	intralobar nephrogenic rests
INPC	International Neuroblastoma Pathology Committee
INSS	International Neuroblastoma Staging System
IT	immature teratomas
ITGCN	intratubular germ cell neoplasia
JCML	juvenile chronic myelomonocytic leukaemia
kb	kilobase
KS	Klinefelter's syndrome
LAN	linker-arm-modified nucleotide
LDH	lactate dehydrogenase
LDHL	lymphocyte depletion HL
LFS	Li Fraumeni syndrome
LOH	loss of heterozygosity
LPHL	lymphocyte predominance HL
LR	late relapse
MCHL	mixed cellularity HL
MD	myotonic dystrophy
MDM2	murine double minute two
MEN	multiple endocrine neoplasia
M-FISH	multicolour FISH
MGB	minor groove binder
MGCT	malignant germ cell tumours
MKI	mitosis-karyorrhexis index
MPNST	malignant peripheral nerve sheath tumour
MRD	minimal residual disease

MRI	magnetic resonance imaging
MRP	multidrug resistance-associated protein
MRT	malignant rhabdoid tumor
MSI	microsatellite instability
MT	mature teratomas
NF-1	neurofibromatosis type1
NFQ	non-fluorescent quencher
NF	neurofilament
NGF	nerve growth factor
NHL	non-Hodgkin lymphoma
NIH	National Institute of Health
NLS	nuclear localization signals
NPVM	non-pulmonary visceral metastases
NSE	neuron specific enolase
NSHL	nodular sclerosis HL
NWTS	National Wilms Tumor Study
OLT	orthotopic liver transplantation
OPT	optic pathway tumours
OS	overall survival
PAGE	polyacrylamide gel electrophoresis
PAP	Peroxidase–anti-peroxidase
PAS	periodic acid Schiff
PCAP	placental alkaline phosphatase
PCR	polymerase chain reaction
PGC	primordial germ cells
PGP	protein gene product
PIC	polymorphic information content
PLNR	perilobar nephrogenic rests
PNET	primitive neuroectodermal tumour
PNF	plexiform neurofibromas
POG	Pediatric Oncology Group
pPNET	peripheral PNET
PTCL	peripheral T-cell lymphoma
PTGC	progressive transformation of germinal centers
PXA	pleomorphic xanthoastrocytoma
RB	retinoblastoma
RCT	round cell tumour
RER+	replication error positive
RFLP	restriction fragment length polymorphism
RMS	rhabdomyosarcoma
RTK	rhabdoid tumor of the kidney
RT-PCR	reverse transcriptase polymerase chain reaction
SAM	significance analysis of micro arrays
SAS	sarcoma amplified sequence
SCID	severe combined immunodeficiency
SEER	surveillance, epidemiology, and end-result
SGB	Simpson Golabi Behmel
SIOP	International Society for Paediatric Oncology
SJCRH	St Jude's Children's Research Hospital
SKY	spectral karyotyping
SNPS	short nucleotide polymorphism

STR	short tandem repeats
TCR	T-cell receptor
TdT	terminal deoxytransferase
TRITC	tetraethyl rhodamine isothiocyanate
UBO	unidentified bright objects
UKCCSG	United Kingdom Children's Cancer Study Group
UV	ultraviolet
VEGF	vascular endothelial growth factor
VMA	vanillylmandelic acid
VNTRs	variable number of tandem repeats
WT	Wilms' tumour
XLP	X-linked lymphoproliferative
YST	yolk sac tumour

An introduction to children's cancer and the patient pathway

Ian J. Lewis

Introduction

There has been an explosion of knowledge and enormous progress in the fundamental understanding of the biology of cancer in recent years. This has included the realisation that cancer occurs when normal cellular functions are disturbed leading to a malignant phenotype. Much research has focussed on understanding the types of disturbances that can occur, the contribution that these abnormalities can make to the development and behaviour of particular cancers, and more recently, the recognition that these cellular and genetic abnormalities can provide rational targets for new therapeutic approaches.

Information about the biology of cancers that occur in children has increased in parallel with these more general advances and this book is intended to provide a focus for readers who wish to have an understanding of our current state of knowledge. The purpose of this first chapter is to provide a general overview of childhood cancer for readers who do not consider themselves expert in this field. It is not intended to be comprehensive but rather to put this book into a clinical context.

Cancer arising in children is nearly always unexpected and results in significant burdens on the children themselves, their families, and the wider community. Enormous challenges arise for all who are involved in trying to provide care for the child with cancer and in many ways the practice of paediatric oncology has become a paradigm of true multi-professional and multidisciplinary care. The primary aim of that care is to offer each affected child the best possible chance of survival whilst minimising the physical, psychological, and social costs. Modern convention is that this should be carried out in an atmosphere and environment of support and openness. Key to this is the requirement to provide as much information as possible about the possible causes and behaviour of their specific cancer. It is therefore important that professionals dealing with children and their families can help explain our current state of knowledge about cancer biology. Similarly, it is important that professional scientists working or researching into aspects of specific cancers have a broad understanding of childhood cancer and to what patients and families experience during the quest for cure.

Epidemiology

Society does not expect children to develop cancer and fortunately cancer in childhood is relatively rare with only approximately 1 child in 650 developing cancer before the age of 15 years. Nevertheless, despite major advances in diagnosis and treatment over the past 40–50 years, cancer remains a significant public health problem and a common cause of death in children over the age of 1 year in developed countries.

In contrast to adult malignancy where most cancers are epithelial in origin and are classified by site of origin, cancers occurring in children are histologically very diverse and can occur in many different anatomical sites. This has led to a separate standard system of classification, 'The International Classification of Childhood Cancer', which has 12 main diagnostic groups, most of which are divided into a number of subgroups (Table 1).

Interestingly, age-standardised incidence rates of childhood cancer in different countries and cultures are relatively similar, lying in the range of 75–140 cases per million children. There are however quite marked variations in the incidence of particular types of childhood cancers in different countries and ethnic groups. Acute leukaemias account for around a third of all childhood cancers in the white populations of Europe and North America but are less than half as frequent in Black African populations. Burkitt's lymphoma is by contrast the commonest cancer in much of sub-Saharan Africa whilst being rare in White European children. In the

Table 1 Cancer incidence in children under 15 years of age

Type of malignancy	Percentage of cases	Peak age incidence (years)
Leukaemia	34.2	
ALL	26	2–8
AML	7	
Central nervous system	23.5	
Astrocytoma	8.8	
Medulloblastoma	4.6	
Other	10.2	
Lymphoma	11.0	
Hodgkin's	4.5	>10
Non-Hodgkin's	6.0	
Neuroblastoma	6.0	<3
Kidney	6.0	<5
Wilms'	5.9	
Soft tissue sarcomas	6.0	
Rhabdomyosarcoma	3.8	
Embryonal		<10
Alveolar		>10
Bone tumours	5.0	10–20
Osteosarcoma	3.0	
Ewing's sarcoma	2.0	
Retinoblastoma	2.7	<1
Germ cell tumours	2.3	<5 or >15
Liver	0.8	
Hepatoblastoma		<5
Hepatic carcinoma		
Epithelial/Carcinoma	2.0	
Others	<1.0	

United Kingdom, Hodgkin's lymphoma has a higher incidence amongst children of South Asian origin than amongst white children. There are quite considerable variations in incidence for Ewing's sarcoma with particularly low rates in African, Chinese, and American Black children compared to white children in the United States, Europe, and Australia.

Different childhood cancers also occur at different ages. The embryonal tumours of childhood; neuroblastoma, nephroblastoma (Wilms' tumour), hepatoblastoma, and retinoblastoma occur most commonly in young children under 5 years of age. Osteosarcoma and Ewing's sarcoma are predominantly malignancies of adolescence associated with periods of maximal somatic growth. In White children lymphomas predominate in teenagers whilst occurring at a younger age in South Asians. Acute lymphoblastic leukaemia (ALL) occurs throughout childhood but is most common in children between the ages of 2 and 8 years. These variations signpost that both genetic and environmental factors play roles in the causation of childhood cancer.

Aetiology

All cancers arise as a result of sequential genetic disturbances occurring in target cells in a step-wise manner. The initiating genetic change may be inherited either as a single gene mutation or may be induced by external or environmental agents but requires further genetic events to take place in order to evolve to a true malignant state.

In some childhood cancers as few as two mutations can be sufficient to cause cancer. In other types of childhood cancer, for example, neuroblastoma, multiple genetic events can be identified in advanced cases although how many of these events are necessary to initiate a truly malignant state has not yet been identified.

A small, but important, minority of childhood cancers arises in association with genetic predisposition, some of which can be familial. The retinoblastoma gene *RB-1* on chromosome 13q14 normally acts as a negative regulator of cell division. Deletions or mutations of this gene cause loss of function and predisposes those affected to retinoblastoma, the commonest childhood eye cancer. These genetic abnormalities can be inherited or mutate spontaneously and both gene copies need to have been affected for a cancer to arise. Children with germline mutations of *RB-1* are predisposed to multiple retinoblastoma tumours occurring in both eyes, and also to other tumours such as osteosarcoma, the commonest type of bone tumour arising in children. Despite this, only a minority of retinoblastoma tumours are found in children with germline mutations, the majority occurring sporadically.

Other examples of cancer genetic predisposition abound. These include the Li–Fraumeni syndrome where a range of germline mutations in the *P53* gene on chromosome 17 predispose to a wide spectrum of cancers including adreno-cortical carcinoma in young children, sarcomas, brain tumours, and early onset breast cancer in adults. Neurofibromatosis type 1 (NF1), occurs where mutations of the *NF1* gene on chromosome 17q result in an aberrant neurofibromin protein. The normal protein regulates ras protein activity and mutations result in a varied clinical picture that includes an increased incidence of cancer, most commonly brain tumours.

There are many examples of particular cancers arising in children with specific chromosome anomalies or congenital malformations. Children with Trisomy 21 (Down's syndrome) have a higher incidence of acute leukaemia. Wilms' tumour occurs in children with a range of malformations including aniridia, anomalies of the genito-urinary tract, and certain overgrowth syndromes such as hemi-hypertrophy or Beckwith–Wiedemann syndrome. The genetic basis of these is more complex than just the involvement of a single gene and as an example, a number of gene abnormalities have been identified that are associated with or result in Wilms' tumour. This introductory chapter cannot do more than highlight the issues and direct the reader to the chapter focussing on family genetics and predisposition syndromes or to specific tumour chapters.

The majority of childhood cancers occur sporadically and are not associated with germline mutations or congenital anomalies. It is clear that some environmental factors can either interact with germline genetic defects or initiate novel genetic change that results in cancer. As an example of the former, it is apparent that children with conditions such as hereditary dysplastic naevus syndrome or xeroderma pigmentosum are at particular risk of melanoma at a young age if exposed to ultraviolet radiation. Certain viruses are known to be associated with particular malignancies in children. As examples, Epstein–Barr (EB) virus genetic material is found in Burkitt lymphoma cells and EB virus is also associated with other lymphomas and nasopharyngeal carcinoma. Hepatitis B virus infection predisposes to hepatocellular carcinoma and HIV1 predisposes to Kaposi sarcoma and B-cell neoplasms in children.

Certain drugs can also cause cancer. A class of anti-cancer drugs called topoisomerase 2 inhibitors used for treating a variety of childhood cancers has been shown to initiate a specific genetic defect in chromosome 11q23 resulting in the occurrence of secondary leukaemia. This event appears to be schedule dependent, occurring with greater frequency when patients are exposed to the drug for a prolonged period. Similarly, secondary leukaemia or lymphoma can occur after treatment with alkylating agents. The risk of second malignancies appears to increase when radiation therapy is combined with alkylating agents and this combination can result in a variety of second tumours including sarcomas and breast carcinoma. These most commonly occur within, or adjacent to, the radiation field.

Despite rapidly increasing knowledge about childhood cancers, the cause of the majority of these tumours remain unknown and this is often a source of enormous frustration to affected families that will only be relieved by continued research.

Changes in outcome

There have been major improvements in outcome over recent decades for many childhood cancers (Fig. 1). It has been estimated that in the 1960s in the United Kingdom, only 26% of children diagnosed with cancer survived at least 5 years from diagnosis. This had increased towards 50% by the late 1970s and 65% by the late 1980s. Current evidence is that around 75% of children diagnosed during the 1990s will be living 5 years after diagnosis and that the majority of these will become long-term disease-free survivors.

There are a number of quite complex and interlinked reasons for these improvements. There is no doubt that many of the initial advances in prognosis occurred as a result of the introduction of effective chemotherapy agents and in particular the understanding that successful use of chemotherapy often required the use of a number of drugs in combination in order to overcome chemo-resistance. Perhaps two of the best examples of this approach were improvements in prognosis for ALL and Hodgkin's lymphoma. Concurrently, solid tumours were beginning to be treated in a more coordinated multimodal fashion combining surgery and radiotherapy with the newer chemotherapeutic agents. This approach resulted in some early benefits and improvements in survival, for example, in Wilms' tumour, Ewing's sarcoma, and rhabdomyosarcoma. These early successes contributed to at least two further advances. First, the development of children's cancer centres where expertise in these complex treatment approaches and the associated complications could be developed, where children with these rare diseases could be managed in a supportive environment. Second, the coming together of children's cancer centres into cooperative groups to learn from each other, to develop common treatment approaches and subsequently to develop multicentre and multinational clinical trials aimed at bringing new approaches or treatments rapidly into practice. Many of these cooperative groups came into existence during the late 1960s and 1970s, perhaps led by the formation of the Children's Cancer Study Group (CCSG) in North America and the International Society of Paediatric Oncology (SIOP), which mainly operated trials and studies in Europe.

In the United Kingdom, the Medical Research Council established a national Leukaemia Working Group in 1969. This Group subsequently set up a number of sequential therapeutic randomised trials in both childhood ALL and acute myeloid leukaemia

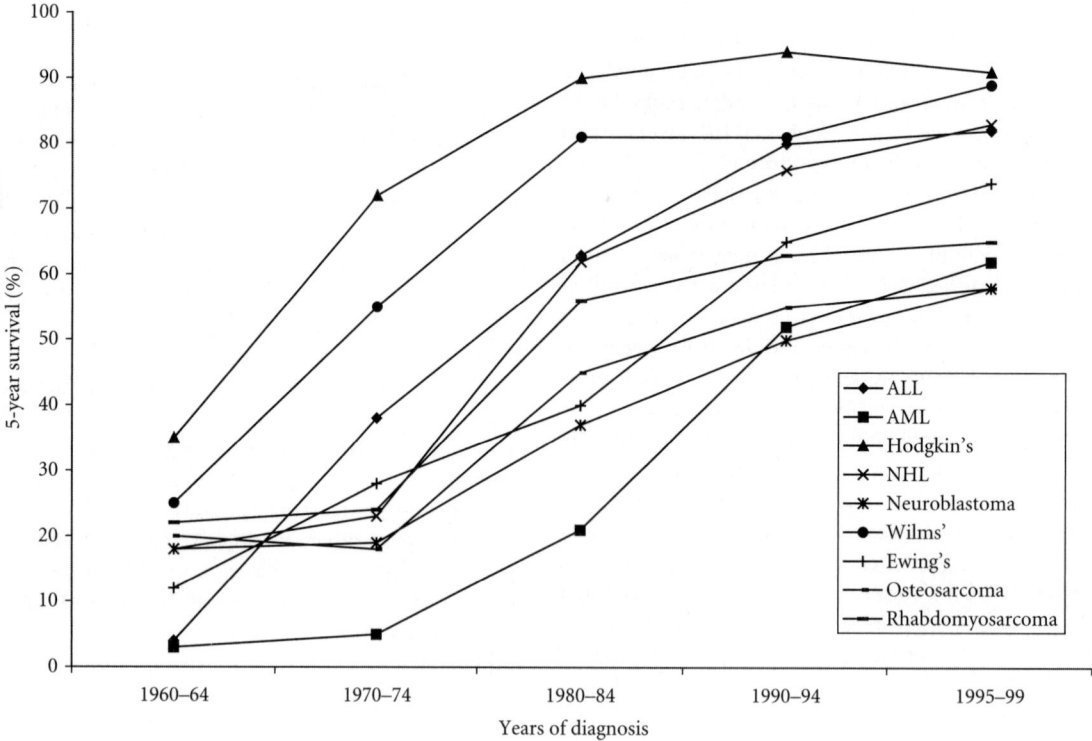

Fig. 1 Trends in 5-year survival rates for childhood cancers.

(AML), which have resulted in major improvements in outcome for both groups of diseases. In 1977, the United Kingdom Children's Cancer Study Group (UKCCSG) was formed and has been the focus of developments in children's solid tumours for 25 years. The UKCCSG now offers a wide portfolio of trials and studies across the broad range of childhood solid tumours and includes subgroups developing new therapeutic agents and studying the biology of these rare cancers. In recent years it has become apparent that very large clinical trials involving hundreds of patients are required if further advances are to be made using current trial methodology. Even trials involving the entire United Kingdom are unlikely to have adequate numbers of patients to allow statistically valid completion in a timely fashion. As a result, clinical investigators from many cooperative organisations including the UKCCSG have been instrumental in coming together and developing multinational studies for a number of tumour groups including randomised trials in neuroblastoma, B-cell lymphomas, osteosarcoma, Ewing's sarcoma, Wilms' tumour, soft tissue sarcomas, and hepatoblastoma. This increase in international collaboration has encouraged a greater common understanding of the cancers, the further development of evidence-based treatment and allowed improvements in treatment to reach patients more rapidly.

The patient pathway

The successful overall management of a child with cancer is complex and grounded in teamwork involving personnel from a variety of medical and allied professions and disciplines within individual professions. The organisation of care is based on the triad of *diagnosis, treatment, and supportive care* (Fig. 2).

It is perhaps easier to understand the processes and potential pitfalls involved if considered from a patient and family perspective. On rare occasions, a child might present through a cancer-screening programme because there is a known genetic or other predisposition but with our current state of knowledge this is very unusual.

The journey nearly always begins when a child develops a particular symptom or symptoms and help is sought

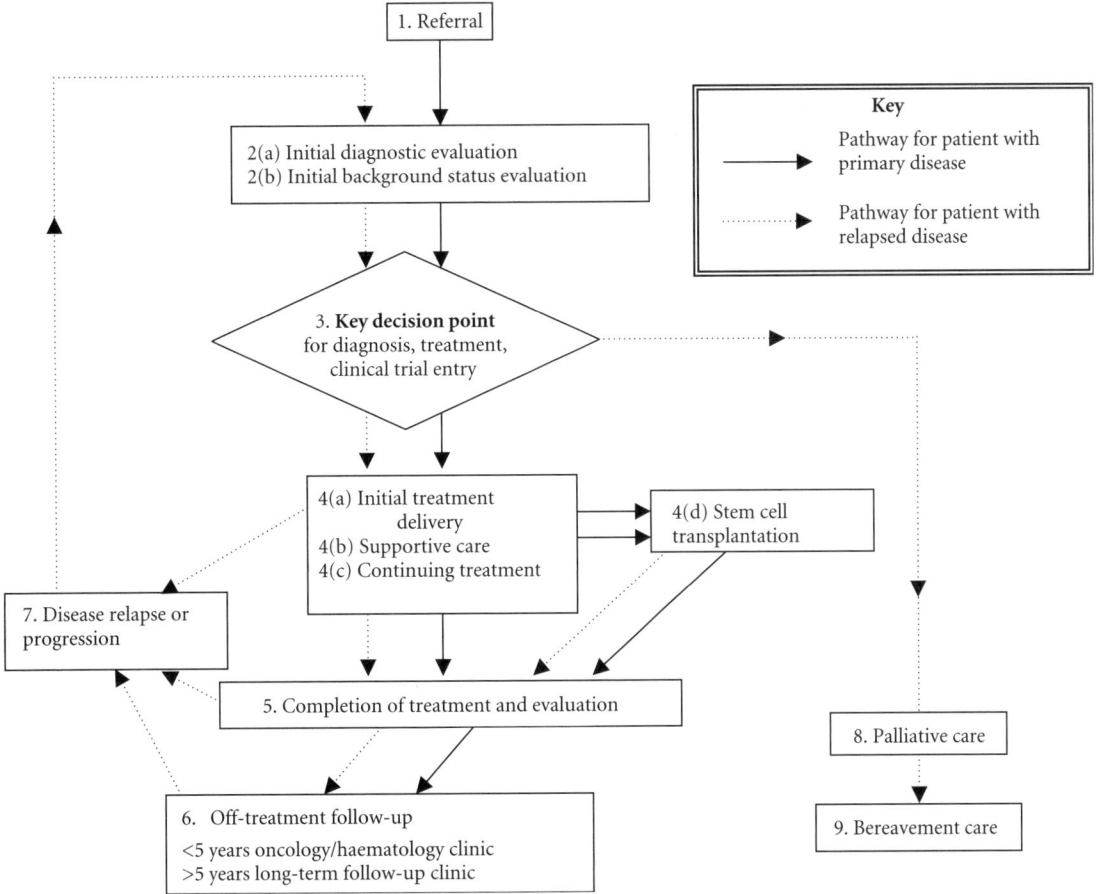

Fig. 2 Patient pathway through disease management stages.

from primary health care professionals. In the United Kingdom this is usually the family General Practitioner. It is beyond the scope of this book to give a full description of the protean ways that cancer can present in childhood but the relative rarity of childhood cancer means that it is quite uncommon for primary care professionals to recognise that cancer is occurring in a particular child at the time of first presentation and a degree of delay in further referral is common.

1. Referral

In the United Kingdom and most of the developed world, nearly all children with cancer eventually reach specialist children's cancer units; however the routes by which they get there are varied and this can potentially have an adverse effect on the outcome.

The pattern of referral from primary care depends on the particular symptoms and physical findings. Children with lethargy, bruising, or enlarged lymph nodes may well be referred for either haematological assessment by peripheral blood evaluation or directly to a local paediatrician for a clinical assessment. Children with pain or loss of function may be referred to a paediatrician but are more likely to be referred to specialists such as ENT, ophthalmic, or orthopaedic surgeons depending on the site of symptoms. Similarly, children with 'lumps' or swellings may be referred to general or specialist surgeons who may or may not have a particular understanding of children's cancer. Children with symptoms that might include headaches with vomiting, weakness, loss of sensation, or unsteadiness are commonly referred to paediatric neurologists or neurosurgeons.

At some stage there is a realisation by the medical team that the child may be suffering from one or other form of cancer and it is usually at this point that referral to the specialist cancer unit is made. Historically, this often happened after a tissue diagnosis had been made by biopsy but it has been increasingly understood that children are best served by referral to a specialist centre when a diagnosis of cancer is suspected so that a full and comprehensive evaluation can take place giving maximum information from minimal interference.

2. Diagnostic evaluation

The families of children suspected of having cancer want and need to know the answers to the questions, 'What is it?', 'Where is it?', 'How has it happened?', 'Is it treatable?', and 'What will the outcome be?'. The children's cancer team also needs to answer these questions in order to be able to respond to the families and plan the most effective treatment. Therefore the aim of the diagnostic evaluation is to establish an accurate pathological diagnosis and the extent of disease in as timely a manner as feasible whilst providing the child and family with clear information and an understanding of the processes involved.

The initial part of the evaluation is clinical. A comprehensive history of symptoms and full examination is a major tool in establishing an accurate differential diagnosis so that investigations can be appropriately targeted. Pallor and fatigue or bruising tends to point towards leukaemia. Bone pain or limping with or without fever can also point to leukaemia but might also indicate Ewing's sarcoma, neuroblastoma, or osteosarcoma, the latter particularly in the presence of a limb mass. Enlarged lymph nodes most commonly occur with infections but in the absence of fever or if persistent and not responding to antibiotics then strongly suggest Hodgkin's lymphoma, non-Hodgkin's lymphoma, or leukaemia. On occasions parents notice a mass or swelling in their child's abdomen. This may indicate Wilms' tumour, neuroblastoma, or a liver tumour. Persistent headaches with vomiting, disturbances of vision, or newly developed unsteadiness may all indicate the presence of a brain tumour. Protrusion of an eye can occur in neuroblastoma, rhabdomyosarcoma, histiocytosis, or leukaemia. These are just a few common examples of typical symptoms but a significant number of children present with less obvious problems so the clinical level of suspicion that a malignancy is present needs to be high. Clearly the child's age is of importance. As already described, certain cancers are more likely to arise at particular ages.

Other aspects of the history can also be of vital importance. A careful family history may reveal a familial predisposition to cancer, for example, retinoblastoma or neurofibromatosis. The past medical history of the child may identify an unexpected predisposition. Down's syndrome is usually obvious to all, but the relationship between some of the overgrowth syndromes such as hemi-hypertrophy or immunodeficiency syndromes and malignancy may not have been brought to the family's attention. An understanding of the social and family background is also essential, not particularly to help with the diagnosis but to put the child into a social context so that the oncology team can provide help and support to the family during the considerable stresses incurred during and following treatment. The clinical examination is essential in providing confirmatory information but also, on occasions, in identifying new signs that aids the establishment of a diagnosis.

The initial investigations should be targeted towards the likely diagnosis and may involve a number of disciplines. The first investigation in children suspected of leukaemia is usually to obtain a blood sample for a blood count and film in order to identify abnormalities or deficiencies in red cells, white cells, or platelets. Children suspected of having solid tumours almost always require radiological evaluation, and a close relationship between the clinical and radiological teams is essential to determine the most appropriate investigations for each child. Plain X-rays, ultrasound, computerised tomography, magnetic resonance imaging, and isotope studies may all be important in determining both the local extent and distant spread of tumours but each possible diagnosis demands a different range of investigations. On occasions, the clinical chemistry laboratory can be of enormous help in trying to establish a timely diagnosis. Some solid tumours produce chemical metabolites that can be used as specific tumour markers. Neuroblastoma, arising from sympathetic nerve cells, produces a range of substances but those most commonly assessed are catecholamine metabolites, which are excreted and can be measured in urine. These metabolites can also be used to monitor treatment and subsequent disease progress. Other tumours, which produce tumour markers that can be measured in serum include germ cell tumours, which produce alpha feto-protein (AFP) and/or beta human chorionic gonadotrophin (BHCG), and hepatoblastoma, which also secretes AFP. Notwithstanding this wide range of helpful initial investigations, for the overwhelming majority of tumours a tissue sample for pathological diagnosis is absolutely essential.

In the relatively recent past, it was very common for the initial evaluation, biopsy, and even treatment to be undertaken prior to referral to a specialist centre. At a time when the tumours were little understood, treatment was rudimentary, and outcomes poor, this approach was perhaps understandable, but the complexities of tumour sub-types and the subtleties of varied treatments based on biological and genetic phenotypes really make this approach unacceptable. Despite this it is not uncommon even nowadays for children suspected of having cancer to have a biopsy undertaken without due consideration being given to the complex technical requirements needed to establish the most accurate pathological diagnosis possible. Specialist children's cancer centres combine the advantages of having access to comprehensive diagnostic facilities whilst at the same time providing an environment where children and their families can be offered appropriate information and support. It is difficult to understand the logic as to why the diagnostic process might be undertaken without these facilities and support.

The process of obtaining the most appropriate and relevant tissue in order to make a pathological diagnosis is a complex multidisciplinary process requiring close collaboration between oncologist, surgeon, diagnostic radiologist, and pathologist. Factors that require consideration include the most likely diagnosis, the site to biopsy, the amount of tissue needed, the method of biopsy, and how the specimens should be handled. For most paediatric cancers, establishing a pathological diagnosis involves a number of techniques in addition to routine microscopy. These include specific immunohistochemical evaluation, determination of cytogenetic anomalies using techniques such as G-banding, fluorescent *in situ* hybridisation (FISH), comparative genomic hybridisation (CGH), and increasingly molecular techniques such as the polymerase chain reaction to analyse tumour DNA or RNA. It has become common practice to request permission from families to store frozen tumour samples in order to take advantage of newer diagnostic methods or prognostic tests as they become available, or to use the tissue for research.

When leukaemia is suspected, tissue samples are obtained by aspirating bone marrow through a hollow needle and by trephine using a cutting needle in order to preserve the marrow architecture. Samples are processed in a variety of ways in order to give maximum microscopic, immunophenotypic, and cytogenetic information and in the majority of cases results are available within hours enabling treatment to commence. These samples allow the haematopathologist to differentiate between the common forms of leukaemia, acute lymphoblastic and acute non-lymphocytic leukaemia (also called AML). This is extremely important as the treatment regimes for these two main diagnostic groups of leukaemia differ markedly. They also enable identification of leukaemic sub-types and these can indicate differences in prognosis that also require different treatment approaches, perhaps indicating the need for a more intensive treatment or even bone marrow transplantation. This can be illustrated by 'Philadelphia chromosome' positive ALL. In these cases the presence of a translocation between chromosomes 9 and 22 results in fusion between 2 genes *BCR* and *ABL*. This phenomenon gives rise to a leukaemia, which is relatively unresponsive to standard therapy and where the recommended treatment involves bone marrow transplantation. Developing this theme further, it has become apparent that understanding some of the apparently more esoteric biological mechanisms has led to treatments that can be targeted at leukaemia-specific abnormalities. An example of this is acute promyelocytic leukaemia, a subtype of AML. This type of leukaemia is characterised by a translocation t(15;17), which involves a re-arrangement of the *RAR-alpha* gene, a retinoic acid receptor gene. It has now been shown that treatment of this particular leukaemic sub-type using all *trans*-retinoic acid (ATRA) is of benefit in reducing complications and improving outcome so that early confirmation of diagnostic sub-type is important.

For solid tumours, the situation in obtaining diagnostic samples is more complex. Where, following radiological evaluation, a tumour appears to be confined to a single site and is thought possible to remove, then surgeons will consider an exploratory operation with a view to complete excision. However, when this approach does not seem feasible then there is often a healthy tension between the different professional groups about the method of biopsy and the quantity of tissue required. The agreed basic premise is to obtain the required amount of tissue with minimum disruption to the child. This has led to the development of minimally invasive techniques such as fine needle aspiration and radiologically guided needle biopsy. Experience however has led to the realisation that whilst these approaches clearly have advantages, questions often arise as to whether the sample is truly representative of the tumour as a whole and the small tumour volumes limit the possibilities of undertaking some of the more complex diagnostic evaluations outlined above. As a result, there has been a resurgence of the view that open, carefully controlled incisional biopsies will provide optimum tissue for diagnosis and prognosis. Nevertheless, decisions about the methods of obtaining diagnostic tissue must be tempered by the clinical status of the child. Examples of clinical situations where the wrong choice of diagnostic approach can be life threatening include children with serious biochemical disturbances such as can occur with high grade Burkitt lymphomas. Similarly, children with major respiratory compromise caused by massive liver involvement reducing diaphragmatic movement as can occur with hepatoblastoma or neuroblastoma. Under these circumstances clinical expediency clearly demands as minimally disruptive approach as possible and these children often require intensive care. There are rare situations where the clinical status of the child is so precarious that it is necessary to consider starting treatment without a tissue diagnosis and in these circumstances treatment is based on clinical, radiological, and biochemical information. Perhaps the commonest of these situations is the diagnosis of brain stem glioma where there is genuine controversy about the role and dangers of biopsy in the face of typical clinical and radiological features.

The importance of an accurate tumour diagnosis cannot be overemphasised. Decisions about treatment regimes and prognostic information for the family are dependent on this process. Whilst conventional tissue staining and light microscopy are of enormous benefit in some circumstances, many paediatric tumours are notoriously difficult to distinguish without the full panoply of diagnostic methodology. Neuroblastoma, rhabdomyosarcoma, lymphoma, and Ewing's sarcoma can all appear as small round blue cells indistinguishable by standard microscopy, yet have markedly differing treatment regimes. Immunocytochemistry can be of major assistance in establishing the correct diagnosis. For example, lymphomas nearly always demonstrate positive reactions to common leukocyte antigen (CD45) but are negative to antibodies that are markers of mesoderm or muscle differentiation. These will nearly always give positive results in rhabdomyosarcoma but are negative in Ewing's sarcoma or pPNETs. Despite being very helpful, there are still areas of overlap as for instance between pPNETs and neuroblastoma, both of which might have similar phenotypic positive results with neurally derived antibodies. In these circumstances, cytogenetic analysis can be key to diagnosis. Ewing's or pPNETs typically exhibit the t(11;22) or a variant whilst neuroblastoma does not. Cytogenetic abnormalities in neuroblastoma include near-triploidy, deletions of chromosome 1p, double minutes, and excess copies of chromosome 17q. These can be of major prognostic significance. Near-triploidy in a baby of less than 1 year with apparently disseminated neuroblastoma indicates that this tumour may spontaneously remit with an excellent long-term outlook. Contrast this with a slightly older infant with similar dissemination in whom the cytogenetic changes include 1p deletion, extra copy of 17q, or double minutes indicative of MYCN amplification. This latter infant has a much worse disease and prognosis requiring very intensive multimodal therapy in order to have a reasonable chance of survival.

In a similar way, cytogenetic methods can help distinguish rarer tumours or variants of common tumours. Synovial sarcoma is a relatively uncommon tumour in the childhood population and may cause diagnostic confusion, however typically this tumour has a t(X;18) translocation. A variety of cytogenetic changes can be found with rhabdomyosarcoma but one particular subtype, known as alveolar rhabdomyosarcoma, typically has a characteristic translocation between chromosomes 13 and 2. This subtype has historically required a more intensive treatment approach. Interestingly, recent experience with a new chemotherapeutic agent, topotecan, has indicated that alveolar rhabdomyosarcoma is more sensitive to this agent than is the commoner embryonal subtype and it might be predicted that further improvements in diagnostic sophistication will lead to more examples of tumour-specific tailored therapies.

It is to be expected that the even newer methods of molecular diagnosis will provide oncologists with helpful information for treatment planning and communicating to patients. To a limited extent this has happened already. Analysis of *MYCN* gene amplification is already used as an indicator of relatively poor prognosis in neuroblastoma and a number of clinical trial protocols take this into account when allocating treatment arms. Reverse transcriptase PCR is now used as a diagnostic adjunct allowing the identification of tumour-specific RNA transcripts that result from specific gene translocations. There are an increasing number of leukaemias and solid tumours where this technology is finding a place for this purpose. Examples abound but include identification of *BCR-ABL* in chronic myeloid leukaemia or Ph positive ALL; *EWS-ETS* transcripts in Ewing's or pPNETs; *PAX-FKHR* variants in alveolar rhabdomyosarcoma and *MLL* gene rearrangements in acute leukaemias. This technology is now increasingly used not only for diagnosis but also for identifying minimal disease or micrometastases, particularly in bone marrow. It appears as though this technology will become a useful adjunct to routine clinical management in many childhood cancers. There have been similar developments using tissue-specific methods for identifying micrometastatic or malignant disease in neuroblastoma, rhabdomyosarcoma, and melanoma. One example that might prove to be of clinical benefit is the identification of tyrosine hydroxylase mRNA in blood or bone marrow as a marker of poor prognosis in neuroblastoma.

3. Key decision point

At the completion of the diagnostic process members of the oncology team should know the pathological diagnosis and have enough information about relevant prognostic factors to enable treatment to be started. The multidisciplinary team should have discussed treatment options and agreed a course of action to be recommended to patients and their families. In most situations, these decisions are relatively uncontroversial. Diagnosis and staging is usually straightforward and protocols or trials exist for most clinical eventualities and these will be offered to families. Not infrequently, the situation may be less clear. It is possible that the pathological diagnosis is unusual or that some of the staging investigations might be inconclusive. Under these circumstances the multidisciplinary team need to come to an agreement about the situation and it is often helpful to take advantage of the informal national or international networks in order to obtain a rapid second opinion or pathological review by acknowledged experts.

At this time, members of the oncology team meet with the family in order to provide the diagnostic information and to discuss treatment options. This is a key meeting. Who is present needs careful thought. It must be remembered that parents and children are experiencing one of the most difficult and frightening times of their lives. Facing a life-threatening illness induces a range of reactions and responses that may include fear, denial, anger, loss, and disbelief. It is unusual for this key meeting to be the first time that the family has met members of the oncology team.

For many patients with solid tumours the process from presentation through investigations including a biopsy to a diagnosis can take a number of days up to several weeks and these patients and families can be well prepared for the discussion. In contrast, children with leukaemia can present acutely and have a comprehensive diagnosis confirmed within 24 h. Under these circumstances families may be much less adjusted and prepared for detailed and difficult discussions.

It is advantageous if all relevant parents and carers can be present at the key discussions. Changes in patterns of family life means that this can vary from a single parent through 'standard' two married parents to one or both biological parents and current partners. Whilst tensions may be apparent, there is clear benefit in all parties hearing the same information at the same time. Single parents should be encouraged to have a trusted partner, friend, or family member with them for support.

Whether the affected child is present at the meeting is a matter for debate. Clearly it is not particularly appropriate for infants or young children under about 7 or 8 years to be present. Equally, it is probably appropriate for most teenagers to be present during the discussion although they need to be given a clear choice in the matter. Some choose not to be present but to have a separate meeting with medical staff. However meetings are structured it is important that children can access clear information in an age-appropriate form.

The person providing the information and leading the discussion from the oncology team needs to be knowledgeable and have a comprehensive understanding of the issues that need to be raised or that might need addressing. In most cases this will be the paediatric oncologist but might be a surgeon or radiotherapist with a particular interest in children's cancer. It is helpful to limit the number of professionals but usually essential for the child's nurse or social worker to be present throughout to help support the family and to provide feedback and reinforcement after the meeting is concluded.

Families need a clear and understandable explanation of the diagnosis and staging. Questions often at the forefront of their minds include 'Is it something we've done?' and 'Is our child going to die?', so a significant period of time needs to be given to listen and respond to the fears of families. Answers need to be as clear as possible but truthful, otherwise trust will be lost. Families require time to hear and adjust to what is being said so it is imperative that enough time is set aside. A balance has to be set between being too simplistic and short or trying to be too comprehensive, thereby overwhelming families with too much information. Different individuals within families have different information thresholds and the members of the oncology team have to judge the appropriateness of continuing. It is not unusual for the key discussion to stretch over two or even three meetings each taking over an hour before it can be considered to be concluded and decisions made.

In addition to information about the disease and staging, it is imperative that families understand the principles of the oncology team's agreed treatment plan, how this has been chosen, how it works, what common side effects are likely to occur and the range of outcomes using this approach. Providing families with written information or tape recording the meetings has been shown to be helpful. It is often necessary to revisit or repeat information as parents often find it difficult to absorb a flood of facts and opinion and can feel overwhelmed.

At the conclusion of the process parents will be asked to give written consent to treatment and the professional team need to be satisfied that the consent is as close to 'informed consent' as feasible. Often, parents will be asked to consent to a range of procedures and this can add to the feelings of confusion and being overwhelmed. Consent may be required for treatment, for entry into a randomised clinical trial, for use of residual biopsy material for research, and on occasions, for other local or national research projects. Families need protection and the pace of requesting these consents needs to be carefully judged. The concept of clinical trials is foreign to many people and raises thoughts of the child being used as an 'experimental' subject. This is rarely the case as most Phase 3 clinical trials are testing current standard treatment with variations that are thought to be of possible advantage and have usually been used extensively in patients who have relapsed. Nevertheless, parents often find agreeing to participation in clinical trials one of the hardest things they are asked to do as they often feel either that the clinician 'knows' which treatment arm is best or that they can choose one particular arm. Parents have to be reassured that refusal to participate in a clinical trial (or any other research) will not harm their child or affect their treatment other than them not having access to any test arm. A helpful convention is for patients who do not participate in clinical trials to be treated on the standard arm.

It is rare for parents to refuse all treatment although there are occasions when particular personal, religious, or cultural views can produce conflict between the family and the oncology team. Examples might include particular religious views that prohibit transfusion of blood products or the use of any treatment that might interfere with 'God's will'. It is possible that parents will change their minds if they build trust in the team but it has to be made clear to parents that the best interests of the child is paramount. In the United Kingdom the courts are very supportive to this view and will override parents if it is demonstrated that they might not be acting in their child's best interests. Conversely, it is also extremely rare now for the oncology team not to offer some form of curative therapy at the time of initial presentation but there are occasions when this might happen. Examples might include children who have very major handicaps or serious medical problems prior to developing cancer where it is felt that the child might not tolerate appropriate intensive therapy or rarely children with such extensive metastatic cancer that treatment could be viewed as futile. Even in these circumstances the views of the family are imperative. Children will always be offered appropriate palliative care.

At the conclusion of this key decision point all involved parties need to have a clear view of each other's understanding and of the agreed path ahead.

4. Treatment

It has already been recognised that treatment delivery involves a number of different disciplines. Medically this involves the paediatric oncologist who has responsibility for prescribing chemotherapy, the radiation. or clinical oncologist who plans radiotherapy, and one or more specialist surgeons depending on the site and type of tumour. As examples, brain tumours will be operated on by neurosurgeons; bone tumours by orthopaedic surgeons; abdominal neuroblastoma or Wilms' tumour by paediatric surgeons and so on. Most children receiving chemotherapy will have venous access established using one or other type of central venous catheter usually inserted into the neck veins and tunnelled under the skin of the chest wall.

The type of treatment experienced by the child varies considerably depending on diagnosis and stage. Some treatments are predominantly surgical and can be completed within short weeks. Examples of this include Stage 1 testicular teratoma or localised synovial sarcoma. Other treatments involve intensive chemotherapy extending over 4–6 months but no surgery or radiotherapy, for example, AML or high grade B-cell lymphoma. In these cases children may have to stay in hospital for many weeks.

The treatment of many solid tumours starts with several courses of chemotherapy to produce a reduction in tumour size following which the primary tumour is removed surgically, is treated with radiotherapy, or receives both. This is usually followed by further chemotherapy courses. Examples of this approach include Wilms' tumour, osteosarcoma, and Ewing's sarcoma. Metastatic disease brings additional challenges in how to treat metastatic sites. This also often involves complex multimodal therapy and may include a very high dose therapy with autologous peripheral blood or bone marrow stem cell rescue. An example of this is treatment for patients with Stage 4 neuroblastoma.

It should be recognised that delivering treatment involves a wide variety of professionals in addition to the medical input. Safe delivery of chemotherapy demands an expert and comprehensive pharmacy service. The pharmacist is a key team member. Similarly, delivering radiotherapy requires expert therapeutic radiographers and medical physicists, surgery requires anaesthetic and operating theatre staff skilled in dealing with sick children and their worried parents. Central to delivering all treatment are paediatric oncology nurses without whom it would be extremely difficult to manage children with cancer successfully. They are involved in monitoring children, giving chemotherapy, supporting the children and their families, and often act as advocates for them.

Whilst nearly all specialised cancer centres undertake the initial diagnostic evaluation, determine the treatment plan, and initiate treatment, much of the continuing treatment and supportive care may be undertaken in collaboration with shared care hospitals nearer to the child's home. It is clear that parents and children want access to the best possible care and are willing to travel long distances to get it. Shared care works best where the teams are seen to be working harmoniously, using identical management guidelines and where the families perceive benefits without sacrificing any quality of care.

5. Supportive care

The successes achieved in improving the outcome for children with cancer would not have occurred without major parallel improvements in supportive care. The successful treatment of a child with cancer is dependent on an interdependence of the many different clinical support teams working within the local complex healthcare environment.

In broad terms, supportive care of the child with cancer can be thought about under two main headings, medical/technical support and psychosocial support. Both of these are dependent on the expertise of the oncology nursing team as outlined above. At the time of initial presentation with cancer, some children can have immediately life-threatening tumour complications requiring complex medical and technical support. Examples include obstruction of the superior vena cava by a number of tumours, most commonly T-cell lymphomas; raised intra-cranial pressure due to brain tumours obstructing the flow of cerebrospinal fluid; spinal cord compression causing loss of limb, bladder, and bowel function by neuroblastoma, Ewing's sarcoma, soft-tissue sarcomas, or lymphoma; and metabolic disturbances, perhaps most commonly the tumour lysis syndrome seen in Burkitt's lymphoma or high white cell count leukaemia, which can lead to renal failure and death. Appropriate management requires close interaction between the oncology team and a number of other teams offering specialised expertise. Most children with these complications will require high dependency nursing and medical care usually within an intensive care environment. The children will require haematological and biochemical monitoring, sometimes very intensively, so close collaboration with the laboratory teams is essential. Children commonly require repeated blood product support with red cell or platelet transfusions so again it is important that the transfusion service is responsive and has a good understanding of each child's needs. Renal failure demands the involvement of the specialist nephrology team and similarly liver failure requires experts in hepatology so that appropriate organ support can be instituted. Raised intra-cranial pressure requires neurosurgical intervention and a neurosurgical opinion is essential for spinal cord compression.

Chemotherapy, radiotherapy, or surgery all bring treatment associated effects. The most commonly recognised side effects of chemotherapy are hair loss, nausea, and vomiting although some of the recently introduced anti-emetics have improved the management of this latter effect in recent years. Whilst these side effects can be demoralising and difficult for some children it is unusual for them to threaten life. More significant side effects include the severe bone marrow suppression seen particularly with some of the more intensive treatment regimes. This often results in severe immune suppression that predisposes to a range of life-threatening infectious complications. Chemotherapy can also cause damage to skin and mucosal layers particularly of the intestine and respiratory tract. This adds to the risk of microbial infection and invasion. It is therefore imperative that paediatric oncologists and their teams are knowledgeable about, and have procedures for, reducing infection, recognising the various types of infection, and treating patients when infection is present or suspected. The involvement of experts in microbiology and their laboratory teams is another crucial element of care.

Cancer and its treatment can commonly cause major debility. This can manifest in numerous ways and these often overlap. The majority of children develop nutritional problems, sometimes as a direct result of the cancer or as a side effect of any or all of the treatment modalities. Dietetic expertise is again vital in monitoring intake, weight, and advising parents and children about nutritional support. Often this support can be provided orally and dieticians with paediatric expertise are invaluable in offering advice that takes the child's age and preferences into account. Not uncommonly, children require more invasive nutritional support via a nasogastric tube, percutaneous gastrostomy, or intravenously. The choice and appropriateness of method again demands close multi-professional collaboration between medical staff, nursing teams, dieticians, pharmacists, and of course parents and children. Physiotherapists have a major role in reducing morbidity from general debility, specific tumour-related disability, or disability following major tumour surgery such as amputation. Similarly they and other allied health professionals such as occupational therapists and speech therapists can reduce morbidity and improve the child's chances of returning to normal activity, for example, following neurosurgery for brain tumours.

Treatment and monitoring of childhood cancer often involves difficult or painful procedures. These include prolonged radiological investigations, bone marrow examinations, and delivering intrathecal medication. For many years these procedures were endured by children whilst awake but advances in anaesthesia has meant that in most cases children can now have repeated brief general anaesthetics. This has meant a major improvement in the quality of care provided but requires close collaboration with anaesthetists as well as good access to appropriate facilities.

It is difficult to be comprehensive in a relatively short chapter such as this but it should be apparent that medical or technical support for children with cancer extends to virtually every department or area in medical institutions. Other groups that should be recognised as being frequently involved include dental departments and pain teams. The coordination of this activity is the responsibility of the paediatric oncologist working in close collaboration with the nursing team and the involved family.

Cancer in children is virtually always unexpected and the diagnosis always has a major psychological impact on all members of the child's family and close acquaintances.

Families come in many shapes and sizes, from different ethnic, religious, and philosophical origins, from varying educational, social, and financial backgrounds, and with widely different understanding of cancer and expectations of the health care system. For all these families the diagnosis of cancer in a child brings feelings of losing control of their lives and constant uncertainty about the eventual outcome. Treatment is often intensive and requires that the child and one or more parents are at the hospital or clinic for prolonged periods. This is often a long distance from home, extended family and friends, school or place of work. Not surprisingly, there can be enormous pressure on marital relationships and major impact on siblings, careers, family finances, and educational attainment. Many families are remarkably resilient but even the most hardy and cohesive families can struggle with some of the implications of prolonged treatment, disfigurement, or disability in a previously well child or the prospect of the child dying of resistant or recurrent disease.

Whilst treatment now offers a very real prospect of long-term disease-free survival for most children, it is axiomatic that successful outcome also incorporates the concept of psychosocial survival, so that, where possible, the children and families can emerge from the treatment process with an intact capacity to resume their normal lives. This aim demands expert early assessment, prevention, and intervention where necessary by a wide range of professionals including social workers, psychologists, teachers, play therapists, psychiatrists, all working in close collaboration with the nursing and medical teams.

Voluntary agencies, charities, and parents' groups can offer enormous support to affected children, their siblings, and families. Increasingly Internet sites and chatrooms are also being used for this purpose.

6. Completing treatment and early follow-up

Families and children see the end of treatment as a very significant milestone on the path to recovery. This is often an exciting time for them but many families feel extremely apprehensive at the thought of losing the perceived 'security blanket' of treatment. In most cases the child will undergo a re-evaluation of both their disease status and organ function. Children with leukaemia will have bone marrow and cerebrospinal fluid examined for evidence of disease and hopefully to confirm remission with normal cellular morphology. Most children with solid tumours will undergo radiological evaluation of their disease status and only have marrow samples if there had been metastatic disease present at diagnosis.

This is a time that requires further discussion between the oncologist and family about what to expect in the future. Once again the principles of honesty and openness apply. Most children completing treatment for cancer will remain in continuous remission and become long-term survivors. Nevertheless it is impossible to make this statement about any individual child, so the threat of relapse hangs over all families and needs to be recognised. Early follow-up is geared to try and identify relapse at a time early enough to enable re-treatment. For most children this will be by regular physical check-ups in combination with radiological examination and tumour marker assessment either at the cancer centre or shared care centre.

7. Relapse

Despite all the improvements in outcome over recent decades around 40% of children with cancer will have a recurrence of their disease. The chance of this happening to any individual is obviously linked to prognostic factors at diagnosis. Children with ALL who have very high white cell counts at diagnosis have a greater risk of relapse than those with low white counts. Children with solid tumours and identifiable metastases have a similarly higher risk. Nevertheless, prognostic factors do little more than provide an indication of risk and do not predict outcomes completely.

The identification of relapse is always devastating for children and families. It is often seen as a time when the hope of cure diminishes or disappears yet for many children further treatment can still offer the prospect of prolongation of life or even cure. Clinical symptoms, laboratory abnormalities or radiological findings suggestive of relapse means that children re-enter the diagnostic component of the patient pathway and in most situations will undergo a further complete evaluation of their disease status as outlined earlier in this chapter. Once again children and families have to go through a decision-making process about future treatment guided and advised by the professional team. Outcomes can vary enormously. Patients with recurrence of localised Hodgkin's lymphoma or neuroblastoma still have a very good prospect of long term survival with conventional therapy. Patients with widely metastatic sarcoma or neuroblastoma have a very poor outlook with conventional treatment. Children with relapsed leukaemia can often achieve second remission with conventional chemotherapy but are more likely to become long-term survivors if subject to high dose treatment and allogeneic bone marrow transplantation.

These factors often make the decision-making processes complex and stressful. Many parents and patients struggle with the issues and wish to pursue treatment at all costs. If conventional treatment offers a reasonable prospect of longer survival then the majority of families will accept this with relief, albeit with greatly heightened anxiety. More problematic are the many occasions when prospects are significantly bleaker or even negligible. Understandably, many families choose to investigate or participate in more experimental treatment programmes. It is children from these families who are often the first recipients of experimental therapies often within the context of Phase 1 or 2 studies. It is therefore imperative that such treatments are carried out within an approved ethical framework and that children and their families receive full information about the possible risks as well as potential benefits as part of the consent process.

8. Palliative care and bereavement

At some point it becomes apparent that treatment is unlikely to provide further prolonged benefit and the focus of care shifts to providing symptom control whilst maintaining good quality survival for as long as possible. This may include the use of palliative surgery, chemotherapy, and radiotherapy depending on particular symptoms and does not just imply pain control. This is an important area of work for the oncology team and demands close relationships and excellent communications between hospital and community teams and the family if children are to receive the best available care. In some areas children's hospices can provide respite and added family and social support.

Following the death of a child, the oncology team will usually offer continued contact with the family in order to provide bereavement support. Often the families maintain contact with oncology units for many years and provide enormous impetus in trying to improve the experience and outcome for new families following in their footsteps. They are often the focus for fundraising ventures and provide much of the capital for clinical and biological research.

9. Long-term follow-up

The majority of children treated for cancer will become long-term survivors and current estimates are that in the United Kingdom around 1 in a 1000 adults are survivors of childhood cancer. Long-term surveillance of these survivors is important in order to be able to assess the impact of both the 'cancer diagnosis' and persistent treatment effects. Surgery can on occasions be mutilating or disfiguring and impact on both function and self-esteem. Examples include amputation of a limb for sarcoma or removal of an eye as part of the treatment of retinoblastoma. Radiotherapy can cause impairment of growth, which might result in an asymmetrical appearance or abnormality in organ function. A common example of the latter is radiotherapy damage to the pituitary during treatment for brain tumours resulting in a need for lifelong hormone replacement. Many chemotherapeutic agents have the potential for permanent or long-standing organ damage as part of the cost of cure. Anthracyclines cause toxicity to heart muscle, which can result in the need for long-term cardiac support or rarely even transplant. Cisplatin can cause hearing loss and renal damage. Many drugs including alkylating agents can impair future prospects of fertility. All of these can impact on the survivors' perspective of the quality of their survival. Long-term follow-up is therefore vital in supporting each individual patient and family and also in understanding the impact of treatment. Future research should be directed at identifying treatments that not only continue to improve the prospects of survival but do so at less personal cost to each child.

Section 1
Methods and Clinical Application

1 | Cells, tissues, and the diagnostic laboratory

Catherine J. Cullinane, Susan A. Burchill, and John J. O'Leary

Introduction

Advances in the histogenesis and molecular cell biology of paediatric cancer have refined and improved the diagnostic process. Good communication with clinical colleagues, knowledge of the types of tumours encountered at particular sites in different age groups, and recognition of the characteristic light microscopic appearances of these neoplasms is essential for correct diagnosis and management. Childhood malignancies however, may appear similar by routine light microscopy often as a non-descript population of small round cells known as round cell tumours (RCT) of childhood (Table 1.1). The application of ancillary investigations such as immunohistochemistry (IHC), electron microscopy (EM), and molecular techniques is used not only to improve the accuracy of diagnosis but also to predict prognosis; this multidiscipline approach increases the amount of material required at diagnosis (1–3).

In histopathology, most tissues are fixed before they are examined microscopically. Fixation is the essential first step in the processing of tissues for accurate diagnosis, the fixation preserving cell and tissue morphology. A wide variety of fixatives are available as no fixative singly or in combination is capable of preserving all cellular components. With the advent of new technologies, such as IHC and molecular pathology, it is now possible to study specimens in greater detail than was previously imaginable. However optimal conditions for fixation may be at the expense of tumour-specific antigens (see immunohistochemistry) and DNA or RNA quality (see section on Tissue cryopreservation) that may provide important diagnostic or prognostic information.

It is essential to be familiar with the recommendations for tissue triaging, documentation of relevant macroscopic features and appropriate sampling and handling of the various types of tumours (4–10). These are included in most paediatric clinical trial protocols and are also discussed in relevant chapters of this book. As the number of diagnostic procedures increases and the amount of diagnostic material is limited, particularly with the increasing trend to perform needle biopsies rather than open biopsy, how best to process material for maximum diagnostic benefit is critical. This may vary from disease to disease, depending on the most clinically useful diagnostic and prognostic tests available, however, for most pathology departments a routine standard working procedure is most desirable (Fig. 1.1).

In Section A of this chapter we consider the diagnostic tissue trail and more recent methods used for the accurate diagnosis of malignancy in paediatric oncology, and in Section B address more specifically the important issues and dilemmas of tumour fixation that arise for the pathologist with an increase in the number of diagnostic methods.

Table 1.1 Small RCT of childhood

Lymphoma/leukaemia
Neuroblastoma
Rhabdomyosarcoma
Tumours of the Ewing's sarcoma family
Wilms' tumour
Desmoplastic small RCT
Small cell osteosarcoma
Synovial sarcoma

Section A—Tissue handling

Fresh tumour should be transferred immediately to the pathology laboratory under sterile conditions, accompanied by a request form with the appropriate clinical details. In the pathology department it is assigned a unique identification number, which will accompany the specimen through the various procedures in the laboratory. When handling fresh human tissues the worker

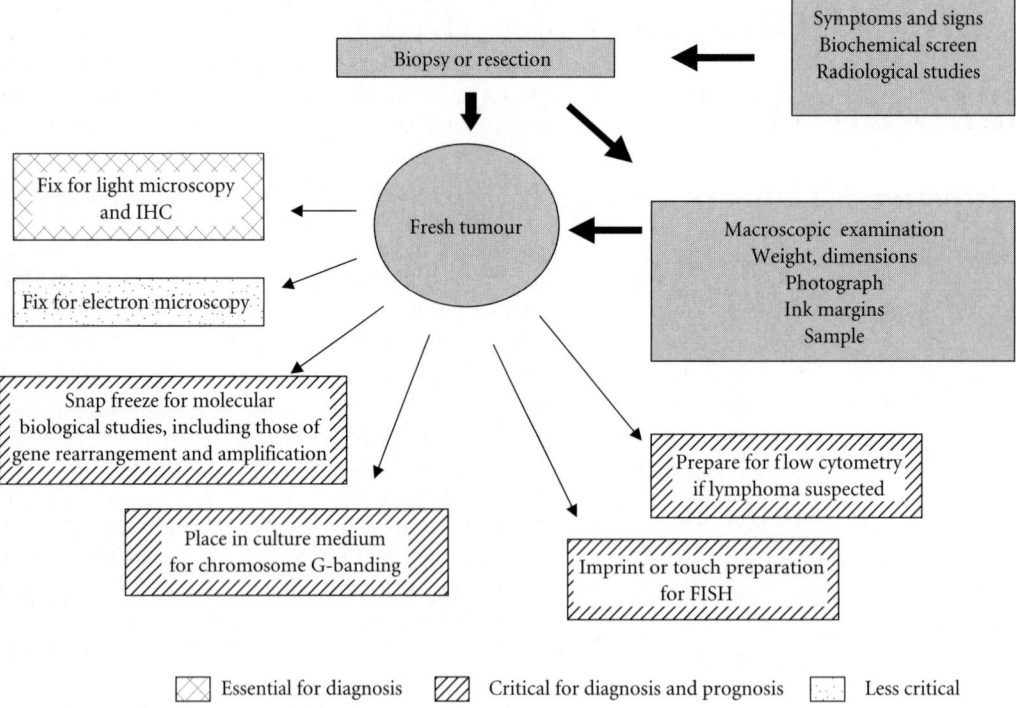

Fig. 1.1 Flow diagram of diagnostic process.

should be aware that the specimen may contain unknown or unrevealed pathogens, for example, hepatitis B, hepatitis C, or HIV, and adopt a working procedure to minimize any risk of infection and contamination of instruments both for themselves and the well-being of colleagues.

The fresh specimen should be given to a designated member of staff (a paediatric pathologist, or a surgical pathologist with a special interest in paediatric tumours), who should have been notified in advance of the arrival of the specimen. The pathologist macroscopically examines the specimen and determines how best it should be divided and handled to satisfy the various investigations required (Fig. 1.1). When the amount of material available is small, that is, needle biopsies or small open biopsies, morphological diagnosis must be the primary objective. If needle biopsies are the only tissue source at diagnosis then multiple biopsies should be taken.

When an excision specimen is received it is orientated and the external surface carefully examined, for example, for penetration of the renal capsule in Wilms' tumour (7). The tumour is measured in three dimensions and weighed. Weight is particularly important in assessment of the malignant potential of adrenal cortical neoplasms (11). The fresh specimen is carefully sliced in two or bivalved avoiding critical margins, permitting sampling of fresh tumour for procedures listed below. The surface and surgical margins are then inked to facilitate the microscopic assessment of extent of infiltration and completeness of excision. A variety of different colored inks may be used, which must be allowed to dry before fixing the specimen. Inspection of the cut surface should include an assessment of the amount of necrosis and documentation of colour and consistency of the mass. The presence of one or more nodules of a softer consistency, which may or may not be haemorrhagic, in a suspected neuroblastoma is critical in the diagnosis of nodular ganglioneuroblastoma (12). Recent evidence of intratumoural biological heterogeneity makes sampling from several sites increasingly important (13).

Photographic documentation is recommended and the photographs should be sent along with any material when central review is requested.

Tissue should be

(1) optimally fixed to retain morphology for examination by light microscopy;
(2) prepared for immunohistochemistry; the fixation method of choice in 1 should consider the effect

of fixation on tumour antigen expression that may be diagnostically and/or prognostically valuable;
(3) fixed for EM;
(4) transported for cytogenetic and cell-cycle analyses;
(5) cryopreserved for assessment of molecular pathology.

1. Light microscopy

Formaldehyde is the most widely used fixative in histopathology for routine paraffin-embedded tissue sections. It is available in a number of commercial solutions, such as 10% formal saline, and is generally called formalin. The aim of the routine histology laboratory procedures is to produce good quality tissue sections on glass slides so that a diagnosis can be made by identification of tumour-specific organelles and cellular patterns following examination under the light microscope. Artefacts due to poor fixation, as well as crush, drying, and heat damage during the operative procedure impact significantly on the quality of the sections, making interpretation difficult. While most procedures are standard, there are variations in the techniques in different laboratories depending on staff preferences. The following is a general outline and greater detail is available in excellent manuals (14, 15).

As routine formalin fixation and processing take time this results in a delay in diagnosis until at least the following day. For more rapid diagnosis a number of different procedures can be employed.

Rapid diagnosis

1. *Frozen section*: A sample of fresh tissue is rapidly frozen and becomes firm as water in the tissue turns to ice and acts as the embedding medium. There are a variety of freezing methods, however commercial rapid freezing products are generally utilized today to minimize cellular damage by the formation of ice crystals. Thin sections (5–10 μm) are cut using a cryostat, which is a refrigerated cabinet that contains a specialized microtome operated from the outside. The temperature in the cryostat is usually kept at −35°C and the tissue block at −10°C for optimal sectioning. The sections are mounted on glass slides, may be fixed briefly in alcohol, and are then quickly stained with haematoxylin and eosin (H&E) or methylene blue depending on the preference of the pathologist. Frozen sections are available throughout the day or night, and the cryostat is often located adjacent to the theatre. It is not a method routinely employed in paediatric tumour diagnosis as it has a number of limitations (16). The quality of the sections is not as good as in routinely processed tissue and as many RCT of childhood require ancillary investigations it is not suitable for diagnosis. However, it can be used to establish that the surgical specimen does indeed contain malignant tumour, although this interpretation itself can be fraught with difficulty, and may be helpful in deciding the appropriate procedures to adopt in a particular case, for example, formalin, B5, zinc formalin, and Bouin's fixation and cell suspension for flow cytometry if lymphoma is suspected (10).

2. *Cytology*: Cytological preparations permit rapid morphological assessment of cells but are limited by lack of architecture (Fig. 1.2). Fine needle aspiration (FNA) is a technique that allows rapid assessment of a patient's lesion in the clinic without the need for anaesthesia or surgical intervention. Cells from the lesion are collected in a needle or aspirated into a syringe and subsequently smeared onto a slide. It is particularly useful for superficial lesions such as thyroid lumps, enlarged lymph nodes, and soft tissue masses (10, 17–19). The technique is not well tolerated by young children and is most often utilized in older teenagers and adults. It has the advantage that inflammatory and benign lesions can be excluded early in patient assessment and those with suspicious or frankly malignant lesions rapidly referred for further investigation and biopsy. It is rarely used as the sole means of diagnosis in paediatric oncology, but may have a role in assessment of metastatic disease and recurrence. Although challenging, there are morphological criteria for specific tumour diagnosis, and aspirated cells can be used for ancillary investigations such as cytogenetics and flow cytometry (18; see later in this chapter). However surgical intervention and biopsy is practically always required to obtain sufficient material.

It is possible to do rapid cytological assessment of a tumour specimen received fresh in the pathology laboratory, including needle biopsies, by means of touch imprints. Making contact between a glass slide and the tumour surface results in transfer of cells onto the slide. Usually 10 or more imprints are made. These can be used for morphological assessment, as well as other studies including immunocytochemistry and fluorescent *in situ* hybridization (FISH). To study the cell morphology the slides are air-dried, and rapidly stained by a Romanowsky method. This consists of methylene blue/azure B and eosin in methanol and includes Giemsa, Leishman, May Grunwald, and Jenner stains. This is the usual procedure for blood and bone marrow smears. Diff Quik or a variety of other commercially available stains are usually used for imprints and fine

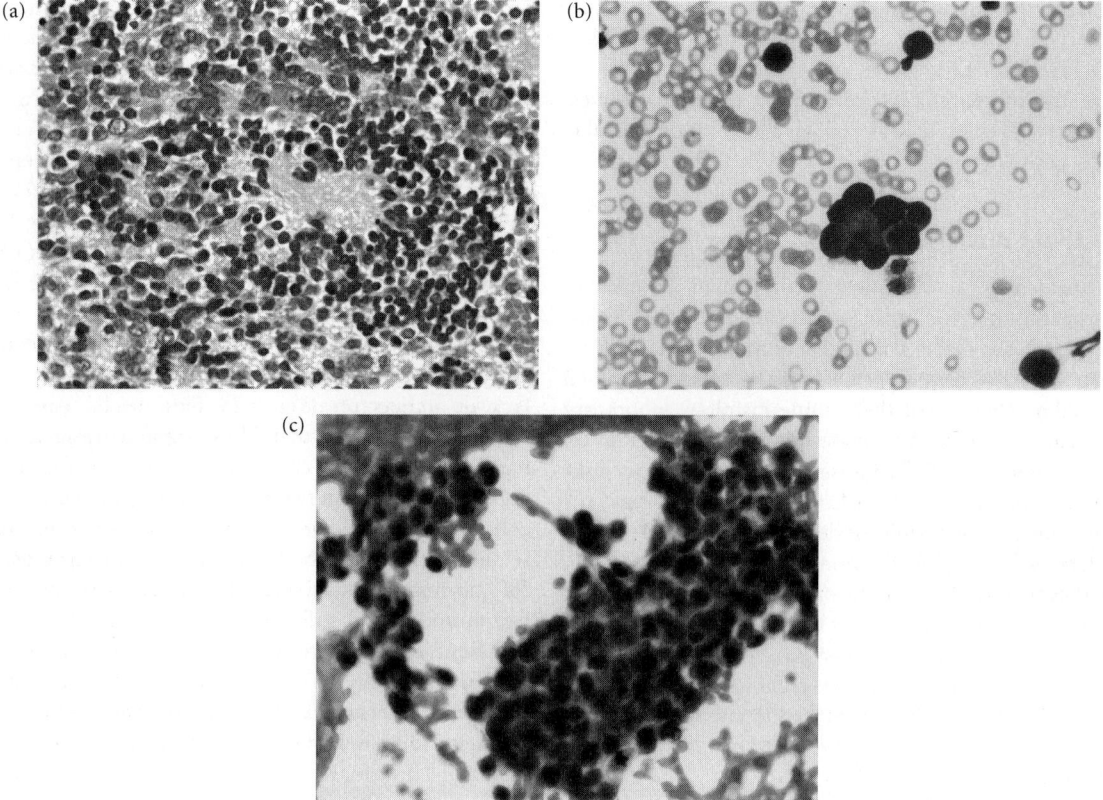

Fig. 1.2 (a) H&E stained section of paraffin wax embedded neuroblastoma, demonstrating nuclear, cellular, and architectural morphology. Note the neural (Homer Wright) rosette with central tangle of neurofibrils. (b) Romanowsky stain (Leishman) of air-dried slide from a malignant effusion (same case as above) with clump of cells with dark nuclei and orientation of cytoplasm centrally forming a structure resembling a rosette. (c) Papanicolaou (PAP) stain of same effusion fixed in alcohol, with clump of dark cells, tending to form a rosette at one edge.

needle aspirates. Slides are also fixed immediately in alcohol (ethanol 95%) and stained by the Papanicolaou technique (PAP stain) which includes haematoxylin, Orange G, and EA 50. H&E or other stains may also be used. A variety of histochemical stains may be used in leukaemia diagnosis such as myeloperoxidase, Sudan black B, oil red O, acid phosphatase, Periodic Acid Schiff (PAS), and naphthol ASD chloroacetate esterase.

3. *Rapid fixation*: Small pieces of tissue (1–2 mm thick) are fixed in alcohol or warm formal saline (40–45°C) for rapid processing, permitting light microscopic examination of cells and tissue architecture in 2–5 h.

Routine diagnosis

Formalin is the fixative of choice but portions of the tumour may be placed in additional fixatives, for example, B5 when lymphoma is suspected. Needle biopsy samples are either placed directly in formalin or placed in a numbered cassette and then immersed in the fixative. Larger biopsies and resection specimens need to be cut into slices to allow optimal fixation throughout the specimen. The larger the specimen the longer it takes to fix. Bone is too hard to cut sections following fixation, therefore the bones must be softened by decalcification, which can take several days to weeks. Large bones are decalcified in mineral acids, usually formic acid, and small bone biopsies in chelating agents, usually EDTA (ethylene diamine tetracetic acid).

Following fixation representative portions or 'blocks' of the tumour are selected for processing. These are placed in numbered cassettes, which accommodate tissue up to 2×2 cm^2 and 3–5 mm thick. With large specimens it is standard practice to take at least one block per centimetre of the greatest dimension and to include resection margins, peripheral and central areas, plus any regions of differing appearance. The sites of the blocks should be documented or noted on a photograph. A block from the region sampled for molecular studies should also be selected and identified separately. In addition adjacent normal tissue should be sampled as well as any lymph nodes.

Following fixation and blocking the tissue undergoes several further procedures before it is suitable for examination under the light microscope. These steps may be automated using a Shandon Hypercentre XP or Shandon Pathcentre. During processing the tissue is embedded in a solid medium to give it support and rigidity so that it can be cut into thin sections (3–5 μm thick) on the microtome, a specialized cutting tool. The embedding medium usually used is paraffin wax. There are several stages in tissue processing: dehydration in increasing concentrations of alcohol, usually ethanol, to remove fixative and water; clearing in a hydrocarbon solvent, usually xylene, which replaces the dehydrating fluid and is miscible with the embedding medium; infiltration with the embedding medium; embedding.

Embedding is usually performed at a commercially available embedding station, for example, Leica EG 1160. This comprises a paraffin wax dispenser, cold plate, and moulds. The tissue block with the surface to be cut face down is placed in a mould, which is filled with molten wax and allowed to solidify on the cold plate. In some circumstances embedding in a medium harder than paraffin wax is necessary in order to provide adequate tissue support to facilitate the cutting of 'semi-thin' sections (<1 μm thick). Semi-thin sections provide greater cytological and nuclear detail and are required in lymphoma/leukaemia diagnosis, they are also used to embed bone marrow trephines that do not require prior decalcification. These harder mediums are plastic resins. Epoxy and methacrylate are the two principal types of resin used. Processing is usually performed manually; from small biopsies semi-thin sections can be available in 1–2 days.

Sections are cut on a microtome. Different types of microtomes are used for paraffin, resin, and EM blocks. With paraffin blocks the ends of successive sections tend to stick together forming a ribbon, which is then floated out onto a waterbath. The sections flatten on the water and creases can be removed by gentle teasing with a forceps. All or selected sections are then mounted, that is, drawn up onto glass slides and allowed to air-dry. In routine practice the sections stick sufficiently to the glass slides, however adhesives are necessary for some procedures.

As the sections are translucent it is necessary to colour the tissue before it can be examined under the light microscope. This is achieved by staining or dyeing the sections. H&E are the standard stains used in diagnostic laboratories. Haematoxylin is a natural dye extracted from the logwood, *Haematoxylon campechianum* that is grown commercially in the West Indies (14). Haematoxylin itself does not stain and must be oxidized to haematein, which acts as the dye. The solution however, is usually known as haematoxylin. In tissue sections it stains the nuclei blue. It is combined with a counterstain, usually eosin, which dyes the cell cytoplasm and other tissue components in varying shades of pink. A wide variety of other stains, often referred to as 'special stains', are available for use in histopathology to demonstrate the various cellular and stromal components in tissues such as proteins, carbohydrates, and collagen fibres (14, 15). With the availability of a wide variety of antibodies to cellular and structural tissue components IHC has largely replaced the need to utilize many of these stains. In current practice H&E staining of tumours is used to determine the nuclear morphology and architectural characteristics. Additional stains still commonly employed include PAS to demonstrate cytoplasmic glycogen, especially useful in Ewing's family of tumours, and reticulin stain to show the architecture in sarcoma and lymphoma. The sections are then covered with a glass-cover slip (fixed in place with nail-varnish or glue) ready for examination under the light microscope.

2. Immunohistochemistry

Although most macromolecules are common to all cell and tissue types, expression of some are specific to particular cell types and/or functions. These so-called molecular markers can be exploited to provide information on tissue structure, integrity, and origin, in addition to pathological or dynamic processes such as proliferation, differentiation, and apoptosis. IHC of tissues or immunocytology (IC) of cells for such molecular markers has been one of the most significant advances in diagnostic pathology over the last two decades. This has been particularly useful in the evaluation of poorly differentiated tumours, and the sub-classification of tumours with similar morphology, for example, use of desmin, myogenin, and MYOD1 to distinguish rhabdomyosarcoma from other small RCT (Fig. 1.3). It is usually necessary to employ a panel of antibodies in the assessment of RCT of childhood; desmin, myogenin, MYOD1, vimentin, MIC2, neural (NSE, PGP9.5,

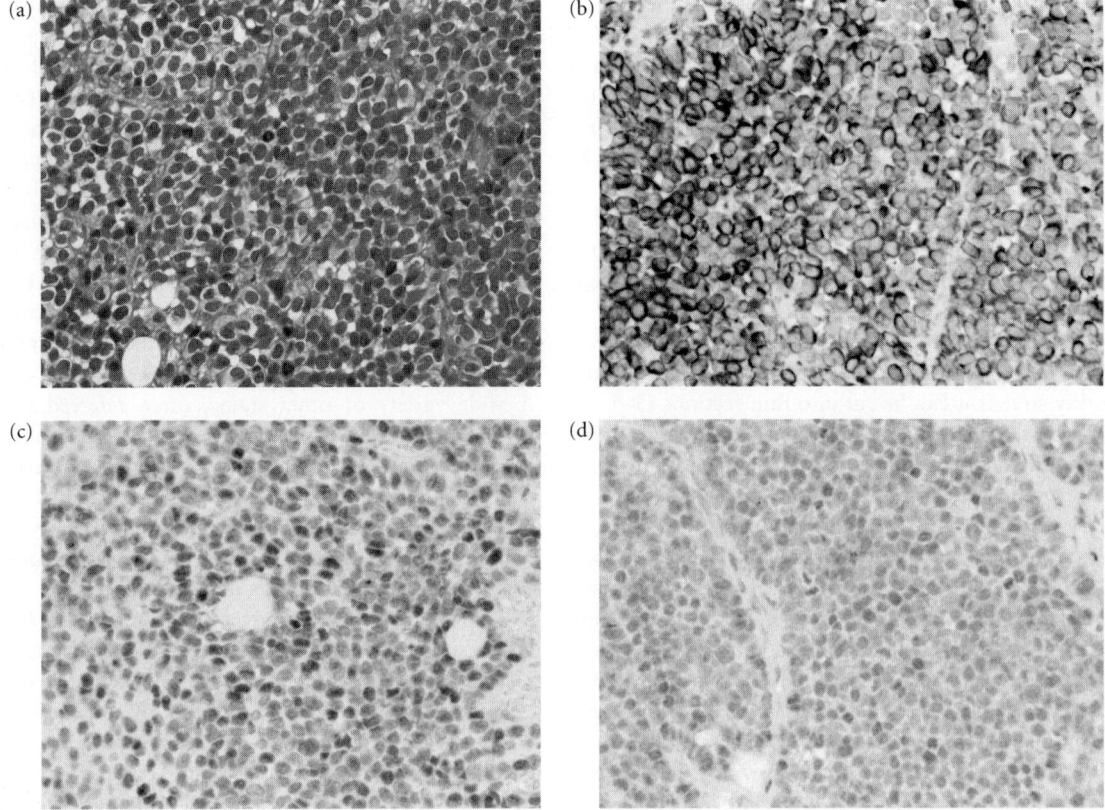

Fig. 1.3 (a) Small RCT (H&E on formalin-fixed paraffin-embedded tissue block), which with the aid of immunohistochemical reactions described below was diagnosed as a rhabdomyosarcoma (solid alveolar type). (b) Desmin antibody positivity in cytoplasm demonstrated by brown colour (ABC method, with DAB as chromogen). (c) MYOD1 positivity in nuclei demonstrated by brown colour (ABC method, with DAB as chromogen). (d) Myogenin positivity in nuclei demonstrated by brown colour (ABC method, with DAB as chromogen). See Plate 1.

synaptophysin, NB84), lymphoid (CD45, CD10, CD3), and epithelial (cytokeratin, EMA). In addition to improving diagnostic accuracy IHC also increases understanding of the relationship between tumours and can provide important prognostic information that may be used to stratify patients for therapy.

The generation of antibodies through immunization of animals with purified antigen or antigen-mixtures (which may be protein, carbohydrate, or lipids) provides a highly specific tool for the recognition of unique antigenic epitopes, many of which are expressed by a limited number of cells and/or tissues. Antisera may contain multiple antibodies to different epitopes of an antigen, that is, polyclonal, or recognize a single antigenic epitope, that is, monoclonal. Both have different advantages and disadvantages, depending on the intended purpose (Table 1.2). Most companies provide data sheets that may help identify the most appropriate antibody for a specific process, for example, IHC, Western blot, enzyme-linked immunosorbent assay (ELISA). To optimize shelf-life antibody stocks are usually stored at 4°C, undiluted or with a protective protein added, that is, bovine serum albumin (0.1% w/v) or foetal bovine serum albumin (10% v/v). Sodium azide (0.1% w/v) may be added to inhibit protein degradation. Most antibodies retain activity for many months when stored in this way. Some antibodies may be stored by freezing, in aliquots to avoid freeze–thawing, although sheep antisera, IgM monoclonal antibodies, and immunoconjugates are particularly susceptible to freeze-damage.

There are three key stages to IHC and IC:

- Specimen preparation
- Binding of antibody
- Detection of bound antibody.

Table 1.2 Advantages and disadvantages of polyclonal and monoclonal antisera used in IHC

Polyclonal		Monoclonal	
Advantages	Disadvantages	Advantages	Disadvantages
Recognise partially denatured epitopes	No reproducible way of generating (immunisation and animal dependent)	Unlimited supply of antibody raised against a single antigenic epitope	Generally not as useful on paraffin-embedded material as polyclonal antisera
Sensitive	May require pre-absorption to improve specificity	Purification of antigen not required	May have reduced sensitivity compared to polyclonal antisera[1]
Form insoluble complexes[2]			Cannot absorb out cross-reactivity

[1] Very antisera dependent.
[2] Useful for immunoprecipitation.

Optimal specimen preparation is essential to retain cellular morphology and antigen expression. Rapid transfer of tissues from surgery to fixation is particularly important for retaining intact RNA (see below), although it is equally important to prevent dehydration of tissues and loss of antigen expression. The primary consideration is the fixation process (see other sections in this chapter). The choice of fixative is usually a compromise between that which preserves cell and tissue morphology and retains the antigens of interest for IHC; optimal conditions for each antibody should be established empirically. Cryopreservation is the optimal method for retaining epitopes, although morphological preservation may be poor. Aldehyde fixation and paraffin wax embedding permits excellent preservation of morphology, but the harsh treatment can irretrievably destroy antigenic epitopes. In many cases the epitopes can be recovered by using antigen-retrieval techniques (Table 1.3), although care must be taken to ensure the retrieval technique does not reveal cryptic or neo-epitopes. Whenever a new antibody is being evaluated it is essential to compare the immunolabelling patterns on paraffin-embedded material after antigen retrieval with those of unfixed cryostat sections. Sections of 4–5 μm are typically prepared from the tissue blocks and mounted onto microscope slides for maximum antibody penetration and ease of handling. Adherence of sections to slides can be increased by using Superfrost slides (BDH) or coating glass slides with 3-aminopropyltriethoxysilane (2% in ethanol v/v) or poly-L-lysine (10% in water plus preservatives).

Optimal IHC is dependent on maximizing the antigen signal to background noise ratio. This is achieved by

Table 1.3 Some common methods of antigen retrieval

Technique	Procedure
Microwave*	Cover sections in citrate buffer (10 mM pH 6), and boil in a microwave. Place on ice
Trypsin	Treat with trypsin (0.1% w/v) in 0.1% calcium chloride pH 7.8 for 10 min at 37°C
Boiling trypsin	Treat with trypsin (0.1% w/v) in 0.1% calcium chloride pH 7.8 for 1 min at 37°C and boil in a microwave as above

Note: Antigen retrieval may be necessary in dewaxed, rehydrated paraffin sections; care should be taken to confirm the retrieval does not expose cryptic-epitopes.
* Some use an autoclave in place of a microwave.

empirical optimization of primary and secondary antibody concentrations; typically primary antibody concentrations are 1–10 μg/ml or up to 1:500 dilution whereas secondary antibodies are diluted to <1 μg/ml or >1:2000 dilution to minimize background. Incubations of 60 min are usually adequate, most frequently at room temperature. Incubation at 4°C, overnight may improve poor specificity. High background staining is most commonly caused by antibody drying on the section during incubations, inadequate washing between incubations, binding to Fc receptors on leukocytes, or endogenous immunoglobulins, endogenous peroxidase, or autofluorescence depending on the detection technique used. These can be minimized by taking a number of simple precautions (Table 1.4). The specificity of antibody binding must be

Table 1.4 Solutions to common background artefacts

Problem	Solution
Antibody drying on slide during incubation	Incubate slides in a sealed container lined with damp paper to humidify
Inadequate washing	Include a detergent in the final wash step e.g. 0.1% (v/v) Tween 20 or Nonident P-40
Endogenous immunoglobulins	Pre-absorption of sera with serum of the same species as the specimen; primary antibody must be raised in a different species to the tissues being labeled
Binding to leukocyte Fc receptors	Pre-block Fc sites with serum from same species as secondary antibody
Endogenous proteins used in the detection process expressed in tissues	Block or destroy endogenous activity or use an alternative detection system. e.g. endogenous peroxidase activity blocked with hydrogen peroxide (0.6% v/v) in methanol or alkaline phosphatase activity destroyed by heating sections at 95°C for 15min*

* These procedures may affect some epitopes or histologies.

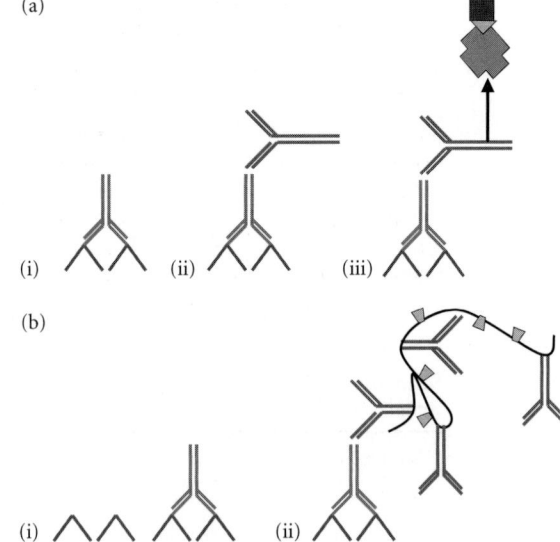

Fig. 1.4 Diagrammatical representation of IHC methods. (a) ABC detection of bound antibody. (i) Primary antibody added to section and incubated. (ii) Biotinylated secondary antibody added. Incubated. (iii) Streptavidin–biotinylated-enzyme complex added. Incubated. (b) The sensitivity of IHC detection can be increased by using a polymer that enables binding of multiple enzyme molecules to a secondary antibody via a dextran backbone, for example, DAKO Envison™ system. (i) Primary antibody added to section. Incubated. (ii) Application of polymer and secondary antibody.

checked by using appropriate positive and negative controls in each experiment. These should include:

(1) a negative no primary antibody control to check non-specific binding of the secondary antibody (ideally an irrelevant primary antibody should be included, isotype matched where appropriate);
(2) a positive tissue to confirm the activity of primary and secondary antibodies;
(3) a negative control tissue to check non-specific binding of the primary antibody. When multi-cellular sections are used this may be a negative cell type readily recognized by its morphology, for example, normal tissue adjacent to a tumour section.

Detection of bound antibody is usually through use of a secondary anti-immunoglobulin antibody raised in a different host species from that of the primary antibody. The sensitivity of detection can be increased by a series of amplification steps (Fig. 1.4). These may include the use of digoxygenin conjugates and antibody reagents (DIG method), avidin (or streptavidin) binding to biotin (ABC method; (20)), peroxidase–antiperoxidase (PAP), or alkaline phosphatase–anti-alkaline phosphatase (APAAP). These use a bridging antibody that binds to the primary antibody but has free-binding sites that bind PAP or APAAP complexes enhancing the detection signal.

There are three key detection systems:

1. Chromogenic where the secondary antibody is conjugated to an enzyme, for example, horseradish peroxidase or alkaline phosphatase, the antibody being detected by precipitation of a coloured reaction product.
2. Fluorescence where the secondary antibody is conjugated to a fluorescent tag, for example, fluorescein-isothiocyanate (FITC) (green fluorescence), tetraethyl rhodamine isothiocyanate (TRITC, red fluorescence), or 7-amino-4-methylcouramin-3-acetic acid (AMCA, blue fluorescence).
3. Colloidal gold particles (10 nm) may be used to bind secondary antibody and visualized under light microscopy or EM. This is most usually the method of choice for transmission and scanning immunoelectron microscopy (21).

For most applications chromogenic or fluorescent detection are the methods of choice; routine IHC usually employs chromogenic detection. This is particularly useful in a diagnostic setting as a permanent record of the staining pattern is the result, unlike immunofluorescence where the signal rapidly fades with time. However recent mountants have been developed that stabilize the immunofluorescence signal (Dako, CA, USA, Fluorescent Mounting Medium). In some cases, for example, cell phenotyping, double- and triple-labelling with multiple antibodies can be a very powerful technique. This is most successful when the primary antibodies are raised in different species and/or different immunoglobulin class, and different fluorochromes and fluorescence microscopy can be used.

One of the concerns for anyone undertaking morphological studies is tissue and antigen preservation. For many years the quality of sections from formalin-fixed, paraffin-embedded tissues was never questioned, however recent studies have shown changes in immunoreactivity in as little as 12 weeks (22, 23). Consequently interpretation of IHC on stored unstained sections should be made cautiously. This appears to be tissue and antigen dependent, although why some antigens are susceptible to change by storage but not others is unclear. Antigen degradation does not appear to be such a problem in uncut paraffin blocks, which suggests exposure of the sections to air may contribute to alteration in the antigen. For routine diagnostic pathology this is unlikely to be a problem, as IHC for patient diagnosis is usually performed on one- or two-day old sections, however for retrospective studies this could be critical. For such studies cryopreserved material may be most useful.

3. Electron microscopy

Glutaraldehyde is the fixative usually employed in diagnostic transmission EM. The fresh tissue is cut into small pieces, usually 1 mm^3, and placed in ice-cold gluteraldehyde for optimal fixation (15). The tissue is postfixed in osmium tetroxide and then dehydrated, embedded in a plastic medium, usually epoxy or acrylic resin, and sectioned on an ultramicrotome. Semi-thin sections (0.5–2 μm thick) are cut initially and stained with basic dyes such as methylene blue, toluidine blue, or a combination of methylene blue and Azur ll for light microscopic examination, to confirm the presence of tumour cells in the block and to assess morphology. The next procedure is to cut ultrathin sections (80 nm thick). These are mounted on copper grids, stained with uranyl acetate followed by lead citrate, and dried. The grid is placed in the electron microscope and the tumour ultrastructure examined.

4. Cytogenetic, DNA, and cell-cycle analysis

Cancer is a genetic disease, and where non-random chromosome abnormalities have been identified these play an important role in the diagnosis of haematological and solid malignancies. Traditionally chromosome analysis is carried out by G-banding of metaphase chromosomes, although FISH (the hybridization of conjugated probes to metaphase chromosomes and visualization of the probe by fluorescent microscopy) is increasingly used (see Chapter 2). For both these techniques tumour material should be taken into tissue culture media and transferred within 24 h to the Cytogenetic Department where viable cells are grown. The main limitation with these techniques is the difficulty obtaining metaphase tumour cells, in the absence of dividing tumour cells these techniques can provide a false normal cytogenetic profile. Adaptations to the FISH technique have overcome such problems, for example, multicolour FISH uses 24 different fluorochromes to paint individual chromosomes of interphase and metaphase cells. This obviates the requirement for dividing tumour cells, as does comparative genomic hybridization. Both these techniques and new developments in the analysis of chromosome abnormalities are described in Chapter 2.

To measure the underlying cell-cycle kinetic features that determine the overall growth rate of cancer cells several methods have been employed including evaluation of cell-cycle stage, exploiting markers of DNA synthesis, counting mitosis, and more recently endogenous markers of proliferation. The term 'growth fraction' (GF) has been proposed to distinguish the cells progressing through the cell-cycle (P) from the non-cycling or quiescent (Q) cells in tumours; $GF = P \div (P + Q)$. The classical autoradiographic techniques based on pulse- or continuous-cell labeling with tritiated thymidine (24) have been largely replaced by flow cytometric methods, as these are less time consuming and overcome the ambiguities in the GF estimation due to radiobiological effects of the precursor radioisotope and the diluting effect of proliferating cells on unlabeled cells. Although flow cytometry is not informative in all tumours, it remains a particularly useful tool in some haematological, for example, acute lymphoblastic leukemia, and solid tumours, for example, astrocytomas, medulloblastomas, neuroblastoma, osteosarcoma, hepatoblastoma (25).

Flow cytometry can be used to measure a number of cellular features including cell size, granularity of cytoplasm, cell viability, cell-cycle (S-phase fraction), DNA content (DNA ploidy), cell surface markers, and enzyme content (26, 27). The flow cytometer hydrodynamically focuses cell suspensions in a sample chamber and passes single cells through a light source, usually using a laser. The light scattered at various angles by the cells is registered by detectors and converted to an electronic signal, which is digitized and analysed by a computer to produce a histogram. The technique allows the analysis of between 5000 and 10,000 cells per second.

The strategies of cell-cycle analysis by flow cytometry can be subdivided into three main categories:

1. Snapshot or static analysis, which can be based on a single measurement of DNA content or multiparameter analysis where DNA content is coupled with a second feature, providing more information on a particular metabolite or molecular trait that generally correlates with progression through the cell-cycle or with cell quiescence. This is the strategy most commonly used in clinical practice.
2. A combination of multiparameter flow cytometry with kinetic measurements; the time lapse static observations as in 1 are combined with the rate of cell progression through the cell cycle.
3. Analysis of DNA replication by simultaneous measurement of BrdU incorporation and DNA content.

The position of a cell in the cell cycle can be estimated based on its DNA content. Because the duration of S and G_2 and M phases is relatively constant, while the duration of G_1 varies, and quiescent (G_0) cells usually have a DNA content equivalent to that of G_1 cells, the sum of cells in S, G_2, and M phases reflects the proliferative potential of the cell population. Nuclear DNA content doubles during S phase and therefore the cell age during S phase can be estimated based on the amount of replicating DNA (increase in DNA content). In contrast, cells in G_1, and cells in G_2 and M, have identical DNA content; equivalent to the DNA ploidy index 1.0 and 2.0, respectively. Under ideal conditions of DNA measurements based on DNA-specific fluorescence, the G_1 and G_2 and M cells therefore would have uniform DNA values. Due to inaccuracies in DNA measurements, the actual data are in the form of G_1 and $G_2 + M$ peaks. Several mathematical methods and computer programs are available to obtain the percentage of cells in G_1, S, and $G_2 + M$ from the flow cytometry histograms (26). This information is clinically useful in some cancers where high rates of proliferation have been correlated with aggressive tumour behaviour (28).

During flow cytometry, any fluorescent dyes the cells contain will be excited by the light beam and the emitted fluorescence intensity quantified using photomultiplier tubes. If antibodies are bound to fluorochromes, antibody staining can readily be detected. Fluorescent dyes, which bind particular cellular components can also be quantified, for example, propidium iodide (a red fluorescent dye, which binds DNA by intercalation). Total DNA content can be measured by red fluorescence per cell; G_2 and M together have twice as much fluorescence as G_1 cells, and S phase cells will have a range of intermediate fluorescence values, giving rise to a characteristic histogram from which the proportions of cells in these phases can be calculated. Tumours are often aneuploid (29), and show an extra fluorescent peak, corresponding to normal diploid cells in the tumour (e.g. lymphocytes, fibroblasts). The major limitation of flow cytometry is that cells need to be prepared in single cell suspensions for analysis. This is easily achieved with blood and other fluids making the analysis of leukaemias and lymphomas relatively simple. Obtaining samples from solid tumours is more difficult as disaggregation of the cells is necessary.

5. Tissue cryopreservation

Tissue samples may be frozen and stored at low temperatures with good preservation for many years if rapidly and appropriately processed (30). Cryopreservation is advantageous as the epitopes of tumour-specific antigens are retained so there is no requirement for antigen retrieval, and RNA and DNA are not chelated to underlying cellular proteins making assays for DNA or RNA markers more reliable and robust. A potential problem with cryopreservation for busy Pathology departments is the speed required to transfer newly dissected material through the freezing process to ensure optimal quality. To minimize degradation of nucleic acids, in particular, RNA, tumour material can be rapidly frozen in liquid nitrogen ($<-200°C$). However loss of ultrastructure and ice-damage frequently occurs as tissues are frozen so rapidly that ice crystals form in the section. This can be overcome by slowing the freezing process by placing the tissue in liquid nitrogen cooled isopentane, this results in rapid freezing but impregnation of the tissue with ice-cold isopentane minimizes crystal formation. Tissue integrity may be further improved by mounting the section, for example, in OCT compound and then freezing through liquid nitrogen cooled isopentane. From material frozen in this way cryosections can be prepared for immunohistology and IHC, laser-capture (see below), or nucleic acid extraction.

Cytogenetic analysis is important for the accurate diagnosis of an increasing number of paediatric malignancies, for example, lymphoma and leukaemia, tumours of the Ewing's sarcoma family, alveolar rhabdomyosarcoma. Genetic anomalies are particularly useful for the accurate diagnosis of tumours with similar histological appearance but which may have atypical clinical presentation, such as the sarcomas and small RCT (Table 1.5). Different techniques have been developed to identify these abnormalities (see Chapters 2 and 3). As the amount of tumour material taken at diagnosis is often small, polymerase chain reaction (PCR) amplification methods are ever more attractive for the increasing number of diagnostic tests.

The analysis of fresh clinical material by reverse transcriptase polymerase chain reaction (RT-PCR) or PCR is relatively straightforward if good quality RNA or DNA respectively can be extracted. Providing there is sufficient material and specimens are rapidly processed or transferred to liquid nitrogen/−80°C freezer this is not usually a problem. Techniques for extracting DNA from fresh tissues are well described in many excellent laboratory manuals (31) and although often long and laborious do produce good quality material, for example, proteinase K digestion for up to 24 h, followed by purification of DNA by extraction using phenol and chloroform. Extraction of un-degraded RNA is more difficult because of its labile nature and the presence of ribonucleases in the specimens. Standard RNA extraction protocols (31) overcome this problem by lysing tissues and cells in guanidium thiocyanate (32), a chemical which denatures ribonucleases. The RNA is then purified by organic extraction and ethanol precipitation (similar to that for DNA extraction) or by sedimentation through caesium chloride. Because RNases are present in the environment, on hands, and on glassware, extraction of RNA requires the use of gloves, sterile plastics and glassware, and RNase-free solutions. Commercial preparations to extract DNA and RNA are readily available; although often expensive these products generally exploit the basic techniques outlined above but often provided in a rapid, user-friendly format.

In contrast DNA or RNA extracted from archived tissue tends to be impure and of low molecular weight. However the sensitivity of RT-PCR and PCR is such that small quantities of degraded nucleic acids may be amplified successfully. Hence PCR can be used for the retrospective analysis of a range of pathological archival material. Improved methods for the isolation of DNA

Table 1.5 Examples of malignancies with characteristic gene translocations and their respective gene fusion transcripts, that can be used as targets for RT-PCR characterization or detection of disease

Malignancy	Translocation	Fusion transcript
Alveolar rhabdomyosarcoma	t(2;13)(q35;q14) t(2;13)(q35;q14)	PAX3-FKHR PAX7-FKHR
Synovial sarcoma	t(X;18)(p11.2;q11.2)	SYT-SSX1 SYT-SSX2 SYT-SSX4
Tumours of the Ewing's sarcoma family	t(11;22)(q24;q12) t(21;22)(q22;q12) t(7;22)(p22;q12) t(17;22)(q12;q12) t(2;22)(q33;q12)	EWS-FLI1 EWS-ERG EWS-ETV1 EWS-E1AF EWS-FEV
Desmoplastic small RCT	t(11;22)(q13;q12)	EWS-WT1
Myxoid chondrosarcoma	t(9;22)(q22;q12)	EWS-CHN
Myxoid liposarcoma	t(12;22)(q13;q12)	EWS-CHOP
Clear cell sarcoma	t(12;22)(q13;q12)	EWS-AFT1
Congenital fibrosarcoma	t(12;15)(p13;q25)	ETV6-NTRK3
Anaplastic large cell lymphoma	t(2;5)(p23;q35) t(2;3)(p23;q21) inv (2)(p23;q35) t(1;2)(q25;p23)	NPM-ALK TFG-ALK ATIC-ALK TPM3-ALK

and even mRNA from archived paraffin-embedded material have now been described (33, 34). The amount of nucleic acid isolated from diminutive and/or archived samples is often small, making it difficult to visualize when the extraction and purification process requires precipitation. Pellet-paint™ NF co-precipitant, a dye-carrier that is co-precipitated with nucleic acids and appears red under normal light, can aid visualization of small nucleic acid pellets (Novagen, United Kingdom).

Although good quality RNA is more difficult to isolate and is less stable than DNA, RT-PCR is increasingly used for the characterization of tumour-specific gene rearrangements or detection of circulating tumour cells. In particular, RT-PCR may be used to design multiplex assays for the characterization of tumours by their genetic abnormalities (35, 36, 37) or tissue-specific RNA profile (38, 39). Amplification by RT-PCR requires the conversion of tumour derived mRNA to cDNA, which is subsequently amplified by PCR for the targets of interest (Fig. 1.5(a)). The position of chromosome translocation breakpoints can vary between tumours and may be scattered across many kilobases of DNA from either chromosome. Splicing exons during transcription of the chimeric gene to generate fusion transcripts usually reduces the length of target nucleic acids to be amplified, improving the efficiency and reliability of the amplification, which can often be achieved with a single primer pair. A second advantage is the broader application of RT-PCR, allowing identification of tissue-specific mRNA. Because of the sensitivity of PCR and RT-PCR, it is susceptible to contamination and false positive results. Consequently stringent laboratory practice and good quality control are essential for its use in a routine diagnostic laboratory (33, 34).

The presence of chimeric fusion products detected by RT-PCR correlates well with conventional G-banding studies, but perhaps more interestingly RT-PCR can be used to identify tumour-specific gene rearrangements in tumours where conventional G-banding has been uninformative, either due to a very complex gene rearrangement or lack of mitotic cells. The use of RT-PCR to detect tissue-specific RNA profiles is less robust that detection of tumour-specific genetic abnormalities, since there is a risk that the RNA sample analysed may contain normal tissues that express the RT-PCR target, for example the use of RT-PCR for myogenin to characterize rhabdomyosarcoma may also detect myogenin expressed by native muscle fibres. In such situations the isolation of tumour mater-ial by laser-capture or microdissection may be particularly useful (Fig. 1.6), ensuring only tumour cells are captured for RNA, DNA, or even

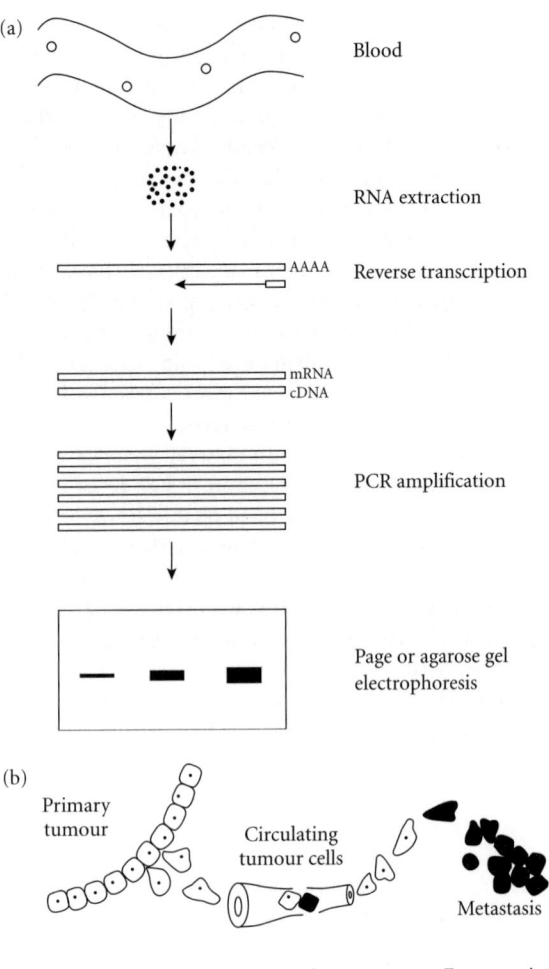

Fig. 1.5 Diagrammatical representation of RT-PCR applied to peripheral blood for the detection of circulating tumour cells. (a) RNA is extracted from peripheral blood, and reverse transcribed into cDNA. cDNA is amplified by PCR to generate double stranded DNA products that can be analysed by separation in an agarose gel, and visualized under ultraviolet (UV)-light after staining with ethidium bromide. (b) Using RT-PCR it is possible to detect 1 tumour cell in up to 1×10^6 normal cells. This approach assumes that non-haemopoietic cells are not normally found in the circulation and requires a target mRNA for amplification by RT-PCR, that is expressed in the tumour cell but not the haemopoietic cells. The presence of tumour cells in peripheral blood does not necessarily mean the tumour cell will go on to metastasize, although dissemination of tumour cells is an essential step for metastasis.

protein isolation and analysis (40–42). This approach can also be useful for the characterization of focal differences within a tumour. Cryostat sections are the most useful sources of tumour material for laser-capture. The

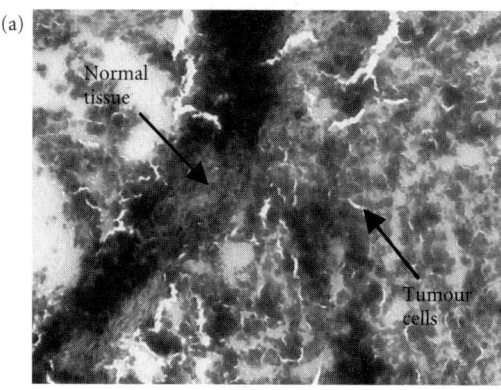 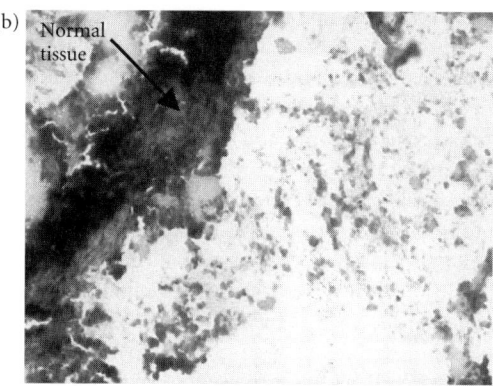

Fig. 1.6 Laser-capture. Tumour sections (7 microns) were stained with H&E and tumour cells were laser-capture microdissected using the PixCell laser-capture micro-dissection system (Arcturus Engineering, Inc., Mountain View, CA); tumour was captured using 2000 pulses of the 30 μm laser beam onto CapSure™ film (Arcturus Engineering Inc.). (a) Tumour before laser-capture micro-dissection. (b) Tumour after micro-dissection of tumour cells, leaving the normal tissue behind.

sections may be stained with H&E to allow identification of cells based on morphology; alternatively sections may be stained with antibodies to isolate cell populations with specific phenotypes. Obviously the small number of cells captured means sensitive methods for the extraction of nucleic acids or proteins from laser-capture cells must be developed. For some of these applications commercial kits are available that work very well, for example, RNA isolated from the laser-captured material using the micro RNA isolation kit from Stratagene, Cambridge, UK.

RT-PCR for tumour- or tissue-specific genes has also been exploited to detect small numbers of tumour cells in cytologically normal bone marrow aspirates and peripheral blood (Fig. 1.5(b)). For metastasis to occur tumour cells must circulate in body fluids. Although the presence of such cells is necessary for metastasis to occur, it is of course not sufficient. However, increasingly the presence of tumour cells detected by RT-PCR is reported to provide clinically significant data that reflects the evolution and management of cancers (43). The molecular detection of these small numbers of circulating tumour cells may ultimately lead to a redefinition of metastatic disease and disease-free, and consequently may change patient management.

Section B—Fixatives

Of the many tissue fixatives available, the most suitable for all the diagnostic and prognostic procedures must be selected. Consequently when deciding which of the

Table 1.6 Categories of fixation* and examples

Fixation method	Examples
Aldehydes	Formaldehyde, glutaraldehyde, acrolein
Oxidising agents	Osmium tetroxide, potassium permanganate, potassium dichromate
Protein denaturing reagents	Acetic acid, methanol, ethanol
Other cross-linkers	Carbodiimides
Physical	Heat, microwave
Unknown mechanisms	Picric acid, mercuric chloride

* According to Baker (44).

many fixatives (Table 1.6) (44) to use, it is essential to know the precise effects of the fixative on the different tissue macromolecules, that is, proteins, nucleic acids. The ideal fixative preserves tissue morphology from osmotic damage and shrinkage (45) and retains *in situ* all tissue components and their characteristics including antigenic epitopes for IHC.

Cytochemical aspects of fixation

1. Protein fixation

The most important reaction in tissue fixation is that which stabilizes protein. The basic mechanism of how this occurs is largely unknown, but in general it appears that fixatives have the ability to form cross-links between different proteins in the cell thereby forming a cellular gel that maintains symmetry within the cell. Thus soluble proteins are fixed to structural proteins, rendering them insoluble and thereby giving the cell added strength.

Aldehydes: Reaction between aldehydes and proteins has long been known and forms the basis of the Cross-link hypothesis (46–49). The reactions which occur are usually mild and the fixation time is relatively short. Cross-links are formed between protein molecules, the reaction centring on the basic amino acid lysine (the residues of which exist on the exterior of the protein molecule). In the case of formaldehyde, the reaction is largely reversible by an excess of water in the first 24 h post fixation. In contrast, glutaraldehyde fixation is more rapid and is irreversible at 24 h. The speed of reaction and the degree of reversibility when treating tissues with aldehyde fixations is pH dependent (proceeding very rapidly in acid pH). Fixation in general denatures protein but for routine diagnostic purposes this is not of great importance. It does however, attain significance in IHC, high resolution EM and molecular pathological techniques. Aldehydes react with basic proteins and alter their iso-electric points. During the process of cross-linking, polymerization occurs and the size of the polymer formed is governed by the pH of the fixative.

Oxidising agents: Little is known about the interaction of oxidizing agents (potassium dichromate, osmium tetroxide, and potassium permanganate) with proteins. It is known that cross-linking occurs with osmium tetroxide, but whether or not this occurs with other agents is unclear.

Mercuric Chloride: When used as a secondary fixative, mercuric chloride has been shown to interact with certain amino acids in proteins, including amino, imidazole, thiol, phosphate, and hydroxyl groups. The reaction with thiol groups has been extensively investigated and it has been shown that dimercaptide is formed. $2R.SH + HgCl_2 = (RS)_2Hg + 2H + 2Cl$. The production of hydrogen ions makes the resulting solutions acidic. In addition, mercuric compounds react with disulphide groups forming reaction products, which may vary with the pH of the reaction.

Microwave fixation: It has been known for a long time that tissues and blood films may be fixed by heating. Cooking is in fact an extreme form of fixation. Until recently, the heat used was relatively uncontrolled, for example, from a Bunsen burner. Microwave ovens can now be used to deliver heat in a uniform manner; microwaves penetrate into the tissues for about 2 cm from the surface. Microwave energy interacts with dipolar molecules causing their oscillation with a frequency of 2450 MHz. Because of this, polar side chains of proteins and water suffer increases in their respective thermal energies, and protein denaturation then ensues. Optimal microwave temperature fixation is approximately 60°C (15). The chief advantages of this system are that the tissue is fixed right through in a very short time, potentially allowing the analysis of cellular processes that proceed quickly. In this way microwaves differ from conventional heating in a water bath, which produces a temperature gradient across the tissue. Microwaving at 45–55°C stabilizes the tissue but does not fix it. It may be stored at 4°C for some time in this state.

2. Nucleic acid interactions

High quality DNA is usually required for PCR work; nevertheless formalin-fixed paraffin-embedded tissue has been successfully used with PCR to detect the presence of viruses or oncogene mutations (51–54). Reaction of nucleic acids and histone proteins with fixatives has not been extensively investigated (55). Fixation of tissues alters the chemical and physical state of DNA and RNA. Little is known however, of the basic mechanism involved but the subject has been reviewed by Hopwood (56). Glutaraldehyde is known to react with histone proteins of chick erythrocyte nuclei; reactivity appears to be confined to F1 histone proteins (57). The interaction between histone and glutaraldehyde and formaldehyde has also been investigated (58). F1 histone proteins react much faster with the aldehydes than any other histone protein group, probably due to the higher lysine content, which is the nidus of aldehyde–protein interactions. The above work suggests that the formaldehyde cross-links histone to DNA whereas glutaraldehyde links histone proteins to one another.

Many fixatives have been used for preservation of nucleic acids but relatively few with the exception of mercury and chromium salts, are known to react with them chemically. Indeed the interaction of mercuric salts with DNA was discovered through preservation of viral DNA sequences with subsequent decrease in the infectivity of the virus. Acidic alcohol fixatives, including Carnoy's are frequently used for nucleic acids. Although largely chemically bland, they are known to extract histone proteins. In prolonged fixation states, acidic alcohol fixatives extract RNA and with continued fixation, DNA.

DNA and RNA normally in their resting/native states do not react with formaldehyde. However, if the fixative solutions are heated to approximately 45°C for DNA and 65°C for RNA, uncoiling of the helices occurs. Similar reactions have been observed with glutaraldehyde (56). At fixation temperatures up to 64°C, no reaction occurred between native DNA (calf thymus or herring roe) and glutaraldehyde. Above 75°C reactions commenced and proceeded more quickly the higher the temperature. A similar reaction held for RNA and glutaraldehyde except that reactions began at 45°C. This selective non-reactivity appears to be related to the structure of the nucleic acids, the hydrogen-bonded structures of which are only broken at relatively high temperatures when purine and pyrimidine bases become available for reactions with aldehyde. Typical thermal transition profiles can thus be created for each particular fixative. Most tissue fixation is carried out at room temperature or 0–4°C where there can be little or no reaction between nucleic acid and fixative.

Amino groups of the nucleosides appear to be involved when and if fixation by formaldehyde takes place with the subsequent formation of methylene bridges. The mechanism and kinetics involved in these reactions have been studied by McGhee and Von Hippel (59–62). Regions of nucleic acids rich in adenosine and thymidine residues are most open to reaction with formaldehyde. This basic mechanism appears as follows: first, base pairs become unstuck due to local thermal fluctuations during fixation, then the exocyclic amino group of adenosine react. This reaction is reversible and the rate of interaction increases in proportion to the pH of the solution.

The denaturing effect of formaldehyde on nuclear chromatin structure has also been investigated (63). Conformational changes seen using circular dichroism in chromatin are due to cross-linkage with histones or between histones. Nucleic acids, being relatively large molecules, are most likely physically entrapped in the tissues following fixation. This non-fixation concept for nucleic acids has been confirmed by Langenberg for viral and yeast RNA (64). The use of more vigorous agents such as chromic-acid formaldehyde has been suggested, as such a mixture of fixatives is believed to stabilize nucleic acids (65). In addition, rapid chilling of tissues before glutaraldehyde fixation for approximately 12 h appears to preserve fragile viral inclusions in various plants. Without cooling, redistribution of viral particles is evident. Cell death, itself temperature dependent, is a very active process and cooling would considerably slow down many metabolic processes while fixation is taking place (66).

The importance of these observations is that, at temperatures normally used for fixation, uncoiling of nucleic acids does not occur. Only when temperatures are elevated does significant degradation of DNA occur. During paraffin wax infiltration or resin embedding, a reaction with any remaining fixative can take place. Adequate washing is therefore required to prevent such a phenomenon.

The question therefore is, how are nucleic acids retained in the tissues following fixation and to what extent do they undergo degradation? From studies, it appears that up to 30% of nucleic acids may be lost during the fixation process. During the cross-linking of proteins and the subsequent polymerization that occurs, it is possible that DNA/RNA becomes trapped in the protein matrix that is formed as a result of the fixation process. This is most likely the principle mechanism by which nucleic acid is retained following fixation.

The alcohol fixatives (ethanol and methanol) are commonly used for nucleic acid fixation and have the added advantage of causing little chemical change. Physical chemistry evaluations show that DNA is largely collapsed (unwound) in ethanol and methanol. It has been estimated that the concentration required for such collapse to occur is approximately 65%. When this denatured DNA is re-hydrated there is considerable reversion to the original state. The presence of salts in the fixative solution is known to be essential for the proper precipitation of nucleic acids.

Like most biological systems, individual fixatives are usually not sufficient for most purposes so usually combinations or mixtures of fixatives are used, the short comings of one being compensated for by another. With some mixtures, the individual components of the fixative cocktail react directly with one another, an example of which are the aldehydes and oxidizing agents. When such mixtures are made, use must subsequently be immediate, otherwise the effective concentration of each of the components will be decreased. Another phenomenon, which has been observed is that cross-linking produced by the mixture is usually less than that produced by the more active of the pair on its own.

Non-tissue factors that influence fixation

1. Buffer and hydrogen ion change

Because fixatives vary, it is natural to expect that the pH of fixatives will vary also. In general, a physiological range of pH is attained by the addition of a suitable buffer. Satisfactory fixation will occur between pH 6 and 8. Outside these limits, ultrastructural changes occur with dissociation of proteins, lipids, etc. Indeed during the agonal stages of cell death, the microenvironment of the cell changes and a reduction of the pH within cells occurs, mediated by anoxia.

A critical fixation pH is required for some morphological assessments. For example, gastric mucosa is optimally fixed at pH 5.5 in keeping with the natural local environment of the stomach. Indeed the idea of selective pH fixation has recently again become popular with the concept that gradual alterations in the pH of fixative solutions may be of advantage in dealing with tissues for EM. Glutaraldehyde, commonly used in EM fixation, is known to selectively polymerize at different pH with subsequent alteration in protein reactive groups and the protein cytoskeleton of the cell.

Some fixatives by their nature will automatically alter the pH of the solution. Acetic acid (a weak acid) will lower the pH, the effect of which is to alter the tertiary and quarternary structures of most proteins, which are usually stable over a limited range of pH. Other acids react similarly. Buffer systems are commonly used in fixation, the most common being Tris, bicarbonate, veronal acetate. When selecting a buffer care should be taken that the chosen buffer will not react with the fixative thereby reducing buffering capacity and fixation effect. If histochemical studies are to be performed, ideally the buffer must not alter enzyme activity or structure.

2. Temperature variations: are they critical?

Traditionally, fixation of routine surgical biopsy material has been carried out at room temperature. For some investigations, such as histochemistry and EM, fixation ideally should be performed at 4°C. At lower temperatures autolysis and diffusion of cellular substances is slowed down and preservation of cellular microarchitecture is more readily achieved. Fixatives in general act more rapidly at higher temperatures. Peracchia (67) has suggested that fixation should ideally be carried out under conditions of increasing temperature, an ideal which immediately appears impractical in busy laboratories. Indeed the interaction of nucleic acids with commonly used fixatives is negligible at temperatures commonly employed for fixation (56). Rapid fixation is achieved with heated formalin (40–45°C). Higher temperatures (60°C) impair tissue morphology.

3. Fixative penetration: a rate limiting step

Fixative penetration into tissue is of paramount importance. The process is usually slow therefore careful attention must be given to the size of the block taken, in order to obtain satisfactory fixation. In 1941 Medawar investigated the basic principles of fixative penetration in tissues, he found the depth of penetration was proportional to the square root of the time immersed (68). Discrete tissues react differently with a particular fixative and also the interaction of cellular subfractions with the fixative governs the diffusibility of the fixative. In general, fixatives with low diffusibility coefficients will give rise to uneven fixation and penetration of the tissues and thus preservation of proteins, nucleic acids, and fats will vary greatly from site to site.

4. Osmolarity of fixative solutions and the importance of fixative concentration

Most fixatives are used in aqueous solutions. More exacting requirements demand the addition of a buffer with special reference to the effect of osmotic pressure exacted by the resulting solution. In general, hypertonic solutions give rise to cell shrinkage; isotonic and hypotonic fixatives result in cell swelling and in general poor fixation.

By varying the osmolarity of the chosen fixative solution, it is possible to alter the structure of membrane systems. The addition of vehicles to fixative solutions (dextrans and polyvinyl pyrrolidone) also plays a part in determining osmolarity. Indeed it is true to say that vehicle osmolarity is usually more important than the total osmolarity of the fixative solution. Vehicle osmolarity should ideally be isotonic with that of tissues in their *in situ* setting. Glutaraldehyde has been investigated for this and it has been found that hypotonic glutaraldehyde solutions produce diffusion of acid phosphatase from lysosomes thus causing chemical changes in the cellular cytostructure (69).

The exact concentration of fixative used in any particular formulation depends not only on fixative effectiveness and solubility, but also invariably on cost. Glutaraldehyde has been extensively researched and has been found to be highly effective when used as a 3% solution but still retains significant activity at lower concentrations. For cellular morphology, staining of tissues varies with the concentration of fixative used.

5. The effect of adding substances on fixatives

Any chosen fixative solution will consist of the fixative agent(s), a buffer, and water. Various substances are sometimes added to produce specific chemical effects. The addition of some salts such as ammonium sulphate and potassium dihydrogen phosphate is known to stabilize proteins. Sodium chloride and sodium sulphate are used in conjunction with mercuric chloride. It has been shown that the sodium chloride in particular increases the bonding of mercuric chloride to the amino group of proteins and possibly also degrades coagulation factors. Tannic acid, used in EM, which is known to enhance fixation of proteins and lipids is also useful in demonstrating microtubules and filaments in the cell cytostructure (70).

6. *The effect of detergents*

The effect of making the cell membrane more permeable and thus allowing fixation of cytosolic components has focused attention on the use of detergents in the fixation processes. These are commonly employed with immunofluorescent techniques where the intracellular localization of substances is critical, many of which with high molecular weights are unable to pass through the cell membrane. Complete removal of the cell membranes by detergents has been used for cell skeletal surveys.

7. *Fixation time: a critical parameter*

The routine practice of many laboratories varies greatly but primary fixation in buffered formalin for 6 h followed by a period in formol sublimate appears to be a popular protocol with some centres. For EM, it is recommended that the submitted tissue be diced and placed in the appropriate fixative for 3 h and then placed in a holding buffer. Formalin fixation is known to proceed rapidly and is largely reversible. If tissues are fixed for 24 h or more in formalin, then most of the formalin can be washed out. Prolonged formalin fixation produces morphometric shrinkage and hardening of the tissues.

Glutaraldehyde on the other hand is shown to exhibit beneficial effects at longer fixation times. Prolonged fixation in aldehydes is known to greatly inhibit enzyme activity and also retards substrate diffusion and cross-linking between protein complexes, which may have implications for molecular pathological techniques on archival material. Oxidizing agents (osmium tetroxide and potassium permanganate) on the other hand degrade the tissues by oxidative cleavage of proteins with the loss of peptides.

8. *Secondary changes in tissues*

Tissue should ideally undergo immediate and complete fixation following removal from the living body. However this ideal is rarely achieved. Primary agonal changes due to anoxia occur during the handling of the tissues. Secondary agonal changes occur during the fixation process, and their extent is governed by individual variables such as the fixative used, fixative concentration, vehicles used in the fixative solution, solution osmolarity, and the tissue itself (70). Until full penetration has occurred, secondary agonal changes will continue. To quantify these changes for various fixatives would be an enormous task.

Time sequences for primary and secondary agonal changes are themselves highly variable. It is known that anoxia causes changes in cellular subfractions after 10 min. An example of this is mitochondrial swelling seen on EM. Within 1 h, enzymes involved in oxidative phosphorylation are lost.

The size of the submitted piece of tissue will directly govern the length of the secondary agonal phase; those cells at the centre undergoing differentially longer secondary agonal changes than those cells at the periphery.

Temperature variations are also important, as primary and secondary agonal changes vary directly with temperature; the hotter the local environment the more rapid the deterioration of the tissues. Indeed at cellular level, the way the individual cell deals with the fixative is dependent both on time and fixative concentration. Following removal from the body, all cells encounter a period at which they are exposed to an increasing gradient of fixative as it diffuses into the tissue. This 'Tidal' concept of fixative penetration dictates that at very low concentration, cells may be able to metabolize some fixatives. One example of this is formaldehyde, which may be metabolized by aldehyde dehydrogenase present in cells. As fixative concentration rises, the local kinetics of the cell alters with protein excess replaced exponentially by fixative concentration. Simultaneously, metabolic pathways will be preferentially lost, with consequent effects on various organelles of the cell microstructure.

9. *Post-fixation: secondary fixation (another fixation tool)*

Several situations warrant the use of two fixatives in succession. The practice in some laboratories is to fix tissues in buffered formaldehyde and then to subject the tissue to further fixation with mercuric chloride, for example, for a period of a few hours. It is observed that tissues are more easily cut and flatten more readily after sublimate post-fixation compared with buffered formaldehyde fixation alone. Staining intensities can be increased by the use of mercuric chloride compounds.

Chemical properties of fixatives

1. The formaldehyde containing fixatives

The aldehydes most commonly used in histopathology are formaldehyde (either by itself or in formulations) and glutaraldehyde. Commercially available formaldehyde is a gas, which is 49% soluble by weight and sometimes called formalin. For routine histological use, it is usually diluted to a 10% solution; pH changes occur during storage due to formation of formic acid and this usually requires buffering. In aqueous solution, formaldehyde exists primarily in its monohydrate form, methylene glycol ($CH_2(OH)$), in equilibrium with monomeric formaldehyde. In addition, low molecular weight polymers are also present. The carbonium ion CH_2OH formed in solutions of formaldehyde appears to be the agent responsible for the majority of the fixative effects of formalin.

Chemically, formaldehyde forms cross-links between protein groups amino peptidyl, thiol, imino, carboxyl, aromatic, amido, and hydroxyl. This interaction is pH dependent and results in the formation of methylene bridges (71, 72). Cross-linking may be abolished by vigorous washing, thus unmasking the reactive groups. The properties of formaldehyde have been assessed by Walker in a monograph in 1964 (73).

The effects on the various tissue components may be summarized as follows:

1. *Nucleic acids*: Formalin is known to block the reactive groups of nucleic acids thereby reducing their stability. During formalin fixation, cross-linking occurs between DNA and histone proteins present in the nucleus thus making DNA more inaccessible to extraction procedures and producing a coupled product.
2. *Carbohydrates*: Formalin fixes glycogen attached to protein very well but has little effect on other carbohydrates.
3. *Lipids*: Preservation is generally good although not all phospholipids are fixed.

In histological and histochemical work, formalin is nearly always used in buffered solutions at or above the neutral point.

2. Glutaraldehyde

This possesses similar physical and chemical characteristics to formaldehyde, the difference being the existence of the second aldehyde group in formaldehyde. Glutaraldehyde has been used extensively as an agent for the modification of proteins for protein linking and thus for fixation. The chemistry of aqueous glutaraldehyde solutions has been reviewed (74, 75). Aqueous solutions consist of approximately 40% free aldehyde, 16% monohydrate, 9% dihydrate, and 70% hemiacetal forms (76). Glutaraldehyde is known to rapidly deteriorate in solution but this is effectively delayed by reducing the pH. Storage at 4°C is recommended with the addition of a few drops of HCl. The reaction of glutaraldehyde with proteins, peptides, and amino acids is analogous to that of formaldehyde since gluraraldehyde is a bifunctional aldehyde. However, the precise mode of action remains to be determined; the cross-linking process produces three dimensional structures, which primarily constitute its action as a fixative.

3. Alcoholic fixatives

The possible singular use of absolute alcohol in tissue fixation is for the preservation of glycogen. Ethanol can preserve some proteins in an undenatured form and is therefore useful in immunofluorescence. The rapid penetration of alcohol in tissues makes it useful in combination with other fixatives, and it may therefore be usefully employed to speed up tissue processing time. Carnoy's fluid is particularly useful for the preservation of nucleic acids in paraffin tissue sections, and has the advantage that it does not interfere with the subsequent use of nucleases if this is so desired by the operator. Methanol and ethanol are the only alcoholic fixatives, which are commonly used in histopathology. Methanol is analogous to water and therefore competes effectively with the latter for hydrogen bonds in proteins, nucleic acids, etc.

The addition of alcohols to a protein solution causes aggregation or precipitation of proteins at or near their isoelectric points. Tertiary structure of proteins is also disrupted primarily due to the interruption of hydrophobic bonds in the protein backbone.

Methacran described in 1970 by Puchtler consists of a mixture of methanol, chloroform, and glacial acetic acid in the proportions 6:3:1 and was especially recommended for the preservation of helical proteins in myofibrils of collagen (77). Retief and Ruchel have presented evidence that a 3:1 mixture of methanol and acetic acid removes almost all H1 histone protein from the nucleus together with a substantial fraction of H2A, H2B, H3, and H4 (78).

4. Picric acid fixatives

The compound 2,4,6-trinitrophenol has long been considered as a single protein precipitant and is now used in a variety of fixative mixtures. It reacts with histone proteins in the nucleus and basic proteins to form crystalline picrates with amino acids. Glycogen preservation is maximal but morphometric volume changes are considerable. In contradistinction to its role as a simple protein precipitant, there is evidence that bonds are created between picric acid and the surface groups of fibrous proteins thus acting as an inter-molecular bonding agent and not functioning totally as a precipitator of protein.

5. Mercuric chloride containing fixatives

Mercuric salts were formerly commonly employed in histological fixative cocktails. The interaction of mercury, and other metallic ions, may be summarized as follows: it combines with the acid groups on protein, especially carboxyl and hydroxyl and phosphoric acid of nucleoproteins. Mercuric ion appears to have a specific and selective affinity for thiol (SH) groups. For histochemical and molecular pathological purposes an important question remains to be answered. Is the reaction of mercuric ion with various tissue components reversible by ordinary processes of tissue embedding, in addition to washing and removal of coarse mercuric precipitates by means of iodine and thiosulphate? It is conceivable that at least some mercuric compounds remain bound where sulphydryl group interaction has occurred, particularly in nucleotides and proteins. This alteration in the conformation symmetry of these molecules may have deleterious effects on PCR and *in situ* hybridization techniques.

Mercuric chloride penetrates tissue poorly and produces considerable tissue shrinkage and thus is used as a combination fixative and rarely used on its own. Indeed Hopwood discussed fully the role of fixation with mercurials and his conclusion was that they are best avoided altogether (47). In contrast, the demonstration of stable peptides like insulin is enhanced by the use of mercuric containing fixatives. Zenker's, Helly's, and B5 solutions contain mercuric chloride.

Nucleic acids and nucleoproteins: what fixative is ideal?

Nucleic acids exist in different forms, and it appears that whatever method of fixation is used the physical properties of nucleoproteins are altered. Chemical reactivity is also changed. Formalin is not a good fixative for nucleic acid and nucleoproteins, its combination with nucleoproteins blocking a large number of reactive groups. Mercuric or chromium salts improve preservation but also inhibit many histochemical reactions.

Precipitant fixatives like alcohol and acetic acid are much more often recommended for preservation of nucleic acids. Unfortunately, ethanol causes irreversible changes in the structure of isolated DNA as measured by the ability of nucleic acids to induce dichroism when stained with a variety of dyes and examined under polarized light (79). Methanol is less active in this respect, possibly because it is a weaker dehydrating agent.

Acid fixatives produce superb morphological preservations by the precipitation of nucleoproteins. If tissues are placed for prolonged periods in acid fixatives, extraction of RNA occurs first, followed by DNA. Therefore, it appears reasonable that prolonged fixation in Carnoy's fixative is best avoided for morphological correlation but may be of value for molecular pathological techniques.

The precise mechanism of formaldehyde interaction with components of chromatin has been studied extensively. Formaldehyde induced histone–DNA crosslinking has been conclusively demonstrated (80, 81).

Marked differences have been noted between formaldehyde and glutaraldehyde in the fixation of histone proteins. Short term treatment of tissues with formaldehyde gives rise to reversible covalent bonds between histones and DNA, while initial treatment with glutaraldehyde induces the production of polymers of F1 histones and oligo polymerization of remaining histone proteins (80).

In 1976, McGhee used formaldehyde as a probe for DNA structure (59, 60). In theory, formaldehyde is capable of replacing protons in the exocyclic amino groups of purines and pyrimidines as well as protons attached to the endocyclic nitrogens of the purine and pyrimidine rings. It was shown that at low formaldehyde concentrations, the product contains a single hydroxymethyl group attached to one of the ring nitrogens on purines and pyrimidines, while at high concentrations a hydroxymethyl adduct existed. Both of these reactions appear reversible. In the sugar backbone of DNA, formaldehyde does not appear to react with hydroxyl groups present in deoxyribose or with the phosphate ester groups of nucleic acids (82). The bi-functional aldehydes, glyoxal and malondialdehyde were investigated for their reactions with DNA (83). Both these aldehydes were found to induce resistance to deoxyribonuclease digestion, suggesting structural alteration of native DNA.

Duration of fixation

Pathology departments aim to give a diagnostic service within 24 h of receiving surgical specimens, for reasons of patient well-being and cost. The duration of fixation is variable. At a minimum this may be 2 h. Prolonged fixation inhibits enzyme and immunological activity although it will still produce satisfactory morphological results. Washing of fixed tissues in running water can restore much activity of some enzymes. There is evidence that if fixation has not exceeded 24 h, much of the formaldehyde may be removed from the tissue by washing. This is largely because the initial reaction, namely the formation of Schiff bases, is reversible by excess water.

Hydrogen ion concentration and buffers

Most fixation is carried out using 0.2 M phosphate-buffered 4% formaldehyde at pH 7.2. Some laboratories use formaldehyde in isotonic saline, which is acidic. Satisfactory fixation occurs between pH 6 and 8. During fixation the cells become increasingly acidic due to anoxia and the alteration in cell metabolism. The pH of the buffer will also have an effect on the molecular conformation of the cellular components and will affect the rate of reaction between protein and aldehyde: at higher pH the reaction proceeds more rapidly. Care must be taken to ensure that the fixative and buffer do not react with each other. The buffers used more commonly in fixation include phosphate, cacodylate, Tris, s-collidine, and veronal acetate.

References

1. Meis-Kindblom JM, Stenman G, Kindblom LG. Differential diagnosis of small round cell tumors. Sem Diag Pathol 1996, **13**, 213–41.
2. Mierau GW, Weeks DA, Hicks MJ. Role of electron microscopy and other special techniques in the diagnosis of childhood round cell tumors. Hum Pathol 1998, **29**(12), 1347–55.
3. Thorner PS, Squire JA. Perspectives in pediatric pathology: molecular genetics in the diagnosis and prognosis of solid pediatric tumors. Pediatr Dev Pathol 1998, **1**, 337–65.
4. Parham DM (ed.). Pediatric neoplasia. Morphology and biology. Lippincott-raven, Philadelphia, 1996.
5. Coffin CM, Dehner LP, O'Shea (ed.). Pediatric soft tissue tumors. A clinical, pathological and therapeutic approach. Williams and Wilkins, Baltimore, USA, 1997.
6. Askin FB, Perlman EJ. Neuroblastoma and peripheral neuroectodermal tumors. Am J Clin Pathol 1998, **109**(Suppl 1), S23–30.
7. Zuppan CW. Handling and evaluation of pediatric renal tumors. Am J Clin Pathol 1998, **109**(Suppl 1), S31–7.
8. Stocker JT, Askin FB (ed.). Pathology of solid tumors in children. Chapman and Hall, Cambridge, UK, 1998.
9. Conran RM. An approach to handling pediatric thyroid and adrenal tumors excluding neuroblastoma. Am J Clin Pathol 1998, **109**(Suppl 1), S73–81.
10. Perkins SL. Work-up and diagnosis of pediatric non Hodgkin's lymphomas. Pediatric Dev Pathol 2000, **3**, 374–90.
11. Cagle PT, Hough AJ, Pysher J, Page DL, Johnson EH, Kirkland RT et al. Comparison of adrenal cortical tumors in children and adults. Cancer 1986, **57**, 2235–7.
12. Shimada H, Ambros IM, Dehner LP, Hata JI, Joshi VV, Roald B. Terminology and morphologic criteria of neuroblastic tumors: recommendations by the International Neuroblastoma Pathology Committee. Cancer 1999, **56**, 348–62.
13. Lorenzana AN, Zielenska M, Thorner, P, Gerrie B, Weitzman S, Squire J. Heterogeneity of MYCN amplification in a child with stroma-rich neuroblastoma (ganglioneuroblastoma). Pediatric Pathol Lab Med 1997, **17**, 875–83.
14. Bancroft JD and Stevens A (eds.) Theory and practice of histological techniques. 4th edn., Churchill Livingstone, 1999.
15. Woods AE, Ellis RC. (ed.) Laboratory Histopathology. A complete reference. 1994 Churchill Livingstone. Updates 1995. Pearson Professional Ltd.
16. Fisher JE, Burger PC, Perlman EJ, Dickman PS, Parham DM, Savell VH et al. The frozen section yesterday and today: pediatric solid tumors—crucial issues. Pediatric Dev Pathol 2001, **4**, 252–66.
17. Layfeld LJ, Reichman A. Fine needle aspiration cytology: utilization in pediatric pathology. Dis Markers 1990, **8**(6), 301–15.
18. Silverman JF, Joshi VV. FNA biopsy of small round cell tumors of childhood: cytomorphologic features and the role of ancillary studies. Diagn Cytopathol 1994, **10**(3), 245–55.
19. Raab SS, Silverman JF, Elsheikh TM, et al. Pediatric thyroid nodules and disease demographics and clinical management as determined by fine needle aspiration biopsy. Pediatrics 1995, **95**, 46–9.
20. Bratthauer GL. The avidin–biotin complex (ABC) method. Methods Mol Biol 1994, **34**, 175–84.
21. Hodges GM, Southgate J, Toulson EC. Colloidal gold—a powerful tool in scanning electron microscope immunocytochemistry: an overview of bioapplications. Scanning Microsc 1987, **1**(1), 301–18.
22. Jacobs TW, Prioleau JE, Stillman IE, Schnitt SJ. Loss of tumor marker-immunostaining intensity on stored paraffin slides of breast cancer. J Natl Cancer Inst 1996, **88**(15), 1054–9.
23. Berteau P, Cazals-Hatem D, Meignin V, de Roquancourt A, Vérola O, Lesourd A et al. Variability of immunohistochemical reactivity on stored paraffin slides. J Clin Pathol 1998, **51**, 370–4.
24. Braunschweiger PG. In: Technique in cell cycle analysis (ed. JW Gray, Z Darzynkiewicz). Humana Press, Clifton, New Jersey, 1987, 47–72.

25. Marshall T, Rutledge JC. Flow cytometry DNA applications in pediatric tumor pathology. Pediatric Dev Pathol 2000, **3**, 314–34.
26. Melamed MR, Lindmo T, Mendelsohn ML. Flow cytometry and sorting. Wiley-Liss, New York, 1990.
27. Darzynkiewicz Z, Crissman HA. Flow cytometry. Academic Press, San Diego, 1990.
28. Bauer KD, Duque RE, Shankey TV. Clinical flow cytometry: principles and application. Williams and Wilkins, Baltimore, 1993.
29. Ross JS. DNA ploidy and cell cycle analysis in cancer diagnosis and prognosis. Oncology 1996, **10**, 867–82 and 887–90.
30. Bratthauer GL. Preparation of frozen sections for analysis. Methods Mol Biol 1994, **34**, 67–73.
31. Sambrook J, Fritsch EF, Maniatis T. Molecular cloning. A laboratory manual, 2nd edn. Cold Spring Harbor Laboratory Press, USA, 1989.
32. Chomczynski P, Sacchi N. Single-step method of RNA isolation by acid guanidinium thiocyanate–phenol–chloroform extraction. Anal Biochem 1987, **162**(1), 156–9.
33. Innis MA, Gelfand DH, Sninsky JJ, White TJ (ed.). PCR protocols. A guide to methods and applications. Academic Press Inc., San Diego, California, 1990.
34. Lo DYM (ed.). Clinical applications of PCR. Methods in molecular medicine. Humana Press Inc., Totowa, New Jersey, 1998.
35. Peter M, Gilbert E, Delattre O. A multiplex real-time pcr assay for the detection of gene fusions observed in solid tumors. Lab Invest 2001, **81**(6), 905–12.
36. Anderson J, Gordon T, McManus A, Mapp T, Gould S, Kelsey A et al. UK Children's Cancer Study Group (UKCCSG) and the UK Cancer Cytogenetics Group. Detection of the *PAX3-FKHR* fusion gene in paediatric rhabdomyo-sarcoma: a reproducible predictor of outcome? Br J Cancer 2001, **85**(6), 831–5.
37. Antonescu CR, Tschernyavsky SJ, Woodruff JM, Jungbluth AA, Brennan MF et al. Molecular diagnosis of clear cell sarcoma: detection of EWS-ATF1 and MITF-M transcripts and histopathological and ultrastructural analysis of 12 cases. J Mol Diagn 2002, **4**(1), 44–52.
38. Gattenlohner S, Muller-Hermelink HK, Marx A. Polymerase chain reaction-based diagnosis of rhabdomyosarcomas: comparison of fetal type acetylcholine receptor subunits and myogenin. Diagn Mol Pathol (June) 1998, 7(3), 129–34.
39. Gilbert J, Haber M, Bordow SB, Marshall GM, Norris MD. Use of tumor-specific gene expression for the differential diagnosis of neuroblastoma from other pediatric small round-cell malignancies. Am J Pathol (July) 1999, **155**(1), 17–21.
40. Emmert-Buck MR, Bonner RF, Smith PD, Chuaqui RF, Zhuang Z, Goldstein SR et al. Laser capture microdissection. Science 1996, **274**(5289), 998–1001.
41. Fend F, Raffeld M. Laser capture microdissection in pathology. J Clin Pathol 2000, **53**(9), 666–72.
42. Craven RA, Banks RE. Laser capture microdissection and proteomics: possibilities and limitation. Proteomics 2001, **1**(10), 1200–4.
43. Burchill SA, Selby PJ. Molecular detection of low-level disease in patients with cancer. J Pathol 2000, **190**, 6–14.
44. Baker JR. Principles of biological microtechnique. Methuen, London, 1960.
45. Jones D. In: Fixation in histochemistry (ed. PJ Stoward). Chapman & Hall, London, 1973, 1–45.
46. Pearse AGE. Histochemistry, theoretical and applied, 4th edn, Vol 1. Edinburgh, Churchill Livingstone (1980).
47. Hopwood D. Fixatives and Fixation; a review. Histochem J 1969, **1**, 323–60.
48. Hopwood D. Theoretical and practical aspects of glutaraldehyde fixation. Histochem J 1972, **4**, 267–303.
49. Peters K, Richards FF. Chemical cross-linking; reagents and problems in studies of membranes structure. Annu Rev Biochem 1977, **46**, 523–51.
50. Login GR, Dvorak AM. Microwave energy fixation for electron microscopy. Am J Pathol 1985, **120**, 230–43.
51. Sheibani K, Wu A, Ben-Ezra J, Battifora H. Analysis of Ha-Ras sequence in DNAs of malignant mesothelioma and pulmonary adenocarcinoma by a sensitive polymerase chain reaction (PCR) method. Lab Invest 1989, **60**, 87A.
52. Shibata D, Forester K, Martin J, Arnheim N, Perucho M. Most human carcinomas of exocrine pancreas contain mutant *c-K ras* genes. Cell 1988, **53**, 549.
53. Shibata DK, Arnheim N, Martin WJ. Detection of human papillomavirus in paraffin embedded tissue using the polymerase chain reaction. J Exp Med 1988, **167**, 225–30.
54. Shibata DK, Martin WJ, Arnheim N. Analysis of DNA sequences in 40 year old paraffin embedded thin tissue sections; a bridge between molecular biology and classical histology. Cancer Res 1988, **48**, 4564–66.
55. Hopwood D. Cell and tissue fixation 1972–1982. Histochem J 1985, **17**, 389–442.
56. Hopwood D. The reaction of glutaraldehyde with nucleic acids. Histochem J 1975, **7**, 267–75.
57. Olins DE, Wright EB. Glutaraldehyde fixation of isolated eukaryotic nuclei. J Cell Biol 1973, **59**, 304–17.
58. Varricchio F, Jamieson G. Reactivity of heterogenous F1 proteins with glutaraldehyde and formaldehyde. Exp Cell Res 1977, **106**, 380–6.
59. McGhee JD, Von Hippel PH. Formaldehyde as a probe of DNA structure. 3. Equilibrium denaturation of DNA and synthetic polynucleotides. Biochemistry 1976, **16**, 3267–93.
60. McGhee JD, Von Hippel PH. Formaldehyde as a probe of DNA structure. 4. Mechanism of the initial reaction of formaldehyde with DNA. Biochemistry 1976, **16**, 3267–76.
61. McGhee JD, Von Hippel PH. Formaldehyde as a probe of DNA structure. 1. Reaction with exocyclic amino groups of DNA bases. Biochemistry 1976, **14**, 1281–95.
62. McGhee JD, Von Hippel PH. Formaldehyde as a probe of DNA structure. 2. Reaction with endocyclic imino groups of DNA bases. Biochemistry 1975, **14**(6) 1297–303.
63. Senior MB, Olins DE. Effect of formaldehyde on the circular dichroism of chicken erythrocyte chromatin. Biochemistry 1975, **14**, 3332–7.
64. Langenberg WG. Glutaraldehyde non-fixation of isolated viral and yeast RNAs. J Histochem Cytochem 1980, **28**, 311–5.
65. Langenberg WG. Chromic acid formaldehyde fixation of nucleic acids of bacteriophage 6 and infectious rhinotracheitis virus. J Gen Virol 1978, **39**, 377–80.

66. Chaw YFM, Crane LC, Lane P, Shapiro R. Isolation and identification of cross-links from formaldehyde treated nucleic acids. Biochemistry 1980, **19**, 5525–31.
67. Peracchia C, Mittler BC. New glutaraldehyde fixation processes. J Ultrastruct Res 1975, **39**(57), ñ 64.
68. Medawar PB. The rate of penetration of fixative. J Royal Microsc Soc 1941, **61**, 46–57.
69. Collins VP, Arborgh B, Brunk U. A comparison of the effect of three widely used glutaraldehyde fixative on cellular volume and structure. Acta Pathol Microbiol Scand. 1977, **a85**, 157–69.
70. Mizuhira V, Shuhashi M, Futaesaku Y. High speed electron microscope autoradiographic studies of diffusible compounds. J Histochem Cytochem 1981, **27**, 143–60.
71. Hopwood D. Fixation and fixatives. In: Theory and practice of Histological Techniques, 3rd edn. Churchill Livingstone, 1990.
72. French D, Edsall JJ. The reactions of formaldehyde with amino acids and proteins. Adv Prot Chem 1945, **II**, 277 onwards.
73. Walker JF. Formaldehyde, 3rd edn. Chapman Hall, London, 1964.
74. Monson P, Pyzo G, Mazarguil H. Etude du mecanisme d'establishment des liasons glutaraldehyde-proteins. Biochemie 1975, **57**, 1281–92.
75. Woodruff EA. The chemistry and biology of aldehyde treated tissue heart valve xenografts in Tissue Heart Valves. Butterworths, London, 1979, 347–63.
76. Korn AH, Feairheller S, Filachione EM. Glutaraldehyde-nature of the reagent. J Mol Biol 1972, **65**, 525–60.
77. Puchtler H, Waldrop FS, Meloan SN, Terry MS, Conner HM. Methacarn (Methanol–Carnoy) fixation. Practical and theoretical considerations. Histochemie 1970, **21**, 97–116.
78. Retief AE, Ruchel R. Histones removed by fixation. Their role in the mechanism of chromosomal banding. Exp Cell Res 1977, **106**, 233–7.
79. White JC, Elmer PC. Fibres of human sodium doeoxyribonucleate and nucleoprotein studies in polarised light by a simple method. Nature (London) 1952, **169**, 15–152.
80. Chalkley R, Hunter C. Histone–Histone propinquity by aldehyde fixation of chromatin. Proc Natl Acad Sci USA 1975, **72**(4), 1304–8.
81. Brutlag D, Schlehuber C, Bonner J. Properties of formaldehyde treated nucleohistone. Biochemistry 1969, 8, 3214.
82. Feldman MY. Reaction of nucleic acids and nucleoprotein with formaldehyde. Prog Nucleic Acid Res Mol Biol 1973, 13, 1–44.
83. Sheibani K, Tubbs RR. Enzyme immunohistochemistry; technical aspects. Semin Diagn Pathol 1984, **1**, 235.

2 | Methods of genetic analysis applied to pediatric cancer

Jane Bayani, Maria Zielenska, and Jeremy A. Squire

Introduction

Genetic technologies have made major advances in recent years, and both the power and sensitivity of methods in molecular biology have been greatly aided by the increasing number of genes discovered as part of the Human Genome Project (1, 2). The fields of genetics and pediatric cancer overlap in many areas, and much of the success in our understanding of genetic defects in childhood tumors has depended on the application of molecular genetic and advanced cytogenetic methodologies. Some of the newest genomics methods used to identify and investigate genes associated with pediatric cancer are presented below. The reader is directed to more comprehensive texts for a full explanation of the methodologies and experimental details (3–6).

Cytogenetics methods

Classical cytogenetic analysis is the cornerstone for many of the recent advancements in molecular cytogenetics. Since the first karyotype from peripheral blood cultures were made in 1959 (7), the wealth of information derived from the study of chromosomes has enabled the identification of recurrent chromosomal aberrations in various diseases, cancers, syndromes and has greatly facilitated an improved understanding of the chromosomal causation of many pediatric cancers. A properly handled specimen can influence the success of any cytogenetics-based assay. All specimens, whether blood, bone marrow, or solid tissue, should be handled using aseptic techniques. Some general considerations include a sterile workspace in a ventilated tissue culture hood. While costly, sterile disposable plastic pipettes, petri dishes, flasks, and disposable scalpel blades are also a wise investment. All tissue culture growth media, antibiotics, and other additives should be used well within their expiry dates and properly stored. The CO_2 incubator should be clean and free of pathogens and fungal spores.

Other texts comprehensively describe various procedures for optimizing the yield and quality of metaphase preparations derived from diverse cell types from cancer cytogenetics samples (5). Briefly, samples in suspension, such as hematologic samples or short-term tumor cultures, can be readily added to the growth medium and allowed to culture in suspension. Solid tumor tissue samples require disaggregation into a single cell suspension. This can be achieved first through manual mincing of the tissue with scalpel blades. Depending on the tissue type, such as brain, manual mincing is sufficient. For other tissues, treatment with enzymes such as collagenase is also required to obtain a single cell suspension. Cells derived from solid tissue samples may grow as an adherent culture, as a suspension, or both. Once in culture, the cells are allowed to divide. Depending on the type of tissue and the quality of the sample, the success of growth in culture will vary. The cells are then arrested at the metaphase stage and fixed using a methanol and acetic acid fixative. These fixed cells are then ready to be applied to clean microscope slides and analyzed. Classical cytogenetic analysis requires the staining of the metaphase cells to reveal their unique banding patterns, typically using Giemsa as the medium (hence the term G-banding Fig. 2.1). The success of banding analysis lies in the overall quality of the starting material, the mitotic activity of the culture, the ability to arrest sufficient numbers of cells at metaphase, and the morphology of the chromosomes themselves (i.e. length and shape).

Fluorescence in situ hybridization (FISH)

Fluorescence *in situ* hybridization is a chromosome-based assay (5) that involves two parts: the chromosome (or interphase) cell target and the labeled probe.

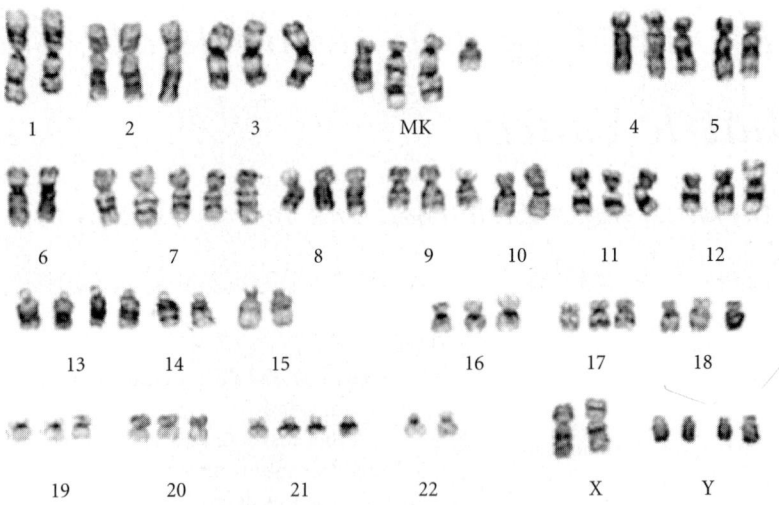

Fig. 2.1 G-banded karyotype of an astrocytoma cell line. Shown is a karyotype of an astrocytoma metaphase cell stained with Giemsa. This cell is hypertriploid with 73 chromosomes present. Structural aberrations as well as over-representation of almost all the chromosomes are indicated. Also present are 4 marker (MK) chromosomes.

Modifications to the basic FISH protocol have spawned two other FISH-based assays: comparative genomic hybridization (CGH) (8) and spectral karyotyping (SKY) (9). Chromosome preparations for FISH involve the same preparations used for banding analysis with little or no pretreatment. The DNA probe used for FISH can be specific for a gene, chromosome segment, or whole chromosome paints (Fig. 2.2(a)). The DNA probe can be derived from cloned sources such as plasmids, cosmids, BACs, or YACs. They can also be DNA fragments extracted through microdissection and polymerase chain reaction (PCR) amplified. Labeling is usually achieved by the incorporation of biotin and/or digoxigenin by nick translation (10–12) and is later detected using a fluorochrome conjugated antibody. More recently, fluorochrome conjugated dNPTs have been more readily available and have been used to "directly" label the DNA probe. This has generally permitted less bench work and cleaner preparations, but at a larger expense as compared to the "indirect" method using biotin or digoxigenin. Once labeled, DNA is quite stable and can be stored at −20°C almost indefinitely. Directly labeled probes generally have a significantly shorter shelf life since the signal from the fluorochrome will degrade over time. For this reason, an indirect approach may be more cost effective and practical. Prior to hybridization, metaphase chromosome spreads are heated briefly to ~75°C with 70% formamide in buffered isotonic saline to denature the DNA. The DNA probe, which has been precipitated with unlabeled Cot-1 DNA to suppress the repetitive sequences, is also heat denatured at ~75°C in a formamide-based hybridization solution to its single stranded state. Following a pre-annealing stage at 37°C for 1 h, the denatured probe is added to the denatured DNA target on the slide and allowed to hybridize at 37°C for at least 24 h. Following the hybridization step, post hybridization washes and hapten detection (if using indirectly labeled probes) is carried out. The slides are counterstained and mounted in an antifade medium to prevent rapid signal quenching. The sites of hybridization are clearly visualized as fluorescent points of light where the probe is bound to chromatin. The versatility of FISH lies in its ability to be used for chromosome targets, interphase nuclei, cells embedded in paraffin section or from a cytological smear. The following section briefly discusses the various sources of target DNA for FISH analysis.

Clinical samples for FISH analysis

Successful FISH depends largely on the initial quality of the patient sample. This presents a technical challenge for the clinical laboratory since the number and scope of applications of FISH is increasing as more commercial probes and hybridization kits become available. In addition, clinicians are becoming more aware of the significant advantages of performing FISH analyses on

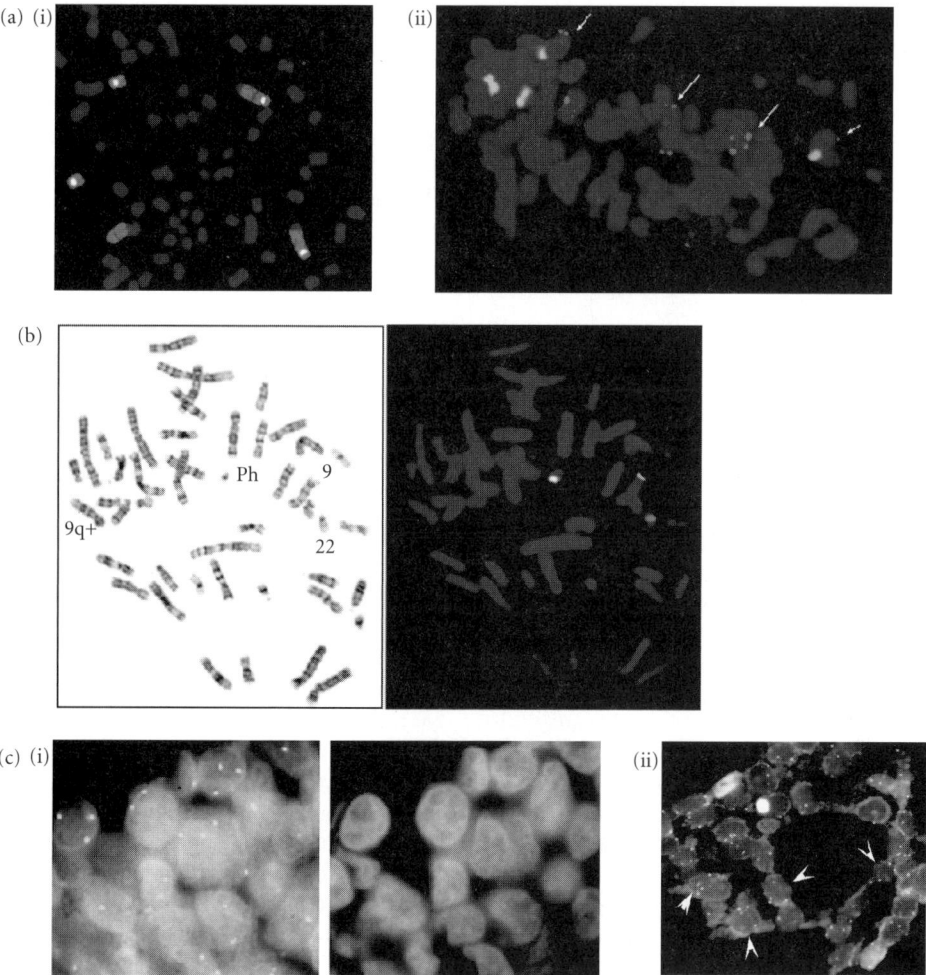

Fig. 2.2 Examples of FISH on metaphase and interphase cells. (a) FISH analysis of a pediatric osteosarcoma. (i) Use of centromere probes and chromosome paints. In this image, a centromere probe for chromosome 8 (green) and a chromosome 8 painting probe (red) were used to examine complex structural rearrangements involving chromosome 8. In this spread there are two normal chromosome 8s (upper left). A pair of abnormal chromosomes (upper right) possess the centromere of chromosome 8, as well as chromosome 8 material, structurally rearranged with some other chromosome. The lower right aberration contains only blocks of chromosome 8 material. (ii) Use of centromere probes and locus specific probes. From the same osteosarcoma sample, rearrangements involving the region of 1p35-p36 are studied using a 1p35-p36 specific probe (red) and a centromere probe for chromosome 1 (green). FISH analysis indicates extra copies of 1p35-p36 over the ploidy number for chromosome 1 as ascertained by the centromere probes. FISH also indicates the translocation of the 1p35-p36 region to other chromosomes. (b) Sequential G-banding and metaphase FISH analysis of a CML specimen, using locus specific probes for BCR and ABL. In this example, G-banding of the spread was carried out to identify the Ph chromosome. FISH using the BCR–ABL probe set was used on the same specimen to confirm the presence of the Ph chromosome and to determine that the derivative chromosome 9 (9q+) also was deleted for the reciprocal fusion signal. (c) FISH on paraffin-embedded material. (i) Interphase FISH analysis on an Ewing's sarcoma specimen using chromosome 8 centromere probes. In this image, chromosome 8 centromere probes were used to examine the ploidy status of an Ewing's sarcoma. The image on the left shows the centromere 8 hybridization under the FITC filter. The corresponding DAPI image to show the cell morphology is also shown. FISH analysis indicates an overall gain of chromosome 8 in most cells. (ii) FISH analysis of a prostate carcinoma sample from paraffin section. In this low power view, a locus specific probe for MYCC (8q24), in red, and centromere probe for chromosome 8, in green, was used to enumerate the number of copies of chromosome 8 and to determine whether amplification of MYCC was present. See Plate 2.

their patient's samples because of the speed, sensitivity, and specificity of FISH techniques (13). Thus, FISH analysis is now being requested from diverse tissue types and results are usually required as fast as possible. This section will review the various types of patient samples used for FISH and describe the commonly used approaches for preparing optimal target slides for FISH in a clinical setting.

Cytogenetic preparations for FISH analysis

Slide quality

Slide quality is one of the most important factors affecting hybridization efficiency and signal intensity. Slides should be evaluated using a phase contrast microscope before hybridization. The cell density should not be too high such that the cells are evenly distributed across the slide. Areas of cell clumping indicate poor slide preparation or sample quality. Under phase microscope, nuclei and chromosome should appear dark gray in color. If they are light gray or very black and refractile they may not hybridize well. Visible cytoplasm surrounding metaphase spreads or interphase nuclei may also adversely affect hybridization and contribute to increased background. It is useful to apply a protease pretreatment, such as Proteinase K, when residual cytoplasmic material is detectable by phase contrast microscopy. Most experienced cytogeneticists acknowledge that the quality of chromosomal preparations for both banding and FISH procedures can be greatly influenced by the drying environment during slide making. Humidity and temperature will significantly influence the rate of fixative evaporation during slide making. The drying time should be well controlled so that when the overall humidity is less than 30% slide making is performed near a steam source or humidifier. In recent years a controlled environmental evaporation chamber developed by Thermotron Inc. (see Appendix) has made for more reproducible slide making and has gained in popularity in clinical laboratories. In our experience the optimal humidity for drying slides for FISH is 55% and we prefer to dry slides at ~25°C so that slides will take approximately 1–2 min to dry.

Slide storage and aging

Once the slide preparations have been made, care must be taken in their storage and aging to ensure future experiments are successful. In contrast to banding procedures where aging for 2–3 days improves the morphology of the sample, FISH could be performed using fresher slides. In general, FISH can be performed the day following slide preparation with aging slides at 37°C overnight in a dry incubator. However, from our experience, 3 h of incubation at 37°C is sufficient. This appears to improve both hybridization efficiency and signal brightness. In general, FISH and chromosome painting should be performed within 2–3 days of making slides. However, FISH will still yield reasonable results several weeks after slides are prepared, provided they are stored at room temperature in a dry atmosphere. Longer storage will lead to slow deterioration of slides. Some investigators feel that this deterioration in signal quality can be prevented if the slides are placed in dry airtight boxes sealed at −70°C for long-term storage. For indefinite storage of patient samples for future retrospective studies, we prefer to store fixed cell pellets in 1.5 ml polypropylene cryotubes at −20°C. Cells stored in fixative should be rinsed in fresh fixative just before making slides, as pH and water content may have changed during long-term storage.

Slides of *in situ* specimens

In many clinical cytogenetics laboratories, an alternative to harvesting a culture into a fixed cell suspension and preparing the cells from solid tumors on slides is to grow the patient specimen directly on the analytical surface to provide *in situ* analysis of individual clones or mosiaics. This is a common practice in prenatal diagnosis where amniocytes or chorionic villi cells are cultured directly on the slide. Solid tumors may also yield more representative cytogenetic preparations when cultured and harvested as attached colonies. To obtain sufficient cells for analysis, primary cultures must contain several large colonies of growth. It should be remembered that colony size and cell density will greatly influence the accessibility of the hypotonic treatment and fixative. Metaphase cells on the peripheral zone of colony growth are often more likely to have less cytoplasmic material yield, better quality FISH signals, and hybridization efficiencies. If cytoplasmic material is apparent throughout a colony of interest when viewed by phase contrast microscopy, then the slide or coverslip should be treated with proteinase K.

Previously G-banded slides

Previously G-banded material is an importance source for FISH analysis (14) (Fig. 2.2(b)). In some situations, it may be necessary to perform FISH on previously G-banded slides. This procedure can be especially important for verifying an inconclusive chromosomal aberration on a specific metaphase cell. In this situation an image of the G-banded metaphase cell of interest should be captured and the microscope coordinates noted. The banded slide is treated with xylene to remove any residual immersion oils from the microscopic work. The slides are destained with methanol and passed through a rehydration series of ethanols. Protease steps, if necessary, can be carried out at this point, and the slides are then dehydrated and ready for denaturation. It is usually possible to obtain FISH results from samples that have been G-banded and stored as stained slides for 1–3 months. For older samples, slide storage variables such as humidity and ambient temperature will greatly influence success. It is thus very important to find out how the sample was prepared and stored. If there are a limited number of slides remaining from the patient sample of interest it is sometimes helpful to use surplus slides from other samples (ideally prepared the same week) to optimize the best experimental conditions with respect to aging and storage.

Other clinical specimens suitable for interphase FISH analysis

Very often only interphase nuclei are present in a clinical sample and special techniques are required to prepare and analyze such specimens for FISH procedures. The unique ability of interphase FISH analysis for documenting cell-to-cell heterogeneity makes interphase FISH particularly important in the analysis of mosaicism, tumor cell heterogeneity, and for monitoring allogeneic transplant engraftments. Similarly, the interphase FISH can be very helpful for the analysis of small samples such as specimens obtained from cytology smears or from needle biopsies. Paraffin blocks are also widely used since most pathology laboratories routinely archive all formalin-fixed paraffin-embedded tissue for future retrospective studies.

Cytological specimens

Routine blood films, cytological smears, cytospin, and tumor touch (or imprints) preparations will usually contain sufficient cells for interphase FISH studies. Often such preparations are "dirtier" than cytogenetic preparations so additional pretreatment steps such as proteinase K treatment are required to reduce background. For cytological preparations cells on the slide should be fixed with a standard cytology fixative and air-dried and then processed usually involving a protease step (such as pepsin or proteinase K) before the general FISH protocol.

Paraffin-embedded specimens

Paraffin-embedded material holds a wealth of material for analysis (Fig. 2.2(c)); however, it can also be technically challenging. Tissue samples such as solid tumors are usually fixed in formalin (a 37% commercially available paraformaldehyde solution) and then embedded in paraffin wax to preserve cell and tissue morphology for histopathological analysis. The success of FISH on paraffin-embedded specimens is directly dependent on the accessibility of the target DNA within the cell nucleus and will be enhanced considerably by the utilization of pretreatment methodologies that increases the efficiency of the hybridization.

To prepare paraffin sections in the most optimum manner, specimens should be fixed as soon as possible upon receipt by the laboratory. They are most commonly preserved in 10% Formalin. Other types of fixatives may be used, however, certain agents alter DNA structure making the samples incompatible with FISH. Furthermore, if specimens are overfixed, the tissue will be dry and brittle, while underfixation may produce soft and malleable tissue. Both these characteristics render sectioning difficult and yield poor subsequent FISH results. A delay in tissue fixation or long incubations in a fixative solution will also lead to weak signals and reduced hybridization efficiencies.

Sections are usually prepared in the histology laboratory. Typically five sections at 5–8 μm on silanated slides will be cut and one Heamatoxalin and Eosin (H&E) stained slide prepared. It helps to view the stained slide prior to the FISH experiment to determine if the section contains tumor or area of tissues of interest. It is useful to get an experienced pathologist to carefully examine the slide, if it is difficult to interpret. Once sections have been prepared, the insoluble wax embedding compound must be removed. Deparaffinization is accomplished by immersing the slides in xylene followed by dehydration in ethanol to prepare the samples for pretreatment. The pretreatment procedure involves a series of incubations in sodium bisulfite (optional), a protein digestion solution, wash buffer, and an ethanol series in order to denature cellular proteins, aid in the removal of nuclear and extracellular matrix proteins, and to remove protein crosslinks caused by formalin fixation. Digestion with a protease such as proteinase K or pepsin further enhances hybridization efficiency by digesting tissue proteins and making the target DNA more accessible for probe entry and subsequent hybridization (15).

Troubleshooting suboptimal FISH results on paraffin sections may be difficult due to the large number of steps occurring between specimen procurement and FISH analysis. Proper preparation, embedding, and sectioning techniques are dependent on the type of tissue under investigation and these steps can introduce many variables to processing. Specimen variability will also introduce difficulties relative to the tissue type and the amount of extracellular and cytoplasmic material present. Certain tissues show greater resistance to protease digestion and prove difficult to analyze by FISH. Difficult samples may benefit from an increased incubation time in the protease solutions or an increased incubation time in sodium bisulfite to increase the permeabilization of the tissue and to enhance the action of the enzyme.

Recently, interphase FISH surveys of formalin-fixed tumor tissue have been greatly facilitated by the use of tissue arrays which contain multiple small circular punches derived from representative areas of a paraffin section of different tumors (16). The arrays can contain hundreds of different tumors represented as a 0.5–2 mm diameter disc of tissue containing several thousand cells which retain all the morphologic features of the original specimen from which the tissue punch was obtained. Tissue arrays should be processed in much the same way as a regular paraffin section as described below.

Isolation of intact nuclei from paraffin-embedded material. One of the drawbacks of using paraffin sections for FISH studies is that statistical methods have to be employed to indirectly estimate whether numerical changes in chromosomal regions of interest have taken place. Statistical inference is not required if FISH is performed on intact nuclei that have been dissected from the region of interest on the section (17).

Criteria for assessing and reporting FISH results

The minimum number of cells or metaphase spreads required to obtain a given result reflects the clinical context of the finding and the limitations of the patient material available for study. With tissue or cells that are hard to obtain, a single abnormal metaphase may be significant. For example, in some situation limited FISH data may be supported by results obtained using quantitative PCR and/or Southern analysis. Prior to enumerating or analyzing FISH results on a patient sample, it is important to carefully assess the overall quality, uniformity, and effectiveness of hybridization. Each hybridized slide should be evaluated for the specificity of the hybridization, the probe signal intensity, and the signal to background noise to determine if the hybridization was optimum for the given analyses. There should be minimal background or nuclear fluorescent "noise." At least 85% of all nuclei in the target area should be easily enumerable. For some applications (such as the detection of chromosomal heterogeneity, disease progression or minimal residual disease), more rigorous analytical sensitivities and hybridization efficiencies are required.

General considerations when selecting cells for FISH microscopy

Generally look at all areas of the slide analyze regions with uniformity in signal strength. Compare the intensity of the background signals to the intensity of the signals in the nuclei or metaphases of interest. The FISH signal intensity should be consistently greater than background intensity in the regions of the slide chosen for analysis. If there are any background signals with an equivalent signals in the nuclei, then your counts will be skewed and the results biased.

FISH signal evaluation and enumeration

Interpretation of interphase FISH is very much dependent on statistical analyses and has inherent technical challenges. The presence of the signal is dependent upon the probe and its fluorescent label successfully entering the cell and hybridizing to the target DNA. The detection of the correct number of signals can be complicated by signals overlapping or splitting. Any background hybridization whatsoever will lead to major complications in interpretation. It is not uncommon to find "monosomy" or "trisomy" in nuclei that reflect technical artifact or "false positive" background signals. Therefore, the accuracy of interphase FISH analysis is dependent upon recognizing these technical issues, correcting them, and standardizing the scoring criteria accordingly.

Analytical sensitivity of interphase FISH assays

Once a particular probe set is made available as a routine "FISH test" as part of clinical service it is important that the laboratory performs assay validation and establishes a database, which will allow reportable range and general laboratory experience with each probe to be established. The analytical sensitivity assay measures the success of a given FISH test in a particular laboratory environment and on a given tissue type. Since there are known differences in the cell populations and tissue types, it is important to use the appropriate positive control tissue for the assessment of analytical sensitivity and for the establishment of the database. Analytical sensitivity analyses are performed by scoring 200 interphase nuclei representing at least 5 normal, preferably male, individuals (pooling of samples on one slide is acceptable). The nuclei are scored for the percentage of nuclei that exhibit the appropriate number of distinct signals.

Statistical consideration concerning interphase FISH analysis of paraffin sections

Due to truncation of the nuclei during sectioning, loss of signal from areas of the nucleus excluded from the target slide will be encountered when enumerating signals after FISH has been performed on paraffin sections. The criteria for determining the significance of loss or gain of signals in interphase nuclei will depend on a number of parameters such as nuclear diameter, age of patient, type of tissue, etc. Readers are referred to some of the scientific literature where suggested cutoff values were adopted from the available literature (18). In our experience with FISH analysis of prostate cancer, chromosomal gains can be identified when more than ~10% of the nuclei exhibit more than two signals. Chromosomal losses have been identified when more than 50% of the nuclei exhibit a reduction of signal number and tetraploidy has been assumed when all chromosomes investigated show signal gains up to four.

Analysis of pediatric hematologic malignancies

Use of the three color fusion (translocation/inversion) probes

If the probes based on green and red fluorescence used for FISH are close to specific translocation breakpoints on different chromosomes, they will appear joined as a result of the translocation generating a "yellow color fusion" signal (14, 19). In Fig. 2.3(a), the detection of a Philadelphia chromosome in interphase nuclei of leukemia cells is achieved by the presence of two double fusion (D-FISH) signals. All nuclei positive for the translocation contain one red signal (BCR gene), one green signal (ABL gene), and two intermediate fusion yellow signal because the 9;22 chromosome translocation generates two fusions: one on the 9q+ and the other on the 22q−. The following general guidelines may be helpful for performing this type of assay.

1. A green and red signal that are juxtaposed but not overlapping should be scored as "ambiguous."
2. Do not score nuclei that are missing a green or a red signal. This assay is looking for the presence or absence of a fusion signal, not the absence of a green or red signal.
3. Atypical signal patterns have been reported and these are now considered to be clinically important (14, 19).

In Table 2.1 some of the commonly used FISH assays in hematologic cancer are presented. In addition to the scientific literature readers are referred to the suppliers web sites (see Appendix), which will provide the most up-to-date listing of currently available probes and the preferred scoring method.

Use of FISH probes in assessing childhood tumors

Gene amplification is one of the mechanisms by which cancer cells achieve over-expression of some classes of oncogenes and involves an increase in the relative number of copies per cell of a gene. This can range from one or two additional copies per cell to extreme examples where over a thousand copies per cell have been reported. Gene amplification can occur in association with the over-expression of oncogenes, thus conferring a selective growth advantage or as a mechanism of acquired resistance to chemotherapeutic agents and to poor prognosis. Gene amplification is highly suited to FISH analytical approaches which have the added benefit of excellent sensitivity and the ability to address cellular heterogeneity (20). Neuroblastoma is characterized by the frequent occurrence of a highly amplified oncogene, MYCN (15, 21). It has been known for many years that the presence of this aberration is strongly associated with poor outcome. More aggressive management is usually required when MYCN is found to be amplified. Examples of metaphase and interphase FISH assays for gene amplification are shown in Fig. 2.3(b). Some of the commonly detected aberrations observed in solid tumors, which are amenable to FISH analysis, are presented in Table 2.2.

Spectral karyotyping

Spectral karyotyping (9, 22) and a related technique called multicolor FISH (M-FISH) (23) are recent applications of FISH technology that overcome some of the shortfalls of classical banding cytogenetics and standard

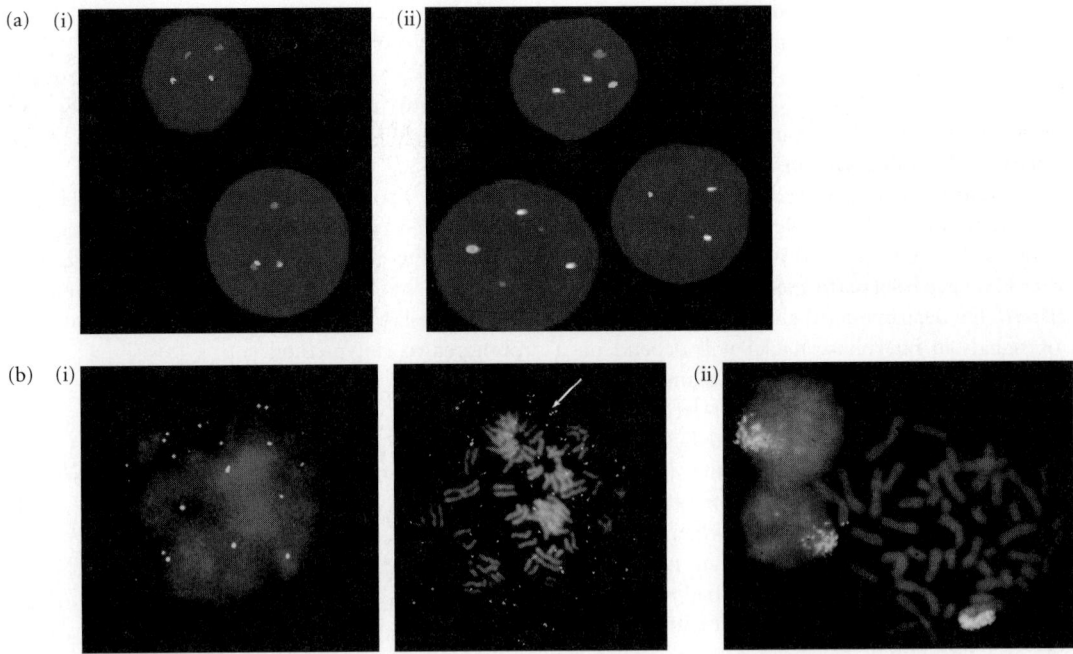

Fig. 2.3 FISH analysis for the detection of translocations and gene amplification. (a) Interphase FISH analysis using locus specific probes for BCR and ABL. (i) A normal interphase cell. Hybridized with the BCR and ABL probes, in this normal cell, two distinct signals for BCR (red) and ABL (green) are present. (ii) A CML interphase cell. Shown in this image is the typical double fusion signal for a positive CML sample as described in the text. (b) FISH analysis of neuroblastoma samples with different patterns of amplification. (i) A neuroblastoma specimen hybridized with a specific probe for MYCN. Shown is an interphase cell and metaphase cell from the same specimen. The hybridization signal pattern in the interphase cell is indicative of double minute chromosomes (left), confirmed by the hybridization of the probe to extrachromosomal bodies in the metaphase cell (right). (ii) A neuroblastoma specimen hybridized with a specific probe for MYCN. In this image, hybridization with the MYCN probe revealed a block of signal in the nucleus characteristic of a pattern of highly amplified sequences inserted into a chromosome, called a homogeneously staining region (HSR). A metaphase cell nearby illustrates the block of amplified MYCN sequences. A normal pair of MYCN signals can be seen on chromosome 2 beside the nuclei. See Plate 3.

FISH assays (reviewed in (24)). In some karyotypes, it is often difficult to determine the identity of a small structural chromosomal aberration with certainty using conventional cytogenetic banding methods alone. The problems that can typically arise in both clinical and cancer cytogenetics are the presence of structural chromosome aberrations with unidentifiable chromosomal regions, or very complex chromosomes (sometimes called "marker chromosomes") in which no recognizable region appears to be present. Confirmation of the cytogenetic origins of such chromosomal aberrations can sometimes be obtained by the judicious application of locus-specific FISH analysis, as discussed above, if the investigator has some general impression regarding a possible identity. However, such an approach is very subjective, risky, and requires some knowledge of the specific loci and available probes likely to be involved in the aberration. A more systematic approach is to use whole chromosomal paints in succession, until the marker chromosome and its constituents can be identified. While this strategy will eventually identify each chromosomal region involved, it is both costly and time consuming and may lead to the depletion of valuable patient samples.

In one experiment SKY permits the simultaneous visualization of all the chromosomes. It is a combination of optical microscopy, high-resolution imaging, and the measurement of spectral emissions by Fourier spectroscopy (25, 26) (Fig. 2.4(a)). The commercial SKY probes are derived from flow-sorted chromosomes that are amplified and labeled using DOP–PCR (27). A 24-chromosome probe cocktail is generated by the combinations of 5 pure dyes, namely Rhodamine, Spectrum-Orange™, Cy5, Cy5.5, and Texas Red. This allows

Table 2.1 FISH analysis of pediatric hematologic malignancies

Neoplasm	Chromosomal location	Probe	Scoring method
CML/pediatric ALL	9q34/22q	BCR/ABL	Color fusion observed in metaphase and interphase
Various leukemias	11q23	MLL	Split signal, metaphase
Various leukemias	5q31	EGFR1	Loss of signal, metaphase/interphase
Various leukemias	7q31	DSS486	Loss of signal, metaphase/interphase
AML M4 EO	Inv(16)	CBFB	Split signal, metaphase
Various leukemias	20q13.2	ZNF217, D20S183	Loss of signal, metaphase/interphase
Various hematologic malignancies	8q24/14q32	MYCC/IgH	Color fusion observed in metaphase and interphase
AML-M1	12p13/21q22 8q22/21q22	TEL/AML1 AML1/ETO	Color fusion observed in metaphase and interphase
AML-M3	15q22/17q21.1	PML/RARA	Color fusion observed in metaphase and interphase
Various hematologic malignancies, often when acceleration suspected	8cen	D8Z1	Enumeration using interphase and metaphase cells
Intersex transplant monitoring	Yp11.3/Xcen	SRY/DXZ1	Enumeration using interphase and metaphase cells

Table 2.2 FISH analysis of solid tumors

Neoplasm	Chromosomal location	Probe	Scoring method
Neuroblastoma	2p24 2p23-24	MYCN LSI N-myc	Interphase, metaphase Amplification
Ewing's sarcoma	11q24/22q12	FLI1/EWS	Color fusion observed in metaphase and interphase
Rhabdomyosarcoma	2q35/13q14	PAX/FKR	Color fusion observed in metaphase and interphase

2^{n-1} or 31 combinations. Thus, each chromosome has a unique spectral "signature," generated by the specific combination of the five pure dyes. For every chromosomal region, identity is determined by measuring the spectral emission at that point. Regions where sites for rearrangement or translocation between different chromosomes occur are visualized by a change in the display color at the point of transition. Examples of the use of SKY are illustrated in Fig. 2.4(b).

The SKY assay follows the basic FISH protocol: a cytogenetic (metaphase) preparation of the patient sample is prepared and denatured to its single stranded state. The 24-chromosome painting probe cocktail is also denatured and applied to the denatured slide. The probe and slide are allowed to hybridize at 37°C for 48 h, after which any unbound probe is washed off. The commercially made probe (Applied Spectral Imaging) consists of both directly labeled and indirectly labeled

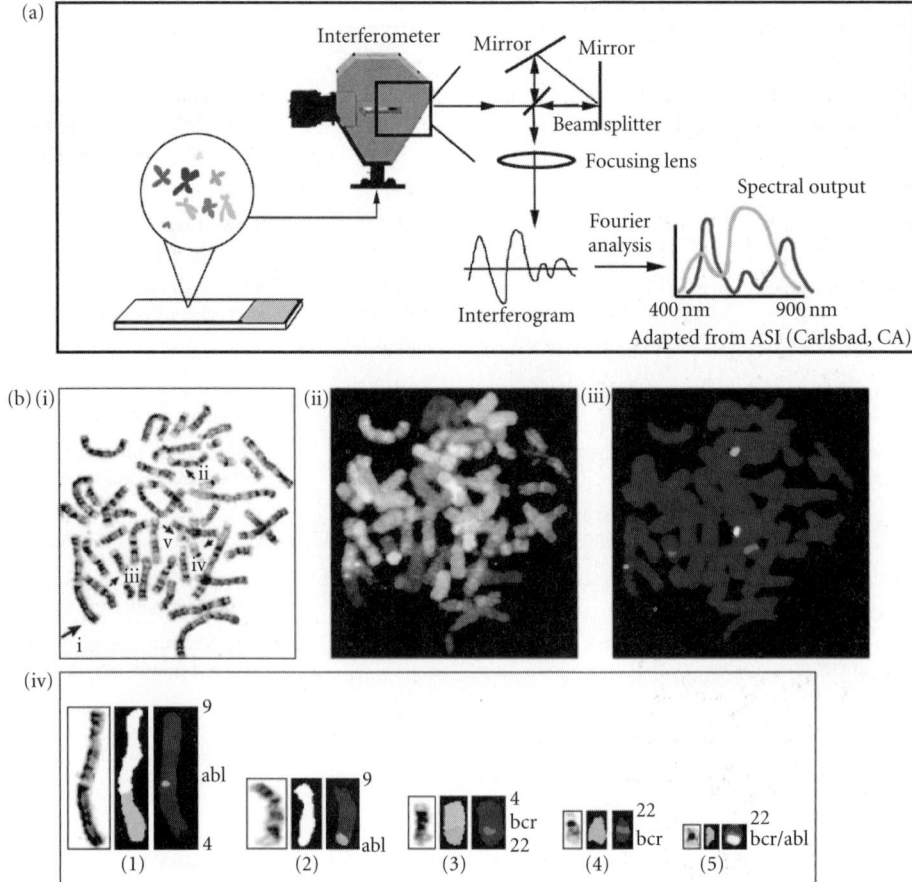

Fig. 2.4 SKY. (a) Schematic representation of image acquisition and conversion. (b) Sequential G-banding, SKY, and FISH analyses of a variant CML specimen. (i) G-banded metaphase of interest. Abnormal chromosomes detected by G-banding are annotated. (ii) SKY analysis of the same metaphase spread. Following a destaining protocol, the 24-color SKY probes are hybridized to the slide. Shown is the Red–Green–Blue (RGB) image of the fluorescent dyes. (iii) FISH analysis using the BCR–ABL probe set. After SKY analysis, the slides are washed, dehydrated, and denatured once more and hybridized to the locus specific probe set. (iv) Identification of abnormal chromosomes by G-banding, SKY and FISH. For each abnormal chromosome, the G-banded image, pseudo-colored (classified) SKY image and FISH image are presented. In this specimen, the hallmark Ph chromosome (5) on the derivative chromosome 22 is present, however, the ABL–BCR translocation usually on the derivative chromosome 9 is not present. SKY analysis confirmed the involvement of chromosome 4 in the translocation process leading to the variant karyotype. See Plate 4.

DNAs, thus antibody incubation is required. Like FISH, the criteria for target slides include specimens that are free of extracellular debris and cytoplasm and are stored in good condition. Previously banded slide materials are also amenable to SKY analysis (14, 28) and are illustrated in Fig. 2.4(b).

Spectral karyotyping has enabled the elucidation of latent structural aberrations that may otherwise have been left undetected by classical cytogenetics or FISH alone. Fan *et al.* (29) described the lower limit for detection to be a chromosomal segment at least 1–2 Mb. Furthermore, the chromosomal origins of all "marker chromosomes" can usually be identified. However, SKY cannot identify specific arm or band locations without generating unique arm specific probes, making the strategic use of analysis subsequent to FISH an extremely powerful cytogenetic tool (22, 24, 28, 30).

The most amenable malignancy to SKY analysis are the hematological malignancies (14, 31–35). Although a number of known chromosomal aberrations have been identified to be specific to certain hematological malignancy, the value of SKY analysis is in the identification of novel recurrent aberrations that may confer a specific phenotype or predict a modified response to treatment or outcome. The study of solid tumors, including sarcomas (36–39), carcinomas (40–42), and brain tumors (43, 44) have also benefited from SKY analysis. Known to be highly aberrant, solid tumors have revealed spectacular karyotypes using SKY analysis. Numerous marker chromosomes, hidden translocations, chromosomal insertions, and additions have been revealed.

Still in its infancy, current studies involve the cataloging of the chromosomal changes as revealed by SKY, then using gene/locus-specific FISH probes to identify recurrent aberrations that may have diagnostic and prognostic significance (14, 28, 39, 45) (Fig. 2.4(b)). Many of the cytogenetic changes are thought to arise as a result of segregation defects during mitosis leading to an increase in the number of numerical changes in the karyotype. SKY analysis provides an opportunity to readily gauge the level of instability or cytogenetic heterogeneity within a tumor population, by giving more information on the number and forms of structural aberrations present.

Comparative genomic hybridization (CGH)

Comparative genomic hybridization is a FISH-based assay that determines the net gain and loss of genomic material in a given DNA sample (8, 46). This comparison between the tumor (or test DNA) and a normal reference DNA sample is visualized against a normal metaphase spread. This is in contrast to standard FISH and SKY analyses where the actual patient material is the chromosomal/interphase preparation on the slide, is the target substrate for hybridization, and is probed with a known DNA probe. The real advantage of CGH over the other FISH-based techniques described above, is that archived DNA samples or DNA extracted from paraffin blocks section (47) can be studied and investigated to identify recurrent genomic imbalances such as amplification or deletion.

For CGH, the slide preparation is a normal metaphase preparation, with the probe being the patient "unknown" sample. In this scheme, DNA is extracted from the tumor and is labeled with biotin. An equal amount normal reference DNA is labeled with digoxigenin. Both normal and tumor DNAs are denatured in the presence of unlabeled COT-1 DNA and allowed to pre-anneal at 37°C for 1 h. A normal metaphase slide preparation is denatured and hybridized with the normal/tumor DNA probe at 37°C for 72 h. The unbound probes are washed off and the haptens are detected with FITC for the biotinlylated tumor DNA, and rhodamine for the digoxigenin-labeled normal DNA. CGH analysis relies on the ratio differences between the tumor and normal along the length of the chromosome. Thus, a increase in green : red ratio indicates that a gain of genomic material in the tumor is present at that chromosomal location. Conversely, a decrease in green : red ratio indicates that a loss of genomic material in the tumor is present at that chromosomal location. However, because CGH is limited by the resolution of cytogenetics metaphase-based, the technique can only detect at best large blocks (>5 Mb) of over- or under-represented chromosomal DNA. This shortcoming is now being addressed by the application of CGH methods to microarray targets (see below). When metaphase CGH is applied and there are no gross chromosomal imbalances, i.e. rearrangements such as inversions or translocations in the sample, then such alterations will escape detection. In addition, the sensitivity of CGH can be compromised when normal cell contamination approaches 40–50% of the test sample.

The CGH technique has been useful in detecting patterns of gains and losses for many pediatric tumor types (36, 39, 43, 44, 48–50). An example is shown in Fig. 2.5(a) in which regions of amplification has been detected, a significant shift in the green : red ratio is present as a peak as shown in Fig. 2.5(a). Shown in Fig. 2.5(b) is an example of CGH analysis of a pediatric osteosarcoma sample where SKY and FISH were used to confirm changes detected by CGH (39), specifically in this case the gain of 1p35-36. Together with standard cytogenetic analyses, FISH and SKY analysis, CGH provides valuable complimentary information on a tumor sample.

Cancer genomics and microarray methods

One of the important high-throughput technologies that has been developed to assess the expression of the increasing number of genes identified by the Human Genome Project is microarray analysis (51). The approach involves the production of DNA arrays on solid supports for large-scale hybridization experiments. Two variants of the microarray or "DNA chip"

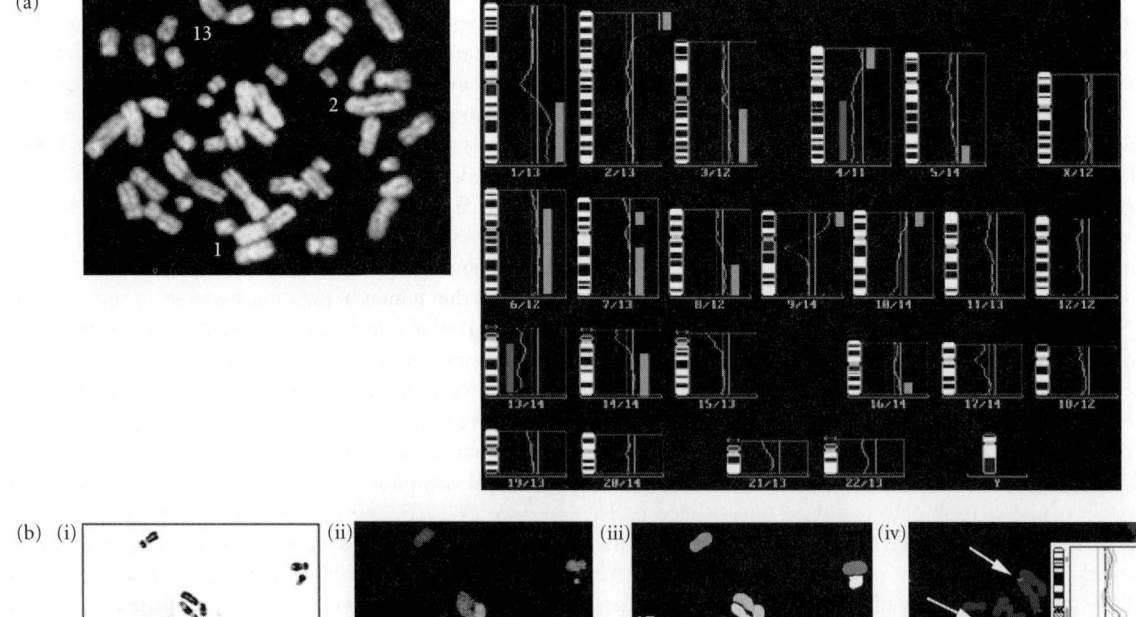

Fig. 2.5 CGH analysis and combined molecular cytogenetic techniques. (a) CGH analysis of a pediatric medulloblastoma. Shown is a normal metaphase spread hybridized with both normal (red) and tumor (green) DNA. An increase in green:red ratio indicates a gain of genomic material as in chromosomes 1 and 2, while a decrease in green:red ratio indicates a loss of genomic material as in chromosome 13. High level of amplification can be seen as bright areas of green as in chromosome 2. The corresponding CGH karyotype is presented with green bars indicating regions of net chromosomal gain and red bars indicating regions of net chromosomal loss. Amplification as in the case of chromosome 2 (2p24) is seen as a spike in the profile. (b) The use of sequential SKY and FISH analysis to confirm CGH findings. In this pediatric osteosarcoma sample (also shown in Fig. 2.2(a)), CGH analysis detected a net gain of the 1p35-p36 region. SKY analysis of metaphase spreads revealed many chromosomal aberrations: (i) inverted DAPI, (ii) RGB image, (iii) classified image, (iv) FISH of the same metaphase using probes for centromere 1 (green) and locus specific probes for 1p35-p36 (red). FISH verified the increased copy number of 1p35-p36 from the expected 3 copies to 6 copies. Both FISH and SKY analysis indicated that the region of 1p35-p36 was translocated to chromosome 17. See Plate 5.

technology exist currently: in one format, DNA probe targets are immobilized to a solid inert surface such as glass and exposed to a set of fluorescently labeled sample DNAs; in the second format, an array of different oligonucleotide probes are synthesized *in situ* on the chip (52). The array is exposed to labeled DNA samples; hybridized and complementary sequences are determined by digital imaging techniques. This approach, in theory allows for the simultaneous analysis of the differential expression of thousands of genes at once and is having a major impact on understanding the dynamics of gene expression in cancer cells (53). Microarrays are also being used to look at copy number changes in CGH-like approach, thus increasing the sensitivity to the gene level, rather than in blocks of >5 Mb of chromosomal material (5).

Expression microarrays

Expression microarray analysis detects differential gene expression using complex populations of RNAs. Cancer results from the accumulation of genetic and epigenetic changes resulting from the altered sequence or expression level of cancer-related genes such as oncogenes or tumor suppressor genes, as well as genes involved in cell cycle control, apoptosis, adhesion, DNA repair, and angiogenesis. Because gene expression profiles provide a snapshot of cell functions and processes at the time of sample preparation, comprehensive combinatorial analysis of the gene expression patterns of thousands of genes in tumor cells, and comparison to the expression profile obtained with normal cells should provide insights concerning consistent changes in gene expression that are associated with tumor cellular dysfunction and any concomitant regulatory pathways. Microarray technology has been widely used in the past 3 years to investigate tumor classification, cancer progression, and chemotherapy resistance and sensitivity.

Manufacturing of microarrays

For both expression microarrays or CGH microarrays, the spotted arrays are manufactured using xyz robots that use hollow pins to deposit cDNA (PCR products) or short oligonucleotides onto specially coated glass microscope slides (54). Spot sizes range between 80 and 150 μm in diameter and arrays that contains up to 80,000 spots can be obtained. Gene sequences to be arrayed are selected from several public databases, which contain resources to access well-characterized genes and ESTs representative of genes of unknown function. The clones chosen are amplified from appropriate cDNA libraries using PCR, and purified before spotting on the solid support.

In addition to their lower price and flexibility in design, spotted arrays (Fig. 2.6(a)) offer the advantage of allowing the simultaneous expression analysis of two biological samples, such as test and control samples. This direct comparison of expression profiles of two biological samples, such as untreated cells compared to treated cells, or normal tissue compared to cancer is an enormous advantage for any pairwise analysis. Furthermore, because these arrays can be spotted with thousands of sequenced expressed genes and ESTs of unknown function, they offer the potential for the discovery of new genes and defining their role in disease. One disadvantage of spotted arrays is that they provide information only on the relative level of gene expression between specific cells or tissue samples as opposed to direct quantification of RNA level.

Affymetrix GeneChips™ are produced by synthesizing tens of thousands of short oligonucleotides *in situ* onto glass wafers, one nucleotide at a time, using a modification of semiconductor photolithography technology (55, 56). Generally, GeneChips are designed with 16–20 oligonucleotides representing each gene on the array. Each oligonucleotide on the chip is matched with almost identical one, differing only by a central, single base mismatch. This allows the determination of the level of non-specific binding by comparison of target binding intensity between the two partner oligonucleotides. The main advantage of Affymetrix GeneChips™ is their ability to measure absolute level of expression of genes in cells or tissues. Their disadvantages, beside their higher costs, include their current inability to compare simultaneously, on the same array, the level of expression of two related biological samples. In addition, oligonucleotide-based microarrays require a priori knowledge of the gene sequences and require complex computational manipulation to convert the 40 feature signals into an actual expression value. More recently, oligonucleotide arrays have been developed that combine some the flexibilities and qualitative advantages associated with the use of synthetic probe arrays, with the benefits of simultaneous analysis afforded by spotted glass array (57).

Target preparation and hybridization

Both total RNA and mRNA can be used for microarray experiments and allow the attainment of high quality data with a high level of confidence. High quality RNA is crucial for successful microarray experiments. One of the current limitations in the routine application of microarray technology to patient samples is sufficient RNA availability. Thus, there has been considerable interest in the development of RNA amplification strategies that facilitate RNA extraction from laser capture microdissected (LCM) samples such as fine needle biopsies. For standard microarray experiments the isolated RNA is reverse-transcribed into target cDNA in the presence of fluorescent (generally Cy3-dNTP or Cy5-dNTP) or radiolabeled deoxynucleotides ([^{33}P]- or [^{32}P]-αdCTP). After purification and denaturation, the labeled targets are hybridized to the microarrays at a temperature determined by the hybridization buffer used. After hybridization, the arrays are washed under stringent conditions to remove non-specific target binding, and air-dried (Fig. 2.6(b)).

Image acquisition and quantification

Microarray image processing employs differential excitation and emission wavelengths of the two fluors to

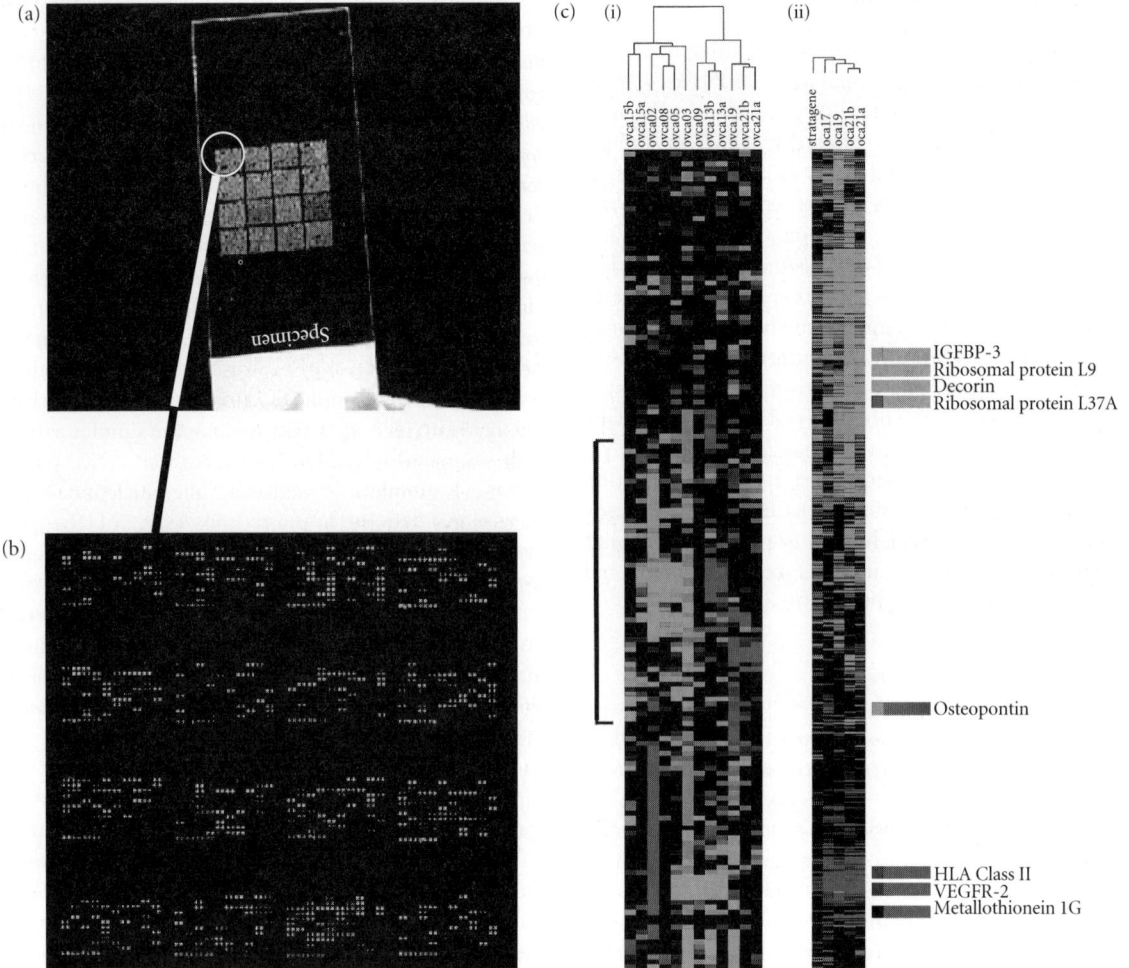

Fig. 2.6 Expression microarray technology. (a) Unhybridized spotted glass array. Shown is a spotted glass array before hybridization. (b) Imaged array post-hybridization. Shown is one quadrant of the array after being hybridized with differentially labeled RNA. In this experimental design, cDNAs found to be over-expressed appear more red, while those found to be under-expressed appear more green. Those with normal or similar levels of expression appear yellow. (c) Cluster analysis. Shown is an example of a cluster analysis and the resulting dendogram, where groupings are based on similarity within the group of tumors. See Plate 6.

obtain a scan of the array for each emission wavelength. These images are then analyzed to identify the spots, calculate their associated signal intensities, and assess local background noise. Most image acquisition software packages also contain basic filtering tools to flag spots such as extremely low intensity spots, ghosts spots (where background is higher than spot intensity), or damaged spots (e.g. dust artifacts). Using these results, an initial ratio of the evaluated channel/reference channel intensity is calculated for every spot on the chip. The products of the image acquisition are the TIFF image pairing and a quantified data file that has not yet been normalized. An excellent assessment of different image analysis methods can be found at http://oz.berkeley.edu/tech-reports/.

Statistical analysis and data mining

Analysis of large gene expression data sets is a new area of data analysis with its own unique challenges. Data mining methods typically fall into one of two classes: supervised and unsupervised. In unsupervised analysis the data is organized without the benefit of external classification information. Hierarchical clustering (58), K-means clustering (59), or self-organizing maps (60) are examples of unsupervised clustering approaches that have been widely used in microarray analysis (58, 61, 62). Supervised analysis uses some external information, such as the disease status of the samples studied. Supervised analysis involves choosing from the entire data set a training set and a testing set, and the construction of classifiers, which assign predefined classes to expression profiles. Once the classifier has been trained on the training set and tested on the testing set, it can then be applied to data with unknown classification. Supervised methods include k-nearest neighbor classification, support vector machines, and neural nets. Tusher et al. (63) recently proposed a strategy called significance analysis of microarrays (SAM) which allows the determination of significantly differentially expressed genes between groups of samples analyzed by expression arrays. We have used this approach to narrow down the analysis to a subset of genes that were also shown to be differentially expressed when analyzed by conventional two-dimensional hierarchical clustering (Fig. 2.6(c)).

CGH microarray

An emerging platform that addresses the shortcomings (described above) of metaphase-target CGH couples the technique to microarray expression technology, and is generally referred to as "microarray CGH." Instead of using metaphase chromosomes, CGH is applied to arrayed short sequences of DNA bound to glass slides and probed with genomes of interest (Fig. 2.7). With sufficient representation on the microarray, this system significantly increases resolution for localizing regions of imbalance. Furthermore, just as with expression microarray screening, the analysis is straightforward and automated.

The manufacturing and imaging of the arrays for CGH is the same as for expression microarrays (as discussed above). The only differences are with regard to the type of analytical and interpretative software required. Quantification of fluorescence intensities requires normalization and establishment of the fluorescence ratio baselines, based on control studies using DNA, with known chromosomal deletions or gains. Often, microarray DNA features are spotted in duplicate or triplicate for assessing result reproducibility. For array CGH, inclusion of genomic clones onto the microarray from regions that are known not to be involved in copy number change are recommended as internal controls for these purposes. In addition, parallel experiments in which differentially labeled normal genomic DNA is compared against itself can serve to establish the specificity of the system. Overall, there is an obvious need for statistical analysis of the conformity of the results (64). Global normalization approaches such as those used in expression microarray experiments may also be used for establishing baseline thresholds (65).

As representation on the microarrays increases in density, data storage (66) and bioinformatics will become an important aspect of the CGH analysis. Furthermore, the increase in resolution will make the task of identifying consensus regions of genomic imbalance amongst samples more challenging. This will necessitate data mining techniques that can handle many data points on multiple dimensions between experiments. Moreover, for cDNA array CGH, in silico determination of chromosomal localizations of cDNA targets is essential for providing a comprehensive ideogram-type schematic of chromosomal copy number changes (65). As microarray CGH technology becomes more prevalent, more standardized informatics and analysis tools will appear.

Validation of microarray findings

One of the most significant challenges facing investigators using microarray analysis is determining which of the plethora of new differentially expressed genes is biologically relevant to the tumor system being studied. Even when rigorous efforts are made to minimize the number of variables in a microarray study, there may be an unmanageable number of differentially expressed genes that will contribute excessive background values. Therefore, combining expression microarray analysis with other approaches, particularly cytogenetics techniques, such as SKY and chromosome and array CGH (51), offers the possibility to focus on significantly smaller subsets of genes of direct relevance to tumor biology (67). Monni and colleagues have recently used a combination of expression arrays and CGH array techniques on breast cancer cell lines, and have identified a limited number of genes that are both amplified and over expressed (68).

Finally, validation of the relative levels of expression obtained from genomic-wide microarray analysis is critical. Several approaches can be chosen, from basic Northern analysis or semi-quantitative reverse

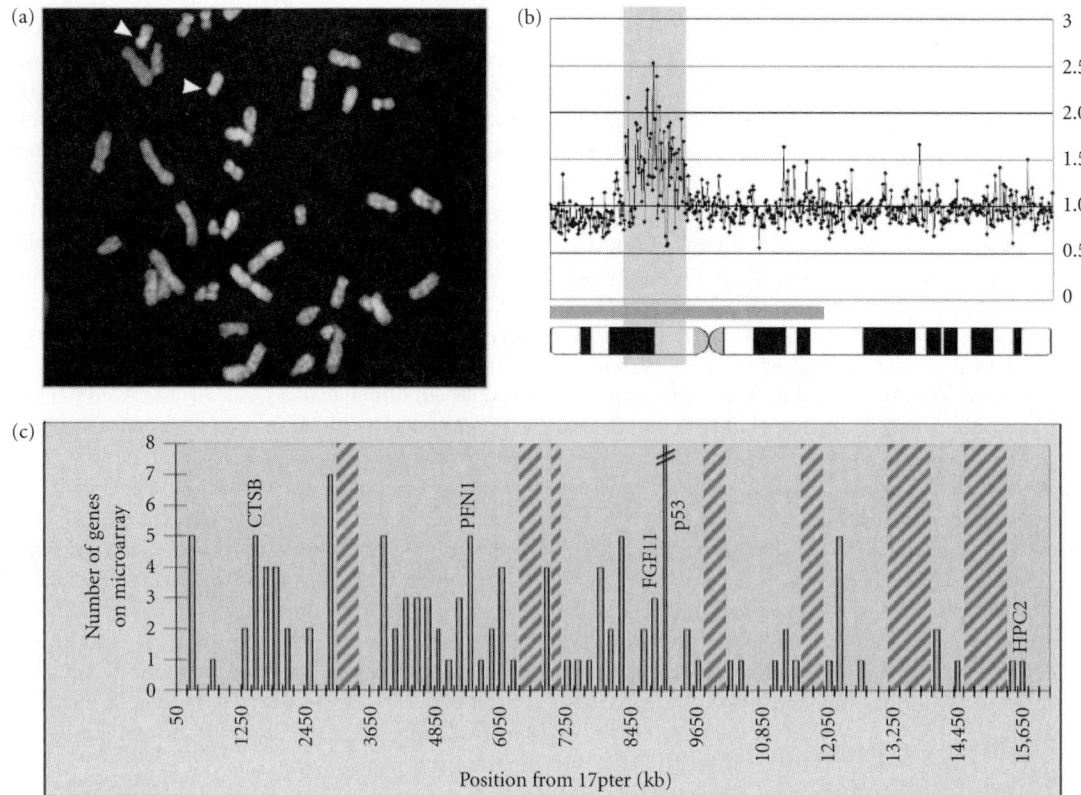

Fig. 2.7 CGH microarray analysis of chromosome 17 in osteosarcoma. (a) Metaphase CGH spread of a pediatric osteosarcoma sample. In this spread, arrow heads point to chromosome 17 where amplification of the p arm was detected. (b) High resolution detection of gene dosage changes at 17p. Chromosome CGH analysis detected the amplification of segments from 17pter to 17q21 (green line). Microarray analysis of the same sample resolved the boundaries of the amplification to 17p12 to 17p11.1 (green shading). The Y-axis represents copy number following normalization. (c) Distribution of genes in the 17p region arrayed on the slide. See Plate 7.

transcriptase PCR (RT-PCR), to *in situ* hybridization using tissue microarrays. Mousses *et al.* (69) have recently analyzed expression levels of a number of candidate genes associated with prostate cancer that they had previously identified using cDNA microarray analysis. Tissue microarrays constructed from 544 histological biopsies were analyzed by ISH using RNA probes and/or antibodies immunohistochemistry (IHC). There was excellent correlation between the cDNA microarray results and the results obtained with ISH and Northern blot analysis. In addition, protein levels assessed by IHC were also consistent with RNA expression levels. Similarly, Dhanasekaran *et al.* (70) have used comparable technologies to confirm over-expression of hepsin and PIM-1 in prostate cancer.

Future applications of profiling techniques

The range of future applications of genomic profiling technologies is enormous. Recent studies in human cancer have demonstrated that microarrays can be utilized to develop a new molecular taxonomy of cancer including clustering of cancers according to prognostic groups on the basis of gene expression profiles. The applications of profiling techniques is not limited only to the analysis of DNA and RNA. Now global analyses of protein profiles of gene expression are being performed using a variety of analytical techniques, including two-dimensional gel analysis, mass spectrometry, and "protein chips" (71). By combing cellular profiling techniques at all levels, the role of drugs, environmental toxins, or oncogenes may be elucidated and regulatory networks and co-expression patterns of cancer cells will be deciphered comprehensively.

Acknowledgments

The authors express their gratitude to Paula Marrano, Elena Kolomietz, Zong Mei Zhang, Jianming Pei, Jana Karaskova, Derek Bouman, Ben Beheshti, Ajay Pandita, Pascale MacGregor, and James D. Brenton for their technical expertise and critical evaluation of this manuscript.

Appendix

Cytogenetics

Thermotron: http://www.thermotron.com/cryogen.html

Imaging systems and optics

Applied Spectral Imaging: http://www.spectral-imaging.com/
Metasystems: http://www.metasystems.de/
Applied Imaging: http://www.aicorp.com/
Zeiss: http://www.zeiss.com/
Chroma: http://www.chroma.com/

FISH probes

Vysis: http://www.vysis.com/
Cytocell: http://www.cytocell.co.uk/
Ventana: http://www.ventanamed.com/
Research Genetics: http://bio.worldweb.net/indorgs/resgen.html
Cambio: http://www.cambio.co.uk/

Microarray

Affymetirx: http://www.affymetrix.com/index.affx
Spectral Genomics: http://www.spectralgenomics.com

Tissue arrays

Tissue array: http://www.tissue-array.com

References

1. Trent RJ. Milestones in the Human Genome Project: genesis to postgenome. Med J Aust 2000, **173**, 591–4.
2. Pennisi E. Human Genome Project. And the gene number is...? Science 2000, **288**, 1146–7.
3. Ausubel F, Brent R, Kingston R, Moore D, Seidman J, Smith J, et al. Current protocols in molecular biology, John Wiley & Sons, Inc., New York, USA, 2001.
4. Dracopoli NC. Current protocols in human genetics, John Wiley & Sons, Inc., New York, USA, 2001.
5. Beatty B, Mai S, Squire J. FISH. A practical approach, Oxford University Press, Oxford, 2002.
6. Schena M. Microarray BioChip Technology, Eaton Publishing, Natick, MA, 1999.
7. Hungerford D, Donnely A, Nowell A, Beck S. The chromosome constitution of a human phenotypic intersex. Am J Hum Gen 1959, **11**, 251.
8. Kallioniemi A, Kallioniemi OP, Sudar D, Rutovitz D, Gray JW, Waldman F, et al. Comparative genomic hybridization for molecular cytogenetic analysis of solid tumors. Science 1992, **258**, 818–21.
9. Schrock E, du Manoir S, Veldman T, Schoell B, Wienberg J, Ferguson-Smith MA, et al. Multicolor spectral karyotyping of human chromosomes [see comments]. Science 1996, **273**, 494–7.
10. Trask BJ. Fluorescence *in situ* hybridization: applications in cytogenetics and gene mapping. Trends Genet 1991, **7**, 149–54.
11. van de Corput MP, Dirks RW, Wiegant WW, Wiegant J, Muhlegger K, Raap AK. Oestradiol, a new hapten for detecting nucleic acid sequences by FISH. Histochem Cell Biol 1997, **108**, 359–64.
12. Pinkel D, Gray JW, Trask B, van den Engh G, Fuscoe J, van Dekken H. Cytogenetic analysis by *in situ* hybridization with fluorescently labeled nucleic acid probes. Cold Spring Harb Symp Quant Biol 1986, **51**, 151–7.
13. Blancato JK. Fluorescence *in situ* hybridization, Humana Press Inc., New Jersey, 1999, 443–72.
14. Markovic V, Bouman D, Bayani J, Al-Maghrabi J, Kamel-Reid S, Squire J. Lack of BCR/ABL reciprocal fusion in variant Ph translocations: use of double fusion signal FISH and spectral karyotyping. Leukemia 2000, **14**, 1157–60.
15. Squire JA, Thorner P, Marrano P, Parkinson D, Ng YK, Gerrie B, et al. Identification of MYCN copy number heterogeneity by direct FISH analysis of neuroblastoma preparations. Mol Diagn 1996, **1**, 281–9.
16. Rummukainen JK, Salminen T, Lundin J, Joensuu H, Isola JJ. Amplification of c-myc oncogene by chromogenic and fluorescence *in situ* hybridization in archival breast cancer tissue array samples. Lab Invest 2001, **81**, 1545–51.
17. van Lijnschoten G, Albrechts J, Vallinga M, Hopman AH, Arends JW, Geraedts J. Fluorescence *in situ* hybridization on paraffin-embedded abortion material as a means of retrospective chromosome analysis. Hum Genet 1994, **94**, 518–22.
18. Qian J, Bostwick DG, Takahashi S, Borell TJ, Brown JA, Lieber MM, et al. Comparison of fluorescence *in situ* hybridization analysis of isolated nuclei and routine histological sections from paraffin-embedded prostatic adenocarcinoma specimens. Am J Pathol 1996, **149**, 1193–9.

19. Kolomietz E, Al-Maghrabi J, Brennan S, Karaskova J, Minkin S, Lipton J, et al. Primary chromosomal rearrangements of leukemia are frequently accompanied by extensive submicroscopic deletions and may lead to altered prognosis. Blood 2001, **97**, 3581–8.
20. Obara K, Yokoyama M, Asano G, Tanaka S. Evaluation of myc and chromosome 8 copy number in colorectal cancer using interphase cytogenetics. Int J Oncol 2001, **18**, 233–9.
21. Pandita A, Godbout R, Zielenska M, Thorner P, Bayani J, Squire JA. Relational mapping of MYCN and DDX1 in band 2p24 and analysis of amplicon arrays in double minute chromosomes and homogeneously staining regions by use of free chromatin FISH. Genes Chromosomes Cancer 1997, **20**, 243–52.
22. Ried T. Images in neuroscience. Spectral karyotyping analysis in diagnostic cytogenetics. Am J Psychiatry 1997, **154**, 594.
23. Speicher MR, Gwyn Ballard S, Ward DC. Karyotyping human chromosomes by combinatorial multi-fluor FISH. Nat Genet 1996, **12**, 368–75.
24. Bayani J, Squire JA. Advances in the detection of chromosomal aberrations using spectral karyotyping. Clin Genet 2001, **59**, 65–73.
25. Malik Z, Dishi M, Garini Y. Fourier transform multipixel spectroscopy and spectral imaging of protoporphyrin in single melanoma cells. Photochem Photobiol 1996, **63**, 608–14.
26. Bell R. Introductory Fourier transform spectroscopy, Academic Press, London, 1972.
27. Telenius H, Pelmear AH, Tunnacliffe A, Carter NP, Behmel A, Ferguson-Smith MA, et al. Cytogenetic analysis by chromosome painting using DOP-PCR amplified flow-sorted chromosomes. Genes Chromosomes Cancer 1992, **4**, 257–63.
28. Bayani J, Pandita A, Squire JA. Sequential G-banding, SKY and FISH provide a refined identification of translocation breakpoints and complex chromosomal rearrangements. Vol. 2000, Elsevier Trends Journal Technical Tips Online, 2000.
29. Fan YS, Siu VM, Jung JH, Xu J. Sensitivity of multiple color spectral karyotyping in detecting small interchromosomal rearrangements [in process citation]. Genet Test 2000, **4**, 9–14.
30. Fleischman EW, Reshmi S, Sokova OI, Kirichenko OP, Konstantinova LN, Kulagina OE, et al. Increased karyotype precision using fluorescence in situ hybridization and spectral karyotyping in patients with myeloid malignancies. Cancer Genet Cytogenet 1999, **108**, 166–70.
31. Mark HF, Gray Y, Mark Y, Khorsand J, Sikov W. A multimodal approach in the diagnosis of patients with hematopoietic disorders. Cancer Genet Cytogenet 1999, **109**, 14–20.
32. Rowley JD, Reshmi S, Carlson K, Roulston D. Spectral karyotype analysis of T-cell acute leukemia. Blood 1999, **93**, 2038–42.
33. Rowley JD. Molecular genetics in acute leukemia. Leukemia 2000, **14**, 513–7.
34. Sawyer JR, Lukacs JL, Munshi N, Desikan KR, Singhal S, Mehta J, et al. Identification of new nonrandom translocations in multiple myeloma with multicolor spectral karyotyping. Blood 1998, **92**, 4269–78.
35. Veldman T, Vignon C, Schrock E, Rowley JD, Ried T. Hidden chromosome abnormalities in haematological malignancies detected by multicolour spectral karyotyping. Nat Genet 1997, **15**, 406–10.
36. Pandita A, Zielenska M, Thorner P, Bayani J, Godbout R, Greenberg M, et al. Application of comparative genomic hybridization, spectral karyotyping, and microarray analysis in the identification of subtype-specific patterns of genomic changes in rhabdomyosarcoma. Neoplasia 1999, **1**, 262–75.
37. Barnard M, Bayani J, Grant R, Teshima I, Thorner P, Squire J. Use of multicolor spectral karyotyping in genetic analysis of pleuropulmonary blastoma. Pediatr Dev Pathol 2000, **3**, 479–86.
38. Zielenska M, Zhang ZM, Ng K, Marrano P, Bayani J, Ramirez OC, et al. Acquisition of secondary structural chromosomal changes in pediatric Ewing sarcoma is a probable prognostic factor for tumor response and clinical outcome. Cancer 2001, **91**, 2156–64.
39. Zielenska M, Bayani J, Pandita A, Toledo S, Marrano P, Andrade J, et al. Comparative genomic hybridization analysis identifies gains of 1p35 approximately p36 and chromosome 19 in osteosarcoma. Cancer Genet Cytogenet 2001, **130**, 14–21.
40. Beheshti B, Karaskova J, Park PC, Squire JA, Beatty BG. Identification of a high frequency of chromosomal rearrangements in the centromeric regions of prostate cancer cell lines by sequential giemsa banding and spectral karyotyping. Mol Diagn 2000, **5**, 23–32.
41. Beheshti B, Park PC, Sweet JM, Trachtenberg J, Jewett MA, Squire JA. Evidence of chromosomal instability in prostate cancer determined by spectral karyotyping (SKY) and interphase fish analysis. Neoplasia 2001, **3**, 62–9.
42. Luk C, Tsao MS, Bayani J, Shepherd F, Squire JA. Molecular cytogenetic analysis of non-small cell lung carcinoma by spectral karyotyping and comparative genomic hybridization. Cancer Genet Cytogenet 2001, **125**, 87–99.
43. Bayani J, Zielenska M, Marrano P, Kwan Ng Y, Taylor MD, Jay V, et al. Molecular cytogenetic analysis of medulloblastomas and supratentorial primitive neuroectodermal tumors by using conventional banding, comparative genomic hybridization, and spectral karyotyping. J Neurosurg 2000, **93**, 437–48.
44. Squire JA, Arab S, Marrano P, Bayani J, Karaskova J, Taylor M, et al. Molecular cytogenetic analysis of glial tumors using spectral karyotyping and comparative genomic hybridization. Mol Diagn 2001, **6**, 93–108.
45. Ning Y, Liang JC, Nagarajan L, Schrock E, Ried T. Characterization of 5q deletions by subtelomeric probes and spectral karyotyping. Cancer Genet Cytogenet 1998, **103**, 170–2.
46. Kallioniemi OP, Kallioniemi A, Sudar D, Rutovitz D, Gray JW, Waldman F, et al. Comparative genomic hybridization: a rapid new method for detecting and mapping DNA amplification in tumors. Semin Cancer Biol 1993, **4**, 41–6.
47. Speicher MR, du Manoir S, Schrock E, Holtgreve-Grez H, Schoell B, Lengauer C, et al. Molecular cytogenetic analysis of formalin-fixed, paraffin-embedded solid tumors by comparative genomic hybridization after universal DNA-amplification. Hum Mol Genet 1993, **2**, 1907–14.
48. Karhu R, Siitonen S, Tanner M, Keinanen M, Makipernaa A, Lehtinen M, et al. Genetic aberrations in pediatric

acute lymphoblastic leukemia by comparative genomic hybridization. Cancer Genet Cytogenet 1997, **95**, 123–9.
49. Rice M, Breen CJ, O'Meara A, Breatnach F, O'Marcaigh AS & Stallings RL. Comparative genomic hybridization in pediatric acute lymphoblastic leukemia. Pediatr Hematol Oncol 2000, **17**, 141–7.
50. Nishizaki T, Harada K, Kubota H, Ozaki S, Ito H, Sasaki K. Genetic alterations in pediatric medulloblastomas detected by comparative genomic hybridization. Pediatr Neurosurg 1999, **31**, 27–32.
51. Pollack JR, Perou CM, Alizadeh AA, Eisen MB, Pergamenschikov A, Williams CF, et al. Genome-wide analysis of DNA copy-number changes using cDNA microarrays. Nat Genet 1999, **23**, 41–6.
52. Bowtell DD. Options available—from start to finish—for obtaining expression data by microarray. Nat Genet 1999, **21**, 25–32.
53. Cole KA, Krizman DB, Emmert-Buck MR. The genetics of cancer—a 3D model. Nat Genet 1999, **21**, 38–41.
54. Schena M, Shalon D, Davis RW, Brown PO. Quantitative monitoring of gene expression patterns with a complementary DNA microarray. Science 1995, **270**, 467–70.
55. Fodor SP, Read JL, Pirrung MC, Stryer L, Lu AT, Solas D. Light-directed, spatially addressable parallel chemical synthesis. Science 1991, **251**, 767–73.
56. Lipshutz RJ, Fodor SP, Gingeras TR, Lockhart DJ. High density synthetic oligonucleotide arrays. Nat Genet 1999, **21**, 20–4.
57. Okamoto T, Suzuki T, Yamamoto N. Microarray fabrication with covalent attachment of DNA using bubble jet technology. Nat Biotechnol 2000, **18**, 438–41.
58. Eisen MB, Spellman PT, Brown PO, Botstein D. Cluster analysis and display of genome-wide expression patterns. Proc Natl Acad Sci USA 1998, **95**, 14,863–8.
59. Tavazoie S, Hughes JD, Campbell MJ, Cho RJ, Church GM. Systematic determination of genetic network architecture. Nat Genet 1999, **22**, 281–5.
60. Tamayo P, Slonim D, Mesirov J, Zhu Q, Kitareewan S, Dmitrovsky E, et al. Interpreting patterns of gene expression with self-organizing maps: methods and application to hematopoietic differentiation. Proc Natl Acad Sci USA 1999, **96**, 2907–12.
61. Alizadeh A, Eisen M, Davis RE, Ma C, Sabet H, Tran T, et al. The lymphochip: a specialized cDNA microarray for the genomic-scale analysis of gene expression in normal and malignant lymphocytes. Cold Spring Harb Symp Quant Biol 1999, **64**, 71–8.
62. DeRisi J, Penland L, Brown PO, Bittner ML, Meltzer PS, Ray M, et al. Use of a cDNA microarray to analyse gene expression patterns in human cancer. Nat Genet 1996, **14**, 457–60.
63. Tusher VG, Tibshirani R, Chu G. Significance analysis of microarrays applied to the ionizing radiation response. Proc Natl Acad Sci USA 2001, **98**, 5116–21.
64. Brazma A, Hingamp P, Quackenbush J, Sherlock G, Spellman P, Stoeckert C, et al. Minimum information about a microarray experiment (MIAME)-toward standards for microarray data. Nat Genet 2001, **29**, 365–71.
65. Beheshti B, Braude I, Marrano P, Thorner P, Zielenska M, Squire JA. Chromosomal localization of DNA amplifications in neuroblastoma tumours using cDNA microarray comparative genomic hybridization. Neoplasia 2003, **5**(1), 53–62.
66. Sherlock G. Analysis of large-scale gene expression data. Brief Bioinform 2001, **2**, 350–62.
67. Bayani J, Brenton JD, Macgregor PF, Beheshti B, Albert M, Nallainathan D, et al. Parallel analysis of sporadic primary ovarian carcinomas by spectral karyotyping, comparative genomic hybridization and expression microarrays. Cancer Res, 2002, **62**(12), 3466–76.
68. Monni O, Barlund M, Mousses S, Kononen J, Sauter G, Heiskanen M, et al. Comprehensive copy number and gene expression profiling of the 17q23 amplicon in human breast cancer. Proc Natl Acad Sci USA 2001, **98**, 5711–6.
69. Mousses S, Wagner U, Chen Y, Kim JW, Bubendorf L, Bittner M, et al. Failure of hormone therapy in prostate cancer involves systematic restoration of androgen responsive genes and activation of rapamycin sensitive signaling. Oncogene 2001, **20**, 6718–23.
70. Dhanasekaran SM, Barrette TR, Ghosh D, Shah R, Varambally S, Kurachi K, et al. Delineation of prognostic biomarkers in prostate cancer. Nature 2001, **412**, 822–6.
71. Haab BB. Advances in protein microarray technology for protein expression and interaction profiling. Curr Opin Drug Discov Dev 2001, **4**, 116–23.

3 | Blots, dots, amplification, and sequencing

John J. O'Leary, Cara Martin, and Orla Sheils

This chapter details some of the technologies used in molecular pathology and their potential uses. The chapter does not aim to provide an exhaustive list of technologies but attempts to highlight important developments, which facilitate molecular diagnostics.

Restriction endonucleases (REs)

Restriction enzymes (REs) are bacterial proteins that cut long, linear DNA molecules into smaller fragments. Restriction endonucleases are a major tool in recombinant DNA technology. A RE recognizes a specific sequence in DNA such as AGCT and cuts DNA wherever this combination of bases occurs in the genome. The enzymes are isolated from bacteria and are named with a three or four letter sequence, usually followed by a roman numeral (eg. *Eco*RI). The prime function of REs is to destroy bacteriophages or other viruses that invade bacteria. Bacteria have developed these enzyme systems to cut the invading DNA sequences of viruses, etc., thereby rendering the virus harmless.

Importantly, the nucleotides of the bacteria's own DNA are methylated to protect them from autodigestion by the bacteria's own REs.

Table 3.1 lists some examples of commonly used REs in molecular biology. The number of cut sites in lambda bacteriophage DNA is given. The hundreds of REs now available provide a very powerful tool in the molecular analysis of DNA molecules (1). The REs are extensively used in restriction fragment length polymorphism (RFLP) analysis and may be used for confirmation of polymerase chain reaction (PCR) products. They are extensively used in cloning protocols.

Southern blot analysis

Southern blot analysis was first described by Edwin Southern in 1975. The technique allows the analysis of DNA fragments from a wide variety of samples (1). The technique proceeds as follows.

DNA is extracted from a clinical sample. Usually 1–5 μg of DNA are required to perform a Southern blot analysis, thereby necessitating the use of fresh/frozen material. This in general precludes archival paraffin wax embedded material and small biopsies.

The extracted DNA is then incubated with a RE (e.g. *Bgl*II). This enzyme cuts the entire human genome into tens of thousands of fragments ranging from 100 to 20,000 bases in size. These fragments are then run on an electrophoretic gel and size sorted. The smallest fragments move most rapidly through the gel. For demonstration of the fragments, the gel is stained with an intercalating DNA dye such as ethidium bromide. The second step involves transfer of the resolved DNA to a solid support, such as nitrocellulose or nylon. Nitrocellulose or nylon binds DNA. To do this, the nitrocellulose paper is placed on top of the gel slab, which is then covered with absorbent paper. DNA is wicked out of the gel by using a transfer solution such as 20 × SSC (sodium chloride, sodium citrate). Overnight transfer is usually achieved. For laboratories performing many blots, vacuum blotting is commonly used.

After blotting the gel, the membrane is now hybridized with a labelled (isotopic or non-isotopic)

Table 3.1 Examples of commonly used restriction endonucleases

Enzyme	Recognition sequence	# sites in bacteriophage lambda
*Bam*HI	G/GATCC	5
*Bgl*II	A/GATCT	6
*Dde*I	C/TNAG	>50
*Eco*RI	G/AATTC	5
*Hind*III	A/AGCTT	6
*Pst*I	CTGCA/G	18

probe, to the region of interest, using a suitable solution called a hybridization buffer. Hybridization is usually carried out in a plastic bag (hybridization bag) or a hybridization oven. The probe is a cloned fragment of DNA that has a complementary sequence to the DNA fragment of interest. During the hybridization, the probe seeks out its complementary sequence. The specificity of binding of the probe to its complementary sequence is called the stringency. The stringency of the hybridization can be varied by adjusting the temperature of hybridization, salt concentration of the hybridization mix, and adding additional agents such as formamide that lower the melting temperature of DNA interactions. After hybridization, the blot is washed and detected. Figure 3.1 shows a Southern blot analysis of lambda DNA, a normal patient DNA, and DNA from the HL 60 cell line (a leukemia cell line) for the myeloperoxidase gene (a reference housekeeping gene), with different enzyme patterns illustrated.

The Southern blot analysis can be used to detect alterations in DNA sequences, by looking for differences in DNA fragments after digestion with a restriction endonuclease. Southern blot analysis has been successfully applied to the analysis of many diseases including sickle cell anaemia, cystic fibrosis, and for the detection of the Philadelphia chromosome (Ph) in chronic myeloid leukaemia.

Northern and Western blots

Northern blot is analagous to Southern blotting except that it analyses RNA molecules (1). Western blot analyses protein (1).

mRNA is an unstable molecule, making Northern blot technically more difficult that Southern blots, even in experienced hands. Northern analysis begins with the extraction of RNA from the cell or tissues. Cells are initially lysed in the presence of strong RNase inhibitors, in order to prevent destruction of endogenous RNA within the cell by ubiquitous RNases present in the environment. Because RNA is labile precautions to reduce its degradation must be taken; all plastics and glass-ware must be sterile, solutions that may contain RNases must be treated with diethylpyrocarbonate (destroys RNAses), and gloves worn at all time (fingers are covered in RNases). Isolation of RNA from crude cell extracts is usually performed by chromatographic separation. mRNA is then electrophoresed in an agarose gel; however unlike the gel for the Southern blot the gel for Northern blot is a denaturing gel, for example, formaldehyde containing gel. Restriction digestion is not required, because RNA molecules are already small compared to their larger DNA counterparts. After electrophoresis, blotting is carried out as for Southern transfer (as described above). Hybridization is then carried out using a labelled probe specific to the mRNA molecule of interest.

Western blotting, is an analogous technique for the analysis of proteins within the cell. Proteins are electrophoresed through a vertical polyacrylamide gel so as to separate the molecules according to size and charge, and are then transferred to a membrane and hybridized with an antibody against the specific protein of interest. Unlike Northern or Southern blots, Western blots can be denaturing or non-denaturing (depending on the application).

Dot and slot blots

Alternative techniques have now developed to short-cut classical transfer techniques described above. Included among these are dot and slot blots (where DNA or RNA samples are applied directly onto a membrane). Commercially available instrumentation using blotting manifolds are available to perform these techniques (e.g. BioRad dot blot apparatus). These are high through put ways of analysing DNA and RNA; once the nucleic acid

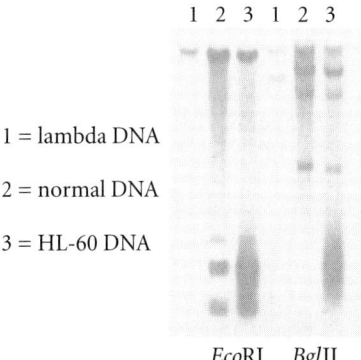

Fig. 3.1 Southern blot autoradiograph. Lambda DNA, normal human DNA, and HL-60(leukaemic) DNA was examined using the myeloperoxidase gene.

has bound to the nitrocellulose membrane it is hybridized and washed as for standard Southern and Northern blots. However using these techniques nucleic acids are not size-separated, and so this information is lost. False positives and high backgrounds can also be a problem, where probes or hybridization conditions are not optimal.

Microsatellite PCR analysis

Microsatellites (also called simple repeat sequence length polymorphisms or short tandem repeat polymorphisms), are defined as arrays of short stretches of nucleotide sequences scattered throughout human DNA, repeated between 15 and 30 times (2–4).

Several authors however distinguish between microsatellites (2-base pair (bp) repeats) and short tandem repeats (STR; 3–5-bp repeats) (5, 6). Microsatellites belong to the family of repetitive non-coding DNA sequences, which are classified as follows:

1. *Satellite sequences:* arrays with repeat sizes ranging from 5 to 100 bp, usually arranged in clusters up to 100 megabases (Mb). These are usually located in the heterochromatin near chromosomal centromeres and telomeres and are not variable in size within populations, as compared with other members of this family (7–9).
2. *Minisatellite sequences:* arrays with repeat sizes of 15–70 bp which range in size from 0.5 to 30 kilobases (kb). Minisatellites are found in euchromatic regions of the genome and are highly variable in repeat size within the population (6, 10).
3. *Microsatellite sequences:* arrays with a repeat of 2–6 bp, highly variable in size, but ranging around a mean size of 100 bp. Microsatellites are found in euchromatin and allele sizes in populations characteristically exhibit multiple size classes distributed about a population mean (11).
4. *Short nucleotide polymorphisms (SNPs):* short nucleotide polymorphic regions scattered throughout the geonome and associated with known/sequenced genes. Each individual has a specific SNP profile, making these markers extremely useful in disease pedigree analysis and linkage studies.

Microsatellites were originally described in eukaryotic genomes as stretches of dT–dG alternating sequences with varying lengths. Subsequently it was shown that these microsatellites could easily be amplified using PCR, particularly of dT–dG and dC–dA dinucleotide repeat microsatellites. Importantly, these repeat sequences showed the Mendelian codominant inheritance of the size polymorphisms.

In order of decreasing abundance, dA, dA–dC, dA–dA–dA–dN, dA–dA–dN, and dA–dG repeats were identified as the most frequent sequence motifs in human microsatellites.

(dC–dA)n microsatellites are estimated to number between 35,000 and 100,000 copies in the human genome—giving a marker density of one microsatellite every 100,000 bp (12). Although widely distributed, microsatellites are not evenly distributed along chromosomes, being particularly under-represented in subtelomeric regions of the genome.

The informativeness (polymorphic information content, PIC) of dinucleotide microsatellites increases with increasing average number of repeats (13). The human genome contains approximately 12,000 (dC–dA)n microsatellites with $PIC > 0.5$ (700 of which have $PIC \geq 0.7$. Tri- and tetranucleotide microsatellites have been identified at a frequency of 1 every 300–500 kb on chromosome X (4). About half of these microsatellites appear to be informative.

The precise function of repeat sequences in the human genome is not known. The initial occurrence of short repeat sequences could be due to chance alone, or they may have arisen as mutations from poly(dA)n sequences at the 3' end of adjacent Alu repeat sequences (12). The selective prevalence of (dC–dA)n repeats can be explained by the methylation of dC residues at the 5' dG–dC 3' sequences normally present in the human genome. Methylated dC residues can be deaminated, producing a transition of dC to dT. This process leads to an abundance of 5' dC–dA 3' motifs in the genome. Subsequent expansion of the repeat sequence may be due to slippage synthesis during DNA replication. This will then create polymorphisms differing by a few repeats each time. Additional sequence motifs may subsequently arise because of mutations of the expanded dC–dA repeats.

It was initially thought that repeat sequences possessed a functional role in the genome, either directly via gene regulation or indirectly as hot spots for recombination (14). CAG tri-nucleotide repeats are transcribed to polglutamine tracts. In addition, DNA binding proteins specific to di- and trinucleotide repeats have been identified and it has recently been suggested that some repeats may act as a site for nucleosome assembly *in vitro* (15).

Microsatellite PCR

PCR amplification of microsatellite DNA sequences follows the basic broad principles of a normal solution phase PCR. Like a standard PCR, the reaction mixture consists of the sample DNA, two primers, four deoxynucleotides, a buffer containing magnesium chloride, and Taq DNA polymerase, combined in a single tube assay.

When performing microsatellite PCR the following should be borne in mind:

DNA template: starting DNA template can be extracted from a wide variety of sources, including formalin fixed tissues, paraffin embedded blocks, cytological smears, and cell aspirates. The extraction protocol used depends largely on the individual investigator, but can include proteinase K digestion followed by phenol–chloroform purification and ethanol precipitation, simple boiling, or chelex treatment of cells and tissues. DNA degradation (due to fixation, etc.) must be considered when one is performing microsatellite PCR. This requires that each assay is optimized for each primer pair under investigation.

Primers: 20 mers are best used for microsatellite PCR with a GC content of 35–55%. The matched GC content of the primers should be within 5%. Additional precautions need to be taken to ensure non-complementarity, no secondary structure, and non-homology with alu repeat sequence, which are often located near microsatellites. Primers should ideally be sited as close to the microsatellite as possible, ensuring optimal amplification. Optimal annealing temperature range 3–12°C above the theoretical Tm values and require empirical optimization. The concentration of primer used varies between 0.1 and 0.3 μM.

dNTPs: deoxynucleotide concentrations between 20 and 100 μM are suitable. These concentrations are lower than standard solution phase PCR, and reflect the specificity and fidelity required for microsatellite PCR.

PCR buffers: the buffer for each assay should ideally be optimized for each assay. Initially it is advisable to prepare six buffers (100 mM Tris–HCl, 500 mM KCl, and 1% Triton-X 100) at two magnesium concentrations (1.5 and 3.0 mM) and three pH values (pH 8.0, 8.5, and 9.0). Simultaneous amplification under the same cycling conditions with these six buffers is a useful aid to optimization. The addition of bovine serum albumin (BSA), glycerol, formamide, and ammonium sulphate have been reported to increase specificity, and should be used if initial optimization is unsuccessful.

Thermocycling: the accurate scoring of allelic fragments can be severely affected by spurious amplification bands, which are due to mis-priming events. High annealing temperatures and short extension times (given that the nucleotide incorporation rate of Taq DNA polymerase is 35–150 nucleotides (nt)/s at 70–80°C, and the size range of allelic fragments is small) are advised. Hot start PCR and heat soaked PCR (invoving incubation of the DNA template at 94°C for 30 min before adding Taq DNA polymerase) are recommended to increase specificity. Touchdown PCR (using high initial annealing temperatures, and reducing by 1–2°C in each successive cycle) has been suggested as a way of bypassing the need to optimize individual PCR thermal cycling conditions.

Detection and scoring of microsatellites: polyacrylamide gel electrophoresis (PAGE) is the usual means to resolve microsatellite PCR amplicons. Specific oligo-probing can also be performed using a specific probe that will only recognize the desired repeat sequence. 'Stutter bands' are often encountered on PAGE gels, making interpretation very difficult in some assays. Stutter bands are additional bands differing by 1–2 bp in size. They arise probably due to slippage synthesis by Taq DNA polymerase (akin to the mechanism that may be involved in the formation of microsatellites in the first place). It is also possible that Taq DNA polymerase fails to read through the repeat sequence, or due to the 3′ terminal addition of nucleotides by Taq DNA polymerase, or due to differences in the migration of (dC–dA)n and (dG–dT)n strands (when both strands are labelled) (16).

There are several methods which can be used for the detection of microsatellite amplicons.

Radioactive methods have traditionally been used for the detection and quantitation of microsatellite PCR, using either a labelled nucleotide triphosphate in the PCR reaction mix (alpha 32) P-dCTP or a single labelled (gamma 32) dATP labelled primer (Fig. 3.2). The primer end labelled approach minimizes additional bands on the gel and facilitates analysis. Products are resolved on sequencing gels, fixed, dried, and autoradiographed, with or without intensifying screens. Pre-flashing of the X-ray film is important to ensure linearity. Optical densitometry is then used for quantitation of PCR products (17).

Non-radioactive methods include ethidium bromide staining (which offers low detection sensitivity; only >10 ng of dsDNA can be detected) and silver staining (with attendant problems of background and non-linear deposition of silver) (17).

Fluorescence analysis offers the most sensitive and reliable method for the detection of microsatellite PCR amplicons (Figs 3.3, 3.4, and 3.5). The advantage of analysing multiple polymorphic markers using an automated DNA sequencer was first described by Skolnick and Wallace in 1988 (18). In 1992, Ziegel et al. reported the use of an automated DNA sizing technology, for genotyping microsatellite loci, using a four colour fluorescence technique (19).

In this method, fluorescent phosphoramidites are linked to the 5' end of one of the primers in a PCR assay. The labels used include FAM (blue), TAMRA (yellow), JOE (green), and ROX (red). In addition, newly introduced fluorescently labelled dNTPs (R110, blue: R6G, green; TAMRA, yellow) can be used to internally label the PCR product.

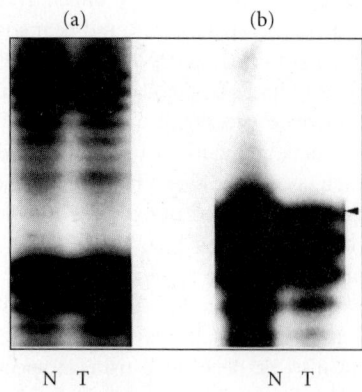

Fig. 3.2 Autoradiograph showing an AI assay in normal (N) and tumour DNA(T) from the same patient. (a) no LOS. (b) LOS in the tumour sample.

Uses of microsatellites and SNPs in pathology

Genome analysis

Restriction fragment length polymorphisms were initially proposed as the DNA markers of choice permitting the reliable detection of genes for dominant

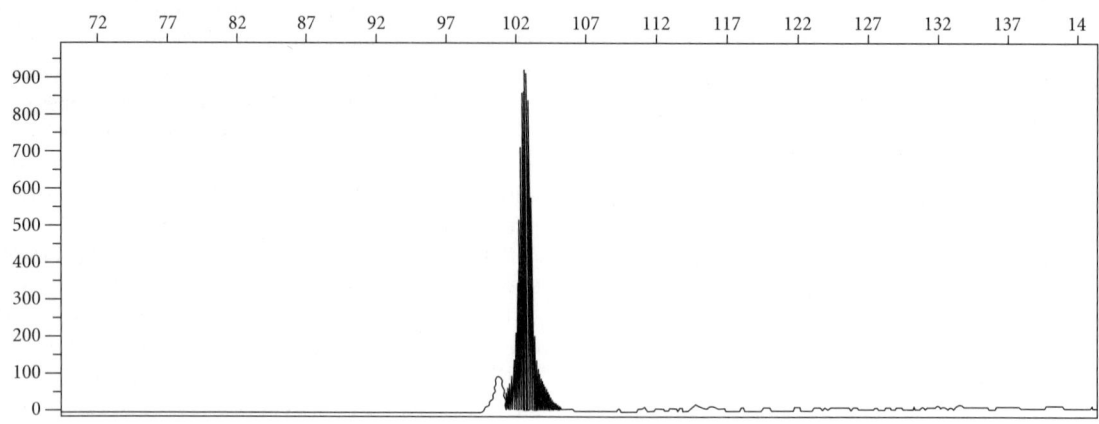

Fig. 3.3 Electrophoretogram of a chromosome 11 microsatellite analysis showing an uninformative homozygous case (one allelic peak).

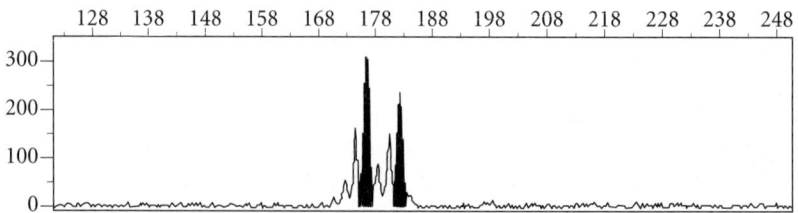

Fig. 3.4 Electrophoretogram of a chromosome 11 microsatellite analysis showing an informative heterozygous case, with two allelic peaks.

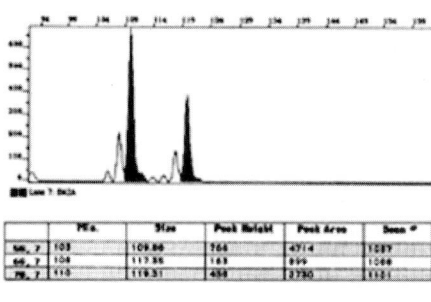

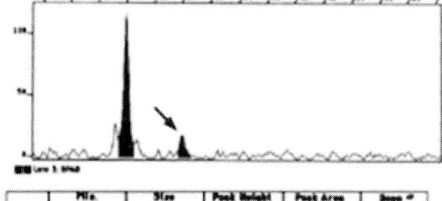

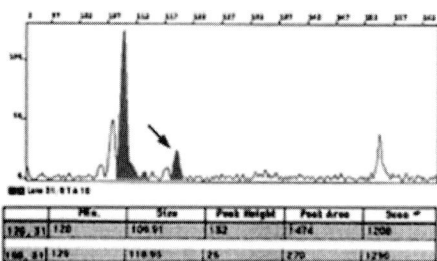

Fig. 3.5 Electrophoretogram of a chromosome 11 microsatellite analysis in normal glandular intra-epithelial neoplasia (GIN) and invasive adenocarcinoma of the cervix. Note the decrease in the size of the allelic peak in the middle and bottom panels, indicating that AI is present both in GIN and the invasive adenocarcinoma.

Table 3.2 Human genome maps

Year	Group	Marker	Loci no.	Resolution (cM)
1981	Keats	Classical	53	16
1987	CRI	RFLP	403	10
1992	Genethon	CA	814	4.4
1992	NIH/CEPH	Mixed	1416	3.0
1994	Genethon	CA	2066	2.9
1994	CHLC	Mixed	5840	0.7
2000	Celera	SNP	?	0.2

diseases. The RFLPs suffer from one major disadvantage, in that they exhibit low heterozygosity. The analysis of RFLPs is also tedious and laborious (see later in the chapter).

The most informative member of this class, VNTRs (variable number of tandem repeats) or minisatellites, tend to cluster at the ends of chromosomes, where telomeric shortening occurs independent of tumourigenesis, as part of the normal ageing process. Minisatellites however give good coverage of centromeric regions of chromosomes, where microsatellites tend to be sparsely distributed. Currently, the number of Genome Database (GDB) marker loci, scorable by PCR with heterozygosities greater than 69%, is in excess of 3000 (see Table 3.2). The current microsatellite map of the human genome gives a 0.7 cM resolution (21). More recently SNP analysis has facilitated completion of the genome mapping project by Celera Corporation USA.

Microsatellites can be used easily for linkage analysis studies. Owing to the enhanced density of microsatellite markers, linkage analysis is now no longer limited to monogenic markers, and has been successfully applied in the study of early onset Alzheimer's disease and in mapping BRCA1 in breast cancer (22–24).

In addition to linkage analysis, allele sharing and association studies can easily be performed using microsatellite PCR, to identify novel disease loci. In allele sharing, one attempts to prove that the inheritance pattern of a chromosomal region is not consistent with random Mendelian inheritance, with association studies testing whether a disease and an allele show correlated occurrences in a defined population. Allele sharing has been successfully applied by Todd et al. in their genome-wide study of type I diabetes mellitus, in which they identified 18 chromosomal regions with evidence for linkage, identifying three new genes involved in diabetes mellitus, IDDM3, IDDM5, and a locus on chromosome 18 (25). Other genes have similarly been identified including apolipoprotein E in Alzheimer's disease and angiotensin converting enzyme in myocardial infarction (17).

Allelic imbalance (AI)/loss of heterozygosity (LOH) studies

Allelotyping of the entire 23 pairs of chromosomes has been performed by Vogelstein et al. in colorectal cancer (26). The AI assays use the Knudson hypothesis of deleted anti-oncogenes. Loss of hereozygosity, the loss of an allelic band in a tumour versus constitutional DNA from the same individual is now universally recognized as indicative of putative tumour suppressor

Table 3.3 Tumours associated with AI/LOH

Breast	1p,1q,3p,6q,11p,11q,13q,16q,17p,17q
Lung	3p,5q,8p,11p,13q,17p
Renal	3p,5q,17p
Colorectal	1p,2p,5q,8p,11q,13q,14q,17p
Gastric	13q,18q
Pancreas	1p,3p,6q,8p,11,17p
Hepatocellular	8p,13q,16q,17p
Cervical	3p,11q,17p
Ovarian	3p,6q,11p,13q,17p
Testicular	3p,11p,17p
Prostate	8p,10q,16q
Melanoma	6q,9p,11p

Table 3.4 Microsatellites associated with disease

Repeat sequence	Association
Mononucleotide Dinucleotide Trinucleotide	HPNCC
Dinucleotide Trinucleotide Tetranucleotides	Various human cancers
CCG	Fragile X syndrome FRAXA FRAXE FRAXF
CAG	Spinal and bulbar muscular atrophy MD Huntington's disease Spinocerebellar ataxia (type 1) RED-1 Machado–Joseph disease Haw River syndrome

genes. Cawkell *et al.* have applied microsatellite PCR technology for the analysis of microdissected tissues from archival paraffin wax embedded material. With small starting amounts of DNA, allelic amplification is difficult to distinguish from allelic loss, and therefore the term allelic imbalance (AI) is used (27).

Individuals are either heterozygous or homozygous at microsatellite loci (see Figs 3.3 and 3.4). The AI is calculated as a ratio; the numerator and denominator being the ratios of the intensities of the two allelic peaks in the tumour and constitutional DNA (Fig. 3.5). At least 30% tumour load is required for AI/LOH assays, although recent reports using flow cytometry suggest a figure as low as 10% tumour cells.

Using such AI/LOH assays, the search is now on to identify novel tumour suppressor genes in many solid/non-solid tumours (Table 3.3).

Microsatellite markers in human disease

Microsatellite expansion in disease

Mutations in repeat sequences may be a common cause of human disease. In myotonic dystrophy (MD) and the fragile X syndrome, expansion of microsatellite repeats has been identified (28). The expansion is linked to parental copy number and that such repeats predispose to mutations. In the fragile X syndrome, expansion of the CCG trinucleotide repeat in the 5′ untranslated region of the FMR1 gene on chromosome X, causes methylation at the CpG residues, both in the repeat region and also in the adjacent FMR1 promoter, effectively stopping transcription of the gene (17). In MD, the degree of expansion of the non-coding 3′ trinucleotide repeat is associated with disease severity and the age of onset. Table 3.4 lists common microsatellite markers, which are associated with disease.

Microsatellite instability (MSI) in human disease

Microsatellite instability was first discovered in the search for causal mutations in hereditary non-polyposis colorectal cancer (HNPCC), an autosomal dominant syndrome, in which there is a predeliction to colorectal and endometrial tumours (29). In HNPCC kindreds, there is linkage to the marker D2S123 on chromosome 2p. In addition, MSI was present throughout the genome. This was represented by microsatellites of varying size. These groups of patients became known as replication error positive (RER+). It is estimated that the total number of mutations at microsatellite loci in RER+ tumour cells could be up to 100-fold that in RER− cells, suggesting a mutation affecting DNA replication, or repair, thereby predisposing to replication errors. Studies in mutator mutants of *Saccharomyces cerevisiae* and *Escherichia coli* showed that mutations in the mismatch repair genes, PMS1, MLH1, or MSH2 and Mut S produced an RER+ phenotype. The mechanism of error is explained by slippage DNA synthesis, whereby DNA polymerases slip on the repeat motif during normal cellular replication, with subsequent correction of the frame-shifts by the mismatch repair complex, thereby predisposing to the RER+ phenotype. Thus was discovered hMSH2, homologous to the yeast MSH2 gene, whose protein product has been shown to be a DNA mismatch binding protein. Other mismatch repair genes involved in the pathogenesis of HNPCC include, hMLH1, hPMS1, and hPMS2. Indeed analysis of sporadic tumours belonging to the HNPCC spectrum also reveals a significant proportion of cases with multiple replication errors. Some small cell lung tumours (with multiple primary sites) are also now shown to demonstrate the RER+ phenotype.

Forensic and population study applications of microsatellites

Population studies reveal that microsatellite alleles segregate in a Mendelian fashion in families (30). The *de novo* mutation rate for tri- and tetranucleotide repeats (STRs) ranges from 2.3 to 15.9×10^{15}. Therefore new mutations are not a significant problem in identity determination. The STRs are therefore ideally suited for use in medical and forensic identification and are admissible in court. Using fluorescent technology as little as 100 pg of DNA target can be used for the direct identification of an individual.

In addition, a number of markers of genetic diversity have been utilized to construct a phylogenetic tree of human populations, in order to understand fully population mobility traits and evolutionary trends. Genetic similarity can be interpreted as evidence of shared ancestry, though most genetic variation in humans exists between individuals within races.

DNA fingerprinting

The establishment of identity in forensic medicine and in paternity cases is extremely important. Fingerprinting has long been the only method of identification of human subjects. Recombinant DNA testing now has the potential to replace conventional hand fingerprinting. Just like the fingerprint, the human genome is different for every individual (except for genetically identical twins). Of the 6 billion bp making up the diploid content of a human cell, one person differs from another by about 3 million bp, or at least 0.5% of the genome. Some of these differences between individuals are due to mutations, thereby affecting the phenotype of the individual, although most mutations are silent with no constitutive effect. Most changes do not occur within coding regions of the genome, and therefore do not affect the phenotype of the individual. These alterations are called *polymorphisms* (incidental variations in the genome, with no affect on gene expression). Many of the polymorphisms that constitute differences in individuals occur in areas called 'spacer DNA'. These are short segments of DNA that repeat a variable number of times (see microsatellites above).

When a sperm or an egg is formed by the process of meiosis, the number of spacer segments in the germ cell changes in a random fashion. A fertilized zygote is formed at the moment of conception by the combination of two haploid genomes (from haploid germ cells) to give a diploid cell. The diploid zygote has different numbers of spacer elements than either of its parents. This forms the basis of DNA fingerprinting.

The human genome is present in every cell of the body, and all cells serve as sources of material for DNA fingerprinting. DNA is very stable: indeed a dried blood sample can be tested many years after a crime.

Several recombinant DNA techniques are useful for DNA fingerprinting, employing both PCR and Southern blot techniques. One technique utilizes VNTRs, typically 6–8 bases in length, repeating 6–20 times. The random nature of VNTRS throughout the genome of an individual gives that individual a unique serial number, akin to a 'bar-code' on the side of a carton of corn flakes. Figure 3.6 illustrates schematically how the mapping pattern of VNTRs from two different individuals can be used in DNA fingerprinting. In this illustration, three different regions with VNTRs are used (A, B, and C). An RE digestion site (indicated by the vertical arrows) on either side of the VNTR, releases the DNA fragments containing that VNTR. More copies of the tandem repeat results in larger DNA fragments being cut. In region A, patient 1 has six repeats, patient 2 has two repeats. In region B, patient 1 has five repeats and patient 2, three. In region C, patient 1 has two repeats and patient 2 has eight. Southern blot analysis of the restriction digest electrophoresis, probed for the VNTR

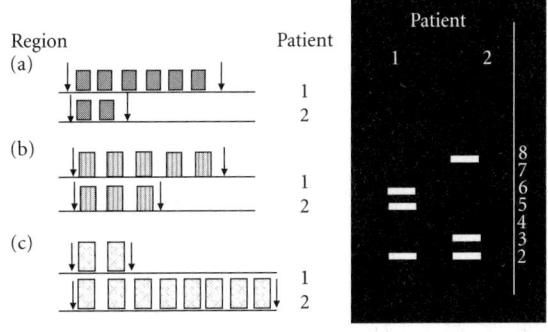

Fig. 3.6 Schematic diagram illustrating a typical DNA fingerprinting assay using the VNTR method.

sequences establishes the banding pattern and size of each band for a particular patient. Figure 3.6, only shows a three region analysis, but in practice many regions (up to a 1000 or more) can be probed for using such a methodology. This increases the specificity of the DNA fingerprint, effectively giving a 'bar-code' result as mentioned previously.

PCR can be used to detect specific site differences in DNA, which also form a unique DNA signature for that individual. PCR methods are now commonly employed to examine variations in regions of the HLA-Dq locus of the human histocompatability system (HLA). Employing PCR means that minute quantities can be used (as little as 100 pg), as compared to Southern analysis, which requires 10 µg, a 10^6-fold difference in starting DNA template concentrations. More importantly, however, PCR can be used with degraded DNA samples, which are often the only means of forensic identification.

DNA fingerprinting is offered by several companies and hospital laboratories worldwide, particularly in the investigation of rape, paternity suits, and forensic identification of human remains.

There are however problems associated with DNA fingerprinting techniques. False DNA left at a crime scene can totally confound a DNA fingerprinting result. In addition, some cosmetics contain human DNA (e.g. shampoos), consequently if hair samples were used for DNA fingerprinting analysis this may make interpretation of the result extremely difficult. In routine histopathology, DNA fingerprinting is sometimes resorted to, to sort out mis-labelled tissue specimens from different individuals, where the diagnosis carries serious implications for one individual.

Taq Man PCR for DNA and RNA amplification

This newly described technique utilizes the 5'–3' endonucleolytic activity of AmpliTaq DNA polymerase (31–33) (Fig. 3.7). The technique allows the direct detection of PCR product by the specific release of a fluorescent reporter molecule during the PCR reaction (34). Taq Man PCR uses a primer pair (as in conventional solution phase PCR) and an internal oligoprobe, called a Taq Man probe. The release of the fluorescent reporter molecule only occurs if target specific amplification occurs, obviating the need to confirm the amplicon following amplification.

Taq Man probe chemistry

The Taq Man probe consists of an oligonucleotide usually 20–30 bases in length with a 5' reporter dye, a 3' quencher dye and a 3' blocking phosphate. The fluorescence reporter dye, for example, FAM (6-carboxyfluoroscein), JOE, or VIC is covalently linked to the 5' end of the oligonucleotide probe. In this system, TET (tetrachloro-6-carboxy-fluoroscein) and HEX (hexachloro-6-carboxy-fluoroscein) can also be used as fluorescent reporter dyes. Each of these reporters is quenched by TAMRA (6-carboxy-tetramethyl-rhodamine) a non-fluorescent quencher (NFQ), which is attached by a LAN (linker-arm-modified nucleotide) to the 3' end of the probe. The probe is chemically phosphorylated at its 3' end, which prevents probe extension during PCR applications. When the probe is intact (linearized), the proximity of the reporter dye to the quencher dye results in direct suppression of the fluorescence from the reporter dye by Forster-type energy transfer (35, 36). During PCR, if the target of interest is present the probe will specifically anneal between the forward primer (primer 1) and the reverse primer (primer 2). Due to the nucleolytic activity of the AmpliTaq DNA polymerase, the probe is cleaved between the reporter and the quencher sequence only if the probe is hybridized to its target.

Importantly, AmpliTaq DNA polymerase does not digest free probe. After cleavage, the shortened probe dissociates from the target and strand polymerization continues. The process occurs in every cycle and does not interfere with the exponential accumulation of product. Cleavage of the oligonucleotide between the reporter and quencher dyes results in a specific increased fluorescence from the reporter that is proportional to the amount of the product that has accumulated.

The specificity of the 5' nuclease assay results from the requirement of the Taq polymerase enzyme for sequence complementarity between the probe and the template, in order that specific cleavage of the probe occurs. Thus the fluorescence signal that is generated is a reflection of the presence of the target sequence of the probe being amplified during PCR. No signal is generated by non-specific amplification. The availablity of spectrally resolvable reporter dyes enables the investigator to use up to three probes in a single reaction, thus performing multiplex Taq Man PCR. Applications for multiple probes include multiplex PCR allelic discrimination, and internal standards.

Increase in fluorescence can be detected using a luminescence spectrophotometer for end-point detection

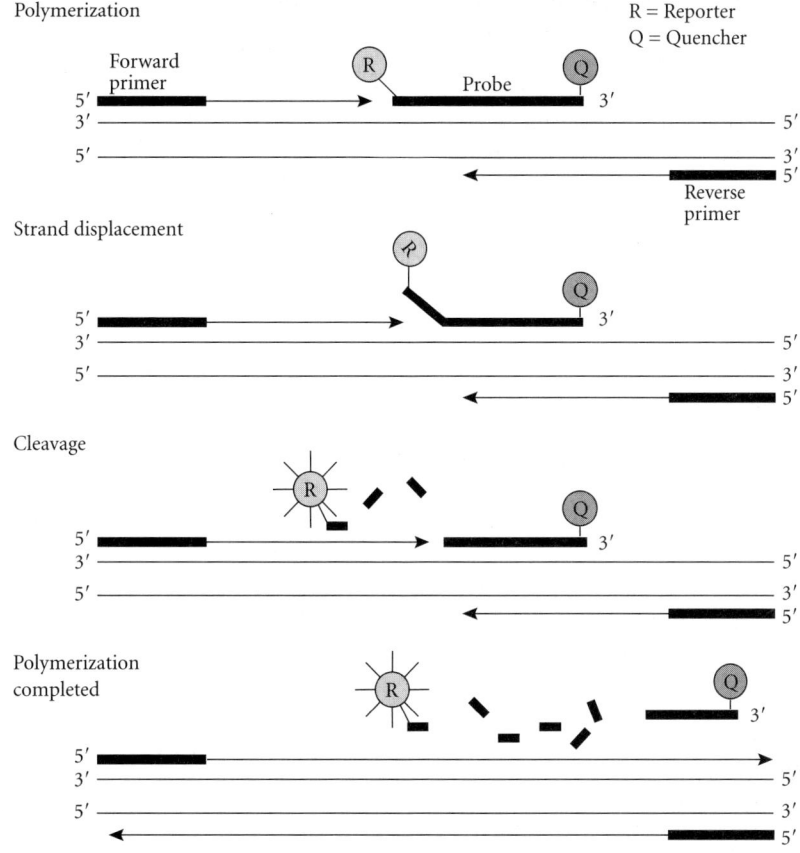

Fig. 3.7 Schematic representation of Taq Man PCR, illustrating the use of a conventional primer pair and a Taq Man probe. The assay utilize the 5′ nuclease activity of Taq DNA polymerase.

(i.e. at cycle 35, 40, etc.). This allows a relatively easy quantitative detection of amplified nucleic acid and is reliable and simple to perform. Detection is achieved using a 96-well plate reader and avoids the complexities of gel electrophoresis followed by ethidium bromide staining or autoradiography.

Real-time amplicon detection can also be achieved using the Applied Biosystems 7700 DNA thermal cycler, which utilizes a laser scanning format to detect increases in fluorescence at defined time points in the thermocycling protocol.

The fact that the fluorogenic probe emits fluorescence if the target sequence is amplified confers great specificity on the reaction without the need for post-PCR hybridization. Fluorescence emission increases in direct proportion to the starting copy number so that the system produces directly quantitative results.

Amplified signals may typically be within the range of 100–1200 bp. Larger signal detection is theoretically possible but has not yet been investigated.

For end-point detection, the luminescence detector is used. The increase in fluorescence is compared to fluorescence of a 'No Template Control'. To normalize for pipetting errors and volume changes that inevitably occur during PCR, the reporter fluorescence is divided by the quencher fluorescence to determine a ratio known as the RQ for each reaction.

The difference between the sample RQ (RQ+) and the No Template Control RQ (RQ−) is called ΔRQ. This difference represents the amplification of the specific product, which has occurred during PCR.

Using the real-time detector (7700), a value called the ΔR_n is derived, using an integrated software package inbuilt in the 7700 DNA thermal cycler. An additional fluorogenic reporter, such as ROX, can be added to the PCR mix, which serves as an internal standard for the reaction.

An advancement in Taq Man chemistry has been the development of minor groove binder (MGB) probes. It has been found that conjugation of an MGB to an oligonucleotide stabilizes nucleic acid duplexes. This causes a dramatic increase in oligonulceotide melting temperature. Such probes have enhanced performance in the 5′ nuclease (Taq Man) assay and allow for shorter probe and amplicon sizes.

Taq Man PCR can also be used for allelic discrimination assays for the detection of cystic fibrosis mutants, viral strain identification, and complex allelotyping reactions (Fig. 3.8). Alleleic discrimination employs two differentially labelled Taq Man probes emitting spectrally different signals (Fig. 3.9). The assay facilitates single copy gene detection and allelic assignment can then be performed using dedicated software.

DNA sequencing

In 1953 the three-dimensional structure of double stranded DNA molecule was unravelled and published by James Watson and Francis Crick (37).

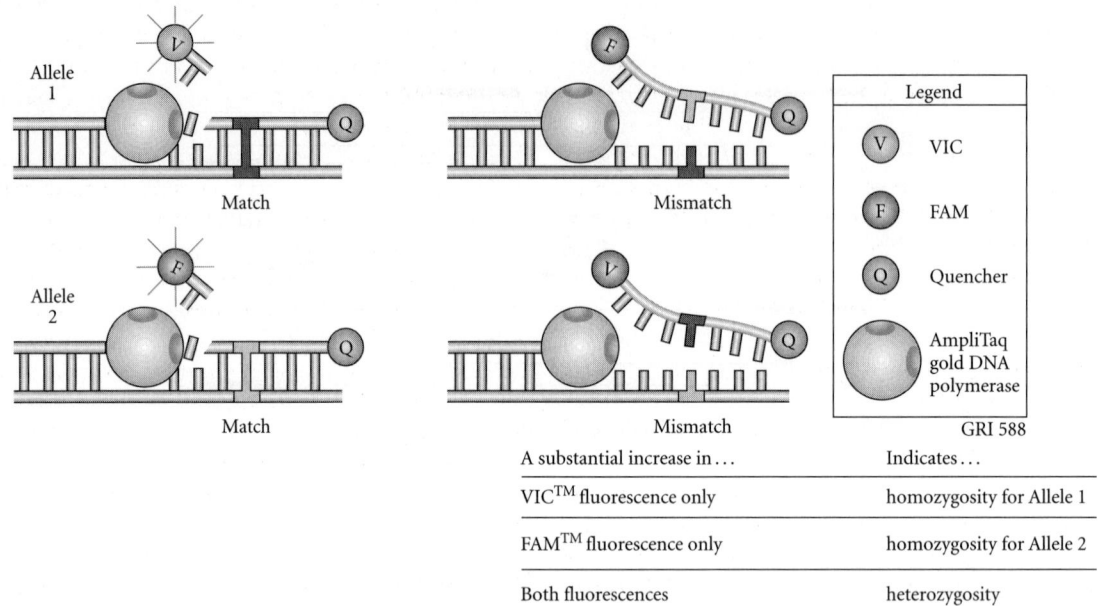

Fig. 3.8 Schematic representation of allelic discrimination Taq Man PCR using a two-colour Taq Man probe system.

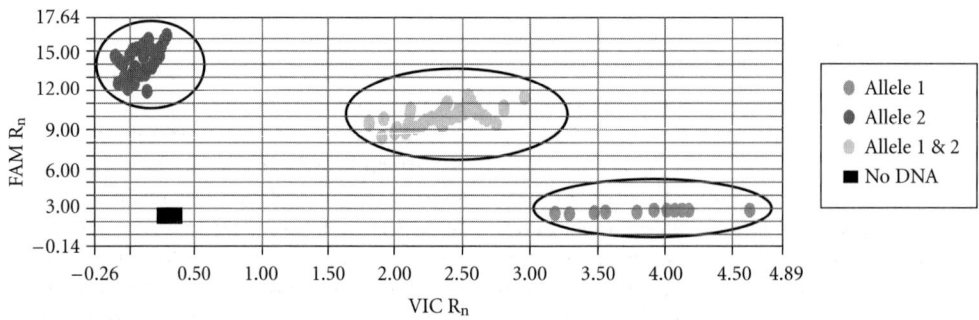

Fig. 3.9 Typical result obtained with a Taq Man allelic discrimination assay.

Since the identity and structure of the molecule responsible for inherited change was discovered the language of the genetic code, based on the four bases, adenine (A), cytosine (C), guanine (G), and thymine (T) has been established.

Chemical sequencing of DNA, the Maxam and Gilbert approach

One of the earliest methods to determine the nucleotide sequence of a fragment of isolated DNA was the chemical sequencing of the DNA strand, more usually referred to as the Maxam–Gilbert technique, published in 1977 (38). In this method isolated single stranded DNA is labelled, generally with a radioisotope marker, at its terminus and is then partially degraded by subjecting the labelled template to a series of base-specific cleavage reactions. Conditions are designed such that only a limited number of each of the cleavage reactions occurs within a given DNA strand. Four different chemical modifications occur in separate reaction tubes with G residues being methylated using dimethylsulfate in one tube, G and A residues being methylated by formic acid, C and T being removed by hydrazine, and C alone being removed by hydrazine in the presence of NaCl. Following each of the specific chemical reactions the template in the tube is treated with piperidine, which then cleaves the DNA where there is a chemically modified or missing base.

Since the starting DNA template is end labelled and the components of the reaction and its kinetics can be closely controlled such that the lengths of the labelled fragments can identify the position of the individual bases the combination of reactions yield a 'ladder' of fragments that vary in size from one another by a single base. This array of cleaved products generated can then be subjected to PAGE to resolve fragments of different lengths and the ladder of radiolabelled products can be then visualized and analysed by autoradiography, the process of exposing the radiolabelled fragments in the gel to X-ray film to produce an image of the fragments. In the early days it was possible to only read some 100 bases from the point of labelling, making the sequencing of long fragments of DNA time consuming and tedious. Since the publication of this method many modifications have been made to optimize both the sequencing chemistry and to improve the spatial separation of the labelled fragments, in some cases the use of 1-m long gel separation systems has enabled the number of bases that can be resolved from a single reaction to approach 600 or more bases.

Sequencing by chain termination, the Sanger methodology

The Sanger (37) or chain termination method of sequencing DNA is now the main workhorse of the major genome initiatives. The principle of this method is simple; an isolated fragment of DNA or entire plasmid, cosmid, or PCR product is denatured to its single stranded form by heat or alkali treatment. A short synthetic oligonucleotide primer is annealed to its complimentary sequence encoded on one of the single stranded templates. The 3' end of the primer/template duplex is then used as the initiation site for polymerase action and a complimentary DNA strand is synthesized using dNTPs as precursors (Figs 3.10 and 3.11).

Chain termination chemistry has been used in conjunction with either labelled oligonucleotide primers or by incorporation of labelled nucleotides during the extension reaction. Early chemistry employed polymerases such as the Klenow fragment of DNA polymerase I or used the bacteriophage derived T7 DNA polymerase or its variants. In more recent times thermostable polymerases such as AmpliTaq DNA Polymerase and its variants have been exploited to carry out the chain termination chemistry by the marriage of chain termination and the PCR process. Such an approach is termed cycle sequencing (Fig. 3.12).

In a standard chain termination sequencing approach four separate synthesis reactions are required. Each of the individual reactions contains a small amount of one of the four dideoxynucleotide triphosphates (ddNTPs). When the growing strand of DNA being synthesized incorporates a specific ddNTP the reaction elongation reaction is terminated since the ddNTP lacks the 3'-hydroxyl group required for further chain elongation. By careful control of the ratio of ddNTP to dNTP in each of the four reactions one achieves a random but low level incorporation of each of the ddNTPs into the growing strands of DNA and creates an array of fragments with a common 5' end, defined by the primer, but terminating at each possible position where the specific ddNTP could have been incorporated. The average length of such chains can be manipulated by altering the ddNTP to dNTP ratios to ensure that all of the products can be easily resolved by PAGE.

By carrying out four reactions, with each of the four ddNTPs present and then resolving the four reactions, A, C, G, and T terminated, side by side on a resolving gel we again produce the characteristic ladder of fragments that enables the sequence to be read. Common labelling strategies include incorporation of radiolabelled dNTPs

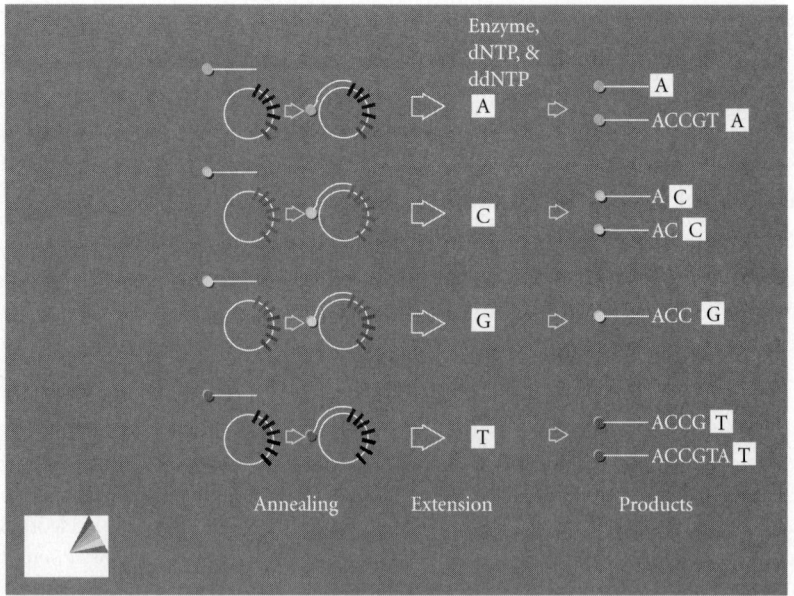

Fig. 3.10 Sanger or chain termination sequencing chemistry employing fluorescent dye labelled primers. Four different dye labelled primers (A, C, G, and T termination) are used in four separate extension and termination reactions. At completion of the reactions the contents of the four tubes are pooled and loaded onto a single lane of a polyacrylamide gel. The ladder of dye labelled products are separated by electrophoresis and detected in real-time.

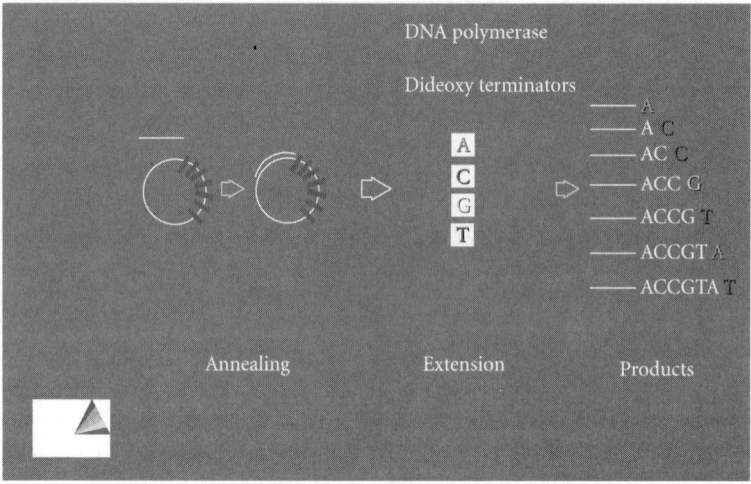

Fig. 3.11 Sanger or chain termination sequencing chemistry employing dye labelled dideoxy terminators. Dideoxy terminators, with each of the four possible ddNTPs being labelled with a different fluorescent dye, are incorporated by a polymerase during the extension phase of the sequencing reaction. The ladder of dye labelled products are separated by electrophoresis and detected in real-time.

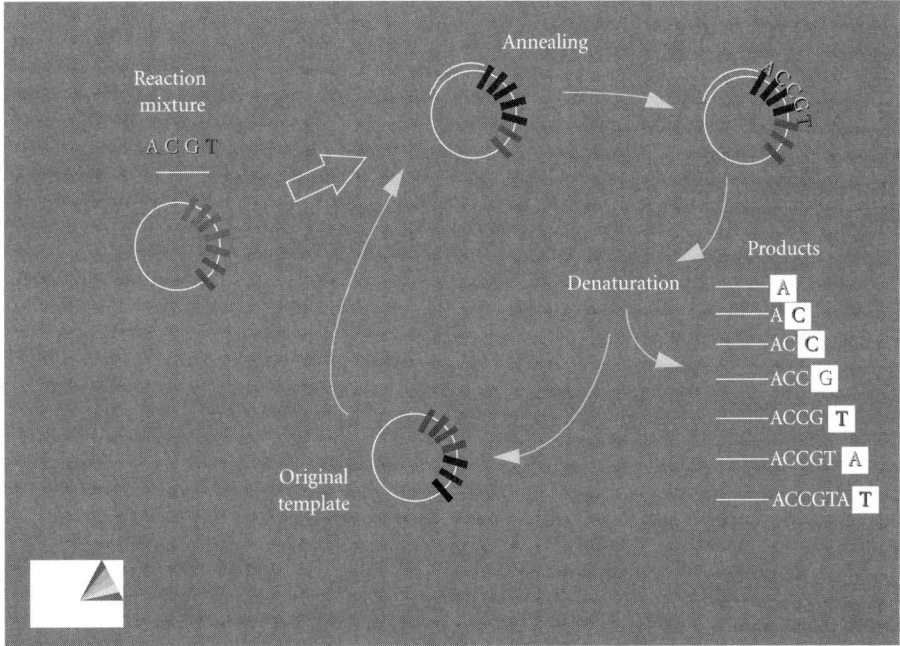

Fig. 3.12 Chain termination cycle sequencing. In a combination of the Sanger chain termination method and the PCR process the original DNA serves as a template for a linear PCR reaction. In each of 25 rounds of PCR cycling a ladder of dye labelled terminated fragments are produced from the templates. Following the extension step the subsequent denaturation then allows the same DNA molecules to serve again as a template for production of more dye-labelled products.

followed by autoradiography or chemiluminescent detection of the terminated products.

Comparative genomic hybridization

Comparative Genomic Hybridization (CGH) is a technique that allows detection of chromosomal copy number changes and provides a global overview of chromosome gains and losses throughout the whole genome of a tumour and it maps the origins of amplified and deleted DNA sequences in normal chromosomes (39). Kallioniemi *et al.* 1992, were the first group to describe CGH as a new chromosome analysis technique (40). Briefly tumour DNA is labelled with a green fluorophore and mixed (1:1) with red labelled normal DNA and hybridized to normal metaphase preparations. The green and red DNA compete for hybridization to their specific locus of origin on the chromosome. The ratio of green to red fluorescence is measured along the chromosomal axis, a ratio of <1 representing a loss and >1 representing a gain of genetic material in the tumour at that specific locus.

Using metaphase chromosomes for hybridization limits the detection of events involving small regions (<10–20 Mb) of the genome. The sensitivity of CGH depends upon the level and size of the copy number changes and contamination of tumour material with normal DNA. A novel technique that is currently being developed is CGH microarray analysis. Microarray CGH enables the analysis of genetic aberrations in cancers with a high resolution and provides the precise locations of the amplified gene boundaries within the chromosome. A number of studies to date have compared array-based CGH with conventional CGH techniques and found the array CGH had a greater sensitivity than conventional metaphase CGH, and a number of a specific oncogenes were amplified or deleted by array CGH that were not detected by metaphase CGH.

The quality of DNA is a very important issue when performing CGH. DNA extracted from fresh or frozen tissue is usually of high molecular weight and is of good quality for labelling purposes. However DNA extracted from formalin fixed, paraffin wax embedded tissues can be quite degraded and may yield low amounts of DNA.

Laser Capture Microdissection is a technique that allows a researcher to procure specific cell types from a given tissue section (41). This technique overcomes the issue of contamination of tumour material with normal DNA and ensures a pure tumour DNA sample. Briefly, to capture cells from fixed tissue, a tissue section is mounted on a glass slide and viewed under an inverted microscope (PixCell II laser capture microdissection system; Arcturus Engineering Inc., Mountain View, CA). A transparent cap, which fits into a microfuge tube, has attached to it a transfer film that is placed directly above the tissue to be examined. The cells of interest (tumour) are then selected by activating a laser beam. Cells that are in the path of the laser beam become focally adhesive and fuse to the transfer film, which is then lifted off for processing. DNA can then be extracted from the sample for analysis. In the majority of instances the DNA yield from microdissected tissue specimens is too small to perform microarray CGH.

In this situation degenerate oligonucleotide-primed (DOP) PCR can be used to amplify the DNA. DOP PCR was first described in 1992 by Telenius *et al.*, and employs a single primer of partially degenerate sequence, which utilizes a low annealing temperature and allows random priming from multiple evenly dispersed sites within a given genome (42). A number of studies have used DOP PCR amplification to amplify genomic DNA from microdissected tumours for use with genomic CGH microarrays. In these instances it was often necessary to perform two rounds of DOP PCR amplification to obtain sufficient DNA to hybridize to the array. The authors also compared microarray CGH results obtained from genomic DNA and DOP PCR amplified DNA from control cell lines with known amplification profiles and comparable results were obtained.

Microarray-based genomic analysis (Genosensor CGH, Vysis, Downers Grove, IL) is a novel technique intended for the rapid examination of human DNA for changes in copy number of specific sequences. The AmpliOnc I microarray contains 58 target DNA clones (P1, PAC, or BAC clones) representing genetic regions that have so far been associated with tumour formation through amplification at the genome level. Similar to conventional CGH tumour DNA and normal control DNA is labelled by nick translation with green and red labelled nucleotides. In the case of DOP PCR amplified DNA there are two methods to label the DNA,

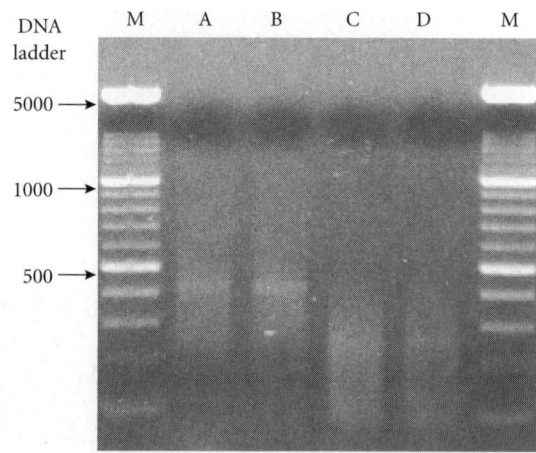

Fig. 3.13 A 1% agarose gel of DOP PCR amplified tumour and control DNA labelled with green and red fluorophores. Two approaches for labelling DNA were compared: (a) direct incorporation of labelled nucleotides during second round DOP PCR amplification (lanes A and B) and (b) nick translation of second round DOP PCR amplified DNA with labelled nucleotides (lanes C and D).

incorporating the fluorescent nucleotides during a second round of DOP PCR amplification or nick translating the 2 round DOP PCR amplified DNA. Several groups have reported on these approaches (5, 6). The authors have found that nick translation to label the DOP amplified DNA is more efficient than direct incorporation of labelled nucleotides during DOP amplification. Figure 3.13 shows an agarose gel of DOP labelled DOP amplified DNA and labelling of DOP PCR amplified DNA by nick translation. The optimum size range of labelled probe for microarray analysis is shorter (300 nt and below) than for conventional CGH (~600–800 nt).

Briefly the microarray CGH assay involves labelling a sample (Tumour) DNA (0.5–1 ug) with a green fluorophore. This is mixed with whole genomic reference DNA (0.5–1 ug) that is labelled with a red fluorophore and co-hybridized to a microarray in the presense of human Cot 1 DNA to suppress hybridization of labelled probe to repeat sequences. Following hybridization and removal of unhybridized probe target spots are counter stained with a blue fluorophore (DAPI IV mounting soliution) and analysed using the Vysis Genosensor™ System. Figure 3.14 shows a CGH array scanned using the Vysis Genosensor™ System and a typical plot of genes amplified in the test sample (Fig. 3.15). The technique allows simultaneous examination of

250 oncogenes/anti-oncogenes known to be amplified/deleted in various human cancers.

cDNA microarray technology

Microarrays are one of the latest breakthroughs in experimental biology, which allow monitoring of gene expression of tens of thousands of genes in parallel and are already producing huge amounts of valuable data (43, 44). The ability to monitor gene expression at the transcript level has become possible due to the advent of DNA microarray technology. A microarray is a glass slide, onto which single stranded DNA molecules are attached at fixed locations (spots). There may be tens of thousands of spots on an array, each related to a single gene. Microarrays exploit the preferential binding of complementary single stranded nucleic acid sequences. There are several variations of microarray technology, each used in a specific way. Many commercial arrays are now available including Affymetrix, Clontech ATLAS arrays, Micromax (Perkin Elmer Life Sciences) to mention a few.

One of the most popular experimental platforms is used for comparing mRNA abundance in two different samples (or a sample and a control). RNA from the sample and control cells are extracted and labelled with two different fluorescent labels, for example, a red dye for the RNA from the sample population and a green

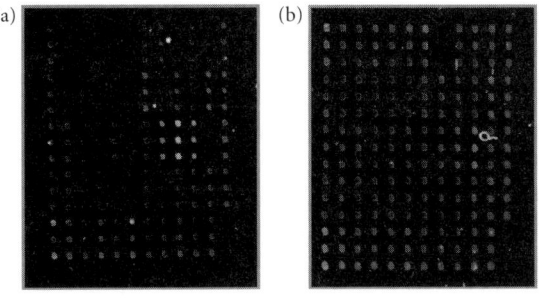

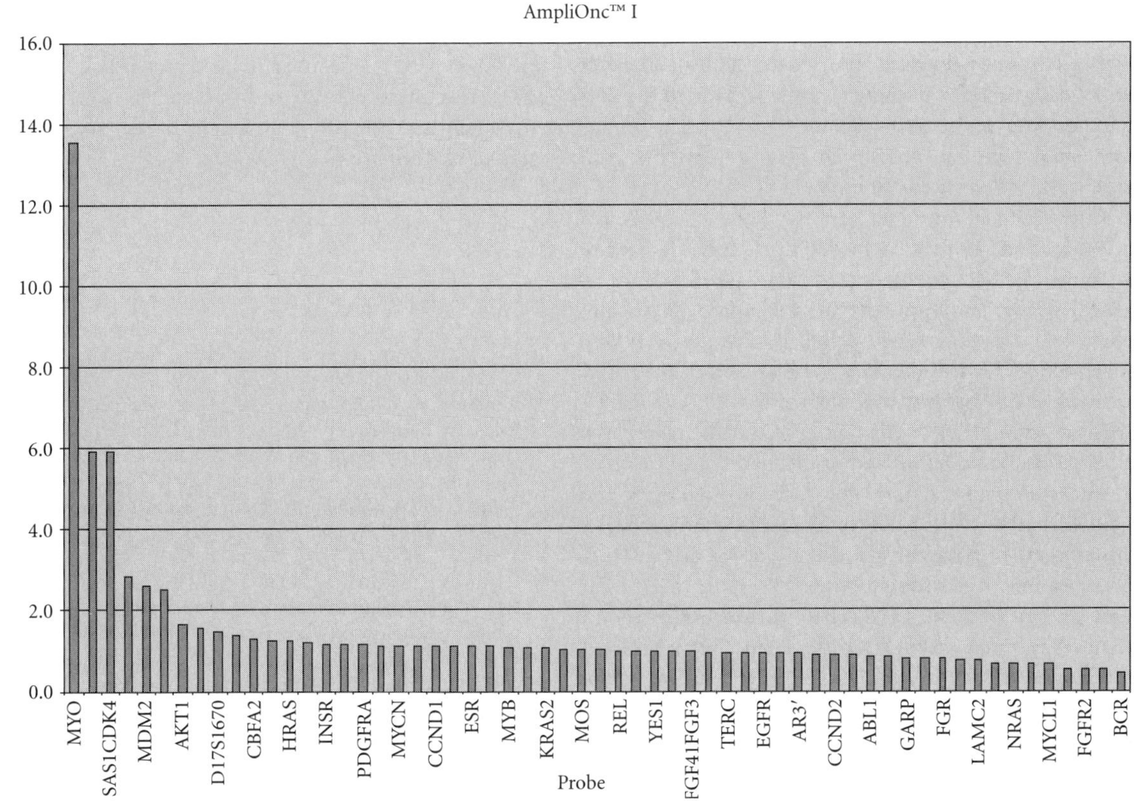

Fig. 3.14 CGH array using nick translated PCR products (a) and DOP labelled PCR products (b). See Plate 8.

Fig. 3.15 Typical result obtained from Vysis CGH array showing gene copy number of defined oncogenes/anti-oncogenes.

dye for that from the control population. Both extracts are washed over the microarray. Gene sequences from the extracts hybridize to their complementary sequences in the spots. To measure the relative abundance of the hybridized RNA the array is excited by a laser. If the RNA from the sample population is in abundance, the spot will be red; if the RNA from the control population is in abundance, it will be green. If sample and control bind equally, it will be yellow. While if neither binds it will not fluoresce and appear black. Thus from the fluorescence intensities and colours for each spot, the relative expression levels of the genes in the sample and control population can be estimated.

The process of differential gene expression analysis with Micromax TSA (Perkin Elmer life sciences) (45) involves total RNA extraction, in parallel from cells or tissues being compared.

The poly A^+ mRNA in each pool, without further purification, is then converted into Fluorescein (FL) and Biotin labelled cDNA using reverse transcriptase and nucleotide analogues, for use as individually traceable gene targets in the assay. These cDNA probes are then mixed and simultaneously hybridized to the microarrays in an overnight incubation.

FL and biotin labelled cDNAs are sequentially detected with a series of conjugate reporter molecules according to the TSA process. Ultimately, each of the two fluorescent reporter molecules (Cyanine 3 or Cyanine 5) are associated with the hybridized genetic material from each of the two starting samples.

The sequential Cyanine 3 and Cyanine 5 TSA detection process follows hybridization and stringency washes. The microarray is first conjugated with anti-FL–HRP. This antibody–enzyme conjugate specifically binds to the hybridized FL labelled cDNA probe. The enzyme portion of the conjugate is horseradish peroxidase, which catalyzes the deposition of cyanine 3 labelled tyramide amplification reagent. The reaction is quick, (less than 10 min) and results in the deposition of numerous Cyanine 3 labels immediately adjacent to the immobilized HRP. Because this is an enzymatic process, the amount of tyramide relative to cDNA hapten (i.e. FL or biotin) is greatly amplified. Prior to the second TSA step, the residual HRP is inactivated. In the second TSA step, streptavidin–HRP binds to the hybridized biotin labelled cDNA probes. The HRP portion of the enzyme conjugate catalyzes the deposition of Cyanine 5 Tyramide. Fluorescence detection takes place in a slide-scanning instrument containing two tuned lasers, which excite both Cyanine dyes at the appropriate wavelengths. A laser detection system is required to scan and report the relative quantity of the two dyes at any given gene spot on the microarray.

Finally, the differential scanning data must be processed by computer imaging software to ascertain and profile the genes of interest identified by the experiment. The Micromax™ system of differential cDNA expression is semiquantitative. It is capable of detecting signal from as little as 0.5 μg of total RNA. It is a ratiometric assay. All results should be interpreted with regard to the relative differences between the samples under analysis. Typical results indicate that any comparative signal (e.g. Cyanine 3 to Cyanine 5 ratio) that is greater than three-fold is considered biologically significant.

By measuring transcription levels of genes in an organism under various conditions, at different developmental stages and in different tissues, we can build up 'gene expression profiles', which characterize the dynamic functioning of each gene in the genome. Although mRNA is not the ultimate product of a gene, transcription is the first step in gene regulation, and information about the transcript levels is needed for understanding gene regulatory networks. The correlation between the mRNA and protein abundance in the cell may not be straight forward, but the absence of mRNA in a cell is likely to imply a not very high level of the respective protein and thus at least, qualitative estimates about the proteome can be based on the transcriptome information.

References

1. Ross DW. Introduction to molecular medicine. Springer Verlag, Berlin, 1996.
2. Litt M, Luty JA. A hypervariable microsatellite revealed by *in vitro* amplification of a dinucleotide repeat within cardiac muscle actin gene. Am J Hum Genet 1989, **44**, 397–401.
3. Tautz D. Hypervariability of simple sequences as a general source for polymorphic DNA markers. Nucl Acid Res 1989, **17**, 6436–71.
4. Edwards A, Civitello A, Hammond HA, Caskey CT. DNA typing and genetic mapping with trimeric and tetrameric tanfem repeats. Am J Hum Genet 1991, **49**, 746–56.
5. Braaten DC, Thomas JR, Little RD, et al. Locations and contexts of sequences that hybridize to poly (dG–dT). (dC–dA) in mammalian ribosomal DNAs and two linked X genes. Nucl Acids Res 1988, **16**, 865–81.
6. Shriver MD, Jin L, Chakraborty R, Boerwinkle E. VNTR allele frequency distributions under the step-wise mutational model: a computer simulation approach. Genetics 1993, **134**, 983–93.

7. John B, Miklos GLG. The eukaryotic genome in development and evolution. Allen & Unwin, London, 1988.
8. Tyler Smith C, Willard HF. Mammalian chromosome structure. Curr Opin Genet Dev 1993, **3**, 390–7.
9. Lohe ARE, Hillike AJ, Roberts PA. Mapping simple repeated DNA in heterochromatin of *Drosophila melanogaster*. Genetics 1993, **134**, 1149–74.
10. Armour JA, Jeffreys AJ. Biology and applications of human minisatellite loci. Curr Opin Genet Dev 1992, **2**, 850–6.
11. Tautz D, Renz M. Simple sequences are ubiquitous repetitive components of eukaryotic genome. Nucl Acid Res 1984, **12**, 4127–38.
12. Beckmann JS, Weber JL. Survey of human and rat microsatellites. Genomics 1992, **12**, 627–31.
13. Weber JL. Informativeness of human (dC–dA)n.(dG–dT)n polymorphisms. Genomics 1990, **7**, 524–30.
14. Hamada H, Seidman M, Howard BH, Gorman CM. Enhanced gene expression by poly (dT–dG).poly(dC–dA) sequence. Mol Cell Biol 1984, **4**, 2622–30.
15. Richards RI, Holman K, Yu S, Sutherland GR. Fragile X syndrome unstable element, p(CCG)n, and other simple tandem repeat sequences are binding sites for specific nuclear proteins. Hum Mol Genet 1993, **2**, 1429–35.
16. Litt M. PCR amplification of TG microsatellites. In: PCR—a practical approach. (ed. MJ McPherson, P Quirke, GR Taylor). Oxford, IRL Press, 85–9.
17. Koreth J, O'Leary JJ, McGee JO'D. Microsatellites and PCR genomic analysis. J Pathol 1996, **178**, 239–48.
18. Skolnick MH, Wallace RB. Simultaneous analysis of multiple polymorphic loci using amplified sequences polymorphisms (ASPs). Genomics 1988, **2**, 273–9.
19. Ziegle JS, Su Y, Corcoran KP, *et al*. Application of automated DNA sizing technology for genotyping microsatellite loci. Genomics 1992, **14**, 1026–31.
20. Cox DR, Green ED, Lander ES, Cohen D, Myers RM. Assessing mapping progress in the human genome project. Science 1994, **265**, 2031–2.
21. Murray JC, Buetow H, Weber JL, *et al*. A comprehensive human linkage map with centimorgan density. Science 1994, **265**, 2049–54.
22. Tomfohrde J, Silverman A, Barnes R, *et al*. Gene for familial psoriasis susceptibility mapped to the distal end of human chromosome 17q. Science 1994, **264**, 1141–5.
23. Goate A, Chartier-Harlin MC, Mullan M, *et al*. Segregation of a missense mutation in the amyloid precursor protein gene with familial Alzheimer's disease. Nature 1991, **349**, 704–6.
24. Hall JM, Lee MK, Newman B, *et al*. Linkage of early onset familial breast cancer to chromosome 17q21. Science 1990, **250**, 1684–9.
25. Davies JL, Kawaguchi Y, Bennett ST, *et al*. A genome wide search for human type I diabetes suspicibility genes. Nature 1994, **371**, 130–6.
26. Vogelstein B, Fearon ER, Kern SE, *et al*. Allelotype of colorectal carcinomas. Science 1989, **244**, 207–11.
27. Cawkwell L, Bell SM, Lewid FA, Dixon MF, Taylor GR, Quirke P. Rapid detection of allele loss in colorectal tumours using microsatellites and fluorescent DNA technology. Br J Cancer 1993, **67**, 1262–7.
28. Brook JD, McCurrach ME, Harley HG, *et al*. Molecular basis of myotonic dystrophy: expansion of a trinucleotide (CTG) repeat at the 3′ end of a transcript encoding a protein kinase family member. Cell 1992, **68**, 799–808.
29. Lynch HT, Lanspa S, Smyrk T, Boman B, Watson P, Lynch P. Hereditary non-polyposis colorectal cancer (Lynch syndromes I & II). Genetics, pathology, natural history and cancer control, Part 1. Cancer Genet Cytogenet 1991, **53**, 143–60.
30. Edwards A, Hammond HA, Jin L, Casket, CT, Chakraborty R. Genetic variation in five trimeric and tetrameric tandem repeat loci in four human population groups. Genomics 1992, **12**, 241–53.
31. Lawyer FC, Stoffel S, Saiki RK, Myambo KB, Drummond R, and Gelfand DH. Isolation, characterization, and expression in *Escherichia coli* of the DNA polymerase gene from the extreme thermophile, *Thermus aquaticus*. J Biol Chem 1989, **264**, 6427–37.
32. Holland PM, Abramson RD, Watson R, Gelfand DH. Detection of specific polymerase chain reaction product by utilizing the 5′–3′ exonuclease activity of *Thermus aquaticus* DNA polymerase. Proc Natl Acad Sci USA 1991, **88**, 7276–80.
33. Lyamichev V, Brow MAD, Dahlberg JE. Structure-specific endonucleolytic cleavage of nucleic acids by eubacterial DNA polymerases. Science 1993, **260**, 778–83.
34. Lee LG, Connell CR, Bloch W. Allelic discrimination by nick-translation PCR with fluorogenic probes. Nucl Acids Res 1993, **21**, 3761–6.
35. Forster VTH. Zwischenmolekulare Energie-Wanderung und Fluoreszenz. Ann Phys (Leipzig) 1948, **2**, 55–75.
36. Lakowicz, Joseph R. 1983. Chapter 10. Energy Transfer. In: Principles of fluorescent spectroscopy. Plenum Press, NY, 303–39.
37. Sanger F, Nicklen S, Coulson AR. DNA sequencing with chain-terminator inhibitors. Proc Natl Acad Sci USA 1977, **74**, 5463–7.
38. Maxam AM, Gilbert W. A new method for sequencing DNA. Proc Natl Acad Sci USA 1977, **74**, 560–4.
39. Weiss MM, Hremsen MAJA, Meijer GA, van Grieken, NCT, Baak JPA, Kuipers EJ, van Diest PJ. Comparative Genomic Hybridization. J Clin Pathol Mol Pathol 1999, **52**, 243–51.
40. Kallioniemi OP, Kallioniemi A, Sudar D, *et al*. Comparative genomic hybridization for molecular cytogenetic analysis of solid tumours. Science 1992, **258**, 818–21.
41. Emmert-Buck MR, Bonner RF, Smith PD, Chuaqui RF, Zhuang Z, Goldstein SR, Weiss RA, Liotta LA. Laser capture microdissection. Science 1996, **274**, 998–1001.
42. Telenius H, Carter NP, Bebb CE, Nordenskjold M, Ponder BAJ, Tunnacliffe A. Degenerate oligonuceotide-primed PCR: general amplification of target DNA by a single degenerate primer. Genomics 1992, **13**, 718–25.
43. Brazma Z, Vilo J. Gene expression data analysis. FEBS 2000, **480**, 17–24.
44. Kononen J, Bubendorf L, Kallioniemi A, Bariund M, Schrami P, *et al*. Tissue microarrays for high-throughput molecular profiling of tumour specimens. Nat Med 1998, **4**, 844–7.
45. Micromax TS labelling and detection kit using fluorescein/biotin TSA. Perkin Elmer (NEN) Life Science Products, Inc.

4 | Familial and predisposition syndromes

Eamonn G. Sheridan and C. Geoffrey Woods

Inherited cancer predisposition syndromes

Genetic cancer predisposition can be inherited as a result of mutations inherited in either dominant or recessive manners.

In paediatric practice the issue of inherited predisposition has an impact on the following areas:

1. Congenital malformation syndromes where cancer risks are increased. This refers especially to the DNA repair disorders.
2. Familial cancer syndromes caused by highly penetrant genes in which children are at risk in childhood. Possibly 5–10% of childhood cancers are a consequence of mutations in such genes. These figures are an estimate only and may underestimate the true frequency. Highly penetrant cancer predisposition syndromes such as Li Fraumeni syndrome (LFS), neurofibromatosis (NF), Beckwith Wiedemann syndrome (BWS), and multiple endocrine neoplasia (MEN), cause a minority of childhood cancers. Low penetrance genes are likely to be of more importance clinically, but at present little is known about such mechanisms.

DNA repair disorders

1. DNA repair disorders are individually rare.
2. Suspected diagnoses should always be confirmed by laboratory tests, which are reliable, before the full phenotype has evolved.
3. Disorders are autosomal recessive, prenatal diagnosis is usually available but mainly should be arranged with specialist centres, prior to pregnancy.
4. Many of the disorders are cancer prone, but can also be hypersensitive to chemo and radiotherapy.

Introduction

Over the past 30 years a number of rare DNA repair disorder phenotypes were delineated, for example, Bloom syndrome, ataxia–telangiectasia (AT), and Fanconi anaemia. In each phenotype it was hypothesized that the underlying defect was an inability to repair a particular type of DNA damage. For a number of these disorders this hypothesis was supported by cytogenetics studies using DNA damaging agents; these tests detected the so-called chromosome breakage syndromes. More recently a number of the genes causing these phenotypes have been discovered, confirming that often one phenotype may have more than one genotype, for example, xeroderma pigmentosa.

Work has also progressed on discovering how each specific different type of DNA damage repair occurs and how the cell monitors the integrity of its DNA. This has led to a more complete understanding of the normal function of each gene (and how such repair genes often have other cellular functions, such as in transcription), how the malfunction of the gene causes a particular DNA repair disorder phenotype, and whether there are any new therapeutic strategies possible. This chapter deals only with the more common DNA repair disorders.

Bloom syndrome

This condition was first described by Bloom in 1954 in his paper 'Congenital telangiectatic erythema resembling lupus erythematosus in dwarfs' (1). The major clinical features of this condition are pre- and postnatal growth retardation, a thin triangular face, and a telangiectatic rash in sun exposed areas, particularly on the cheeks. Birth weight is typically under 2.5 kg at term. Postnatal growth retardation continues giving an average adult height in males of approximately 151 cm and in females, 144 cm. The resultant short stature is proportionate with borderline microcephaly. Because of the growth retardation, children may be investigated, often extensively, for causes of failure to thrive (2). A telangiectatic rash develops on the face in a butterfly distribution and later on the backs of the hands and other sun exposed areas. The onset of this rash is usually within the first six months of life but may be delayed in darker skinned children. The telangiectasia probably reflects sun-sensitivity and progresses to erythema, excoriation, and premature ageing changes. The face is usually triangular with an apparently long or large nose and little subcutaneous fat.

Clinical immunodeficiency occurs in less than half of the individuals and is usually only a problem in the first decade of life. However, a greater proportion have *in vitro* immunoglobulin deficiency, particularly hypo-IgA and IgM, as well as specific deficiencies in the production of antibodies to common pathogens. Fertility is normal in females but probably all males are infertile. Intelligence is normal. The major complication of Bloom syndrome is a substantially increased incidence of malignancies. It has been said that Bloom syndrome is the most cancer prone syndrome known to man. The cancer spectrum mirrors that seen in the normal population, with leukaemias developing at an average age of 22 years and other solid tumours, particularly of the breast and gastrointestinal tract at 35 years (3).

Whilst the diagnosis of Bloom syndrome can be suspected clinically, the condition is probably not characteristic enough for laboratory confirmation to be omitted. The differential diagnosis includes Dubowitz syndrome, Russell–Silver syndrome (including maternal chromosome 7 uniparental disomy), chromosome anomalies, foetal alcohol syndrome, and Rothmund–Thomson syndrome. In only Bloom syndrome, does such cytogenetic analysis show an increased rate of sister-chromatid exchanges. An increase in spontaneous chromosome breaks also occurs. The cytogenetic laboratory test for sister-chromatid exchange is simple to perform and reliable. Sister-chromatid exchanges are normal events occurring during mitosis. Homologous chromosomes exchange identical chromosome segments, the situation being somewhat similar to that occurring in meiosis, except in that situation the exchange is between the paired maternally derived and paternally derived chromosomes and the resultant exchange segments, are not necessarily homologous. Sister-chromatid exchanges occur at a rate of 4–10 per cell division normally. This rate is increased by at least sixfold, commonly tenfold, in Bloom syndrome. Given the reliability, specificity, and sensitivity of the test, it is unlikely that gene mutation analysis will take over in the diagnosis of Bloom syndrome in the foreseeable future. Prenatal diagnosis has rarely been performed. Therefore, it should be carried out by a centre with previous experience and a combination of techniques should be used, that is sister-chromatid exchange rate and mutation detection, or linked polymorphic markers.

There is no treatment available for the growth retardation seen in Bloom syndrome. The children do not respond specifically to growth hormone or to increased calorific intake. Immunodeficiency should be treated symptomatically with the occasional child needing prophylactic antibodies and gammaglobulin injections for a limited period. Given the range of cancers that occur in Bloom syndrome, it is difficult to know how to screen for these and hence a paediatric oncologist should be involved. Whilst bone marrow transplantation may remove the risk of leukaemia, it would not remove the risk of developing other cancers and, therefore, has not been used to-date.

Bloom syndrome is an autosomal recessive disorder. The condition is extremely rare, anecdotally <1 case per million, the exception being the Ashkenazi Jewish population where the carrier frequency is approximately <1%. The gene causing Bloom syndrome was found to be located on chromosome 15q21.3 (4). The actual gene was discovered by the exploitation of the increased rate of sister-chromatid exchange seen Bloom syndrome. Occasional cell lines were present in affected individuals, which appeared to be 'cured'. It was reasoned that this was because the patient had two different mutations in the Bloom's gene and that a sister-chromatid exchange had separated these, hence producing a 'healed' gene and a gene with two mutations. Such a cell line would be expected to have no increase in sister-chromatid exchange, as this is the finding in parents of affected children who are obligate carriers. By analysis of such cell lines a 2 centimorgan region (approximately 2 million base pairs of DNA) was delineated. A gene within this region proved to be the cause of Bloom syndrome and was found to be a member of a group of proteins known as the RecQ helicases. Such protein helicases are capable of unwinding DNA and RNA. Another gene in the same family of proteins is known to cause Werner syndrome (a rare recessive disorder causing growth retardation with accelerated ageing). The proteins are hypothesized to interact with topoisomerases within the cells; proteins which are involved in untangling DNA. Quite how this causes growth retardation, increased sister-chromatid exchanges and the increased predisposition to cancer, is not yet understood.

Ataxia–telangiectasia (Louis-Bar syndrome)

Whilst initially reported by Madame Louis-Bar in 1941, it was Boder and Sedgwick in the United States, who were responsible for describing and bringing to medical attention this condition (5). The principal clinical features of AT are a progressive complex neurodegeneration, bulbar telangiectasia, variable immune deficiency, and an increased predisposition for lymphoreticular malignancies (6). The majority of children present within the first 5 years of life with motor delay. This is sometimes initially considered to be cerebral palsy until the progressive nature of the disorder overcomes the chronological increase in motor ability. Truncal ataxia develops first, but is soon followed by limb ataxia, dysarthria, and later dystonia, chorea, weakness, and sometimes spasticity. The face is typically rather impassive with emotions shown in an exaggerated manner. Eye movements are usually abnormal by the age of 3 years and involve a dyspraxia of rapid saccadic eye movements, both in the vertical and horizontal fields of vision. (A very similar eye movement disorder is seen in Cogan's ocular motor apraxia. However, this is a disorder, which improves during the first decade, as opposed to AT, and only horizontal saccades are involved.) The bulbar telangiectasias are occasionally present at birth but usually develop within the first 3 years of life. They may only present in the lateral canthi of the eyes and are characterized by an increased and constant size and tortuosity of bulbar vessels, which do not cause irritation, do not bleed, and are not sun-sensitive. An increase in severity and frequency of upper and lower respiratory tract infections is seen in most affected individuals. Approximately a quarter of patients have more significant immunodeficiency.

Referral to a paediatric immunologist, prophylactic antibiotics, pneumovax, and immunoglobulins should all be considered in such cases. Reduced fertility is expected, although one affected woman has borne children (who were normal). AT is a malignancy prone condition. The risk is initially for lymphoreticular malignancies and later for adenocarcinomas. The risk of developing a malignancy has been estimated to be 1% per year.

Clinical diagnosis of AT can be difficult to make in the first 5 years of life. However, in children over the age of 8 the condition is clinically distinct. The diagnostic laboratory test is an increased level of chromosome breakage, following ionizing irradiation. Typically 0.5 and 1 grey gamma rays are used and a 6–10-fold increased breakage is found compared to controls. The breaks are randomly distributed. There is also an increased incidence of spontaneous chromosome breakage and specific translocations involving the T-cell receptor genes on chromosomes 7 and 14. These findings are not pathognomonic and are identical to those seen in the much rarer Nijmegen breakage syndrome (borderline microcephaly, moderate to severe immune deficiency, increased incidence of lymphoreticular malignancies, autosomal recessive). They may also be present in other rare chromosome breakage syndromes. Therefore, the diagnosis of AT should be made by a combination of clinical and laboratory investigations. Whilst alpha-fetoprotein (AFP) is often raised in the condition and immunoglobulins IgA and G, particularly, IgG 2 and 4 subgroups are deficient, these findings are not as sensitive as ionizing irradiation and certainly not as specific.

Prenatal diagnosis is available, but should only be carried out in centres with a specialist interest and previous experience. At present chromosome breakage analysis at amniocentesis has been shown to be reliable. Doubt remains for chorionic villus sampling (CVS); we know of one case where a false negative result was obtained. A further proviso is that prenatal diagnosis should not be performed without the radiosensitivity of the index case in the family being tested by the laboratory that will carry out the prenatal diagnosis. With the advent of the discovery of the *ATM* (ataxia–teleangiectasia mutated) gene, linkage analysis by CVS will probably become the prenatal diagnosis method of choice in the foreseeable future.

Variant AT: approximately 10% of individuals with AT have a later onset and slower disease progression of the condition. Such individuals exhibit less sensitivity to ionizing irradiation and they may be less cancer prone. In some cases the sensitivity to ionizing irradiation can only be shown in fibroblasts, lymphocyte testing is normal. The majority of variant AT is caused by *ATM* gene mutations. However, one Asian family has been described with variant AT not linked to the AT gene.

There is no curative treatment available for AT. Whilst bone marrow transplantation may reduce the risk of lymphoreticular malignancies, it would not be expected to affect the neurodegeneration and risk of other cancers seen in the condition. There are a number of practical measures, which are helpful, for example, the use of a ruler when reading line by line, and further advice can be gained from the Ataxia–Telangiectasia Society. Treatment from immune deficiency is symptomatic, as outlined in Bloom syndrome. Screening for lymphoreticular malignancies is again problematic because of the sensitivity to irradiation and radiomimetic drugs seen in AT. This can lead to death, significant tissues burning, or in the case of cerebral irradiation, encephalopathy. Routine use of X-rays, such as to detect fractures of limb or skull bones, is not contra-indicated in AT. Guidelines have been produced by the Department of Health (UK) on this matter and are available from the Ataxia–Telangiectasia Society.

Ataxia–telangiectasia is a single gene autosomal recessive disorder. Initial cell line fusing experiments had suggested that there would be at least four genes (genotypes) that could cause AT (phenotype). However, this proved erroneous. Linkage in AT was initially found in a Pennsylvanian Amish family by Gatti on chromosome 11q23 (7). Subsequent work by the United Kingdom, the United States, and Israeli groups refined the position of the gene and, eventually, found an extremely large hitherto unknown gene, which was called *ATM* (8). The gene seems homologous to a group of phosphatidylinositol-3 kinases involved in the signal transduction, meiotic recombination, and cell cycle controls. Mutations in the *ATM* gene have been found in all of the four apparent groups of AT. The inferred function of the gene is in the coordination of DNA damage recognition, repair, and preventing progression of DNA replication until such damage has been successfully repaired.

ATM gene mutation carriers (AT heterozygotes, that is, parents and two-thirds of the siblings of affected children) are reported to have an increased risk of cancer. Epidemiological studies had suggested that female heterozygotes had an increased risk of developing breast cancer. Furthermore, it was suggested that mammography may be deleterious in this population because of increased radiosensitivity. This is a vexed field but recent re-analysis of the British data has not shown a significantly increased risk of breast cancer in known AT heterozygotes. Furthermore, AT heterozygotes have not been shown to respond adversely clinically to irradiation and only subtle experiments can show an increased ionizing irradiation sensitivity in them as a group. The Department of Health (UK) has advised that women under the age of 50 should only have mammography symptomatically. They should enter the National Breast Screening Programme at 50 and should avoid unessential X-rays.

Fanconi anaemia

The condition was first described by Fanconi in 1927 in three siblings, who developed pancytopaenia (9). Subsequent work has helped to define the other features of the disease and, in particular, the variety of congenital anomalies seen, the increased risk of acute non-lymphoblastic leukaemia, and the chromosome breakage. The latter feature was particularly marked after the use of bifunctional alkylating agents (which can covariantly cross linked daughter DNA strands). It later became obvious that the Estren–Dameshek syndrome of autosomal recessive congenital pancytopaenia is part of the Fanconi anaemia spectrum. Whilst the chromosome breakage and probably the pancytopenia are universal, features of Fanconi anaemia, congenital abnormalities, dysmorphic features, and growth retardation are not. This has lead to difficulties, both in recognizing cases where there are no or minimal clinical features before the onset of pancytopenia and, conversely, failure to recognize that some children with multiple severe congenital malformations actually have Fanconi anaemia (10). Furthermore, with regard to the congenital anomalies, there is not only an interfamilial but also an intrafamilial variability. That is, the features of one child with Fanconi anaemia do not predict how the next child may be affected.

Proportionate short stature is seen in at least three-quarters of individuals. Unusual café-au-lait patches (i.e. with irregular outline) are seen in about three-quarters of individuals. Radial ray and renal anomalies each occur in about 60% of cases. The radial ray anomalies can be anything from mild thumb hypoplasia to absent thumbs and radial club hands. Radial ray defects are usually asymmetric. Renal anomalies extend from duplex collecting systems to horseshoe kidneys, through to renal aplasia. They are usually, however, asymptomatic. Microcephaly with mild mental retardation is seen in about a quarter of cases. Microcephaly, however, does not predict mental retardation. Microphthalmia, which is usually unilateral, is seen in about a third of cases. Vision, however, is not affected. Unusually shaped ears and deafness is seen in about one in eight cases, as is congenital heart disease.

Approximately one-quarter of all cases of Fanconi anaemia have no abnormal clinical features. A host of other rare, but significant, malformations can occur, including tracheooesophageal fistula, choanal atresia, anal atresia, cloacal anomalies, and duodenal atresia. Two useful features, which help distinguish Fanconi anaemia from other conditions, are the growth retardation and the (usually unilateral) microphthalmia. The onset of pancytopenia is typically around the age of 7 years, although it has been described at birth and also in the 20s. There is usually an initial reduced platelet count and a slow progression to pancytopenia thereafter. Some patients achieve a plateau phase for a considerable length of time, whilst others develop pancytopenia relatively quickly. There is an increased incidence of acute non-lymphoblastic leukaemia with a mean age of diagnosis at 15 years in individuals who have not received a bone marrow transplantation (11).

Clinical diagnosis of Fanconi anaemia before the onset of pancytopaenia, remains difficult. The differential diagnosis includes VATER syndrome, Holt–Oram syndrome, IVIC syndrome, chromosome abnormalities, Baller–Gerold syndrome, Russell–Silver syndrome, Aase syndrome, etc. Not all children with an apparent phenocopy will have the condition and, in other individuals, the diagnosis will be missed because of their lack of or excessive features. Therefore, laboratory testing should be considered in all siblings of an affected individual, all individuals with congenital anomalies within the Fanconi anaemia spectrum, and in all individuals who develop unexplained pancytopenia. The laboratory diagnosis is made by finding an increased incidence of chromosome breaking following the use of alkylating agents, such as nitrogen mustards, mitomycin C, and diepoxybutane. An increased incidence of spontaneous chromosome breakage is seen, as are unusual cruciate exchange figures between non-homologous chromosomes. False negatives have been described in Fanconi anaemia (this has variously been ascribed to a temporal increase in sensitivity to these agents, the use of inactive agents, and some patients may be sensitive to one alkylating agent but not another). An increased incidence of alkylating agent chromosome breakage has also been reported in some other rare syndromes, incorporating either dwarfism or leukaemia, but not pancytopenia. If there are any doubts about the cytogenetic diagnosis, either a repeat sample or testing of another tissue, such as skin, or use of a different alkylating agent is mandatory.

Prenatal diagnosis is possible. Auerbach has reported a large series using Diepoxybutane (12). Prenatal diagnosis should only be performed after confirming that the index case is sensitive to the alkylating agent used and performed in centre with previous experience. Treatment of the congenital anomalies in Fanconi anaemia is symptomatic. Growth retardation does not respond to growth hormone and, anecdotally, this may be contra-indicated. Pancytopenia responds, at least temporarily, to androgens and steroids in about half of the cases. However, many become resistant to this treatment, as well as develop side-effects, such as virilization and, possibly, hepatic malignancies. Ultimately, pancytopenia can only be treated by bone marrow transplantation, for which modified protocols have been developed.

Whilst Fanconi anaemia is a variable phenotype, it also shows genetic heterogeneity. There is good evidence for five separate Fanconi anaemia genes, cytogenetic groups A to E. So far only one gene has been cloned, the Fanconi group C gene on chromosome 9q22.3 (13). Preliminary mutation analysis shows both a wide spectrum of mutations present in the *FAC* gene, and also that this gene accounts for 10% of all Fanconi anaemia. An apparently homologous gene has been found in mice. Studies are currently under way to determine how the *FAC* mutations cause the disease phenotype. At present there seems no clinical method of differentiating Fanconi anaemia group C from other Fanconi anaemia types, except by finding a more specific gene mutation.

Xeroderma pigmentosa, Cockayne syndrome, and trichothiodystrophy

These three conditions are discussed together because of clinical overlaps and that they are caused by mutations of excision repair pathway genes. Cleaver showed in 1968, that xeroderma pigmentosa could be caused by a defect in repair of ultraviolet (UV) damaged DNA (14). The predominant feature of xeroderma pigmentosa is a much increased sensitivity to UV light, present in sunlight (15). The skin is normal at birth but develops progressive atrophy, irregular pigmentation (e.g. freckles at abnormally young ages, or in racially pigmented skin), telangiectasia, and later, keratoses, basal cell, and squamous cell, carcinomas. Other kinds of skin malignancy can occur, but more rarely. Usually tumours occur by 3 or 4 years of age and most patients die of malignancy in the second and third year; such is the sun-sensitivity that tumours of the tongue can occur. Terminal malignancies are not present to excess. Photophobia is also an early finding, as is recurrent conjunctivitis, keratitis, and keratoconus.

A subgroup of individuals with xeroderma pigmentosa developed the de Sanctis–Cacchione variant (16). This variant can occur in any of the different genotypes of xeroderma pigmentosa, but it is most frequently in group B. Also it does not run true in families, that is, one child may have xeroderma pigmentosa alone and the next child the de Sanctis–Cacchione variant. The reasons for this are unknown. The clinical features are those of xeroderma pigmentosa, as well as progressive microcephaly, mental retardation, cerebellar ataxia, areflexia, growth retardation leading to dwarfism, and hypogonadism. It has a considerable phenotypical overlap with Cockayne syndrome.

The major clinical features of Cockayne syndrome are progressive leucodystrophy, progressive microcephaly, and progressive growth retardation. The majority of patients present between the ages of 3 and 5 years. Many children present with sensorineural deafness, initially masquerading as mild developmental delay, later growth deficiency, particularly with loss of adipose tissue, becomes apparent, as well as the characteristic facial appearance with sunken eyes. A retinal pigmentary dystrophy and/or optic atrophy and/or cataracts develop sometime in the first two decades. In the first decade there is often sun-sensitivity, giving rise to sunburn with little sun exposure. However, the atrophic changes seen in xeroderma pigmentosa do not occur, nor do skin cancers. Usually from the second decade onwards the thickness of the skin is sufficient to prevent the sun-sensitivity. The most helpful findings are intracranial calcification, particularly of the thalami, and the distinctive facial appearance. The majority of patients end up severely handicapped and short statured. Rare cases present in the neonatal period (sometimes called COFS syndrome) and also later onset or slowly progressive variants have been described (17).

Trichothiodystrophy is an extremely rare disorder and is characterized by brittle hair, ichthyosis, short stature, and sometimes a distinctive facial appearance, microcephaly and mental retardation, and sun-sensitivity. The natural history of the disorder has not been well documented and there does not appear to be an excess of skin or other malignancies.

The diagnosis of the three conditions, xeroderma pigmentosa, Cockayne syndrome, and trichothiodystrophy, is made by the characteristic clinical features. For xeroderma pigmentosa, the definitive laboratory investigation is the fibroblast survival following UV irradiation. Lymphocyte cytogenetic studies are normal. Cockayne syndrome can usually be diagnosed by clinical findings backed up by abnormal findings, sensorineural hearing loss, and particularly intracranial calcification, best detected by MRI.

Gene mutation and cellular defect tests, as outlined below, in Cockayne syndrome, are only available via research laboratories. Trichothiodystrophy would, again, be suggested by the clinical phenotype, although other disorders, which involve mental retardation and brittle hair, such as argininosuccinicaciduria, Menkes syndrome, and citrullinaemia need to be considered. The specific test for trichothiodystrophy is a specialist UV irradiation survival study and gene analysis. Some cases of the Pollitt syndrome (also known as TAY, IBIDS, BIDS) who have brittle hair with low soft content and trichorrhexis nodosa, short stature and mental retardation plus or minus ichthyosis, and sun-sensitivity have trichothiodystrophy, others do not seem to.

There is no successful treatment available for xeroderma pigmentosa, apart from severe avoidance of sun exposure, the wearing of clothes, which cast a heavy shadow, hats with a wide brim, barrier creams, and early excision of suspected malignancies. There is no successful treatment for Cockayne syndrome. Growth retardation has not been shown to respond to growth hormone, however hearing aids and removal of cataracts may be of benefit. There is no treatment available for trichothiodystrophy.

Genetics

All three conditions are autosomal recessive and are found in all racial groups, xeroderma pigmentosa being more common than Cockayne syndrome and the very rare trichothiodystrophy, which has an incidence of probably <1 per million. The primary defects in this group of disorders involve various components of the excision repair pathway, as outlined in the section on DNA repair. That is, xeroderma pigmentosa can be caused by mutations in a number of genes involved in excision repair. As noted above a number of these genes will also have additional functions in the transcription complex producing messenger RNA from DNA. The diagnosis of an excision repair defect can usually be made by measure of 'unscheduled DNA synthesis'. The fourth step of nucleotide excision repair can be assayed by the use of tritiated thymidine in place of normal thymidine in growth media of the test cells. The amount of radioactive thymidine incorporated into the DNA, is a measure of the amount of nucleotide excision repair that has been performed.

The majority of the genes causing xeroderma pigmentosa groups A to G and variant xeroderma pigmentosa, have been located and most cloned (18). They are all highly homologous, either in terms of DNA sequence or activity of genes of similar function in mice, bacteria, and yeast. Given the number of genes, the complexity in determining the xeroderma pigmentosa groups, and the spectrum of mutations found in the genes, mutation hunting for causative genes is not routinely available. Cockayne syndrome cells are hypersensitive to UV light, though this is not as marked as in the excision repair deficiency of xeroderma pigmentosa cells. The specific defect is in the preferential repair of mutations in transcribed genes, rather than in general excision repair. The diagnostic findings are failure of recovery of RNA synthesis following UV irradiation, but normal excision strand repair. Two genotypes can cause Cockayne syndrome, both genes have been cloned and are involved in the coupling of transcription and repair. Individuals with trichothiodystrophy are either photosensitive or not. A wide range of excision repair defects has been shown in cells from individuals with trichothiodystrophy. Mutations in some individuals have been found in the *XPD/ERCC2* gene. This gene is a helicase and part of the transcription factor complex TFIIH. This complex is both involved in transcription and the recruitment of the excision repair pathway. It seems that mutations in the *XPD* gene neither affect the excision repair pathway recruitment giving rise to xeroderma pigmentosa type D, nor the transcription and function of TFIIH giving rise to trichothiodystrophy.

DNA damage

DNA is subject to both exogenous mutagens and endogenous mutagenesis. Endogenous mutagenesis is the inevitable consequence of a large complex molecule present in a metabolically active environment. Specific mutagens are depurination, which occurs because of the reaction of DNA in water, the effect of oxygen and free radicals, and errors caused by DNA replication. Cells have built up sophisticated mechanisms to minimize the effects of this ongoing mutagenesis with an emphasis on repairing DNA mutations before DNA is replicated and a mutation becomes 'fixed' in the genome. Depurination has been estimated to occur in 10,000 bases per day per cell (19). Other DNA hydrolysis reactions occur at a lesser rate, approximately 100-fold slower than depurination. These products, as well as those from deamination reactions, all have specific repair pathways. The most important reaction of this type is deamination of cytosine, which has a 5-methyl group attached to it. 5-methylation of cytosine is used by cells to mediate gene expression control. Whilst mutations of bases produce uniquely different products to aid the cells and their repair, 5-methylcytosine's deamination product is thymidine. Therefore, if spontaneous deamination of 5methylcytosine occurs, thymidine is produced and a mutation has occurred that will get copied by DNA polymerase at replication.

Reactive oxygen species have been estimated to introduce 20,000 DNA mutations per cell per day. Whilst it has been estimated that oxygen free radicals can cause more than 70 different chemical alterations to DNA, the damage is often limited by a large number of repair mechanisms, as well as systems for minimizing the amount of free radicals present within cells. It is thought that ionizing irradiation causes most of its deleterious effects through the production of free radicals. DNA replication has a very high fidelity. However, both occasional mistakes are made by the DNA polymerases (despite their proof-reading abilities) and also polymerase complex skips areas of DNA in which there is a mutation present. Both these regions and any mutations introduced by DNA polymerase, are detected and repaired by specific post-replication repair mechanism, detailed below. General mutations in genes in this pathway cause the autosomal dominant predisposition to bowel cancer, known as hereditary non-polyposis colon cancer (HNPCC) (20). Exogenous DNA mutants have been classically divided into UV irradiation, ionizing irradiation, and alkylating agents. UV irradiation can cause a number of specific base changes, as well as cross-link bases together. Ionizing irradiation, as noted above, is thought to generate the majority of its mutational load by free radical production. Alkylating agents either mutate DNA bases, or cause cross-linking between DNA strands. A wide variety of other DNA damaging agents, both natural and man made, are known, many are used as chemotherapeutic agents.

DNA repair

The DNA double helix seems to have evolved so that mutations, even as small as individual base damage, are easily recognized. Such recognition is usually by a change to the physical structure of the DNA double helix. Also, with one exception, mutations in each base produce specific intermediates, which can be recognized and repaired back to the original base. The one exception to this being 5-methylcytosine, as noted above. Not only is DNA a very well designed molecule for showing mutations, there are also a number of different pathways involved in DNA repair. Furthermore, these pathways are coordinated with other functions of the cell, in particular, the gene transcription and the cell cycle. For obvious reasons, a cell will pause in its attempts to replicate until all DNA damage has been repaired. Similarly, after a cell has replicated its DNA, there is a process of checking that the replication fidelity has been accurate.

DNA repair can now be classified into four groups: (a) specific base change repair mechanisms; (b) excision repair pathway; (c) recombinational repair; (d) post-replication repair. For many individual base mutations, glycosylase has evolved to detect and remove the damaged base. Specific DNA polymerase, then ligase, repair the removed base. The excision repair pathway has been widely studied and, although complex, is capable of repairing a wide variety of types of DNA damage. Many of the proteins involved in excision repair have other functions. Whilst this pathway can repair any type of DNA, it goes preferentially and actively to the transcribed gene. This is because of the activities of the transcription complex TFIIH. This is involved in transcription, but should transcription halt, it is also involved in the recruitment of the excision repair pathway protein. When the repair is complete, the same transcription complex then recruits back the genes required to continue transcription. A number of the genes in the excision repair pathway are components of the TFIIH complex (21).

The cell uses a combination mechanism, that is, it is able to combine DNA from one chromosome into that of another. This process is used in meiosis, mitosis, and DNA repair. It is particularly of use where the original chromosome has damaged both DNA strands, or has been involved in a double strand DNA break. This mechanism involves proteins, which can detect three DNA strands (involving q proteins and DNA dependent protein kinase, the cause of autosomal recessive severe combined immunodeficency syndrome (SCID)), proteins that actually re-combine the DNA strands together (for instance the rec proteins ABC), as well as the DNA polymerase complex, as in stage IV of excision repair. Post-replication repair occurs immediately after DNA polymerase has produced a daughter strand using one of the bases in DNA strands as the template. Before the newly synthesized daughter strand is methylated, any DNA mutations are detected and repaired by a process, which is almost identical in *Escherichia coli* bacterium to man. When a mutated base is detected, a second protein is recruited, which then recruits in an endonuclease that nicks the DNA and then DNA polymerase (delta or gamma) to synthesize the new correct daughter DNA strand. Following this process, DNA is methylated.

Autosomal dominant cancer predisposition syndromes

1. Dominant predisposition to childhood cancer is rare.
2. The phenotype is defined by an increased incidence of cancer in families. This is only identifiable by taking a careful family tree.
3. The second cancer risk in these conditions is high.

The concept that cancer predisposition could be handed down in families is not a new one. Paul Broca published the pedigree of his wife's family in 1866; ten women in four generations were affected by breast cancer. In 1948 Lionel Penrose observed a familial tendency to breast cancer in UK families. An inherited tendency to gastric cancer was reported in the family of Napoleon Bonaparte. A biological basis for these reports became clearer in the 1980s, and the concept of cancer predisposition syndromes inherited in an autosomal dominant manner was established. This remains the dominant theory in the field of inherited cancers. The genetic basis for inherited breast and ovarian cancers; mutations in the *BrCa1* and *BrCa2* genes were established in the early 1990s. This has made a huge impact on the public perception of cancer and cancer risk.

Estimates of the inherited component to adult cancer are usually of the order of 5%, a considerable proportion of the overall burden. In contrast there is little evidence for an inherited genetic component to the common cancers of childhood. It is possible that 5–10% of childhood cancers are a consequence of mutations in such genes. These figures are an estimate only and may underestimate the true frequency. Highly penetrant cancer predisposition syndromes such as LFS, MEN, and Beckwith Weidemann syndrome, cause a minority of childhood cancers. Low penetrance genes are likely to be of more importance clinically, but at present little is known about such mechanisms. This is not the case for the rarer embryonal tumours including Wilms' tumours, retinoblastomas, neuroblastoma, and hepatoblastoma. Genetic factors, albeit usually not inherited factors, frequently play a role in the development of these lesions.

High penetrance genes and familial cancer syndromes

These syndromes are characterized by a high incidence of specific cancers within families. There may be no non-neoplastic features of the syndromes. This means that diagnosis is based upon the recognition of the pattern of cancers in the family and can only be done if a careful family history is taken. Several of these syndromes confer a high risk of malignancy in childhood. Their importance in clarifying our understanding of cancer generally has been far greater than their clinical importance. All inherited familial cancer syndromes are a consequence of inherited mutations in tumour suppressor genes apart from MEN type 2.

Li Fraumeni syndrome

In 1969 Li and Fraumeni reported on a survey of 280 medical records and 418 death certificates of children with rhabdomyosarcoma. They identified five families in which there was a sibling with a sarcoma (22). Subsequent reports of similar families resulted in the recognition of a characteristic phenotype of sarcoma (S), breast and brain tumours (B), leukaemia, lung and laryngeal cancer (L), and adrenocortical cancers in childhood (A). This was designated the SBLA syndrome. Diagnostic criteria for the LFS are: a proband with sarcoma at age less than 45; a first degree relative with any cancer at age less than 45; another first or second degree relative with cancer at age less than 45 or sarcoma at any age. Li Fraumeni Like (LFL) families conform to the following criteria: a proband with childhood cancer or sarcoma, brain tumour or adrenal cortical tumour under age 45 years with one first or second degree relative with a typical LFS cancer (sarcoma, brain, breast, adrenal cortical cancer, or leukaemia) at any age, and another first or second degree relative with any cancer at age less than 60.

Tumour spectrum

The target organs for malignant transformation in LFS are limited. In childhood adrenal cortical tumours, bone and soft tissue sarcomas, brain tumours, and haematological malignancies occur most frequently (23). There are few figures for the age specific penetrance for germline *TP53* mutation carriers, thus precise age specific cancer risks cannot be given. The study by Kleihues *et al.* confirmed the clinical impression that there was specific age associated risks, even though statistical significance could not be achieved (23).

The mean age of onset of osteosarcomas and soft tissue sarcomas is 16, similar to that for sporadic lesions. However rhabdomyosarcomas occur almost exclusively in young children with a mean age of onset of 5.9 years. Central nervous system (CNS) tumours in *TP53* mutation carriers show two peaks, the first in children aged less than 10 years, the second in adults in the third and fourth decades. Adrenocortical tumours in LFS occur almost exclusively in early childhood, mean age 4.9 years. This is in striking contrast to sporadic adrenocortical lesions whose peak is beyond age 40 years. Any child with an adrenocortical lesion should be regarded as a potential *TP53* mutation carrier. The risk of childhood cancer in LFS has been estimated as about 20% overall (24).

Second cancer risk

A high risk of second malignancy is a well-recognized feature of LFS (25, 26). A recent analysis of 24 families with LFS identified 200 family members with cancer. Overall 15% of the total developed a second cancer, and 4% a third cancer. The cumulative risk of second cancer was 57% at 30 years after first diagnosis (27). The risk of second cancers among probands with sarcoma was even higher, 64% at 20 years and 100% at 30 years. The highest relative risks overall were for survivors of childhood cancers with a relative risk of 83 in the 0–19-year age group. The majority of the cancers were of the LFS type, among those aged 0–19 years the most common second cancers were soft tissue sarcomas and osteosarcomas. In a series of children with adrenocortical tumours, not all known to be *TP53* mutation carriers, 3/18 (17%) developed a second tumour. All three arose at sites within the irradiation treatment field.

Clinical aspects of LFS

From the clinical point of view a diagnosis of LFS has profound implications for the original proband and their family. In affected children the risk of a second cancer is very high. The majority of such children will be treated with the therapeutic modalities most suited to their malignancies. It is known that *TP53* mutant cells are extremely radiosensitive, however there is also data to suggest that the risk of second sarcomas is particularly associated with previous irradiation (27). Although the risk of second malignancies is high no simple strategy for screening has so far been proposed. Since the major risk in childhood is for second sarcomas the best clinical option is probably to arrange easy access to appropriate diagnostic services, and encourage a policy of early referral for review. For siblings of affected children the overall risk of cancer to age 20 years is 10%. The range of lesions can be anticipated, adrenocortical tumours, sarcomas and brain tumours. Again no simple screening policy has ever been suggested (26, 28). Adrenocortical tumours might be identified early by screening for abnormal androgen production found in over 90% (29). However, this remains conjectural. An awareness of the signs and symptoms of possible malignancy in potential gene carriers and early referral for assessment is again probably the best policy clinically.

Penetrance of *TP53* mutation carriers has always been regarded as extremely high with estimates of 90% reported (30). Mean age at diagnosis of first tumour was 28 years (31). Mutations in 11 of 14 cases of apparently sporadic childhood adrenocortical tumour were detected by Varley *et al.* (31). In the families of these children there were no other cases of childhood cancer and the overall incidence of malignancy appeared low. In this series all but two of the children had germline mutations at codons 152 or 158. In series of LFS families with cases of childhood adrenocortical tumour a variety of other mutations were identified. It is thus possible that there are low penetrance *TP53* alleles, particularly associated with isolated cases of childhood adrenocortical tumour.

Molecular genetics

TP53 gene is a tumour suppressor gene that is encoded by 20 kilobases (kb) of genomic DNA. The gene consists of 11 exons, the first is non-coding. There are five functional domains with little variation (32). Domain I is responsible for transactivation properties, while the remaining Domains II–V make up the core DNA-binding domain (28). The majority of reported *TP53* mutations are missense mutations. Most *TP53* mutations have been reported within exons 5–8, which reside in the core DNA-binding region of the gene. There are hotspots at codons 175, 248, and 273. *TP53* gene was first identified as a protein that complexes to the large T antigen of SV40 (33). TP53 protein is a tetramer, it is regarded as the 'guardian of the genome', and plays a vital role in DNA repair and apoptosis (34). Normal TP53 protein responds to DNA damage in one of two ways: (a) transcriptionally activates the downstream targets (*p21, MDM-2, GADD45, Bax, IGF-BP,* and *cyclin-G*) to repair the DNA or (b) commits the cell to apoptosis. Cell cycle arrest depends on the interaction with the retinoblastoma gene pathway.

Germline mutations in the *TP53* gene were identified as the biological basis for the LFS syndrome (35). Up to 70% of families with classic LFS have *TP53* mutations identifiable by current techniques. In the same series 22% of LFL families harboured a *TP53* mutation. Germline mutations in *hCHK2*, a cell cycle G2 checkpoint kinase, were recently identified in one LFS and in two further LFL families (36). This confirms the genetic heterogeneity of LFS, hitherto suspected but never confirmed. Uptake of predictive testing is still relatively low (37, 38). Protocols have been established for such testing and are similar to those used for *BrCa1* and *BrCa2* mutation testing (39, 40). Genetic testing of children in such cases is fraught with problems, each case must be assessed on its own merits.

Multiple endocrine neoplasia

Diagnostic criteria have been developed for both MEN1 and MEN2. MEN1 is defined as a case with endocrine tumours in two of the three component systems; parathyroid, gastrointestinal tract endocrine system, and anterior pituitary. MEN2 is similarly defined as a case with the development of tumours in two of the component systems; thyroid C cells, anterior pituitary, and adrenal cortex. Cases may also be identified with medullary thyroid cancer alone in the context of a family history of the disorder. MEN is characterized by the development of tumours in two or more endocrine glands. MEN1 involves the parathyroid, anterior pituitary, pancreatic islet cells, and adrenal cortex. The tumours do not necessarily develop simultaneously. The majority of MEN1 is inherited. In the largest British series there were 36 isolated cases compared with 220 inherited cases in 62 families (41). Non-endocrine features of MEN1 are facial angiofibromas, lipomas, and collagenomas.

MEN2 involves the thyroid C cells, adrenal medulla, and parathyroid. MEN2 is further subdivided into MEN2a, MEN2b, and familial medullary thyroid cancer (FMTC). The biological basis for all of these disorders is germline mutations in the *RET* proto-oncogene. MEN2b is differentiated from MEN2a by the presence of associated developmental anomalies. Gene carriers have a characteristic facies with prominent lips and nodules on the tongue and conjunctivae. There is thickening of the corneal nerves and there may be hyperplasia of the intrinsic autonomic ganglia of the intestine leading to disordered gut motility, which presents as failure to thrive, constipation, or diarrhoea. There is often a Marfanoid habitus with associated skeletal abnormalities. FMTC denotes families in which the only manifestation is medullary thyroid carcinoma.

Tumour spectrum
MEN1

The tumour spectrum in MEN1 is wide. Parathyroid hyperplasia occurs in 95% of cases. Enteropancreatic neoplasia results in gastrinomas, insulinomas, and oversecretion of pancreatic polypeptide in about 40% of cases. VIPomas and glucagonomas occur but are far less common. Foregut carcinoid tumours, thymic, bronchial, or gastric in origin occur in only a minority of cases. Anterior pituitary lesions, particularly, prolactinomas occur in about 15–18% of all cases. The vast majority behave in a benign manner; only the anterior pituitary lesions and less commonly the pancreatic lesions exert any local mass effect; distant metastases are rare (41).

MEN2

The hallmark of MEN2 is medullary thyroid carcinoma, arising from the C cells of the thyroid. These are truly malignant lesions, early metastases locally within the neck and then to more distant sites are common even with tumours of less than 10 mm diameter. Phaeochromocytoma also occurs. Parathyroid hyperplasia or adenoma are common but frequently asymptomatic.

Clinical aspects
MEN1

The majority of patients with MEN1 present with hyperparathyroidism, Zollinger–Ellison syndrome or prolactinomas. Primary hyperparathyroidism is the commonest presenting feature in all series (42). Penetrance in this condition is high but not 100% and is age related. At-risk individuals should undergo screening by means of non-ionized calcium, parathyroid hormone, and prolactin estimation. In the UK study penetrance was 7% at age 10 and 52% at age 20 after biochemical screening. The earliest case in this series were two 8-year olds who presented with primary hyperparathyroidism (41). The youngest patient in a French study of 220 gene carriers was a boy of 6 years with an insulinoma. Of the 36 individuals in the UK study affected at age less than 18 years, the majority presented with hyperparathyroidism (41). However 17 had evidence of other lesions including 6 with anterior pituitary tumours and 6 with insulinomas. Biochemical screening has been advocated from age 5 years at six-monthly intervals until age 30 years to identify those at risk and facilitate their management (44). The treatment of MEN1 tumours is primarily surgical with hormonal support as required. Thus the major role for the paediatrician in the management of these families is to ensure appropriate screening takes place and to provide easy access to diagnostic services for symptomatic children.

MEN2

MEN2a is the commonest type; it accounts for about 65% of all MEN2. Associated development anomalies have not been recorded in MEN2a, however several families have been described in which Hirschsprung's disease is inherited with MEN2a. An unusual scaly rash with the features of lichen amyloidosis has been described in a small number of families. The non-endocrine features of MEN2b have been described above and are quite characteristic. As is the case with MEN1 penetrance in MEN2 is age related, and again biochemical screening for medullary thyroid carcinoma will reveal asymptomatic gene carriers. By age 20 years only 3% of patients will present clinically (45). The most useful primary screening tool prior to DNA screening was the pentagastrin stimulation test, which reveals 70% of gene carriers by age 20 years and 95% by age 30 years. Once a gene carrier is identified the management is total thyroidectomy with parathyroid preservation or autotansplantation to the forearm. The rationale is that surgery prior to the development of symptoms greatly reduces the risk of recurrent or persistent medullary thyroid carcinoma (46).

Genetic basis of MEN
MEN1

MEN1 is caused by germline mutations in the *menin* gene on chromosome 11q13. Mutations have been identified in over 90% of affected individuals. One family has been described, which met the criteria for MEN1 but which was not linked to 11q13. This family had two cases with acromegaly, not a feature of MEN1. The *MEN1* gene contains 10 exons and encodes a ubiquitously expressed 2.8-kb transcript. The predicted 610-amino acid protein product, termed *menin*, exhibited no apparent similarities to any previously known proteins. The amino acid sequence of *menin* offers no clue to the function or subcellular location of this putative tumour suppressor. Studies using immunofluorescence, Western blotting of subcellular fractions, and epitope tagging demonstrated that *menin* is located primarily in the nucleus (47). There are two nuclear localization signals (NLSs), located in the C-terminal region of the protein. Of the known disease-associated mutations, none of the 22 missense and 3 in-frame deletions affect the putative NLS sequences. However none of the truncated menin proteins resulting from the 43 known frameshift/nonsense mutations would retain both the NLSs. The precise nuclear role(s) of *menin* remain obscure.

In the largest UK study of MEN1 47 mutations were identified in 63 unrelated MEN1 families (195 affected and 396 unaffected members) accounting for 85% of all families. There were 12 nonsense mutations, 21 deletions, 7 insertions, 1 donor splice site mutation, and 6 missense mutations. Four hotspots were identified accounting for 25% of all mutation, however the rest of the mutations were distributed throughout the gene. Six polymorphisms that had heterozygosity frequencies of 2–44% were also identified and more than 10% of the mutations arose de novo, and four mutation hotspots accounted for more than 25% of the mutations. Age-related penetrance of MEN1 was 7%, 52%, 87%, 98%, 99%, and 100% at 10, 20, 30, 40, 50, and 60 years of age, respectively (44). Similar results were reported in a large French study of the disorder (43). Thus far no genotype phenotype correlations have been reported.

MEN2

The vast majority of families with MEN2 and its variants have mutations in the *RET* oncogene on chromosome 10q11.2. The gene consists of 21 exons spanning approximately 55 kb of genomic DNA. There are 3 main alternatively spliced forms of the 1072–1114 amino acids. Most of the mutations in MEN2a and FMTC are in one of the five cysteine codons of the extracellular domain. Out of 184 families, 160 with MEN2a and phaeochromocytoma have mutations in codon 634, while codon 609, 611, 618, and 620 are more commonly involved in non-phaeochromocytoma families. Most cases of MEN2b are caused by the methionine-to-threonine mutation at codon 918 in exon 16 of *RET*. All families segregating both MEN2 and Hirschsprung's disease have mutations in either cys609, cys618, or cys620.

Clinical implications
The range of *RET* mutations resulting in MEN2 is small. DNA testing is therefore the standard of care of MEN2 families. Once the causative mutation has been identified then testing can be offered to at risk family members. Increasingly the tendency in clinical practice is to offer testing to young children. Gene carriers can then be offered thyroidectomy at an early age. As the risk of adrenal disease is generally low prophylactic adrenalectomy is not advised. In MEN1 biochemical screening from age 8 years has been the standard of care. As mutations are scattered throughout the *MEN1* gene DNA testing is more of a challenge than for MEN2. However again, once a mutation has been identified at-risk family members can be offered a predictive test. Since the likelihood of disease in childhood is low DNA testing is often not offered until adulthood, biochemical screening being preferred.

Central nervous system tumours

Malignant CNS tumours occur in neurofibromatosis type 1 (NF-1), Gorlin syndrome, and von Hippel Lindau syndrome. However the incidence of childhood tumours in these disorders is low. The major exception to this is the development of hypothalamic/chiasmatic tumours in children with NF-1. Although this is again infrequent any child with NF-1 who presents with visual disturbance or symptoms and signs of raised intracranial pressure needs urgent investigation.

Deletions and monosomy of chromosome 22 have been observed at high frequency in CNS rhabdoid tumours. Based on the identification of overlapping deletions of a region within 22q11 it was proposed that loss or inactivation of a tumour suppressor gene on chromosome 22 was responsible for the initiation of rhabdoid tumours. The *INI1* gene, which maps to 22q11, was recently identified by a positional cloning strategy as the target for putative loss of function mutations in these tumours (48). We have recently demonstrated that inherited germline mutations of the *INI1* gene can be the cause of rare familial cases of rhabdoid tumour (49).

Neurofibromatosis-1

NF-1 is a common autosomal dominant disorder that affects about 1/3000 individuals (50). The disorder was first described by von Recklinghausen in 1882 and its hereditary nature was demonstrated by Preiser and Davenport in 1918. The distinction between peripheral NF (NF-1) and central NF (NF-2) was not clearly made until cohort studies in the 1950s. NF-1 is characterized by multiple café-au-lait spots and associated cutaneous findings of neurofibromas (PNF), plexiform neurofibromas, and axillary or inguinal freckling. Other manifestations include an increased risk for optic glioma, osseous lesions, and learning disability. The diagnosis rests on clinical grounds; according to the National Institutes of Health (NIH) consensus criteria the diagnosis can be made in an individual who has two or more of the following features (51):

(1) six or more café-au-lait macules over 5 mm in greatest diameter in prepubertal individuals and over 15 mm in greatest diameter in postpubertal individuals;
(2) two or more neurofibromas of any type or one PNF;
(3) freckling in the axillary or inguinal regions;
(4) optic glioma;
(5) two or more Lisch nodules (iris hamartomas);
(6) a distinctive osseous lesion such as sphenoid dysplasia or thinning of long bone cortex with or without pseudarthrosis;
(7) a first-degree relative (parent, sib, or offspring) with NF-1 as defined by the above criteria.

The disorder is highly penetrant with no cases of non-penetrance in over 200 families studied (50, 52–54). No case of non-penetrance has ever been documented with mutation analysis or linkage and full clinical evaluation. The NIH diagnostic criteria are both highly specific and highly sensitive in adults with NF-1 (55). However, they may not be fulfilled in young children with no family history, many of the features do not develop until later (50, 55, 56). The disease is apparent in almost all affected individuals by age 8 years and in 100% by age 20 years (57). Family history is frequently lacking, as the new mutation rate is extremely high, only 50% of cases have a family history (50, 52, 54). Estimates of the new mutation rate vary from 1 in 7800 to 1 in 2300 gametes. More than 80% of new mutations arise on the paternal chromosome (58, 59). Cases resulting from gross genomic deletions account for only 5% of NF-1, conversely these tend to arise on the maternal chromosome (59, 60).

NF-1 associated malignancy
Although neoplasia is common in NF-1 most associated tumours are benign and the majority of individuals with

NF-1 will not develop a primary malignancy either in childhood or later life (61–63). The true malignancy risk remains unclear. A follow-up study over a period of 42 years in Denmark revealed a relative risk of between 1.5 and 4.0 for all cancers (62). The study was hospital based, so was subject to ascertainment bias. When the study was expanded to include relatives with NF-1 not identified in hospital records the relative risks declined. No tumours were specific for NF-1. CNS tumours were over represented accounting for 47% of all malignancies, about one-third of these were optic gliomas.

Cancer in children with NF-1

Studies of malignancy in children with NF are plagued by the same biases as those in adults. The early literature over-reports the incidence of malignancy as it tends to deal only with hospitalized children. Rates in these early reports suggest a malignancy rate of about 19% but with wide variation (64–67). More recent studies reveal lower rates of cancer of the order of 5–8% (50, 68, 69). The list of malignancies seen in children with NF-1 is growing and some of these are undoubtedly chance occurrences. Evidence of an increased risk in children with NF-1 exists for malignant schwannoma, neurofibrosarcoma, rhabdomyosarcoma, and astrocytoma, including optic pathway glioma, and some myeloid leukaemia (67–71). The clear message from these studies is that the cancer risk for NF-1 sufferers is not greatly increased over that seen in the general population. The malignant phenotype seen in NF-1 shares features seen in other heritable cancer systems:

(1) a tissue restricted pattern of primary malignancies in neural crest and myeloid lineages;
(2) early age of onset;
(3) multiple primary tumours.

CNS tumours

Gliomas are a well known complication of NF-1. They tend to occur in the brainstem, cerebellum, and along the optic pathway. While medulloblastomas and ependymomas have been reported, meningiomas do not seem to occur more frequently in NF-1 (61).

Optic pathway gliomas

Symptomatic tumours were seen in 2 out of 135 patients in the South Wales study (50). They have been reported in up to 15% of NF children overall (72). More recently 176 children with NF-1 were assessed by neuroimaging (73). Out of 176 children, 33 were found to have an optic tract glioma, at a median age of 4.2 years. No tumour was identified in a child over 6 years of age. The majority (25/33) of these children were asymptomatic at the time of diagnosis, and 21/33 had no eye signs on examination. The six children with signs alone had unrecognized decreases in their visual acuity. All of the symptomatic children were aged less than 6 years, two had precocious puberty. Five children had rapidly progressing proptosis, all five had no vision in the affected eye. Progression was seen in only three children with mean follow up of 2.4 years. Apparent differences in the mode of presentation between children with NF-1 optic pathway tumours (OPT) and non-NF-1 OPT were documented in a follow-up study by the same group (74). Precocious puberty appeared to occur more commonly in children with NF-1 OPT, who also more commonly had isolated and bilateral optic nerve tumours, compared with the more frequent chiasmal lesions seen in non-NF-1 OPT. Progressive disease was also far more common in non-NF-1 OPT.

Magnetic resonance imaging (MRI) is now the investigation of choice for optic pathway gliomas, however its routine use for screening has not been shown to improve prognosis, as the majority of children will have non-progressive lesions. Annual ophthalmoloigcal review has been suggested as a mode of screening with colour testing, visual field assessment, acuity, fundoscopy, and lit lamp exam (75). Early treatment of children with tumours of the chiasm or optic nerve pathways does not appear to influence outcome. Debulking surgery may have a role. Radiotherapy may result in stabilization or regression in 80% of patients, however outcome is no better than in patients who do not receive radiotherapy (74, 76).

Brain stem gliomas

Brain stem gliomas occur in a minority of children with NF-1. In contrast as many as 60% of children have unidentified bright objects (UBOs) on MRI. Until recently these lesions were often confused, however their MRI appearances are quite distinct. Unlike gliomas UBOs are not contrast enhancing lesions and do not cause mass effects or brainstem enlargement (77). In a study of 17 children with brainstem gliomas with a median age of 8.4 years, 15 were symptomatic, 6 had cranial nerve lesions, 5 had dysarthria, and 7 of children had hydrocephalus, all requiring shunting. The majority of tumours (14/17) were seen in the medulla (77).

Pollack identified 21 patients with median age 9.5 years—11 were symptomatic and 5 had hydrocephalus (78). In the Molloy series 14 of 17 patients did not progress with mean follow-up of 63 months (77).

Out of the 21 patients studied by Pollack et al. 11 remained stable (78). In the latter group only one asymptomatic patient was identified who needed treatment. There appear to be distinct parallels with OPT. On the whole these lesions run a more benign course than in children with sporadic tumours. Again screening is unlikely to identify lesions, which will require treatment and must be regarded as of dubious benefit.

Plexiform neurofibromas
These are complex lesions that may diffusely involve nerve, skin, muscle, connective tissue, and vascular elements. They consist of a proliferation of cells in the nerve sheath extending across the length of a nerve and involving multiple nerve fascicles. They may be congenital and are almost invariably present by age 4 or 5 (Huson SM, personal communication). They are common lesions, occurring in 26.7% of the patients in the South Wales study (79). Usually they were small and asymptomatic. Any area of the body may be involved; when a limb is involved it may result in isolated overgrowth. They can arise form the cranial nerves, most commonly the trigeminal resulting in proptosis, and there may be associated sphenoid wing dysplasia (80). Visceral involvement has been documented by Tonsgard et al. (81). Twenty per cent of individuals over the age of 16 years had thoracic PNF, 44% had abdominal or pelvic lesions. Schorry assessed 240 children and identified 9 thoracic lesions by MRI, only three of these were symptomatic (82). Both superficial and visceral PNFs may grow at any time during life. Rapid growth is common in early childhood after which lesion may stop or may continue steadily. Growth may occur in any plane of the nerve; there may be increasing soft tissue asymmetry and local invasion. Myelopathy may result if a paravertebral tumour extends into the spinal canal.

Treatment is extremely challenging, particularly with regard to timing. Complete resection is difficult with even small lesions, leaving the potential for regrowth. Prophylactic resection of asymptomatic tumours is hard to justify. Needle et al. reviewed the outcome of 121 patients who underwent surgical resection with median follow-up of 6.8 years (83). Forty-four per cent of tumours recurred, this was particularly common with children aged less than 10 years, residual tumour after surgery and location on head, neck, or face. Chemotherapeutic regimens and radiotherapy have been used in PFN, but formal study of their use has been reported.

Malignant peripheral nerve sheath tumour (MPNST) may arise in a pre-existing PNF. In a hospital-based series of 68 NF patients with PNFs only 2 developed MPNST (84).

Leukaemia
Juvenile chronic myelomonocytic leukaemia (JCML) and monosomy 7 syndrome (Mo7) occur at increased frequency in NF-1 in childhood. Approximately 10% of all children with these disorders have NF-1 (70, 85). The relative risk of children with NF-1 is of the order of 200–500.

Overgrowth syndromes

Generalized patterns of overgrowth are associated with increased risks for a variety of malignancies. There are particular risks of Wilms' tumour, brain tumours, and neuroblastomas (86, 87). These associations do help in identifying a group of children at particular risk who might benefit from specific management protocols. However children with recognizable syndromic causes of overgrowth may well be identified and afforded appropriate intervention. The most easily recognizable syndromic causes of overgrowth are Simpson Golabi Behmel (SGB) and BWS.

Simpson Golabi Behmel syndrome
First described in the two male sons of sisters by Simpson in 1975, SGB is characterized by generalized overgrowth, a distinctive facies (large protruding jaw, widened nasal bridge, upturned nasal tip), enlarged tongue, and broad, short hands and fingers. Polydactyly, neonatal teeth, supernumerary nipples, and cardiac defects are also seen. Visceromegaly, earlobe creases, hernias, and neonatal hypoglycaemia are other features, which are shared with BWS, however the two syndromes are clinically and molecularly distinct. SGB is inherited in an X linked manner, so is only rarely seen in females. The tumour risk in SGB is difficult, to quantify but instances of embryonal tumours are well recorded, particularly Wilms' tumour (88). Hepatoblastoma has also been described in SGB.

SGB is caused by mutations in the *GPC3* gene on Xq26. *GPC3* encodes a putative extracellular proteoglycan. It is selectively expressed in embryonic mesodermal derivatives and is felt to play a role in growth control in these tissues (89). It appears to form a complex with insulin like growth factor-2 (IGF-2) and might thereby modulate IGF-2 action. Over expression of IGF-2 is thought to be the cause of BWS, another overgrowth syndrome.

Beckwith Wiedemann Syndrome
Beckwith Wiedemann syndrome (BWS) is characterized by generalized overgrowth, large tongue, omphalocele,

Table 4.1 Clinical features of BWS

Major features	Minor features
Positive family history (one or more family members with a clinical diagnosis of BWS or a history or features suggestive of BWS)	Polyhydramnios
	Prematurity
	Neonatal hypoglycaemia
Macrosomia (traditionally defined as height and weight >97th%)	Facial nevus flammeus
	Hemangioma
Anterior linear ear lobe creases/posterior helical ear pits	Characteristic facies, including midfacial hypoplasia and infraorbital creases
Macroglossia	
Omphalocele	Cardiomegaly/structural cardiac anomalies/rarely cardiomyopathy
Visceromegaly involving one or more intra-abdominal organs including liver, spleen, kidneys, adrenal glands, and pancreas	Diastasis recti
	Advanced bone age
	Monozygotic twinning
Embryonal tumour (e.g. Wilms' tumour, hepatoblastoma, rhabdomyosarcoma) in childhood	
Hemihyperplasia defined as asymmetric overgrowth of region(s) of the body	
Adrenocortical cytomegaly	
Renal abnormalities including structural abnormalities, nephromegaly, nephrocalcinosis	
Cleft palate (rare)	

neonatal hypoglycaemia, and ear creases or pits. There is predisposition to embryonal tumours particularly Wilms' tumour, hepatoblastoma, neuroblastoma, and rhabdomyosarcoma. The condition is diagnosed on the basis of the clinical findings. Possibly 1% of patients have a chromosomal abnormality involving 11p15.

Clinical features
No consensus diagnostic criteria exist for BWS, however the combination of three major and one minor feature would be accepted as making the diagnosis in most cases (Table 4.1).

Course of BWS
Polyhydramnios, prematurity, and increased birth weight are seen in 50% of cases of BWS (90). Neonatal mortality is common mainly due to complications of prematurity associated with omphalocoele, macroglossia, neonatal hypoglycaemia, and, rarely, cardiomyopathy (91). Although generalized overgrowth and a large tongue are seen in most cases at birth, the development of these features postnatally has been reported (92). Growth normally slows by age 7 or 8. Most cases of neonatal hypoglycaemia are mild and transient, however, it can persist (93). Delayed onset of hypoglycaemia is occasionally observed. Hypothyroidism and polycythemia have also been reported. Anterior abdominal wall defects including omphalocoele, umbilical hernia, and diastasis recti are common (91, 94). Hemihyperplasia (hemihypertrophy) if seen, is generally present from birth, but may become more apparent with time. It may be segmental (95). Renal medullary dysplasia, nephrocalcinosis, cystic changes, and generalized enlargement are well-documented features of BWS (96). Developmental delay is rare in BWS, but has been seen with chromosomal abnormalities (97).

The estimated risk for tumour development in children with BWS is 7.5%. This increased risk for neoplasia seems to be concentrated in the first 8 years of life. In patients with BWS who are older than 8 years, tumour development is uncommon.

Management of BWS
The multisystem nature of BWS is such that review by numerous specialists may be necessary. Surgical management of macroglossia and abdominal wall defects

may be required. Orthopaedic input may be needed if limb length discrepancies are marked. The possibility of renal abnormalities and nephrocalcinosis should be borne in mind. Cardiomegaly is well reported but usually resolves without specific treatment (93). Cardiac assessment may be valuable to document lesions and prevent any unnecessary intervention.

Screening policies
The risks of Wilms' tumour have led to the establishment of screening protocols (98, 99) Abdominal ultrasound every 3 months until age of 7 years and six-monthly thereafter until growth is complete are recommended. It has been suggested that serial AFP to detect hepatoblastoma, and periodic chest X-ray, and urinary vanilylmandelic acid (VMA) assays for neuroblastoma should be performed, but have not been incorporated into most screening programmes (92).

Molecular genetics of BWS
It is well known that genes at the 11p15 locus are involved in BWS. Complex alterations of imprinted genes at 11p15 have been identified. Imprinting is an epigenetic phenomenon whereby there is differential modification of genes such that only one parental allele is expressed (100). A number of differentially expressed genes have been implicated in BWS. *IGF2* encodes a paternally expressed growth factor. Biallelic expression has been observed in some BWS patients and in sporadic Wilms' tumours (101, 102). *p57KIP2* (*CDKN1C*) is a cyclin-dependent kinase inhibitor involved in BWS (103). It has tumour suppressor activities and acts as a negative regulator of fetal growth. There is incomplete paternal imprinting resulting in preferential maternal expression. Five to ten per cent of patients have mutations. Preliminary data suggest that *p57KIP2* mutations are found more frequently in cases with omphalocoele, cleft palate, and positive family history. Not all familial cases are due to *p57KIP2* mutations (104–106).

KVLQT1/KVLQT1-AS codes for a voltage gated potassium channel. It is maternally expressed, and in two patients with translocations disrupting the *KVLQT1/KVLQT1-AS* locus biallelic expression of IGF-2 was found (107, 108). *KCNQ1OT1 is* another imprinted gene at the 11p15 locus, expressed only from the paternal allele. A recent study suggests that tumours are only seen in patients with methylation of h19 and are not seen in patients with isolated methylation of KCNQ1OT1 (106).

Clinical genetics of BWS
One percent or less of patients with BWS have a cytogenetically detectable translocation or inversion of a maternal chromosome 11 or a cytogenetically detectable duplication of a paternal chromosome 11 involving band 11p15. Fluorescent *in situ* hybridization (FISH) studies can be used to clarify the position of a chromosome 11 translocation or inversion and to confirm duplications of chromosome 11. Eighty-five per cent of patients will have no family history and will be karyotypically normal. A proportion of these cases will have paternal uniparental disomy for 11p15, and small numbers will have mutations in the *p57KIP2* gene. There are well-documented occurrences of unaffected mothers carrying such mutations and two cases of unaffected fathers passing on such mutations (104, 109, 110). Clearly in such cases the risk of recurrence is as high as 50%. In cases with a positive family history, between 30% and 50% will have a *p57KIP2* mutation. When the mutation is maternally inherited the recurrence risks is 50%, when it is paternally inherited the recurrence risk is high but the exact figure remains unclear. When no *p57KIP2* mutation is identified the recurrence risk is 50% but impossible to further define.

Other syndromes associated with Wilms' tumours
WAGR syndrome
Aniridia is seen in 1/70 children with Wilms' tumour; put another way, 1/3 children with aniridia will develop a Wilms' tumour (111). WAGR syndrome describes children with the constellation of Wilms' tumour, aniridia, genito-urinary abnormalities, and mental retardation. These children have a cytogenetic deletion of 11p13. This is a contiguous gene defect, the aniridia resulting from the loss of the *Pax 6* gene, the Wilms' tumour from loss of the *WT-1* gene. Mutations in the *WT-1* gene are seen in about 10–15% of sporadic Wilms' tumours (104).

Denys Drash Syndrome (DDS)
Denys Drash syndrome is another dysmorphic syndrome associated with Wilms' tumours. DDS is characterized by ambiguous genitalia and a progressive nephropathy. Some cases of DDS will present with normal male genitalia but most will have ambiguous genitalia or female genitalia. The vast majority of such cases will have a normal male karyotype. The internal findings are much more complex and frequently not concordant with the external genitalia. Renal involvement is twofold: a progressive nephropathy and Wilms' tumour. The nephropathy classically occurs in the first year of life. Renal biopsy shows diffuse mesangial sclerosis. In the review by Mueller of cases in the literature 95% of cases had the nephropathy and 80% of the children had Wilms' tumour (112). It is caused by constitutional mutations of the *WT-1* gene (112).

Wilms' tumours have also been seen in NF-1, LFS, and Perlman syndrome.

Other syndromal associations with malignancy

The presence of cancer and a congenital anomaly in the same child is unexpected and may be the consequence of a shared genetic aetiology. Children with trisomy 21 are at increased risk of acute leukaemias and there is an excess of embryonal tumours in children with overgrowth syndromes. Certain other dysmorphic syndromes do appear to be associated with increased cancer risk: there appears to be an excess of sarcomas in children with Rothmund Thomson syndrome. Children with Rubinstein Taybi syndrome appear to have an excess of cancers, particularly brain tumours, especially medulloblastomas (51).

References

1. Bloom D. Congenital telangiectatic erythema resembling lupus erythematosus in dwarfs. Am J Dis Child 1954, **88**, 754–8.
2. German J, Bloom D, Passarge E. Bloom's syndrome. VII. Progress report for 1978. Clin Genet 1979, **15**(4), 361–7.
3. German J. Bloom's syndrome. XX. The first 100 cancers. Cancer Genet Cytogenet 1997, **93**(1), 100–6.
4. Ellis MA, German J. The molecular genetics of Bloom syndrome. Human Mol Genet 1996, **5**, 1457–63.
5. Boder E. Ataxia telangiectasia: some historic clinical and pathological observations. BDOAS 1975, **11**(1), 255–70.
6. Woods CG, Taylor AMR. Ataxic telangiectasia in the British Isles: the clinical and laboratory features of 70 affected individuals. Q J Med 1992, **82**, 169–79.
7. Gatti RA, Berkel I, Boder E. Localization of the ataxia–telangiectasia gene to chromosome 11q22-23. Nature 1988, **336**, 577–9.
8. Savitsky K, Bar-Shira A, Gilad S, et al. A single ataxia–telangiectasia gene with a product similar to a PI-3 kinase. Science 1995, **268**, 1749–53.
9. Fanconi G. Familiäre infantile perniziosaartige anämie. Z. Kinderheilk 1927, **117**, 257.
10. Kwee ML, Kuyt LP. Fanconi anaemia in the Netherlands. In: Fanconi anaemia (ed. TM Schroeder-Kurth, AD Auerbach, G Obe). Springer Verlag, Berlin, 1989, 18–33.
11. Hebell W, Frederick W, Kohne E. Therapeutic aspects of Fanconi anaemia. In: Fanconi anaemia (ed. TM Schroeder-Kurth, AD Auerbach, G Obe). Springer Verlag, Berlin, 1989, 47–59.
12. Auerbach AD, Ghosh R, Pollio PC, Zhang M. Diepoxybutane test for pre-natal and post-natal diagnosis of Fanconi anaemia. In: Fanconi anaemia (ed. TM Schroeder-Kurth, AD Auerbach, G Obe). Springer Verlag, Berlin, 1989, 71–82.
13. Strathdee CA, Gavish H, Shannon WR, Buchwald M. Cloning of cDNAs for Fanconi anaemia by function and complementation. Nature 1992, **356**, 763–7.
14. Cleaver JE. Defective repair replication of DNA in xeroderma pigmentosa. Nature 1968, **218**, 652–6.
15. Kramer KH, Slor H. Xeroderma pigmentosa. Clin Dermatol 1984, **2**, 33–69.
16. de Sanctis C, Cacchione A. L'idiozia xerodermia. Riv Sper Freniatr 1932, **56**, 269.
17. Nance MA, Berry SA. Cockayne syndrome: a review of 140 cases. Am J Med Genet 1992, **42**, 68–84.
18. Arlett CF, Lehmann AR. Xeroderma pigmentosa, Cockayne syndrome and trichothiodystrophy: sun-sensitive to DNA repair defects in skin cancer. In: Genetic pre-disposition to cancer (ed. RA Eeles, BAJ Ponder, DF Easton, A Horwich). Chapman & Hall, London, 1996, 185–206.
19. Lindahl T, Nyberg B. Rate of depurination of native deoxyribonucleic acid. Biochemistry 1972, **11**, 3610–18.
20. Lynch HT, Smyrk T. Hereditary non-polyposis colorectal cancer. Cancer 1996, **78**, 1149–67.
21. Svejstrup JQ, Wang Z, Feaver WJ, Wu X, Bushnell DA, et al. Different forms of TFIIH for transcription in DNA repair. Cell 1995, **80**, 21–8.
22. Li FP, Fraumeni JF. Rhabdomyosarcoma in children: an epidemiologic study and identification of a familial cancer syndrome. J Nat Cancer Inst 1969, **43**, 1364–73.
23. Kleihues P, Schauble B, zur Hausen A, Esteve J, Ohgaki H. Tumors associated with p53 germline mutations: a synopsis of 91 families. Am J Pathol 1997, **15**, 1–13.
24. Lustbader ED, Williams WR, Bondy ML, Strom S, Strong LC. Segregation analysis of cancer in families of childhood soft-tissue-sarcoma patients. Am J Hum Genet 1992, **51**, 344–56.
25. Birch JM, Blair V, Kelsey AM, Evans DG, Harris M, Tricker KJ et al. Cancer phenotype correlates with constitutional TP53 genotype in families with the Li–Fraumeni syndrome. Oncogene 1998, **17**, 1061–8.
26. Malkin D, Friend SH, Li FP, Strong LC. Germ-line mutations of the p53 tumor-suppressor gene in children and young adults with second malignant neoplasms. N Engl J Med 1997, **336**, 734.
27. Hisada M, Garber JE, Fung CY, Fraumeni JF Jr, Li FP. Multiple primary cancers in families with Li–Fraumeni syndrome. J Nat Cancer Inst 1998, **90**, 606–11.
28. Varley JM, Evans DGR, Birch JM. Li–Fraumeni syndrome: a molecular and clinical review. Brit J Cancer 1997, **76**, 1–14.
29. Driver CP, Birch J, Gough DC, Bruce J. Adrenal cortical tumors in childhood. Pediatr Hematol Oncol 1998, **15**, 527–32.
30. Lebihan C, Moutou C, Brugieres L, Feunteun J, Bonaiti-Pellie C. ARCAD: a method for estimating age dependent disease risk associated with mutation carrier status from family data. Genet Epidemiol 1995, **12**, 13–25.
31. Varley JM, McGown G, Thorncroft M, James LA, Margison GP, Forster G et al. Are there low-penetrance TP53 alleles? Evidence from childhood adrenocortical tumors. Am J Hum Genet 1999, **65**, 995–1006.
32. Soussi T, Caron de Fromentel C, May P. Structural aspects of the p53 protein in relation to gene evolution. Oncogene 1990, **5**, 945–52.
33. Lane DP, Crawford LV. T antigen is bound to a host protein in SV40-transformed cells. Nature 1979, **278**, 261–3.

34. Lane DP. Cancer. p53, guardian of the genome. Nature 2 July 1992, **358**, 15–16.
35. Malkin D, Li FP, Strong LC, Fraumeni JF Jr, Nelson CE, Kim DH et al. Germ line p53 mutations in a familial syndrome of breast cancer, sarcomas, and other neoplasms. Science 1990, **250**, 1233–8.
36. Bell DW, Varley JM, Szydlo TE, Kang DH, Wahrer DCR, Shannon KE et al. Heterozygous germ line hCHK2 mutations in Li–Fraumeni syndrome. Science 1999, **286**, 2528–31.
37. Varley JM, McGown G, Thorncroft M, Santibanez-Koref MF, Kelsey AM, Tricker KJ et al. Germ-line mutations of TP53 in Li–Fraumeni families: an extended study of 39 families. Cancer Res 1997, **57**, 3245–52.
38. Schneider KA, Patenaude AF, Garber JE. Testing for cancer genes: decisions, decisions. Nat Med 1995, **1**, 302–3.
39. Eeles RA. Predictive testing for germline mutations in the p53 gene: are all the questions answered? Eur J Cancer 1993, **29A(10)**, 1361–5.
40. Birch JM, Heighway J, Teare MD, Kelsey AM, Hartley AL, Tricker KJ et al. Linkage studies in a Li–Fraumeni family with increased expression of p53 protein but no germline mutation in p53. Br J Cancer 1994, **70**, 1176–81.
41. Trump D, Farren B, Wooding C, Pang JT, Besser GM, Buchanan KD et al. Clinical studies of multiple endocrine neoplasia type 1. QJM 1996, **8**, 653–69.
42. Marx SJ, Agarwal SK, Kester MB, Heppner C, Kim YS, Skarulis MC et al. Multiple endocrine neoplasia type 1: clinical and genetic features of the hereditary endocrine neoplasias. Recent Prog Horm Res 1999, **54**, 397–438.
43. Giraud S, Zhang CX, Serova-Sinilnikova O, Wautot V, Salandre J, Buisson N et al. Germ-line mutation analysis in patients with multiple endocrine neoplasia type 1 and related disorders. Am J Hum Genet 1998, **63**, 455–6.
44. Bassett JH, Forbes SA, Pannett AA, Lloyd SE, Christie PT, Wooding C et al. Characterization of mutations in patients with multiple endocrine neoplasia type 1. Am J Hum Genet 1998, **62**, 232–44.
45. Mathew CG, Easton DF, Nakamura Y, Ponder BA. Presymptomatic screening for multiple endocrine neoplasia type 2A with linked DNA markers. The MEN 2A International Collaborative Group. Lancet 1991, **337**, 7–11.
46. Skinner MA, Wells SA Jr. Medullary carcinoma of the thyroid gland and the MEN 2 syndromes. Semin Pediatr Surg 1997, **6**, 134–40.
47. Guru SC, Goldsmith PK, Burns AL, Marx SJ, Spiegel AM, Collins FS et al. Menin, the product of the MEN1 gene, is a nuclear protein. Proc Natl Acad Sci USA 1998, **95**, 1630–4.
48. Versteege L, Sevenet N, Lange J, et al. Truncating mutations of hSNF5/INI1 in aggressive paediatric cancers. Nature 1998, **394**, 203–7.
49. Sevenet N, Sheridan E, Amram D, Schneider P, Handgretinger R, Delattre O. Constitutional mutations of the hSNF5/INI1 gene predispose to a variety of cancers. Am J Hum Genet 1999, **65(5)**, 1342–8.
50. Huson SM, Compston DAS, Clark P, Harper PS. A genetic study of von Recklinghausen neurofibromatosis in South East Wales. I. Prevalence, fitness, mutation rate and effect of parental transmission on severity. J Med Genet 1989, **26**, 704–11.
51. National Institutes of Health. Neurofibromatosis. Conference statement. National Institutes of Health Consensus Development Conference. Arch Neurol 1998, **45**, 575–8.
52. Crowe FW, Schull WL, Neel JV. A clinical pathological and genetic study of multiple neurofibromatosis (ed. Charles C Thomas), Springfield, IL, 1956.
53. Riccardi Vm, Lewis RA. Penetrance of von recklinghausen neurofibromatosis: a distinction between predecessors and descendants. Am J Hum Genet **42**, 1988, 284–9.
54. Riccardi VM. Neurofibromatosis: phenotype, natural history, and pathogenesis, 2nd edn. Johns Hopkins University Press, Baltimore, 1992.
55. Korf BR. Diagnostic outcome in children with multiple café au lait spots. Pediatrics 1992, **90**, 924–7.
56. Friedman JM, Birch PH. Type 1 neurofibromatosis: a descriptive analysis of the disorder in 1,728 patients. Am J Med Genet 1997, **70**, 138–43.
57. Obringer AC, Meadows AT, Zackai EH. The diagnosis of neurofibromatosis-1 in the child under the age of 6 years. Am J Dis Child 1989, **143**, 717–19.
58. Upadhyaya M, Shaw DJ, Harper PS. Molecular basis of neurofibromatosis type 1 (NF1): mutation analysis and polymorphisms in the NF1 gene. Human Mutat 1994, **4**, 83–101.
59. Lazaro C, Gaona A, Ainsworth P, et al. Sex differences in mutational rate and mutational mechanism in the NF1 gene in neurofibromatosis type 1 patients. Hum Genet 1996, **98**, 696–9.
60. Upadhyaya M, Ruggieri M, Maynard J, Osborn M, Hartog C, Mudd S, Penttinen M, Cordeiro I, Ponder M, Ponder BA, Krawczak M, Cooper DN. Gross deletions of the neurofibromatosis type 1 (NF1) gene are predominantly of maternal origin and commonly associated with a learning disability, dysmorphic features and developmental delay. Hum Genet 1998, **102**, 591–7.
61. Hope DG, Mulvihill JJ. Malignancy in neurofibromatosis. Adv Neurol 1981, **29**, 33–55.
62. Sorenson SA, Mulvihill JJ, Nielsen A. Long term follow up of von Recklinghausen neurofibromatosis: survival and malignant neoplasms. N Engl J Med 1986, **314**, 1010–15.
63. Poyhonen M, Niemela S, Herva R. Risk of malignancy and death in neurofibromatosis. Arch Pathol Lab Med 1997, **121**, 139–43.
64. Fineman JL, Yakovac DA. Neurofibroamtosis in childhood. J Pediatrics 1970, **76**, 339–46.
65. Cole WG, Meyers NA. Neurofibromatosis in childhood. Aust NZ J Surg 1978, **48**, 360–5.
66. Crawford AH. Neurofibromatosis in children. Acta Orthop Scan (Suppl) 1986, **218**, 1–60.
67. Blatt J, Jaffe R, Duetsch M, Adkins AD. Neurofibromatosis and childhood tumours. Cancer 1986, **57**, 1225–9.
68. Matsui I, Tanimura M, Kobayashi N, Sawada T, Nagahara N, Akatsuka J. Neurofibromatosis type 1 and childhood cancer. Cancer 1993, **72**, 2746–54.
69. Shearer P, Parham D, Kovnar E, Kun L, Rao B, Lobe T, Pratt C. Neurofibromatosis type 1 and malignancy: a review of 32 pediatric cases treated at a single institution. N Engl J Med 1994, **330**, 597–601.
70. Bader JL, Miller. Neurofibromatosis and childhood leukaemia. J Pediatr 1978, **92**, 925–9.

71. Stiller CA, Chessells JM, Fitchett M. Neurofibromatosis and childhood leukaemia/lymphoma: a population-based UKCCSG study. Br J Cancer 1994, 70, 969–72.
72. Lewis RA, Gerson LP, Axelson KA, Riccardi VM, Whitford RP. von Recklinghausen neurofibromatosis, incidence of optic glioma. Ophthalmology 1984, 88, 348–54.
73. Listernick R, Charrow J, Greenwald M, Mets M. Natural history of optic pathway tumors in children with neurofibromatosis type 1: a longitudinal study. J Pediatr 1994, 125, 63–6.
74. Listernick R, Darling C, Greenwald M, Strauss L, Charrow J. Optic pathway tumors in children: the effect of neurofibromatosis type 1 on clinical manifestations and natural history. J Pediatr 1995, 127, 718–22.
75. Ferner RE. Clinical aspects of neurofibromatosis 1. In: Neurofibromatosis type 1; from genotype to phenotype (ed. M Upadhyaya, DS Cooper). Bios Scientific, Oxford, UK.
76. Danoff BF, Kramer S, Thompson N. The radiotherapeutic management of optic gliomas of children. Int J Radiat Oncol Biol Phys 1980, 6, 45–50.
77. Molloy P, Sutton L, Yachnis AT, et al. Brainstem neoplasms. Med Pediatr Oncol 1995, 24, 379–87.
78. Pollack IF, Shultz B, Mulvihill JJ. The management of brainstem gliomas in patients with neurofibromatosis 1. Neurology 1996, 46, 1652–60.
79. Huson SM, Harper PS, Compston DAS. von Recklinghausen neurofibromatosis: a clinical and population study in South Wales. Brain 1998, 111, 1355–81.
80. Korf BR. Plexiform Neurofibromas. Am J Med Genet (Semin Med Genet) 1999, 89, 31–7.
81. Tonsgard JH, Kwak SM, Short MP, Dachman AH. CT imaging in adults with neurofibromatosis-1: frequent asymptomatic plexiform lesions. Neurology 1998, 50, 1755–60.
82. Schorry EK, Crawford AH, Egelhoff JC, et al. Thoracic tumors in children with neurofibromatosis-1. Am J Med Genet 1997, 74, 533–7.
83. Needle MN, Cnaan A, Dattilo J, et al. Prognostic signs in the surgical managementof plexiform neurofibroma— The Children's Hospital of Philadelphia experience, 1974–1994. J Pediatr 1997, 131, 678–82.
84. Waggoner DJ, Towbin J, Gottesman G, Gutmann DH. Clinic-based study of plexiform neurofibromas in neurofibromatosis 1. Am J Med Genet 2000, 92, 132–5.
85. Niemeyer CM, Arico M, Basso G, Biondi A, Cantu Rajnoldi A, Creutzig U, Haas O, Harbott J, Hasle H, Kerndrup G, Locatelli F, Mann G, Stollmann-Gibbels B, van't Veer-Korthof ET, van Wering E, Zimmermann M. Chronic myelomonocytic leukemia in childhood: a retrospective analysis of 110 cases. European Working Group on Myelodysplastic Syndromes in Childhood (EWOG-MDS). Blood 1997, 89, 3534–43.
86. Yeazel MW, Ross JA, Buckley JD, Woods WG, Ruccione K, Robinosn LL. High birth weight and the risk of the specific childhood cancers: a report from the Childrens Cancer Group. J Pediatr 1997, 131, 671–6.
87. Suminoe A, Matsuzaki A, Kinukawa N. Rapid somatic growth after birth in children with neuroblastoma: a survey of 1718 patients with childhood cancer in the Kyushu-Okinawa district. J Pediatr 1999, 134, 178–84.
88. Neri G, Gurrieri F, Zanni G, Lin A. Clinical and molecular aspects of the Simpson–Golabi–Behmel syndrome. Am J Med Genet 1998, 79, 279–83.
89. Pilia G, Hughes-Benzie RM, MacKenzie A, Baybayan P, Chen EY, Huber R, Neri G, Cao A, Forabosco A, Schlessinger D. Mutations in GPC3, a glypican gene, cause the Simpson–Golabi–Behmel overgrowth syndrome. Nature Genet 1996, 12, 241–7.
90. Elliott M, Bayly R, Cole T, Temple IK, Maher ER. Clinical features and natural history of Beckwith–Wiedemann syndrome: presentation of 74 new cases. Clin Genet 1994, 46, 168–74.
91. Pettenati MJ, Haines JL, Higgins RR, Wappner RS, Palmer CG, Weaver DD. Wiedemann–Beckwith syndrome: presentation of clinical and cytogenetic data on 22 new cases and review of the literature. Hum Genet 1986, 74, 143–54.
92. Chitayat D, Friedman JM, Dimmick JE. Neuroblastoma in a child with Wiedemann–Beckwith syndrome. Am J Med Genet 1990, 35, 433–6.
93. Elliott M, Maher ER. Beckwith–Wiedemann syndrome. J Med Genet 1994, 31, 560–4.
94. Weng EY, Moeschler JB, Graham JM Jr. Longitudinal observations on 15 children with Wiedemann–Beckwith syndrome. Am J Med Genet 1995, 56, 366–73.
95. Hoyme HE, Seaver LH, Jones KL, Procopio F, Crooks W, Feingold M. Isolated hemihyperplasia (hemihypertrophy): report of a prospective multicenter study of the incidence of neoplasia and review. Am J Med Genet 1998, 79, 274–8.
96. Borer JG, Kaefer M, Barnewolt CE, Elias ER, Hobbs N, Retik AB, Peters CA. Renal findings on radiological follow up of patients with Beckwith–Wiedemann syndrome. J Urol 1999, 161, 235–9.
97. Slavotinek A, Gaunt L, Donnai D. Paternally inherited duplications of 11p15.5 and Beckwith–Wiedemann syndrome. J Med Genet 1997, 34, 819–26.
98. Beckwith JB. Nephrogenic rests and the pathogenesis of Wilms' tumor: developmental and clinical considerations. Am J Med Genet 1998, 79, 268–73.
99. Clericuzio CL, D'Angio GJ, Duncan M, et al. Summary and recommendations of the workshop held at the First International Conference on Molecular and Clinical Genetics of Childhood Renal Tumors, Albuquerque, New Mexico, 14–16 May 1992. Med Pediatr Oncol 1993, 21, 233–6.
100. Barlow DP. Imprinting: a gamete's point of view. Trends Genet 1994, 10, 194–9.
101. Weksberg R, Shen DR, Fei YL, Song QL, Squire J. Disruption of insulin-like growth factor 2 imprinting in Beckwith–Wiedemann syndrome. Nat Genet 1993, 5, 143–50.
102. Steenman MJ, Rainier S, Dobry CJ, Grundy P, Horon IL, Feinberg AP. Loss of imprinting of IGF2 is linked to reduced expression and abnormal methylation of H19 in Wilms' tumour. Nat Genet 1994, 7, 433–9.
103. Hatada I, Ohashi H, Fukushima Y, Kaneko Y, Inoue M, Komoto Y, Okada A, Ohishi S, Nabetani A, Morisaki H, Nakayama M, Niikawa N, Mukai T. An imprinted gene p57KIP2 is mutated in Beckwith–Wiedemann syndrome. Nat Genet 1996, 14, 171–3.

104. Lee MP, DeBaun M, Randhawa G, Reichard BA, Elledge SJ, Feinberg AP. Low frequency of *p57KIP2* mutation in Beckwith–Wiedemann syndrome. Am J Hum Genet 1997, **61**, 304–9.
105. Steenman M, Westerveld A, Mannens M. Genetics of Beckwith Wiedemann Syndrome associated tumours: common genetic pathways. Genes Chromosomes Cancer 2000, **28**, 1–13.
106. Bliek J, Maas SM, Ruitjer JM, Hennekam RCMM, Alders M, Westerveld A, Mannens MMAM. Increased tumour risk for BWS patients correlates with aberrant H19 and not KCNQ1OT1 methylation: occurrence of KCNQ1OT1 hypomethylation in familial cases of BWS. Hum Mol Genet 2001, **10**, 467–71.
107. Jones JI, Clemmons DR. Insulin-like growth factors and their binding proteins: biological actions. Endocr Rev 1995, **1**, 3–34.
108. Brown KW, Villar AJ, Bickmore W, Clayton-Smith J, Catchpoole D, Maher ER, Reik W. Imprinting mutation in the Beckwith–Wiedemann syndrome leads to biallelic IGF2 expression through an H19-independent pathway. Hum Mol Genet 1996, **12**, 2027–32.
109. O'Keefe D, Dao D, Zhao L, Sanderson R, Warburton D, Weiss L, Anyane-Yeboa K, Tycko B. Coding mutations in p57KIP2 are present in some cases of Beckwith–Wiedemann syndrome but are rare or absent in Wilms' tumors. Am J Hum Genet 1997, **61**, 295–303.
110. Hatada I, Nabetani A, Morisaki H, Xin Z, Ohishi S, Tonoki H, Niikawa N, Inoue M, Komoto Y, Okada A, Steichen E, Ohashi H, Fukushima Y, Nakayama M, Mukai T. New *p57KIP2* mutations in Beckwith–Wiedemann syndrome. Hum Genet 1997, **100**, 681–3.
111. Haber DA. Wilms' tumor in the genetic basis of human cancer (ed. B Vogelstein, KW Kinzler). McGraw Hill, New York, 1998.
112. Mueller RF. The Denys Drash syndrome. J Med Genet 1994, **31**, 471–7.

Section 2
Childhood Cancers

5 | Leukemia

Sheila Weitzman and Jeremy A. Squire

Leukemia is the commonest cancer in children, comprising 25–30% of malignant disease in this population. From being universally fatal, today the cure rate of patients with acute lymphoblastic leukemia (ALL) has reached approximately 75% and that of acute myeloid leukemia (AML) approximately 40%. The improvement in survival has occurred as a result of improvements in methods of diagnosis and classification, a better understanding of leukemia cell biology and of the various clinical and biological prognostic factors, which dictate therapy. Further significant improvements in survival however, will require new approaches to therapy. Better understanding of the leukemic cell at the molecular level will ultimately allow therapy to be selectively directed at specific molecular targets on the malignant cell.

Classification of childhood leukemia

All leukemias appear to arise from a mutational event, which results in an arrest in maturation, followed by clonal proliferation of an early hematopoetic precursor cell (1). ALL occurs as a result of clonal proliferation of lymphoid precursors and accounts for 80% of pediatric leukemia, while AML and chronic myelocytic leukemia (CML) comprise 17% and 3%, respectively. Chronic lymphocytic leukemia (CLL), is almost never diagnosed in the pediatric age range.

Epidemiology

ALL is the commonest cancer of children, with an annual incidence in North America of approximately 4.4 cases/100,000 White children below the age of 15 years (2). In the White child there is a characteristic 3–5-year old age peak, which is absent in the Black child leading to an overall lower incidence of ALL in Black children. This peak is just starting to be seen at a lower level in Black children in developed countries, suggesting an environmental influence.

Unlike ALL, the annual incidence of AML is constant from birth through the first 10 years, followed by a slight peak in adolescence. AML does not show a predelicting for any racial group. A 20% cumulative increase in the reported incidence from 1973 to 1991 (3) may be due to improved diagnosis or reporting, or may be due to increased exposure of child or parents to environmental hazards such as pesticides or ionizing radiation. Non-ionizing radiation in the form of low-energy electromagnetic fields has also been implicated in childhood leukemia, but reports have been inconsistent and lack plausible biological mechanisms.

Drugs such as the topoisomerase II inhibitors result in secondary AML usually of the M4 and M5 subtype. Similarly, the alykylating agents, which produce deletions or losses of chromosomes, particularly 5 and 7, are associated with a risk of myelodysplasia and myeloid leukemias. Therapeutic doses of ionizing radiation are associated with an increased risk of AML, whereas radiogenic ALL has mainly been associated with Japanese survivors of the atomic bomb who were less than 20 years old at the time of exposure (4). Some constitutional genetic defects such as trisomy 21 (Down's syndrome, DS) ataxia–telangectasia, Bloom's syndrome, and Fanconi's anemia have been linked to an increased incidence of leukemia, as have germ-line $p53$ mutations (Li–Fraumeni syndrome). ALL is the commonest form of leukemia in DS children over the age of 3, whereas megakaryoblastic leukemia predominates in the younger Down's patients (5). Bloom's syndrome is usually associated with AML but ALL does occur, while Fanconi's syndrome is more commonly associated with acute myelomonocytic leukemia, and ataxia–telangectasia with T-ALL. Patients with congenital disorders of myelopoeisis such as Kostmann's disease (severe congenital neutropenia), Schwachmann's syndrome, and Diamond–Blackfan anemia are at risk of developing AML. Children with neurofibromatosis type1 (NF-1) have an increased risk of developing myeloid malignancies and the *NF-1* gene may function as a tumor suppressor gene in these malignancies (6). Children with various congenital immunodeficiency syndromes have an increased risk of developing lymphoid malignancies, predominantly lymphomas, but ALL may occur. Thirty percent of ALL patients have low immunoglobulin levels at diagnosis, but whether this precedes or is secondary to the leukemia, is unclear.

There is a 2–4-fold increased risk of ALL in siblings as compared to the normal population and a high concordance in young identical twins, thought to be due to sharing of cells through the placental circulation. In the majority of cases however, the etiology of leukemia remains unknown, reflecting the complexity of the genetic mechanisms that provide the biological "targets" for leukemogenesis (7).

Infant leukemia differs from that of older children in clinical, morphologic, immunologic, and genetic presentation. Unlike childhood leukemia where ALL is four times commoner than AML, the ratio in infants is approximately 1:1 (8). Infant AML typically presents with M4 and M5 morphology, high blast counts, organomegaly, and extramedullary involvement with leukemia cutis and CNS involvement (8). There is a striking female preponderance in the infant, whereas the male predominates in older ALL patients. About 60% of infant AML and 80% of infant ALL is associated with MLL gene rearrangements (see later). Identical rearrangements are seen after therapy with DNA topoisomerase inhibitors and it has been hypothesized that maternal exposure to naturally occurring topoisomerase inhibitors, particularly in the diet, may be causally related to infant leukemia (9).

Acute lymphoblastic leukemia

The extraordinary improvement in survival in childhood ALL began with the development of single agent chemotherapy that induced remissions and prolonged life, but did not cure. Development of combinations of agents started the process toward cure, soon followed by the introduction of central nervous system (CNS)-directed therapy. Evaluation of the results of multi-institutional trials allowed recognition of a group of patients at high risk for relapse and intensification of therapy for this group of patients boosted cure rates, and ushered in the era of "risk-adapted" therapy. The major technologic advances that coincided with the therapeutic advances, has allowed significant refinement of the risk-stratification criteria.

Modern treatment protocols for ALL are based on an accurate clinical and biologic characterization of patients at the time of diagnosis. This enables the "tailoring" of therapy to the risk of relapse, allowing for intensification of therapy for those at high risk and, equally importantly, a reduction in intensity of therapy and thereby toxicity, for those at lesser risk. In support of this "risk-adapted" approach is the fact that in recent years, treatment has emerged as the most important risk factor for survival (10).

Clinical risk factors

As therapy for ALL improved, it became clear that children could be divided into lower, standard, and high-risk groups based on a combination of clinical and biologic criteria. Today a very-high-risk group is being proposed in addition. Different cooperative groups used different clinical criteria to define the risk groups, but criteria common to all included the age of the child, the white cell count at diagnosis, the presence or absence of sanctuary disease, the tumor burden, and the cell of origin.

Age

Infants younger than 12 months of age at diagnosis, and particularly those less than 6 months of age, do poorly in all series. Infant ALL is often associated with other high-risk features such as high leukocyte counts, a higher incidence of organomegaly, CNS disease, CD10 negativity, and 11q23 (*MLL* gene) rearrangements, all of which are known to predict a poor response to therapy. Infants without 11q23 abnormalities and whose blasts are CD10 positive have an outcome comparable to older children, with 67% EFS at 3 years compared to 13% for those with *MLL* rearrangements (11).

Children over the age of 10 years at diagnosis have also been shown to be at higher risk, and intensification of therapy in this group has resulted in significant improvements in survival.

Leukocyte count

Early studies showed an almost linear relationship between increasing white cell counts and the risk of failure. Review of collapsed data from the Pediatric Oncology Group

(POG) and the Children's Cancer Group (CCG), showed that patients who were between 1 and 9.99 years of age with leukocyte counts $<50 \times 10^9$/l, had an 80.3% 4-year event-free survival (EFS), compared to 66.9% for those with leukocyte counts $>50 \times 10^9$/l, and 41.1% for those who were both >10 years and had leukocyte counts $>50 \times 10^9$/l. Participants at a National Cancer Institute (NCI) sponsored conference to standardize risk groups, agreed that age >10 years and leukocyte counts $>50 \times 10^9$/l should define the high-risk group (12).

Changes in other parameters of the blood count are also considered to be of importance, although they are not generally used for risk-group allocation. A hemoglobin of >100 g/l at diagnosis is felt to indicate a poorer prognosis. One explanation is that a more aggressively dividing blast population will reach the level necessary for clinical presentation (10^{10} cells) before the red cell population falls below the 100 g/l mark. By contrast, the much shorter half-life of platelets (9 days) means that a low platelet count merely reflects a high tumor burden and thus also a poorer prognosis.

Other indicators of tumor burden such as the degree of hepatosplenomegaly and of lymphadenopathy, as well as the presence of a mediastinal mass, are also felt to denote a higher relapse risk. These manifestations of the "lymphoma syndrome" are however no longer used as independent criteria to dictate therapy.

Gender

The prognostic value of gender varies between studies. Some studies report no difference in outcome by gender (5) while others show a higher relapse rate for boys (1, 13). This difference may be explained by the 10% risk of testicular leukemia in boys as well as by differences in the metabolism of chemotherapy. There also appears to be a gender difference in the ability to tolerate certain therapies, with females demonstrating greater sensitivity to the deleterious effects of cranial irradiation than their male counterparts.

Sanctuary disease

As well as testicular disease, involvement of other sanctuary areas such as the CNS increases the risk of failure and mandates a more intensive treatment protocol. The occurrence of CNS leukemia at diagnosis is relatively uncommon, occurring in less than 5% of pediatric ALL patients (14). Recent studies suggest that CNS disease status at diagnosis should be reported using the following definitions: CNS-1 (no blast cells), CNS-2 (<5 wbcs/μl with blast cells), and CNS-3 (>5 wbcs/μl with blast cells or cranial nerve palsy). An adverse prognosis for CNS-2 patients has been described by investigators from POG and the St Jude Chidren's Research Hospital (SJCRH) but not by CCG and this issue will be further evaluated in the current ALL studies (12).

Response to therapy

Response to therapy is considered to be one of the most important indicators of prognosis. The number of peripheral blasts following 7 days of steroids was found to be independently prognostic in early B-lineage ALL and in T-cell ALL (15), while investigators from CCG showed the importance of the number of residual marrow blasts at day 7 and day 14, with the day 7 count being a more sensitive predictor of response in higher risk patients (16). The adverse prognostic significance of a slow early response could be eliminated by intensification of therapy however (17) underlining the importance of this evaluation.

With the refining of the biologic criteria for risk allocation, certain of the clinical criteria are no longer considered to be independently prognostic. Thus in the POG studies for example, the age and white cell count dictate the induction therapy (3 versus 4 drug), but the finding of favorable cytogenetics may allow "promotion" of the patient to a lower risk group, just as a slow response to therapy would dictate a very-high-risk group. All the criteria, clinical and biological are therefore considered in the final risk allocation.

Biologic factors

At a biologic level, ALL is a heterogenous disease that varies in the cell lineage of leukemic blasts, their degree of cellular differentiation, and in their underlying genetic abnormalities (18).

ALL may be broadly classified into disease of T- or B-cell origin. Approximately 85% of pediatric ALL is of B-lineage and 15% T-lineage. B-lineage ALL is further subdivided into four distinct subtypes: early B-lineage, pre-B-cell ALL, and mature B-cell ALL. A newly described subtype, transitional B-cell ALL is seen in 1% of patients. Subclassification of T-ALL according to the stage of thymocyte differentiation appears to also be of prognostic significance (10, 23).

Light microscopy

Blast cells are easy to recognize microscopically and the diagnosis of childhood leukemia is made on examination

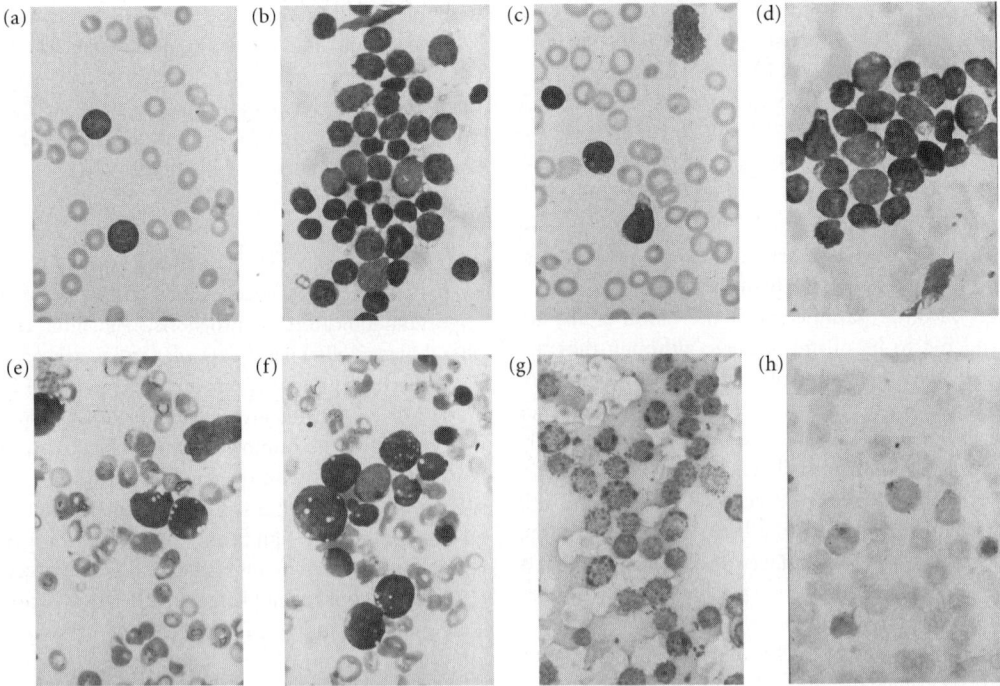

Fig. 5.1 (a) Peripheral blood smear. ALL, L1 subtype. These blasts, as shown here, are characterized by a uniform population of cells with a high nuclear:cytoplasmic ratio, homogeneous nuclear chromatin, and indistinct nucleoli. The L1 blast may have absent or small, indistinct nucleoli and variable cytoplasmic vacuolization. (b) Bone marrow aspirate smear. ALL, L1 subtype. Small homogeneous blasts are evident in this hypercellular specimen. (c) Peripheral blood smear. ALL, L2 subtype. As shown here, the L2 subtype is morphologically heterogeneous. These large cells have a variable nuclear:cytoplasmic ratio, heterogeneous nuclear chromatin, and one or more prominent nucleoli. Nuclear cleavage and indentation are common, and cytoplasmic vacuolization may be present in the L2 blast. Note the adult lymphocyte and smudge cell. (d) Bone marrow aspirate smear. ALL, L2 subtype. The heterogeneity of the L2 blast is seen in this hypercellular specimen. Note the "punched out" nucleoli and variability in size. (e) Peripheral blood smear. ALL, L3 subtype. These blasts are large cells with moderately abundant, vacuolated, basophilic cytoplasm; finely stippled, homogeneous nuclear chromatin; and prominent nucleoli. The L3 blast usually has one or more prominent nucleoli. (f) Bone marrow aspirate smear. ALL, L3 subtype. This specimen shows the vacuoles and the finely stippled nuclei typical of the L3 blast. (g) Bone marrow aspirate smear. ALL. The PAS stain is positive in approximately 50% of ALL cases and is characterized by large fuchsia aggregates or blocks on a clear cytoplasmic background. (h) Bone marrow aspirate smear. T-cell blasts have clusters of cytoplasmic granules that are demonstrated by staining for acid phosphatase. (Reproduced with the permission of The Upjohn Company Inc.)

of Romanowsky stains of blood and bone marrow smears. Differentiation of lymphoid and myeloid blasts can usually be made morphologically, but is always confirmed using other techniques.

The French/American/British (FAB) classification divides ALL blasts into three subtypes, L1, L2, and L3, based on light microscopic features (Fig. 5.1) (1). L1 is the commonest subtype in children representing 85% of childhood ALL, while L2 is the predominant subtype in adults. The L3 subtype (less than 5% of cases), has been shown to be characteristic of B-ALL. The distinction between L1 and L2, originally thought to be prognostic, has not proved to be useful, and there is no correlation of these latter subtypes with immunologic markers.

Cytochemistry

Cytochemical evaluation of leukemic blasts is usually done using myeloperoxidase or Sudan black, Periodic Acid Schiff (PAS), chloroacetate esterase (specific esterase), and nonspecific esterase (NSE) stains. PAS block positivity is seen in ALL and should be distinguished from the discrete granules which may be seen in normal blood cells. Myeloperoxidase and Sudan black positivity is seen in myeloblasts while the positive NSE stain, which is inhibited by fluoride, characterizes monoblasts (19). These stains will therefore usually distinguish ALL from AML and monoblasts from myeloblasts, but most laboratories will confirm the diagnosis with immunophenotyping and chromosomal studies.

In some cases biochemical analysis of the activity of certain enzymes may be useful. Terminal deoxytransferase (TdT), an enzyme not found in normal lymphocytes, is found in the lymphoblasts of all but mature B-cell ALL. TdT determination is thus useful in differentiating lymphocytes from lymphoblasts in the cerebrospinal fluid (CSF). Acid phosphatase positivity, usually demonstrated as focal paranuclear concentrations, can differentiate T-cell from non-T-cell ALL (3).

Immunophenotype

Differences in the expression of surface membrane and cytoplasmic antigens are used to classify leukemias. Virtually all known single antigens as well as immunoglobulin and T-cell receptor gene rearrangements lack lineage specificity however, and the immunophenotypic classification is based on the pattern of reactivity to multiple antibodies. A panel of lineage-associated antibodies is thus used to classify ALL into immunologic subtypes, which reflect the cell of origin and the stage of lymphoid differentiation at which the malignant transformation occurred.

B-lineage ALL

Early B-cell ALL

The majority of childhood ALL, and those associated with the best prognosis, are of early B-lineage, characterized by the presence of the B-lineage antigens CD19 and CD22 and the absence of expression of cytoplasmic or surface immunoglobulin (Ig). Most also express CD10, the lineage-independent common ALL antigen (CALLA), as well as HLA-DR(Ia) antigen. CD10 expression is present on leukemic cells of both T- and B-lineage and its role in leukemic cell proliferation and differentiation is uncertain. Nearly half of infants with ALL, and 10% of older children (>10 years of age) do not express CD10. This lack, which likely represents a more immature early pre-B ALL, is associated with pseudoploidy, high leukocyte counts, and a poorer prognosis (3). Among the immunological subtypes of ALL, early B-cell cases are more likely to have features predictive of a good outcome such as favorable age and lower leukocyte counts, and the 4-year EFS for this group is approximately 80%.

Pre-B ALL

The presence of CD20 plus Cig denotes a later stage in B-cell development, and characterizes the pre-B ALL subtype, which makes up approximately 30% of B-precursor ALL. The prognosis for patients with pre-B-ALL appears to depend on the presence or absence of the commonly associated t(1;19) translocation. Patients with blasts that are CD20+, Cig+, Sig−, and that lack t(1;19), appear to fare well on standard-risk chemotherapy protocols while those that are t(1;19) positive require more intensive therapy for cure (20). Myeloablative therapy with stem cell replacement does not appear to be necessary for these children, however.

Transitional pre-B cell ALL

This is a newly characterized subtype occurring in approximately 1% of ALL cases. The hallmark is the expression of Igµ heavy chains on the cell surface without light chain expression. Transitional B-cell disease has an excellent outcome with conventional anti-metabolite-based chemotherapy (21).

Mature B-cell ALL

It is diagnosed by the presence of Ig heavy and light chains on the surface of the cell (Sig+), in addition to the B-lineage surface antigens CD19, CD22, and CD20. B-ALL occurs in less than 5% of patients, and morphologically is often FAB L3. The blast cells usually show the chromosomal translocations typical of Burkitt's lymphoma (see section on Genetic factors). Some cases of mature B-cell ALL do not show L3 morphology and have lymphoma-like features and particular karyotypic abnormalities such as 6q−, 14q+, t(11,14), or t(14,18) (21).

Patients with mature B-cell disease, once thought to have a very poor prognosis, now have cure rates in excess of 80% with short but very intensive chemotherapy regimens designed to reflect the very rapid growth rate of cells with this phenotype (22). B-ALL is the first leukemia to be treated by protocols designed specifically for its unique features.

T-lineage ALL

T-lineage leukemia, comprising ~15% of childhood ALL, is diagnosed by the presence of the T-cell markers CD3, CD7, CD5, or CD2. Immunophenotyping with monoclonal antibodies to T-cell antigens that correspond to different stages of normal intrathymic differentiation, has shown that in general T-ALL consists of cells in the early to intermediate thymocyte stage and that patients with pro-T-ALL (CD7+, CD2−, CD1−, CD4−, CD8−) have a significantly worse prognosis than those with intermediate [CD7+, (CD2+ or CD5+), CD3−] or mature T-ALL (CD7+, CD2+, CD5+, CD3+) (23). Patients with CD10 negative T-lymphoblasts also fare significantly worse (10) while those with blasts that are CD2+ (E-rosette positive) have a better outlook (23).

T-cell ALL is commonly associated with several poor prognostic features, namely male sex, older age, a high leukocyte count, CNS+ disease, and the presence of a mediastinal mass. Recent studies suggest that the inclusion of high-dose methotrexate, high-dose cytarabine, and l'asparaginase have improved the EFS for T-ALL to around 70% (23). Investigators from CCG found that children with T-ALL who presented without other adverse features (4% of childhood ALL) had a comparable survival to B-lineage ALL, and that the T-cell phenotype was not independently prognostic (12). Other study groups continue to treat all T-ALL patients on specific T-cell protocols regardless of age and leukocyte count.

A new and promising targeted therapy for T-lineage leukemia are the deoxyguanosine analogs which appear to be selectively toxic to T-cells. Compound 506U78, a prodrug derivative of Ara-G(9-β-D-arabinofuranosylguanine) has been shown to achieve toxic levels of Ara-GTP in T-lineage leukemic cells and its use is being studied in pediatric T-cell malignancies (23).

Mixed-lineage leukemia

Myeloid-associated antigens have been reported in up to 24% of childhood ALL cases and lymphoid-associated antigens in up to 50% of childhood AML. Leukemic blasts coexpressing T and B and myeloid markers have also been reported (24, 25). No marker is absolutely lineage specific, for example, CD19, CD2, and CD4 may be found in 50% of certain subtypes of AML. It has been suggested that two or more markers of a different lineage need to be present for the diagnosis of a mixed-lineage leukemia. Most recent studies show that the expression of "myeloid-associated" antigens on ALL blasts does not alter prognosis and that this type of leukemia responds well to contemporary risk-directed therapy (26). Similarly lymphoid-positive AML patients should be treated on AML protocols but some patients who fail AML therapy have been shown to respond to therapy for ALL (24).

Immunoglobulin and T-cell receptor (TCR) rearrangements and lineage specificity

Molecular studies of rearrangements between the variable (V), diverse (D), joining (J), and constant (C) regions of the *Ig* and *TCR* genes are useful in identifying clonality of leukemia. An orderly pattern of rearrangement takes place so that the Ig heavy chain μ gene is the first to rearrange, followed by the κ, and then the λ light chain gene. *Ig* and *TCR* gene rearrangements are not always lineage specific. Ig μ gene rearrangements are found in 10–20% of T-cell ALL while *TCR* rearrangements are found in at least as many B-lineage ALL cases (3). In contrast to heavy chain gene rearrangements, light chain rearrangements appear to be restricted to B-cells, with only a few exceptions (20). Gene rearrangement findings should therefore be used in conjunction with immunophenotyping.

Genetic factors

More than 90% of ALL cases have specific clonal chromosomal abnormalities (27). These chromosomal changes include rearrangements such as translocations (Fig. 5.2(a)) and inversions, gains, and losses of whole chromosomes and partial deletions. Many of these changes, especially the reciprocal translocations, have been well characterized molecularly and are thought to have a central role in leukemogenesis (27). Many of the

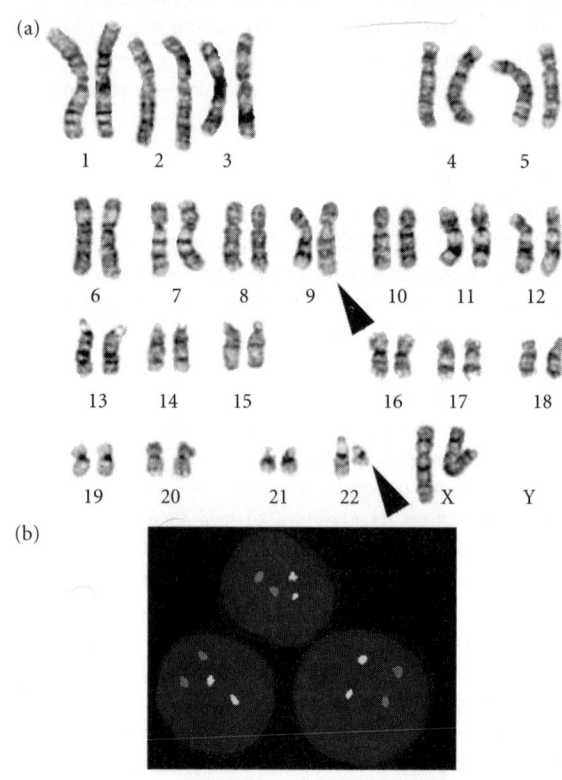

Fig. 5.2 (a) G-banded analysis of CML. The rearranged chromosomes are indicated with arrows. (b) Interphase FISH analysis of CML (for technical details see Chapter 2) The Philadelphia chromosome is detected in interphase nuclei in leukemia cells by the presence of two double fusion signals (yellow), along with the *BCR* gene (red) and the *ABL* gene (green). The nuclei are counterstained with a blue DNA-specific fluorecent dye. See Plate 9.

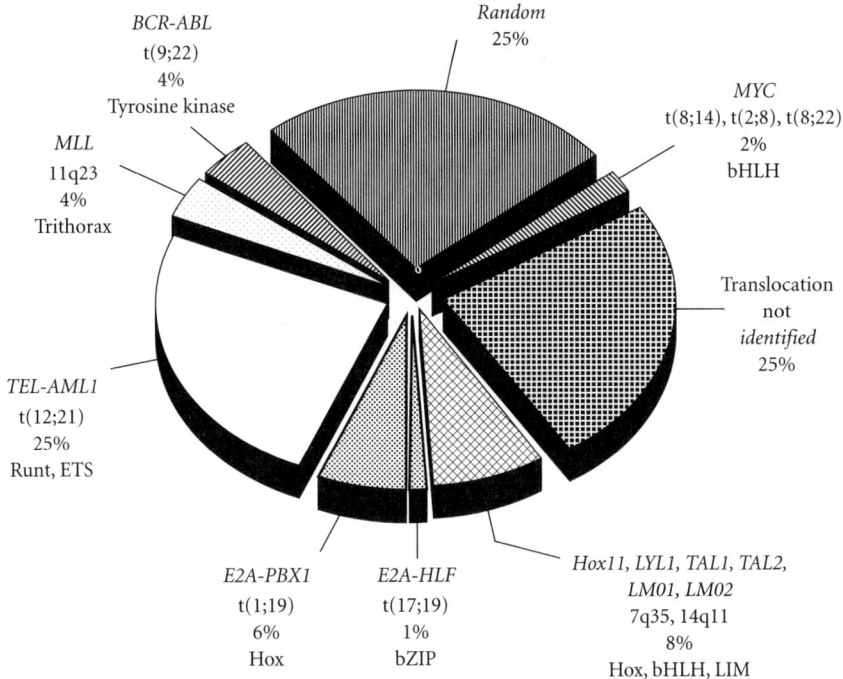

Fig. 5.3 Frequency of recurrent chromosomal aberrations in pediatric ALL. (Reproduced with the permission of Dr. T. Look.)

clinically important genetic changes may be missed by routine karyotyping and may only be detectable at the molecular level. By combining cytogenetic and molecular findings, one can classify 75% or more of ALL cases into prognostic and therapeutically relevant subgroups (27, 28) (Fig. 5.3).

Chromosome number

The chromosome number (or DNA content) per leukemic cell is of significant prognostic importance (29). Hyperdiploid ALL, characterized by the presence of >50 chromosomes per cell, and corresponding to a DNA index of >1.16, accounts for 25% of childhood ALL and carries an excellent prognosis with cure rates of better than 80%. The biologic basis may stem from the ability of hyperdiploid blasts to accumulate increased amounts of methotrexate and its metabolites, as well as the increased propensity of these cells to undergo apoptosis (10).

A clear correlation exists between these nonrandom chromosomal anomalies, the blast cell biologic properties, and the clinical features. Hyperdiploidy (>50 chromosomes) is preferentially seen in children between 1 and 9 years of age, as is the favorable translocation t(12-21) (see below). Approximately 60% of the hyperdiploid cases have additional structural abnormalities, but no consistent abnormality has been identified (18). Patients with "near-tetraploid" (>65) and those with 47–50 chromosomes (DNA index >1 but <1.16) have an intermediate prognosis. By contrast the loss of whole chromosomes, most commonly chromosome 20, resulting in hypodiploidy (<45 chromosomes per cell), results in a significantly poorer response to therapy (10).

Trisomy 4 and 10

Investigators from POG have shown that trisomy of both chromosomes 4 and 10 identifies a subgroup of patients with a very favorable EFS of 96.6% at 4 years, regardless of the DNA index, age, or white cell count (30). In current trials, POG uses this finding to "promote" standard-risk patients to the good-risk group and high-risk patients to the standard-risk group. This criterion has not yet been accepted by the other study groups, however.

Structural chromosomal abnormalities

Pseudodiploid ALL overall has been shown to have a poorer prognosis, with some of the structural abnormalities being of particular significance.

E2A-PBX1

The t(1;19)(q23;p13) translocation is seen in 6% of pediatric ALL and 25% of pre-B cases (31). It generates the transcription factor E2A/PBX1. The resulting fusion protein contains the transcriptional activation domains of E2A linked to the DNA binding domain of PBX1, and is predicted to activate the transcription of genes normally regulated by PBX1 (18). Patients with ETA/PBX1 exhibit other poor prognostic features such as high leukocyte counts and high lactic dehydrogenase (LDH) levels. Although this translocation resulted in a poorer outcome in patients with cytoplasmic Ig-positive, CD20 positive, pre-B ALL, the prognostic importance was lost when therapy was intensified (32). The t(1;19) also occurs in 1–6% of early B-lineage ALL. In these cases neither E2A nor PBX1 are involved and the prognosis is excellent without intensified therapy (33). In contrast to some other minimal residual disease (MRD) studies, the continued detection of the E2A-PBX1 transcript at the end of consolidation therapy did not predict for poorer survival (34).

Translocations that involve core binding factor

Core binding factor (CBF) is a heterodimeric transcription factor that has been shown to play a critical role in the activation of genes important in hematopoetic development. CBF consists of two components, CBFα (also known as AML1) and CBFβ. Chromosomal translocations involving one or other of the two subunits of CBF is associated with both ALL [t(12;21)] and AML [t(8;21), inv(16)] (18).

TEL-AML 1 fusion gene t(12;21)

The translocation t(12;21), which results in the fusion of the 5′ portion of the *TEL* gene to the *AML1* (*CBFα*) gene, is the commonest genetic abnormality in childhood ALL, accounting for about 25% of B-precursor cases (35). The translocation requires molecular techniques for detection and is detected by standard karyotyping in less than 0.05% of ALL. TEL-AML1 expression is associated with an excellent prognosis with EFS estimates of 90–100%. Although the prognostic impact of t(12;21) is independent of age and leukocyte count (35), it is unclear whether it can be used as an indication to reduce therapy. It appears to identify a subset of ALL patients who have a favorable prognosis when treated with appropriate chemotherapy (31). The reason for the favorable outcome in cases with this fusion protein is unknown but the presence of the t(8;21) translocation, which results in AML1(CBFα)/ETO (Eight Twenty One) fusion transcript seen in 8–10% of pediatric AML is also associated with a favorable response to therapy.

MLL gene rearrangements in ALL

Structural arrangements involving chromosome 11q23, are seen in 4–6% of pediatric ALL and approximately 80% of cases of infant ALL (36). In the majority of cases the 11q23 target is a gene designated *MLL* (mixed-lineage leukemia), which spans 100 kb at band 11q23. In total over 25 different reciprocal translocations affecting MLL are present in AML and ALL but the most frequent 11q23 abnormalities in ALL are the t(4;11) and t(11;19). *MLL* encodes a transcription factor containing various DNA binding domains, a transcriptional repressor region, and a region homologous to mammalian DNA methyltransferase. The translocation breakpoints are clustered in an 8.3-kb region, such that some of the functional domains of *MLL* are replaced by sequences encoded by the partner gene. Several partner genes have now been characterized. None appear to be closely related at the structural and functional levels, except for AF10 and AF17 at bands 10q23 and 17q21, respectively, and AF9 and ENL at bands 9p21 and 19p13.3, respectively. Most of the partner genes analyzed so far encode putative transcription factors.

In infants and children over 10 years of age at diagnosis, *MLL* gene rearrangements are associated with a significantly poorer outcome, with long-term EFS rates of less than 20% despite intensive therapy (37). The leukemic blasts in infants are of early B-lineage and are CD10 (CALLA) negative and in addition often express the myelomonocytic marker CD15. The mixed phenotype has led to proposals that 11q23 abnormalities transform an undifferentiated stem cell with the ability to differentiate along both myeloid and lymphoid pathways. The prognosis for children between 2 and 9 years of age with t(4;11), t(11;19), or other translocations involving *MLL* is significantly better than that of infants and of children >10 years of age (31).

BCR-ABL fusion gene

The t(9;22)(q34;q11) translocation resulting in the BCR-ABL fusion gene is seen in 3–5% of cases of childhood ALL, and is associated with older age, higher leukocyte count, and a higher incidence of CNS disease at diagnosis (38). Acute leukemias with this translocation often have an early B-cell or pre-B phenotype but may on occasion have T-cell phenotype. Although cytogenetically indistinguishable from the BCR-ABL transcript found in CML, the latter produces a 210-kDa fusion protein, which is distinct from the 190-kDa protein produced by the ALL translocation. Both proteins have increased tyrosine kinase activity but p190 may have comparably higher transforming potential. ALL patients with this translocation have significantly lower rates of complete remission (75%) and of disease-free survival (<10%) (3). Recent studies have suggested that patients with t(9;22) positive ALL who present with leukocyte counts of less than 25×10^9/l (39) or with disease that responded well to initial prednisone therapy (40) had an approximately 73% and 55% 4-year EFS, respectively, suggesting that stem cell transplants should be reserved for those patients with high leukocyte counts at diagnosis or a poor initial response. A novel treatment approach utilizing a tyrosine kinase inhibitor that shows selectivity for the abl-protein tyrosine kinase has just entered clinical trials in children.

B-ALL

The t(8;14)(q24;q32.3), found in 80% of Burkitts leukemia/lymphoma, brings the *C-MYC* oncogene on chromosome 8 under the control of Ig-gene regulatory sequences on chromosome 14, eventually leading to inappropriate expression of the MYC protein product. This nuclear regulatory protein interacts with other cellular proteins to influence the expression of many genes involved in cellular proliferation. Nearly all of the 20% of cases remaining contain the t(8;22)(q24;q11) or t(2;8(p12;q24), which aligns *C-MYC* with the λ and κ light chain genes respectively (28).

T-ALL and the translocations involving T-cell receptor (TCR) gene

The chromosomal regions 14q11 and 7q35 contain the loci for the *TCR-α/δ* and *TCR-β* genes, respectively. Chromosomal translocations involving the *TCR* genes occur in approximately 50% of T-cell ALL. The most common nonrandom abnormality is t(11;14)(p13;q11) seen in 7% of patients, which fuses the *TCR α/δ* gene to a gene involved in transcription regulation. The t(1;14(p32-p34;q11) translocations occurs in 3% of cases and results in the *TAL1* gene, a basic helix–loop–helix protein that binds DNA and controls transcription, being markedly overexpressed. Recent studies suggest that *TAL1* can be activated by interstitial deletions without cytogenetic abnormalities and that this gene is the most commonly involved protooncogene in T-cell ALL, affecting up to 25% of pediatric cases (3, 41). Non-TCR gene alterations are also frequently seen indicating the biologic diversity of T-lineage ALL.

Tumor suppressor genes

Inherited mutations of the *p53* tumor suppressor gene occurs as part of the Li–Fraumeni syndrome. *p53* inactivation is seen in 1–2% of B-precursor and T-ALL at diagnosis and about 25% of recurrent T-ALL, suggesting that *p53* inactivation plays a role in development of resistant disease (28).

Homozygous deletions of *p16*, a cyclin dependent kinase inhibitor, have been detected in 20–30% of B-precursor ALL and 70–80% of T-ALL suggesting an important role for this tumor suppressor in these leukemias (28).

Risk-adapted therapy has been shown to significantly improve survival in childhood ALL. Based mainly on modern molecular genetic techniques, a new classification has been proposed, which divides patients into four risk groups in an attempt to further refine therapy and improve both the cure rate and the quality of survival (Table 5.1).

Acute myeloblastic leukemia

Acute myeloblastic leukemia is the second most common form of childhood leukemia and has the worst prognosis of all childhood cancer with 5-year survival rates of approximately 37% (42). The diagnosis of AML is sometimes preceded by a myelodysplastic syndrome—a preleukemic phase lasting weeks to months, characterized by a low level of one of the normal blood cells resulting in refractory anemia, neutropenia, or thrombocytopenia. Bone marrow examination is usually hypercellular and abnormal. Occasionally a hypoplastic marrow is seen that later develops into an acute leukemia (1). The FAB group differentiated AML from myelodysplastic syndromes, by defining AML when 30% or more of the bone marrow cells are blast cells.

Classification of AML

Utilizing morphologic, cytochemical, and immunophenotypic data, the updated FAB classification groups AML into eight subtypes, M0–M7 (Table 5.2), based on the appearance of the leukemic cell—myeloblastic, monoblastic, erythroblastic, and megakaryoblastic—as well as the degree of differentiation of the majority of the cells (43). The commonest subgroup is the M2 subtype, acute myeloblastic leukemia with differentiation, followed by acute myelomonoblastic leukemia (M4) and acute monoblastic leukaemia (M5). Eighty percent

Table 5.1 Risk groups in ALL

Risk group	Features	% of ALL patients	Proposed treatment	Est. 5-year EFS%
Low-risk	Hyperdiploid (DI > 1.16)	20–25	Conventional antimetabolite	80–90
	TEL/AML fusion—t(12;21)	20		
Intermediate	Age 1–9 wbc < 50×10^9/l No genetic risk features	15	Intensified antimetabolite	80
High	ETA/PBX—t(1;19), pre-B	25% of pre-B	Intensified therapy	70–80
	T-cell ALL—t(11;14), t(1;14), TAL del Male predominance, older, hyperleukocytosis	15	Intensified therapy ? anti-Tcell (506U78)	70
	Age <1, >10 Wbc >50, no genetic risk features	15	Intensified therapy	60–70
Very high	BCR/ABL—t(9;22), wbc > 25, or slow response	3	Allogeneic transplant in 1st remission ?anti-abl tyrosine kinase	25–35
	MLL rearrangement CD10−, infant, hyperleukocytosis	7	Allogeneic transplant in 1st remission	20–30
	Hypodiploidy (<45) and near haploidy	1	Intensified therapy, ?transplant	20–30
	Induction failure	2	Allogeneic transplant in 1st remission	
B-ALL 80	C-MYC/Ig μ gene—t(8;14) C-MYC/Ig λ gene—t(8;22) C-MYC/Ig κ gene—t(2;8) FAB L3, B phenotype	2–3	B-cell protocol	80

Adapted from ref. 27 and 28 with permission.

of children less than 2 years of age however, will have either M4 or M5 AML.

M0

The M0 subtype, comprising 2% of AML, consists of blasts with minimal myeloid differentiation. M0 AML requires immunologic diagnosis as the blasts resemble lymphoblasts and histochemically do not stain as myeloid cells (10). The blasts express at least one myeloid specific marker such as CD13, CD33, or CD11b and do not express lymphoid markers. M0 blasts almost always express CD34 and HLA-DR and may express CD7 or CD4. Expression of CD7 and CD34 indicate a very early stage of myeloid differentiation and is associated with a worse prognosis (44).

M1

Acute myeloid leukemia without differentiation comprises 10–18% of childhood AML. The blasts are morphologically poorly differentiated with occasional Auer rods, and immunophenotypically are very similar to M0. They usually express CD13, CD33, and HLA-DR.

M2

Acute myeloblastic leukemia with differentiation is the commonest subtype of AML accounting for about 27–29% of cases. Compared to M1 there is a reduced percentage of blasts, with more CD15 and less CD34. HLA-DR, CD13, and CD33 are expressed and Auer rods tend to be prominent. Expression of CD19 occurs in the context of M2 morphology and t(8;21) (see later).

M3

Acute promyelocytic leukemia comprises 5–10% of childhood AML. Morphologically the blasts are hypergranular with bundles of Auer rods. A hypogranular variant of M3 (M3v) is also seen with few granules and infrequent Auer rods. HLA-DR is usually negative, CD13, CD15, CD33 are usually present and CD2 may be expressed.

Table 5.2 FAB classification of childhood AML

FAB	% of AML	Features	Immunophenotype	Cytochemistry	Chromosome
M0	2%	Blasts with minimal myeloid differentiation	CD34 often, TdT, HLA-DR+ at least 1 of CD33, CD13, CD11b, occ CD7, or CD4	neg	del(5), del(7)
M1	10–18%	Poorly differential blasts Occasional Auer rods blasts >90% of nonerythroid	CD33++, occ CD34, CD34++ some CD15 HLA DR+	MP/SB+, CAE− NSE−	
M2	27–29%	>10% maturing granulocytic Prominent Auer rods Chloromas may be present	CD33++, CD13, HLA-DR+ less CD34, more CD15 occ CD19	MP/SB+, CAE NSE−	t(8;21)(q22;q22) (AML-ETO) others inc +8
M3	5–10%	Hypergranular promyelocytes, bundles of Auer rods Microgranular M3v variant— few granules, scanty Auer rods Both variants may show RARα-PLM and respond to ATRA Coagulopathy + fatal hemorrhage	CD33++, CD13+, CD9+, HLA-DR−, CD15++	MP/SB+, CAE+, NSE−	t(15;17)(q22;q21 (RARα-PML) 90% of APL t(11;17)-occ t(5;17)-occ trisomy 8
M4	16–25%	Monoblasts (>20% nonerythroid) Myeloblasts 80% AML <2 years = M4, M5	CD34+, CD33++, CD14++ CD15++, CD13++, HLA-DR	MP/SB+, CAE+ NSE+, NSE inhib by FL	MLL rearranged: t(9;11)(p22;q23) t11;19)(q23;p13) t(10;11)(p12;q23)
M4Eo	subtype	AMML with >5% dysplastic eosinophils favorable prognosis	Above plus CD2+		inv(16) t(16;16) —CBFβ-MYH11
M5	13–22% <2 years = 55%	Monoblastic M5a >80%monoblasts M5b <80%monoblasts Infants <2 years, high counts Extramedullary Poorer prognosis	Less CD34 than M4 CD33++, CD13++, CD15++, HLA-DR, CD14++ Minority = M5 classical profile CD33++, CD34−, CD13−	MP/SB−, CAE− NSE+, NSE inhib by FL	MLL rearranged: T(9;11)(p22;q23) T(11;19)(q23;p13) T(10;11)(p12;q23)
M6	1–3%	Erythroleukemia Dysplastic erythropoesis Megaloblastic features	HLA-DR+, CD34 Poss CD13+, CD33++ Abs to glycophorin	Erythroblasts = PAS+, AP− myeloblasts = MP/SB +, NSE−	
M7	4–8% >2 years 1% <2 years 7–20%	At least 30% megakaryoblasts myelofibrosis Blue cytoplasm, blebs on membrane, cell clustering EM-platelet peroxidase granules common in DS <3 years of age	CD61(GpIIIa Platelet ag) CD41 (GpIIb-IIIa) Factor VIII-rel ag CD33++, CD13+	AP+ MP/SB−, CAE− NSE+	Tristomy 21— good prognosis t(1;22) in non-Downs = poor outcome

AP = acid phosphatase, NSE = nonspecific esterase, MP = myeloperoxidase, SB = Sudan black, CAE = chloroacetate esterase (specific test) Fl = fluoride.

The identification of APL conveys unique therapeutic and prognostic implications. This leukemia is a medical emergency as up to 10% of hemorrhagic deaths are seen despite modern therapy, due to a disseminated intravascular coagulopathy which is associated with the release of procoagulants from dying promyelocytes. In an Italian study the M3v subtype accounted for 25% of pediatric APL, and was characterized by severe bleeding problems and a high leukocyte count in contrast to most of their patient with M3 who presented with low white cell counts (45). APL is associated with chromosomal translocations which result in disruption of the RARα gene locus on chromosome 17, and is the paradigm for specific targeted therapy (see section on Genetics of AML)

M4

Acute myelomonoblastic leukemia (M4), 16–25% of AML, is a mixture of myeloblasts and monoblasts in which the minority cell type represents at least 20% of the total. The subtype M4E0 shows myelomonocytic differentiation plus abnormal bone marrow eosinophils and CD2 positivity and is associated with abnormalities of chromosome 16 [inv(16) and t(16;16)], and a favorable prognosis.

M5

Acute monoblastic leukemia comprises 12–22% of AML in the older child and around 55% in the under-2-year old. It resembles M4 immunophenotypically, although M4 is more often CD34+. Important feature are the presence of CD13+, CD33+, HLA-DR+, CD14+, CD15+. The presence of CD33+ with CD13− and CD34− is highly correlated with M5 but is seen in a minority of patients.

M6

Erythroleukemia is rare, 1–3% of childhood AML, with CD34+, HLA-DR+, and possibly CD13+ and CD33+. Antibodies to glycophorin demonstrate erythroid differentiation. Cytogenetically two major subgroups of M6 AML are found, patients with complex karyotypes usually involving chromosomes 5 and 7 and a poor prognosis, and those with simple or undetectable abnormalities with a more favorable prognosis (46).

M7

A relatively new addition, acute megakaryoblastic leukemia, accounts for 4–8% of all childhood AML, 1% in the older child and up to 20% in the infant. It is diagnosed when more than 30% of nonerythroid cells are megakaryoblasts with characteristic morphologic features such as basophilic cytoplasm, blebs on the plasma membrane resembling budding platelets, and a tendency to cell clustering. The diagnosis is made by demonstrating platelet peroxidase granules on electron microscopy, and by monoclonal antibodies specific for platelet antigens CD61 (GP III a) and/or CD 41(Gp IIb–IIIa). Care must be taken to exclude a false positive reaction due to platelet adherence to blasts. M7 is the commonest form of leukemia in the Down's Syndrome (DS) patients less than 3 years of age and is associated with frequent presentation with myelodysplasia and frequent dyserythropoeisis in bone marrow with coexpression of T-cell antigen CD7 on blast cells (47). DS children with M7 have a markedly superior outcome to non-DS patients. Occurrence of M7 in non-DS patients is associated with acquired trisomy 21 in up to 24% and with t(1;22)(p13;q13) in approximately one-third of childhood M7 AML. The t(1;22) occurs almost exclusively in very young children with massive organomegaly and a poor outlook (46).

Clinical features of AML

Clinical presentation is similar to ALL, but AML is more likely to present with gum hyperplasia, associated with monoblastic phenotypes, and with myeloblastomas (chloromas, granulocytic sarcomas), localized collections of leukemic cells occuring at any site including extradural, bone, skin, and orbit. Myeloblastomas tend be associated with FAB M2 and the t(8;21)translocation (48). Disseminated intravascular coagulopathy can occur with any leukemia but is most commonly associated with FAB M3. Eighty percent of infants present with M4 and M5 AML and are more likely to present with high white cell counts and extramedullary leukemia (49). CNS involvement in AML is seen in approximately 4% of patients (compared to 3% for ALL) (1) but is commoner in children <2 years of age in M4 and M5 AML.

Clinical risk factors

In AML, risk factors have been much more difficult to identify due to lack of effective therapy for more than 50% of the patients, but some groups can be distinguished.

Age

Age at diagnosis does not seem to be as important as in ALL, but most studies have suggested that children <2 years at diagnosis have a poorer relapse-free survival (50). The FAB M4 and M5 subtypes, and extramedullary leukemia (other than CNS), both of which are particularly common in the young child have also been found to impact adversely on survival (50).

White cell count

A leukocyte count over $100 \times 10^9/l$ at diagnosis occurs in 20% of children with AML, and is associated with a lower remission rate and a poorer prognosis. This is only partially due to the increased risk of the hyperleukocytosis syndrome with leukostasis, intravascular plugging, hemorrhagic infarcts particularly in the brain and lung, somnolence, seizures, hypoxemia, coma, and death. Due to the higher blast mean cell volume, AML patients are at greater risk of hyperleukocytosis than patients with ALL.

Secondary AML

Acute myeloid leukemia, which is preceded by myelodysplasia has a poorer prognosis, as has AML, which is secondary to therapy given for a previous malignancy. Other clinical feature such as race, sex, organomegaly, and the duration of prodromal symptoms do not appear to affect the outcome.

Down's syndrome

Children with DS, constitute more than 10% of all AML cases. Most have FAB M7 morphology and the majority present before 3 years of age, often following an antecedent myelodysplastic phase with myelofibrosis and thrombocytopenia. DS AML responds very favorably to adequate chemotherapy with EFS rates of 68–100% when patients are treated with current intensive protocols (51). Myeloblasts from DS patients have been shown to be significantly more sensitive to both cytarabine and daunorubicin, compared to blasts from non-DS patients, and a recent study demonstrated that DS blasts show increased transcript levels of two genes localized on chromosome 21, cystathione-synthetase, which may increase sensitivity to cytarabine and superoxide dismutase, which appears to be associated with increased apoptosis after exposure to apoptosis-inducing agents (52).

Neonates with DS may present with a transient myeloproliferative syndrome, which may be very difficult to distinguish from true leukemia. Clinical and hematological recovery occurs within 4–8 weeks although the blasts cells have been shown to be clonally derived (53), and to express increased levels of the gene transcripts described above in DS AML blasts. Up to 30% of DS patients with transient MPS present later with M7AML.

Biology of AML
Immunophenotypic analysis

The ability of flow cytometry to identify myeloid versus lymphoid differentiation approaches 98%. The value of immunophenotyping of AML is mainly in the differentiation from ALL in the less than 20% of cases in which morphology and cytochemistry are inconclusive, as well as in the recognition of the morphologically difficult FAB M0 and M7 subtypes.

Genetics of AML

Chromosomal rearrangements have been identified in up to 80% of AML patients (54). Cloning of chromosomal translocation breakpoints has identified mutant genes that are causally implicated in the establishment of the leukemic clone and the pathogenesis of AML, and that may serve as targets for specific novel therapies. Large studies have also shown correlations between specific recurrent chromosomal abnormalities, clinical characteristics, and outcome (Fig. 5.4). Patients with a normal karyotype had a favorable outcome with a 53.8% 4-year overall survival (OS) in a recent large POG study (54) (Table 5.3).

AML 1 (CBFα)/ETO

The t(8;21) (q22;q22) translocation is among the most frequent cytogenetic abnormalities in AML. It is present in approximately 12% of pediatric patients (54) and 15% of adults (55), and results in the fusion of the *AML1* (*CBFα*) gene on chromosome 21 to the *ETO* gene on chromosome 8. It is thought that the resulting fusion protein may dominantly inhibit the ability of the *CBFα* (*AML1*) gene to direct normal maturation and development of hematopoetic cells (18).

Forty-six percent of children with AML M2 show the presence of AML1/ETO fusion transcript. It appears to confer a relatively favorable outcome with $45.1 \pm 7.7\%$ of children with t(8;21) in the POG study surviving disease free at 4 years (54). The authors speculated that the improvement in survival compared to previously reported studies in children (56) may be due to the addition of high-dose cytarabine to the therapy. The AML1/ETO protein may be detected by reverse transcriptase polymerase chain reaction (RT-PCR) for as long as 10 years after complete morphologic and cytogenetic remission, and RT-PCR analysis of AML1/ETO for detection of MRD is probably of little value (57, 58).

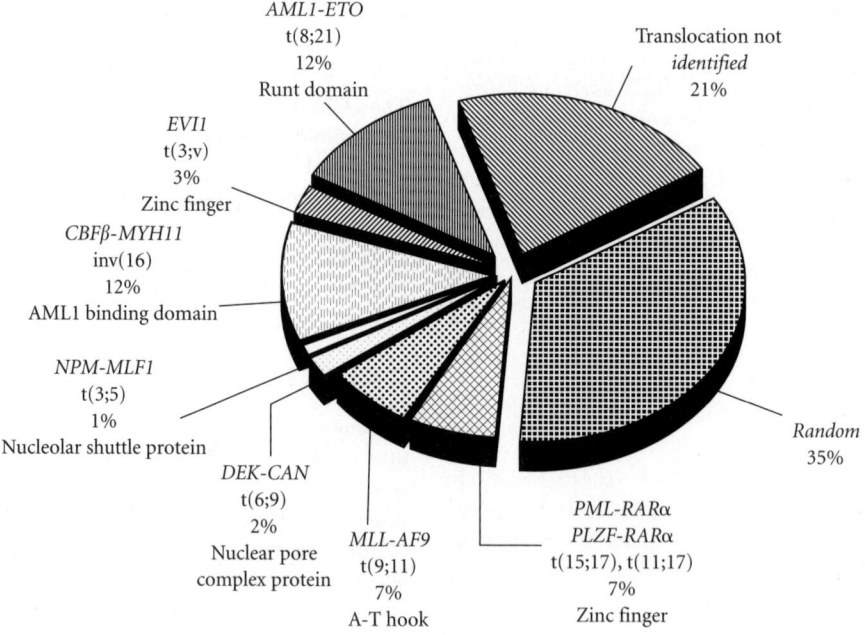

Fig. 5.4 Frequency of recurrent chromosomal aberrations in pediatric AML. (Reproduced with the permission of Dr. T. Look.)

Table 5.3 Prognostic features in childhood AML

Adverse factors
  High WBC count (>100 × 10⁹)
  Secondary AML, prior MDS
  Monosomy 7(7q−)
  FAB M5
  FABM7 with t(1;22), non-Down's
  >1 course to CR
  Multidrug resistance positivity

Possible positive factors
  M1 with Auer rods
  t(8;21)
  t(9;11)
  t(15;17)/M3
  inv(16)/M4Eo

Adapted from Golub T, Weinstein H. Acute myeloid leukemia. In: Principles and practice of pediatric oncology, 3rd edn. (ed. Pizzo and Poplack), with permission.

inv(16)(p13;q22)

The inv(16)(p13;q22) and the variant translocation t(16;16), which are found in 6–12% of childhood AML, result in the formation of a fusion gene consisting of the 5′ portion of the CBFβ fused to a variable amount of the 3′ portion of the smooth muscle myosin heavy chain gene *MYH11*. The CBFβ-MYH11 fusion protein has been shown to directly repress AML1-mediated transcription, and introduction of this fusion gene into murine embryogenesis results in a lethal phenotype (18, 59).

Inv(16)(p13;q22)/t(16;16(p13;q22) are nonrandomly associated with AmoL-M4Eo with bone marrow eosinophilia, abnormal eosinophils, or both (46). In the POG study this group of patients had the best 4-year EFS (58.2%). The OS was 75% suggesting that salvage post relapse is frequently possible and transplant may not be necessary in this subgroup (54).

RARα rearrangements

Acute promyelocytic leukemia (FAB M3) accounts for approximately 10% of childhood leukemia and in more than 90% of cases the t(15;17) translocation, which fuses the retinoic acid gene (*RARα*) on chromosome 17 to the *PML* gene on 15, is found. This occurs in both FAB M3 and the microgranular variant M3v and results in the formation of a PML-RARα fusion protein in all patients. The reciprocal transcript RARα-PML is found in approximately two-thirds of patients. RARα functions as a transcription factor that regulates the expression of a large number of target genes, some of which are critical for normal myeloid cell differentiation. PML on the other hand functions as a tumor suppressor and is an essential component of apoptotic signaling pathways. Other translocations involving the RARα locus such as t(11;17), which fuses the *PLZF* gene to *RARα*, or t(5;17), which fuses *NPM* to *RARα* may occasionally result in the APL phenotype (60). These patients do not express the *RARα-PML* fusion gene however, and do not respond to all *trans* retinoic acid (ATRA).

MLL gene rearrangements

11q23 abnormalities are found in about 15% of children with AML. The most common translocations are t(9;11), t(6;11), and t(11;19) although more than 15 other genetic alterations are known. All involve the *MLL* gene (see above). Only a few examples with translocations or inversions of 11q23 exhibit phenotypes other than M4 and M5 (47). Overall 50–70% of infants with AML have 11q23 abnormalities. 11q23 abnormalities are common in secondary leukemias particularly following therapy with DNA-topoisomerase inhibitors. Children with 11q23 AML associated with t(9;11)(p22;q23) are said to have a better prognosis than AML patients with other 11q23 rearrangements (47), but this was not seen in the POG study in which patients with any type of 11q23 abnormality had a 4-year OS of 23.8% (54).

Abnormalities of chromosome 7 and 5

Monosomy 7 has been observed in about 5% of childhood AML. It is thought to lead to the loss of a putative suppressor gene on 7q and is associated with a poor prognosis. Monosomy 5 occurs very infrequently in childhood AML. Abnormalities of chromosomes 5 and 7 are much commoner in adult AML, and are thought to result from exposure to leukemogenic agents (54).

Many other less common chromosomal translocations are seen in childhood AML, including t(3;5), t(6;9), t(8;16), t(3;21), and t(16;21). Recurrent abnormalities also included acquisition of extra chromosomes of which trisomy 8 is the commonest, followed by acquired trisomy 21. These are most commonly seen in association with other chromosomal abnormalities.

Therapy

AML is recognized to be a heterogenous group with a variety of phenotypes, which tend to be associated with specific cytogenetic abnormalities and significantly different outcomes (61). At the present time however, with the exception of APL (FAB M3) and DS patients, all AML patients continue to be treated on the same protocols with neither FAB subtype nor cytogenetics being used for treatment assignment.

In the early 1970's, the addition of anthracyclines and cytarabine, resulted in improvement in the cure rate of AML to about 37%, and efforts since then have resulted in only minor improvements. Remission induction rates of 75–85% also lag behind that seen in ALL and was achieved by significantly higher treatment intensity resulting in major morbidity and even mortality (62, 63). Emerging insights into the molecular basis of AML will hopefully allow stratification of therapy in a similar strategy to that which has proved successful in ALL.

Acute promyelocytic leukemia

The paradigm for specific molecular-targeted therapy is APL (FAB M3) in which pharmacological doses of ATRA have been shown to reverse the inhibitory activity of PML-RARα and to induce the growth arrest of leukemic promyelocytes and their terminal differentiation. The fusion protein associated with t(15;17) may be found in the hypergranular and hypogranular forms of APL and when present predict response to ATRA therapy and a good survival. APL due to the other variant translocations does not respond to ATRA and has a correspondingly poorer prognosis.

Nearly all cases treated with ATRA achieve CR, but resistance develops quickly and the combination of ATRA with chemotherapy is required to achieve long-term survival. Forty to fifty percent of patients receiving ATRA develop the retinoic acid syndrome, a cardiorespiratory distress syndrome with interstitial pulmonary infiltrates, pleural or pericardial effusions, hypoxemia, and hypotension with otherwise unexplained weight gain. Addition of chemotherapy to ATRA, particularly in patients with high white cell counts at diagnosis, plus the use of dexamethasone at the earliest symptom appears to have reduced the incidence of fatal ATRA syndrome to 1–1.5% (64). The addition of ATRA to chemotherapy has greatly improved the survival of patients with APL from 30% to 40% to close to 80% at 2 years.

In patients resistant to ATRA, low doses of arsenic trioxide has been effective in inducing remission in patients with APL, without significant myelosuppression. This activity appears to be limited to *RAR-PML* expressing cells as the only 2 of 53 APL patients that did not achieve CR with AS_2O_3 had *RAR-PML* negative disease (65). Other subtypes of AML are also resistant to low-dose AS_2O_3 (65). AS_2O_3 appears to induce apoptosis through generation of reactive oxygen radicals, particularly hydrogen peroxide (H_2O_2) and it is postulated that the RARα-PML fusion protein results in decreased activity of H_2O_2-scavenging enzymes (66).

Novel therapies for AML

Differentiating agents
ATRA therapy in APL has been the prototype of this approach. It is hoped that as the molecular mechanisms underlying the different forms of leukemia are better understood, agents will be found that will be able to repeat the ATRA success in other subtypes of leukemia.

Immunotherapy
Antibody therapy
CD33 is expressed on the majority of early myeloid cells and by more than 90% of AML (55). It is not expressed by most immature hematopoetic cells or non-myeloid cells and therefore appears to be an ideal target for antibody therapy.

CD33 is not however a receptor for an obligate growth or survival factor, nor does its binding provide a signal for cell death or differentiation, thus the unbound antibody alone only has been unsuccessful in inducing more than a transient decrease in blast cells (67).

Immunotoxins
Various AntiCD33–toxin conjugates have been developed to try to improve the efficacy of targeted antibody therapy. The most promising results to date have been with an antiCD33–calicheamicin conjugate (CMA-676), which produced complete elimination of blasts from blood and bone marrow in 20% of patients entered onto a phase 1 trial in adults (68). The immunoconjugate is being considered for use in an upcoming Children's Oncology Group AML protocol.

Radiolabelled antibodies are also being tried with the addition of ^{131}I to anti-CD33 antibody. Because of unacceptable myelosuppression when used alone, the ^{131}I-anti CD33 conjugate is now being tried in the pretransplant setting, and new radiolabels with shorter half-lives and shorter path lengths are under investigation (55).

Conclusion
AML accounts for less than 20% of childhood leukemia but more than 30% of deaths. Little progress has been seen in the survival from AML over the past decade. The one major exception to this has been the marked improvement in the survival from APL with the addition of ATRA and more recently Arsenic Trioxide to the treatment, based on the molecular characteristics of the blasts.

Biologic findings in childhood AML are significantly correlated with response to therapy and outcome. The most favorable subgroups are M3 AML treated with retinoic acid, DS patients with M7 AML, and M4Eo AML patients with inv(16)/t(16;16). It appears that these patients do well with currently available therapy without stem cell transplantation. AML patients with t(8;21) have a relatively favorable prognosis as do patients with normal karyotypes.

The worst prognosis appears to be associated with *MLL* gene rearrangements and certain rare translocations such as t(1;22) M7 AML. Children with monosomy 7 AML arising de novo or secondary to previous chemotherapy, also fare badly and all of these patients require more effective therapies than currently available.

As the understanding of the molecular biology of AML improves, future treatment strategies will hopefully be developed, which will be aimed at specific molecular targets on the many different leukemic cell types collectively called AML.

Minimal residual disease studies in childhood leukemia

Detection of MRD in pediatric patients with leukemia has been shown to significantly correlate with the risk of relapse in some but not all subgroups. Recent studies from the European Cancer—childhood cooperative group, SJCRH, and the Dana Farber Cancer Institute (DFCI) suggest that detection of MRD is a powerful and independent prognosticator in childhood ALL. In the European study, multivariate analysis showed that compared to immunophenotype, age and white cell count at diagnosis, the presence or absence and level of residual disease were the most powerful independent prognostic factors (69). In the SJCRH study, using flow cytometric techniques capable of detecting 1 leukemic cell per 10^4 normal cells, and applicable to 80% of patients, those who had high MRD levels (>0.1%) at the end of induction or at week 14 of continuation did particularly poorly (70). In the DFCI study of paired bone marrow and peripheral blood samples, using a quantitative PCR analysis of clonal rearrangements of *IgH, TCR-α/δ,* and *TCR-β*, peripheral blood was shown to be an adequate source for MRD detection and quantification in childhood ALL, allowing for frequent routine monitoring of MRD in this population (71). In APL patients, *RARα-PML* as detected by RT-PCR, has also been used to detect MRD. The finding of the fusion protein in the occasional long-term survivor has cast doubt on the usefulness of this assay in clinical practice. A large Italian trial however has suggested that PCR positivity on two successive samples during follow-up of therapy, is sufficiently prognostic for relapse that therapy should be started based on this finding alone, before the onset of overt relapse (60).

Not all MRD detected by RT-PCR has proved to be prognostic however. Detection of the TEL-AML fusion protein at the end of induction was not associated with a poorer survival in a POG study (34) and as described above the AML1-ETO protein may be detected after 10 years of complete remission (57). It also remains to be demonstrated that intensification of therapy for MRD alters prognosis. Clearly MRD studies are in their infancy and much work remains to be done in this field.

Chronic myelocytic leukemia

It is a clonal myeloproliferative disorder of a pluripotent hematopoetic stem cell. CML accounts for about 3% of childhood leukemia and is characterized by the presence of large numbers of myeloid cells in all stages of maturation. The term chronic no longer has implication for the duration of the disease but designates a form of myeloid leukemia that shows a considerable degree of differentiation in the abnormal cell line. The majority of cases of CML in childhood are similar to adult CML and carry the Philadelphia (Ph+) chromosome. This chromosome results from a balanced translocation between the long arms of chromosomes 9 and 22, resulting in the *bcr-abl* fusion gene that expresses a fusion protein, which is 210 kDa long and has altered tyrosine kinase activity (72). Although very similar in morphologic appearance, the form of leukemia previously known as juvenile CML has been renamed chronic monomyelocytic leukemia (CMML) and is considered to be a form of myelodysplasia/ myeloproliferation.

Clinical features

Chronic myelocytic leukemia is usually seen in older children and adolescents but it has occasionally been reported in infants. The onset is generally insidious with gradual development of extreme hepatosplenomegaly, which is sometimes found on routine examination. Joint pain and/or effusions may be present. Extramedullary manifestations such as myeloblastomas (chloromas) are often found. The chronic phase of the disease has a median duration of 3–5 years when treated with conventional agent and an invariable progression to an accelerated phase of 3–6 months duration and finally to a phase of blast crisis and death.

Special features

A mild normochromic, normocytic anemia, marked leukocytosis with a "left shift," and thrombocytosis is usually found. The median wbc in children ($\sim 250 \times 10^9/l$) is higher than that seen in adults (73). All stages of myeloid differentiation are present in blood and bone marrow. Eosinophilia and basophilia are constant features. A low leukocyte alkaline phosphatase activity in neutrophils is useful in distinguishing CML from inflammatory conditions giving a leukemoid reaction. Increase in vitamin B12 levels and B12-binding protein, LDH, and uric acid are seen. In the course of transformation to the acute blastic phase, cytogenetic changes are often seen, the commonest being duplication of the Ph chromosome, trisomy 8, trisomy 19, and isochromosome 17q (74).

Therapy

For many years Busulfan was the therapy of choice for CML. Frequent and serious adverse effects included irreversible cytopenia and pulmonary, hepatic, and cardiac fibrosis. Hydroxyurea has since shown to produce a significantly longer median disease-free survival but despite good clinical responses, no cytogenetic remissions were obtained and the disease progressed inevitably to blast crisis and death. Studies with interferon-α have been shown to produce complete and partial clinical remission in 7–81% and 6–50% of cases, respectively and complete and partial cytogenetic remission in 0–38% and 0–16% of cases (72), with a complete cytogenetic response being defined as the absence of Ph+ metaphases, and partial response as 1–34% Ph+ metaphases. Interferon combined with chemotherapy, usually hydroxyurea or cytosine arabinoside, appears to achieve a clinical remission within 1–3 months. There is evidence of a dose–response relationship with doses of 4–5 million units/m^2/d of interferon producing better responses than lower doses. Better results are obtained in young patients who are treated early, who have less advanced disease, and who have favorable features such as low or normal platelet counts, a low percentage of peripheral and marrow blasts, a non-palpable spleen, and a good hematologic response to therapy.

Most studies document an association between cytogenetic response and improved survival. Patients in cytogenetic remission may have the bcr/abl transcript measurable by RT-PCR but the significance of PCR positivity is as yet unknown. PCR and Southern blot methods are commonly used to detect *BCR/ABL* rearrangements. In addition a double fusion fluorescence *in situ* hybridization (D-FISH) BCR/ABL probe can also be used to monitor residual disease in CML using interphase nuclei (75). The D-FISH probe also reveals the locations of 3'*ABL* and 5'*BCR* as well as 5'*ABL* and 3'*BCR* on either metaphase or interphase chromosomes (Fig. 5.2(b)).

A retrospective German study of 75 pediatric CML patients showed an overall 12-year survival probability of 27%, while the survival for patients undergoing allogeneic bone marrow transplant (BMT) was 42%, rising to 62% for those in whom the BMT was done within the first 3 years from diagnosis (76). The transplant related mortality was 21%, similar to other studies in which the mortality ranges from 20% to 40% with the lower figure being seen in younger patients. Survival curves appear to plateau after 3–7 years suggesting that young patients particularly with matched sibling donors may be cured (72).

Most patients undergo BMT after initial therapy with chemotherapy and interferon, and one study has suggested that more than 6 months of interferon therapy increases the risk of Graft Versus Host Disease. It appears that BMT offers a better chance for survival than prolonged interferon but side-effects are a problem.

Young patients with a matched sibling donor should probably be offered early transplant. The optimal therapy for patients without sibling donors remains uncertain. Improved understanding of the leukemic cell at the molecular level has allowed for studies of MRD, and donor leukocyte infusions have induced remission in CML patients with evidence of MRD following allogeneic BMT (77). Development of the BCR/ABL tyrosine kinase inhibitor imatinib mesylate has opened a new era of targeted therapy for CML. This drug has proved to be safe and effective in CML (78). Whether this drug, above or in combination, can replace BMT in pediatric CML remains to be determined.

Conclusion

Molecular analysis in childhood leukemia has improved our abilities to diagnose disease, to assign patients to optimal therapy, and to monitor the response to therapy. Detection of MRD by molecular techniques, could in the future allow augmentation of therapy only for those patients at risk for relapse.

In a few subgroups, namely APL and mature B-cell ALL, biologic studies have permitted therapy based on the molecular characteristics of the tumor cells and this specific therapy has been shown to significantly impact on survival.

The challenge is to apply our expanding knowledge of the metabolic pathways underlying leukemia cell formation, metabolism, and death to the development of novel targeted therapy that can be administered safely and effectively to all patients.

References

1. Gustaffson G, Lie SO. Acute leukemias. In: Cancer in children, clinical management, 4th edn. (ed. PA Voute, C Kalifa, A Barrett). Oxford University Press, London, 1998, 99–118.
2. Cortes JE, Kantarjian HM. Acute lymphoblastic leukemia. A comprehensive review with emphasis on biology and therapy. Cancer 1995, **76**, 2393–2417.
3. Ries LAG, Miller BA, Hankey BF, *et al*. SEER cancer statistics review 1973–1991. National Cancer Institute publication, #NIH-2789, 1994.
4. MauerAM. The leukemias of childhood. Practice of Pediatrics **5**, 1–30, 1987.
5. Pui C-H. Childhood leukemias. New Engl J Med 1995, **332**, 1618–29.
6. Shannon K, O'Connell P, Martin G, *et al*. Loss of the normal *NF1* allele from the bone of children with type 1 neurofibromatosis and malignant myeloid disorders. N Engl J Med 1994, **330**, 597–601.
7. Greaves MF. Aetiology of acute leukemia. Lancet 1997, **349**, 344–9.
8. Chessels JM. Leukemia in the young child. Br J Cancer 1992, **66**, 554–7.
9. Ross JA. Epidemiologic studies of childhood leukemia: where do we go from here. Med Ped Oncol 1999, **32**, 65–7.
10. Pui CH, Sallan S, Relling MV, Masera G, Evans WE. International Childhood Acute Lymphoblastic Leukemia Workshop: Sansalito, CA, 30 November–1 December 2000. Leukemia 2001, **15**, 707–15.
11. Dordelmann M, Reiter A, Borkhardt A *et al*. Prednisone response is the strongest predictor of treatment outcome is infant acute lymphoblastic leukemia. Blood 1999, **94**, 1209–17.
12. Smith M, Arthur D, Camitta B, *et al*. Uniform approach to risk classification and treatment assignment for children with acute lymphoblastic leukemia. J Clin Oncol 1996, **14**, 18–24.
13. Sather H. Statistical evaluation of prognostic factors in ALL and treatment results. Med Pediatr Oncol 1986, **14**, 158.
14. Bleyer WA, Poplack DG. Prophylaxis and treatment of leukemia in the central nervous system and other sanctuaries. Semin Oncol 1985, **12**, 131–48.
15. Pui CH, Gaynon PS, Boyett JM, Chessells JM, Baruchel A, Kamps W. Outcome of treatment in childhood acute

lymphoblastic leukemia with rearrangements of the 11q23 chromosomal region. Lancet 2002, **359**, 1909–15.
16. Steinherz PG, Gaynon PS, Breneman JC, *et al.* Cytoreduction and prognosis in acute lymphoblastic leukemia—the importance of early marrow response: report from the Children's Cancer Group. J Clin Oncol, 1996, **14**, 389–98.
17. Nachman JB, Sather HN, Sensel MG, *et al.* Augmented post-induction therapy for children with high risk acute lymphoblastic leukemia and a slow response to initial therapy. N Engl J Med 1998, **338**, 1663–71.
18. Downing JR. Molecular pathology of childhood leukemia. In: ASCO Educational Book (ed. Perry MC). Lippincott, Williams and Wilkins, Baltimore, MD, 1999, 417–31.
19. Hurwitz CA, Mounce KG, Grier HE. Treatment of patients with acute myelogenous leukemia: review of clinical trials of the past decade. J Pediatr Hematol/Oncol 1995, **17**, 185–97.
20. Pui C-H, Behm FG, Crist WM. Clinical and biologic relevance of immunologic marker studies in childhood acute lymphoblastic leukemia. Blood 1993, **82**, 343–62.
21. Sullivan MP, Pullen DJ, Crist WM, *et al.* Clinical and biologic heterogeneity of childhood B-cell acute lymphoblastic leukemia: implications for clinical trials. Leukemia 1990, **4**, 6–10.
22. Reiter A, Schrappe M, Tiemann M, Ludwig WD *et al.* Improved treatment results in childhood B-cell neoplasms with tailored intensification of therapy: A report of the Berlin-Frankfurt-Munster Group Trial NHL-BFM 90. Blood 1999, **94**, 3294–306.
23. Uckun FM, Sensel MG, Sun L, *et al.* Biology and treatment of childhood T-Lineage acute lymphoblastic leukemia. Blood 1998, **91**, 735–46.
24. Pui C-H, Raimondi SC, Rivera GK, *et al.* Myeloid-antigen expression in childhood acute lymphoblastic leukemia. N Engl J Med 1991, **325**, 1378–9.
25. Kuerbitz SJ, Civin CI, Krischer JP, *et al.* Expression of myeloid-associated and lymphoid associated cell-surface antigens in acute myeloid leukemia of childhood: a Pediatric Oncology Group study. J Clin Oncol 1992, **10**, 1419–22.
26. Borowitz MJ, Shuster JJ, Land VJ, *et al.* Myeloid-antigen expression in childhood acute lymphoblastic leukemia. N Engl J Med 1991, **325**, 1379–80.
27. Pui C-H. Acute lymphoblastic leukemia. Pediatr Clin N Am 1997, **44**, 831–46.
28. Rubnitz JE, Look AT. Molecular genetics of childhood leukemia. J Pediatr Hematol/Oncol 1998, **20**, 1–11.
29. Trueworthy R, Shuster J, Look T, *et al.* Ploidy of lymphoblasts is the strongest predictor of treatment outcome in B-progenitor cell acute lymphoblastic leukemia of childhood: a Pediatric Oncology Group study. J Clin Oncol 1992, **10**, 606–13.
30. Harris MB, Shuster JJ, Carroll A, *et al.* Trisomy of leukemic cell chromosomes 4 and 10 identifies children with B-progenitor cell acute lymphoblastic leukemia with a very low risk of treatment failure: a Pediatric Oncology Group study. Blood 1992, **79**, 3316–24.
31. Rubnitz JE. The impact of molecular diagnostics on the evaluation and treatment of childhood leukemia. In: ASCO Educational Book (ed. Perry M.C). Lippincott, Williams and Wilkins, Baltimore MD, 1999, 435–9.

32. Uckun FM, Sensel MG, Sather HN, *et al.* Clinical significance of translocation t(1,19) in childhood acute lymphoblastic leukemia in the context of contemporary therapies: a report from the Children's Cancer Group. J Clin Oncol 1998, **16**, 527–35.
33. Privitera E, Kamps MP, Hayashi Y, *et al.* Different molecular consequences of the 1;19 chromosomal translocation in childhood B-cell precursor acute lymphoblastic leukemia. Blood 1992, **79**, 1781–88.
34. Hunger SP, Fall MZ, Camitta B, *et al.* E2A-PBX1 chimeric transcript status at the end of consolidation is not predictive of treatment outcome in childhood acute lymphoblastic leukemia with a t(1,19)(q23;p13): a Pediatric Oncology Group study. Blood 1998, **91**, 1021–28.
35. Rubnitz JE, Downing JR, Pui C-H, *et al. TEL* gene rearrangement in acute lymphoblastic leukemia: a new genetic marker with prognostic significance. J Clin Oncol 1997, **15**, 1150–7.
36. Rubnitz JE, Link MP, Shuster JJ, *et al.* Frequency and prognostic significance of HRX rearrangements in infant acute lymphoblastic leukemia: a Pediatric Oncology Group study. Blood 1994, **84**, 570–3.
37. Pui C-H, Carroll AJ, Raimondi SC, *et al.* Childhood acute lymphoblastic leukemia with the t(4;11)(q21;q23): an update. Blood 1994, **83**, 2384–5.
38. Crist W, Carroll A, Shuster J, *et al.* Philadelphia chromosome positive childhood acute lymphoblastic leukemia: clinical and cytogenetic characteristics and treatment outcome: a Pediatric Oncology Group study. Blood 1990, **76**, 489–94.
39. Ribeiro RC, Broniscer A, Rivera GK, *et al.* Philadelphia chromosome-positive acute lymphoblastic leukemia in children: durable responses to chemotherapy associated with low initial white cell counts. Leukemia 1997, **11**, 1493–6.
40. Schrappe M, Arico M, Harbott J, *et al.* Philadelphia chromosome-positive (Ph+) childhood acute lymphoblastic leukemia: good initial steroid response allows early prediction of a favorable treatment outcome. Blood 1998, **92**, 2730–41.
41. Bernard O, Lecointe N, Jonveaux P, *et al.* Two site specific deletions and t(1;14) translocation restricted to human T-cell leukemias disrupt the 5 part of the *tal-1* gene. Oncogene 1991, **6**, 1477–88.
42. Landis SH, Murray T, Bolden S, Wingo PA. Cancer statistics 1998. CA Cancer J Clin 1998, **48**.
43. Cheson BD, Cassileth PA, Head DR, *et al.* Report of the National Cancer Institute-sponsored workshop on definitions of diagnosis and response in acute myeloid leukemia. J Clin Oncol 1990, **8**, 813–19.
44. Jennings CD, Foon KA, Recent advances in flow cytometry: application to the diagnosis of hematologic malignancy. Blood 1997, **90**, 2863–92.
45. Rovelli A, Biondi A, Rajnoldi AC, *et al.* Microgranular variant of acute promyelocytic leukemia in children. J Clin Oncol 1992, **10**, 1413–18.
46. Martinez-Climent JA, Garcia-Conde J. Chromosomal rearrangements in childhood acute myeloid leukemia and myelodysplastic syndromes. J Pediatr Hematol/Oncol 1999, **21**, 91–102.
47. Zipursky A, Thorner P, De Harven E, *et al.* Myelodysplasia and acute megakaryoblastic leukemia in Down's syndrome, Leuk Res 1994, **18**, 163–71.

48. Tallman MS, Hakimian D, Shaw JM, et al. Granulocytic sarcoma is associated with the 8;21 translocation in acute myeloid leukemia. J Clin Oncol 1993, **11**, 690–.
49. Ebb DH, Weinstein HJ. Diagnosis and treatment of childhood acute myelogenous leukemia. Ped Clin N Am 1997, **44**, 847–62.
50. Grier HE, Gelber RD, Camitta BM, et al. Prognostic factors in childhood acute myelogenous leukemia. J Clin Oncol 1987, **5**, 1026–32.
51. Lange BJ, Kobrinsky N, Barnard DR, et al. Distinctive demography, biology, and outcome of acute myeloid leukemia and myelodysplastic syndrome in children with Down syndrome: childrens Cancer Group studies 2861 and 2891. Blood 1998, **91**, 608–15.
52. Taub J, Huang X, Matherly LH, et al. Expression of chromosome 21-localizing genes in acute myeloid leukemia: differences between Down syndrome and non Down syndrome blast cells and relationship to *in vitro* sensitivity to cytosine arabinoside and daunorubicin. Blood 1999, **94**, 1393–400.
53. Zipursky A, Brown E, Christensen H et al. Leukemia and/or myeloproliferative syndrome in neonates with Down Syndrome. Semin Perinatol 1997, **21**, 97–101.
54. Raimondi SC, Chang MN, Ravindranath Y, et al. Chromosomal abnormalities in 478 children with acute myeloid leukemia: clinical characteristics and treatment outcome in a cooperative Pediatric Oncology Group study-POG 8821. Blood 1999, **94**, 3703–16.
55. Appelbaum FR, Gilliland DG, Tallman MS. The biology and treatment of acute myeloid leukemia. Educational book, American Society of Hematology meeting, 1998, 15–43.
56. Martinez-Climent JA, Lane NJ, Rubin CM, et al. Clinical and prognostic significance of chromosomal abnormalities in childhood acute myeloid leukemia de novo. Leukemia 1995, **9**, 95–101.
57. Chang KS, Fan YH, Stass SA, et al. Expression of AML1/ETO fusion transcripts and detection of minimal residual disease in t(8;21)-positive acute myeloid leukemia. Oncogene 1993, **8**, 983–8.
58. Saunders MJ, Tobal K, Liu Yin JA. Detection of t(8;21) by reverse transcriptase polymerase chain reaction in patients in remission of acute myeloid leukemia M2 after chemotherapy or bone marrow transplantation. Leuk Res 1994, **18**, 891–5.
59. Castilla LH, Wijmenga C, Wang Q, et al. Failure of embryonic hematopoesis and lethal hemorrhages in mouse embryos heterozygous for a knocked-in leukemia gene CBFβ-MYH11. Cell 1996, **87**, 687–96.
60. Lo Coco F, Diverio D, Falini B, et al. Genetic diagnosis and molecular monitoring in the management of Acute promyelocytic leukemia. Blood 1999, **94**, 12–22.
61. Kalwinsky DK, Raimondi SC, Schell MJ, et al. Prognostic importance of cytogenetic subgroups in de novo pediatric acute non-lymphoblastic leukemia. J Clin Oncol 1991, **8**, 75–83.
62. Woods WG, Kobrinsky N, Buckley JD, Lee JW, et al. Timed-sequential induction therapy improves post-remission outcome in acute myeloid leukemia: a report from the Childrens's Cancer Group. Blood 1996, **87**, 4979–89.
63. Ravindranath Y, Yeager M, Chang MN, et al. Autologous bone marrow transplantation versus intensive consolidation chemotherapy for acute myeloid leukemia in childhood. N Engl J Med 1996, **334**, 1428–34.
64. Fenaux P, Chastang C, Chevret S, et al. A randomized comparison of all *trans* retinoic acid (ATRA) followed by chemotherapy and ATRA plus chemotherapy and the role of maintenance therapy in newly diagnosed acute promyelocytic leukemia. Blood 1999, **94**, 1192–200.
65. Niu C, YanH, Sun HP, et al. Treatment of de novo and relapsed acute promyelocytic leukemia patients with arsenic trioxide. Blood 1998, **92**, 678a.
66. Jing Y, Dai J, Chalmers-Redman RME, et al. Arsenic trioxide selectively induces acute promyelocytic leukemia cell apoptosis via a hydrogen-peroxide-dependent pathway. Blood 1999, **94**, 2102–11.
67. Scheinberg DA, Lovett D, Divgi CR, et al. A phase 1 trial of monoclonal antibody M195 in acute myelogenous leukemia: specific bone marrow targeting and internalization of radionucleide. J Clin Oncol 1991, **9**, 478–90.
68. Sievers EL, Applebaum FA, Spielberger RT, et al. Selective ablation of acute myeloid leukemia using an anti-CD33 calicheamicin immunoconjugate. Blood 1997, **90**, 504a.
69. Cave H, Van der Werff Ten Bosch J, Suciu S, et al. Clinical significance of minimal residual disease in childhood acute lymphoblastic leukemia. N Engl J Med 1998, **339**, 591–8.
70. Coustan-Smith E, Behm FG, Sancho J, et al. Sequential monitoring of minimal residual disease in childhood acute lymphoblastic leukemia. Blood 1999, **94**, 2780a.
71. Donovan JW, Poor C, Bowers D, et al. Concordance of MRD results in matched bone marrow and peripheral blood samples indicate that peripheral blood could be a sole sample source for MRD detection in pediatric acute lymphoblastic leukemia. Blood 1999, **94**, 2781a.
72. Silver RT, Woolf SH, Hehlmann R, et al. An evidence-based analysis of the effect of Busulfan, Hydroxyurea, Interferon and allogeneic bone marrow transplantation in treating the chronic phase of chronic myeloid leukemia: developed for the American Society of Hematology. Blood 1999, **94**, 1517–36.
73. Homans AC, Young PC, Dickerman JD, Land ML. Adult-type CML in childhood: case report and review. Am J Pediatr Hematol Oncol 1984, **6**, 220–4.
74. Altman AJ. Chronic leukemias of childhood. In: Principles and practice of pediatric oncology, 3rd edn (ed. Pizzo and Poplack). Lippincott-Raven, Philadelphia, 1997, 483–504.
75. Dewald GW, Wyatt WA, Juneau AL, Carlson RO, Zinsmeister AR, Jalal SM et al. Highly sensitive fluorescence *in situ* hybridization method to detect double BCR/ABL fusion and monitor response to therapy in chronic myeloid leukemia. Blood 1998, **91**, 3357–65.
76. Creuzig U, Ritter J, Zimmerman M, Klingebiel T. Prognosis of chidren with chronic myeloid leukemia. A retrospective study of 75 patients. Klin Padiatr 1996, **202**, 236–41.
77. Collins RH, Shpilberg O, Drobyski WR, et al. Donor leukocyte infusions in 140 patients with relapsed malignancy after allogeneic bone marrow transplantation. J Clin Oncol 1997, **15**, 433–44.
78. La Rosée P, O'Dwyer ME, Druker BY. Insights from pre-clinical studies for new combination treatment regimens with the Bcr/Abl kinase inhibitor imatinib mesylate (Gleevic/Glivic) in chronic myelogenous leukemia: a translational perspective. Leukemia 2002, **16**(7), 1213–19.

6 | Lymphoma

Mary V. Gresik

Lymphomas are malignancies of the immune system and may derive from any of a number of stages in lymphocyte differentiation, accounting for their heterogeneous histologic appearance and the inordinate number of complex classification systems that continue to proliferate. Despite the large number of lymphoma subtypes seen in adults, only three types are seen commonly in children—Burkitt, lymphoblastic, and large cell lymphoma. The low grade B lymphomas, so common in adults, are not seen in the pediatric age group with very rare exceptions. The types of lymphoma seen in children are all of high grade, but paradoxically may be more amenable to conventional chemotherapy than those disorders seen in adults. Hodgkin lymphoma (HL) in children is similar to the disease seen in adults, with a predominance of nodular sclerosis and mixed cellularity subtypes in most centers. In addition to these three major types of non-Hodgkin lymphoma (NHL) and HL, children may also present with a number of lymphoproliferative disorders, generally in the setting of congenital or acquired immunocompromise. As in the adult, a number of benign lesions may mimic NHL and HL and deserve consideration in the differential diagnosis of malignant lymphoid diseases in children.

Epidemiology, incidence, prognosis

Lymphomas, including both HL and NHL, are the third most common malignancies in the pediatric population and make up 10% of all cancer in this age group. Approximately 60% of cases are NHL and 40% HL (1).

Although the reasons are not clear, the incidence of lymphomas in children in the United States has been increasing since 1973 (2). Figures for the United States in 1994 show an annual incidence rate of 8.4 per million children for NHL and 6.6 per million for HL. The incidence rate varies with age, sex, and race, with NHL being 2–3 times more common in boys than girls and twice as common in Whites than Blacks. The incidence of HL is greater in males than females until puberty when the rate for females surpasses males. HL is rare below the age of 5 years. As with NHL, the incidence of HL in Whites is higher than in Blacks (3).

There is considerable geographic variation in the incidence of lymphomas, with Burkitt lymphoma occurring more commonly in tropical Africa and New Guinea, where Epstein Barr virus (EBV) and malaria are thought to play a role in the pathogenesis. There is a wide variation in the incidence of NHL worldwide with a tendency for higher numbers in Mediterranean countries and lower numbers in Japan (4).

This geographic variation also occurs with HL with a higher incidence in Central and South America and the Middle East. As with NHL, rates of HL are low in East Asia. Throughout the world, HL tends to be very rare below 5 years of age. An overall male predominance is seen in most countries. The peak incidence of HL varies worldwide with a peak in late childhood–early adulthood in western countries, and a peak in the 5–9 year age group in developing countries (4).

Abnormalities of the immune system, especially in T cell mediated immunity, pose an increased risk for the development of lymphomas. Congenital immunodeficiencies such as ataxia telangiectasia, Wiskott–Aldrich syndrome, severe combined immunodeficiency (SCID), and X-linked lymphoproliferative syndrome (XLP), as well as AIDS and patients receiving immunosuppressive medications, all have an increased incidence of lymphoma.

The survival of children with NHL and HL has improved over the past 20–30 years, as newer combinations of chemotherapeutic agents have been introduced and supportive measures such as blood component therapy and cytokines (erythropoietin and granulocyte/monocyte colony stimulating factors) have been added to treatment protocols. The challenge remains to minimize complications of treatment and decrease the incidence of second malignancies in long-term survivors of childhood lymphoma.

Clinical presentation and natural history

Non-Hodgkin lymphomas in children frequently present in extranodal sites, while Hodgkin lymphoma is a nodal or mediastinal disease similar to that seen in adults. As a general rule, Burkitt lymphoma presents below the diaphragm (outside endemic African areas) and lymphoblastic lymphoma presents above the diaphragm. Burkitt lymphoma in Africa is seen in the jaw and bones, while in the United States involvement of the gastrointestinal tract, especially the ileocecal region, gonads, and kidneys is common. Bowel obstruction is a common presenting symptom in these patients. Bone marrow involvement with leukemic extension and central nervous system (CNS) involvement may be seen with Burkitt lymphoma. The peak age for presentation is 7 years in the African (endemic) type and 11 years in the sporadic type, with a male predominance (2–3:1) in both (5). Because of the rapid growth rate of these tumor cells, tumor lysis syndrome and hyperuricemia are common. The tumor lysis syndrome occurs when potassium, phosphates, and purines are released into the blood from dying cells, from either spontaneous tumor necrosis or after chemotherapy. Urine flow must be maintained and measures must be taken to keep phosphates and urates soluble (alkaline urine) or renal failure may ensue. Surgical resection along with combination chemotherapy and intrathecal therapy have resulted in a 70–80% cure rate. Relapses tend to occur within the first year, and patients who remain disease-free for one year may be considered cured (6).

Lymphoblastic lymphoma presents with a mediastinal mass in 50% of patients, often with pleural effusions and/or a superior vena cava syndrome. Males are affected more often (2.5:1) and the peak age is in the second decade. Bone marrow involvement with a leukemic distribution is common. The distinction between lymphoblastic lymphoma and T cell acute lymphoblastic leukemia (ALL) is somewhat arbitrary, but many cooperative groups use the figure of >25% bone marrow involvement to define leukemia. While the two entities—ALL and lymphoblastic lymphoma—are very similar in presentation, morphology, and prognosis, several groups have demonstrated subtle differences in the immunophenotype suggesting that T cell ALL may be derived from a more primitive cell (7). As with ALL, CNS and gonadal involvement are common with lymphoblastic lymphoma. Although less common than the T cell type, lymphoblastic lymphoma may be of B cell lineage, representing the tissue counterpart of early precursor B ALL. Early stage B precursor LBL is treated with the same protocols as the more common T cell type. When treated on high risk leukemia protocols, these patients may achieve a high complete response rate, and have a near 90% 3-year survival if they have localized disease (6, 8).

Large cell lymphomas are a diverse group of lymphomas which may present in lymph nodes, mediastinum or extranodally. Similar only in the large size of the lymphoma cell nuclei, they may be of B or T cell types. Like Burkitt lymphoma and lymphoblastic lymphoma, they are of high grade and exhibit a rapid growth rate. Large cell lymphomas comprise 15–30% of NHL in children. As a group they tend to have a high complete response rate (90%) and a 5-year disease-free survival rate of 70%. Some studies have demonstrated a better prognosis for those patients with purely cutaneous anaplastic large cell lymphoma (ALCL) (9).

Primary mediastinal large B cell lymphoma represents a distinct type of large cell lymphoma seen in children and young adults with a female predominance. The mediastinal location of this tumor and the extensive sclerosis associated with it results in a clinical presentation of airway compromise or superior vena cava syndrome (10).

Anaplastic large cell lymphoma is also a distinct subtype of large cell lymphoma characterized by CD30 positivity and a t(2;5) cytogenetic abnormality. It may present in childhood and in adults with a systemic or primarily cutaneous distribution. The cutaneous form appears to be more indolent than the systemic form. Cures of early stage systemic lesions have been reported, but late relapses may occur (9).

Hodgkin lymphoma in children as in adults generally presents in lymph nodes or the mediastinum, but may have extranodal extension. Painless adenopathy is the most common presentation with B symptoms present in 30% of patients (11). Bone marrow involvement in children with HL is very uncommon (12). While complete remission and 5-year survival rates in HL are high (90% in low stage disease, 75% in advanced staged disease), there is an increased risk of second malignancies, including acute myelogenous leukemia, NHL, and solid tumors in the range of 20% at 20 years (13). Other late sequelae include growth retardation, infertility, cardiac and pulmonary disease (14).

Etiology

Lymphomas, like most neoplasms, arise in a genetically altered cell at some stage in its development. In some instances, this genetic alteration is facilitated by a viral agent. Examples of this phenomenon include the role of HTLV I and II in T cell proliferation allowing for the development of adult T cell lymphoma/leukemia, and EBV resulting in B cell proliferation which may lead to the genetic abnormalities associated with Burkitt lymphoma. Lymphomas also arise with increased frequency in patients with immunodeficiencies, especially of T cell type.

Patients with congenital immunodeficiencies such as SCID, Wiskott–Aldrich syndrome, ataxia telangiectasia, and XLP all have an increased risk of lymphoma, as do patients with acquired immunodeficiency such as AIDS and transplant recipients. A common factor in all these patients is defective T cell regulation, allowing uncontrolled B cell proliferation, increasing the risk for a genetic alteration in these cells.

The role of radiation in the development of lymphomas is not clear. There were no definitive increases in lymphoma in atomic bomb survivors (15). There does appear to be an increased risk of NHL as well as leukemia in patients with HL treated with combined radiation and chemotherapy. The exact role of radiation and chemotherapeutic agents in these patients is not clear.

Classification

Because of their varied appearance and clinical behaviors NHLs have been a source of confusion for both clinicians and pathologists. The many attempts to create a meaningful classification scheme have not helped clarify this situation. Over the last 50 years lymphoma classifications have evolved from being based solely on morphology, to those based on immunophenotype or prognostic implication. The newest classifications for lymphomas the Revised European–American Lymphoma classification (REAL) (16) and the closely related World Health Organization (WHO) classification (17) define specific lymphomas by a combination of morphology, immunophenotype, cytogenetic abnormalities, and clinical presentation.

Despite these modifications and advances in our knowledge about lymphomas, none of the classifications is helpful in dealing with the spectrum of pediatric lymphoma. Pediatric lymphomas represent a small subset of lymphomas, distinctly different in clinical features and biology from the majority of adult lymphomas. Lymphomas in children often present in extranodal sites, are high grade, and are frequently leukemic in distribution. Adult lymphomas, in contrast, are generally nodal, many are low grade, and are rarely leukemic, although they may involve the bone marrow.

The types of NHL seen in the pediatric population include: Burkitt lymphoma (40–50%), lymphoblastic lymphoma/leukemia, T or B cell types (30%), and large cell lymphoma (15–30%) which includes diffuse large B cell lymphoma, peripheral T cell lymphoma (PTCL), and ALCL (6). All other types of lymphoma are extremely rare in the pediatric population. A comparative table of classification of pediatric NHLs is seen in Table 6.1.

There has been much controversy over the years concerning the significance of Burkitt versus non-Burkitt histology. The histologic features used to distinguish the two types are subtle and poorly reproducible even among experts. The non-Burkitt type is said to have greater variability in nuclear size and shape, more cytoplasm, and more prominent nucleoli. A study of pediatric cases from the Pediatric Oncology Group (POG) failed to show any significant differences between the two subtypes and concluded that the distinction between Burkitt and non-Burkitt morphology was clinicopathologically irrelevant in children (18).

Most lymphoblastic lymphomas are of T cell type, but occasionally may be of precursor B cell phenotype. Both types appear similar histologically. Earlier reports on morphology defined two subtypes, convoluted and nonconvoluted, as defined by the appearance of the nuclear contour. Clinical studies have failed to demonstrate any difference in behavior in these two subtypes (19, 20).

In contrast to the confusion generated by the proliferation of lymphoma classifications, HL as defined by Rye conference based on the classification of Lukes and Butler remains the standard (Table 6.2). HL with its four traditional subtypes is included in the REAL and WHO classifications, suggesting that the Reed Sternberg cell (RSC) in HL is derived from a lymphocyte and that HL should be considered as a distinct subtype of lymphoma. Nodular sclerosis HL (NSHL) and mixed cellularity HL (MCHL) are the types seen most commonly. Lymphocyte predominance HL (LPHL) may be seen in children, but is uncommon in all age groups. Lymphocyte depletion HL (LDHL) is very rare in childhood.

Table 6.1 Childhood NHLs—comparisons of classifications

Classification	Burkitt lymphoma	Lymphoblastic lymphoma	Large cell lymphoma
Rappaort	Undifferentiated	Poorly differentiated, diffuse (original) Lymphoblastic (revised)	Histiocytic, diffuse (original) Diffuse large cell (revised)
Lukes and Collins	Small, noncleaved follicular center cell	Convoluted T cell	Large cleaved/noncleaved follicular center cell B-immunoblastic sarcoma T-immunoblastic sarcoma
Kiel	Burkitt	T cell lymphoblastic	Centroblastic Immunoblastic Anaplastic B and T cell
Working Formulation	Small noncleaved	Lymphoblastic	Large cell, follicular and diffuse Immunoblastic
REAL	Burkitt	Precursor B or T lymphoblastic	Large cell, follicular and diffuse Immunoblastic
WHO	Burkitt	Precursor B or T lymphoblastic	Diffuse large B cell Peripheral T cell Anaplastic large cell

Table 6.2 Classification of HL

Lymphocyte predominant
Nodular sclerosis
Mixed cellularity
Lymphocyte depletion

Staging

The evaluation of a child with lymphadenopathy is a common problem in pediatric practice. There is an excellent recent review of the work-up of children with lymphadenopathy by Perkins et al. in *Seminars in diagnostic pathology* (21). While many cases of lymphadenopathy in children are caused by infectious agents, drug reactions, and autoimmune disorders, and may resolve with appropriate antibiotic therapy, if malignancy is a consideration in the differential diagnosis, a lymph node biopsy is warranted. In most instances an excisional biopsy is desirable, but on occasion fine needle aspirate (FNA) may yield diagnostic material. Limited numbers of cells are available from an FNA, but may be sufficient for culture and limited immunophenotyping by flow cytometry. While additional studies such as cytogenetics or electron microscopy may be performed on aspirated material, additional aspirates must be performed to obtain adequate numbers of cells (22). Primary diagnosis of most pediatric lymphomas, including HL may be made on FNAs. However, sampling error, especially in HL where the diagnostic cells are a minor component of the lesion, makes close follow-up of the patient necessary. Persistent or progressive lymphadenopathy warrants an excisional biopsy.

Once a diagnosis of a lymphoid malignancy is made, a staging work-up is initiated. In addition to a complete history and physical exam, the work-up includes a complete blood count, serum chemistries to evaluate liver and renal function, radiologic studies including chest X-ray, computed tomography (CT) of the chest and abdomen, bone marrow examination, and a lumbar puncture with cerebrospinal fluid (CSF) cytology. A gallium scan is done in patients with HL. Staging laparotomy for NHL has not been found to be useful, but may be helpful on occasion in the evaluation of patients with HL when there are questionable findings on the abdominal CT or gallium scan. Institutions participating in cooperative group studies may perform additional chemistry studies such as total proteins, albumin, amylase, calcium, phosphorus, quantitative immunoglobulins, and a number of viral serologies as directed by the study protocols.

The clinical and pathologic information obtained from the staging work-up will enable the clinician to determine the stage of the disease and appropriate therapy. The Ann Arbor staging system, useful in adult lymphomas is not helpful in dealing with pediatric lymphoid

Table 6.3 Staging of childhood lymphoma (St Judes) (1)

Stage I	Single nodal or extranodal site (excluding mediastinum and abdomen)
Stage II	Single extranodal site with regional node involvement
	Two or more nodal areas (same side of diaphragm)
	Two extranodal sites +/− regional node involvement
	Primary GI tract tumor +/− mesenteric node involvement
Stage III	Two extranodal sites on opposite sides of the diaphragm
	Two or more nodal sites (both sides of diaphragm)
	All primary intrathoracic tumors
	All extensive primary intra-abdominal disease
	All paraspinal or epidural tumors
Stage IV	Any of the above with central nervous system or bone marrow involvement

Table 6.4 Ann Arbor staging system for HL (11)

Stage I	Single nodal region or single extranodal site (IE)
Stage II	Two or more lymph node regions (same side of diaphragm)
	Localized extranodal site plus one or more lymph node regions (same side of diaphragm) (IIE)
Stage III	Lymph nodes on both sides of diaphragm
	With splenic involvement (IIIS)
	With localized extranodal site (IIIE)
	Or both (IIISE)
Stage IV	Disseminated involvement of one or more extranodal sites
	A = absence of symptoms
	B = presence of fever, night sweats, or unexplained weight loss (>10% body weight in preceding 6 months)

neoplasia with its high incidence of extranodal disease. A system developed by Murphy (1) (Table 6.3) is more helpful in the staging of pediatric patients. The Ann Arbor system is used to stage children with HL (Table 6.4).

Histopathologic features, immunohistochemistry, differential diagnosis

The three common types of NHL in children are all high grade lymphomas with a rapid growth rate. Consequently numerous mitotic figures and tingible body macrophages producing a starry sky pattern may be seen in all three types of lymphoma, although it is most commonly associated with Burkitt lymphoma. A comparison of the histologic features of the three common types of pediatric NHL is shown in Table 6.5.

Burkitt lymphoma exhibits a diffuse monomorphic proliferation of medium-sized lymphocytes, with small amounts of deeply basophilic cytoplasm on Giemsa-stained touch preparations or aspirate cytologic preparations. Many cases show cytoplasmic vacuoles (Fig. 6.1(a)) which are positive with neutral lipid stains such as Oil Red O. In tissue sections the cytoplasm is not as prominent and the classic starry sky pattern is frequently present (Fig. 6.1(b)). The cells have been categorized as small noncleaved lymphocytes. Their size is determined by comparison to a histiocyte nucleus. Burkitt cells have nuclei that are similar or slightly smaller than histiocyte nuclei (Fig. 6.1(c)). The cells in Burkitt lymphoma are fairly monomorphic in size and shape with irregularly distributed nuclear chromatin and 2–5 small nucleoli. In the so-called non-Burkitt type there is more heterogeneity in cell size and nucleoli tend to be fewer and more prominent. Immunohistochemistry demonstrates B cell marking (CD20) with light chain restriction. Terminal deoxynucleotidyl transferase (TdT) is negative in Burkitt cells.

The differential diagnosis for Burkitt lymphoma includes both lymphoblastic lymphoma and large cell lymphoma. The cells of Burkitt lymphoma have more cytoplasm than lymphoblastic lymphoma (best appreciated in touch preparations or cytological material), and less cytoplasm than large cell lymphomas. The nuclear chromatin pattern is coarser and nucleoli more prominent than lymphoblastic lymphoma. Distinction between large and small noncleaved cells using the histiocyte nuclear size as a guide may be difficult in tissue not prepared adequately. Large cell lymphomas tend to have larger nuclei with fewer nucleoli than Burkitt cells. Cytoplasmic vacuoles are uncommon in both lymphoblastic or large cell lymphoma. Using immunophenotyping, Burkitt lymphoma is of B cell type, while most lymphoblastic lymphomas are of T cell type. Large cell lymphomas may be of B or T cell types. Lymphoproliferative disorders, especially those driven by EBV may resemble Burkitt lymphoma or large cell lymphoma. These proliferations may be monomorphic or polymorphic as well as mono- or polyclonal, making distinction from high grade B cell lymphoma of either Burkitt or large cell type difficult. The endemic or African form of Burkitt lymphoma is consistently associated with

Table 6.5 Comparison of the histologic features of pediatric NHL

Features	Lymphoblastic	Burkitt	Large cell
Pattern	Diffuse +/− starry sky	Diffuse +/− starry sky	Diffuse +/− starry sky
Cell size	Medium	Medium	Large
Nuclear chromatin	Fine	Coarsely reticulated	Vesicular
Nuclear contour	+/− convoluted	Round	Round/variable
Nucleoli	Inconspicuous	2–5 small	May be prominent
Cytoplasm	Scant	Moderate, vacuolated	Moderate–Abundant
Immunophenotype	Immature T cell	Mature B cell	Mature B, T, null

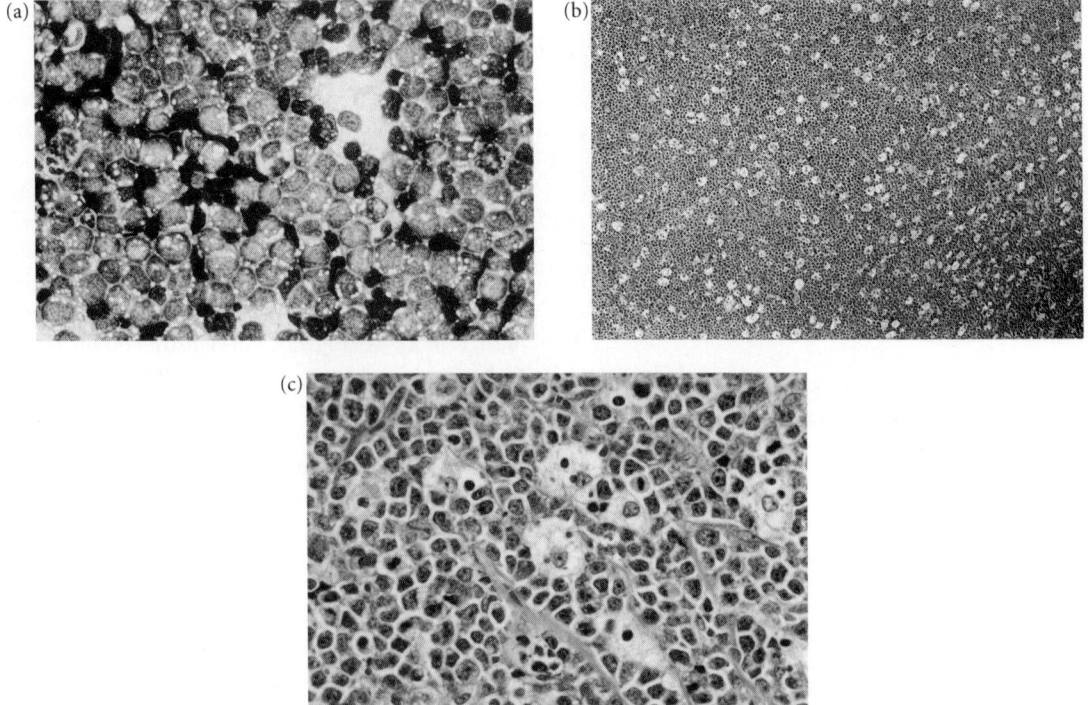

Fig. 6.1 (a) Touch preparation of Burkitt lymphoma. There is a homogeneous population of lymphocytes with a small amount of cytoplasm, fine nuclear chromatin, and prominent vacuoles. Giemsa ×600. (b) Burkitt lymphoma, low power. A starry sky pattern is created by large numbers of phagocytic histiocytes admixed with lymphoma cells. H&E ×100. (c) Burkitt lymphoma, high power. The lymphoma cells are similar or slightly smaller than the nuclei of the histiocytes. H&E ×600.

EBV, but in the sporadic form the association is less frequent (20–80%) (23).

Lymphoblastic lymphoma also presents as a diffuse proliferation of medium-sized cells. On cytologic preparations the cells resemble the lymphoblasts of ALL, having a high nuclear:cytoplasmic ratio and scant amounts of cytoplasm. In tissue sections as in cytologic preparations, the nuclear chromatin is finely distributed with indistinct nucleoli. Some degree of nuclear irregularity or convolution may be seen in most cases (Fig. 6.2(a)).

Mitotic activity is prominent and a starry sky pattern is commonly seen. Immunohistochemistry shows a T cell phenotype (CD3, CD45RO) and TdT positivity in most cases. A small number of lymphoblastic lymphomas are of precursor B cell phenotype.

In addition to Burkitt lymphoma, lymphoblastic lymphoma must be differentiated from T cell ALL and other T cell lymphomas. The distinction between T cell ALL and lymphoblastic lymphoma is somewhat arbitrary. Many cooperative groups define lymphoma as

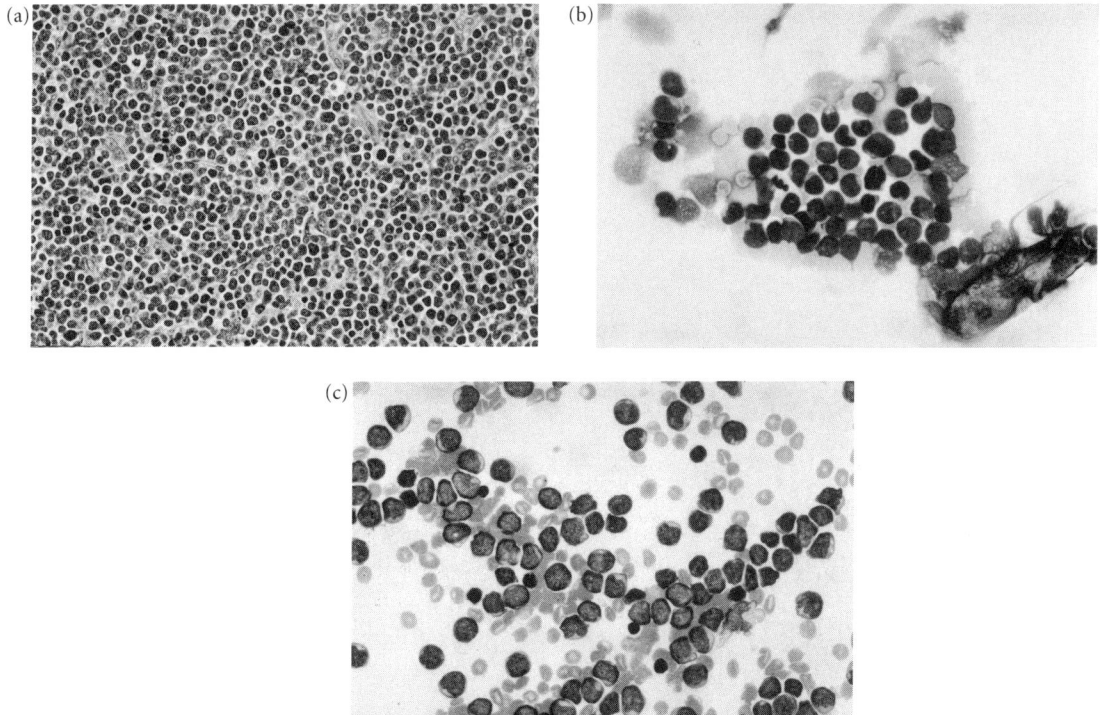

Fig. 6.2 (a) Lymphoblastic lymphoma, high power. There is a diffuse proliferation of medium-sized lymphocytes with a very high N:C ratio. Many of the nuclear contours are irregular. H&E ×400. (b) Lymphoblastic lymphoma, pleural fluid, high power. There is a homogeneous population of lymphoblasts. The cells have a very high N:C ratio and fine nuclear chromatin. Giemsa ×600. (c) Reactive pleural fluid, high power. There is a more heterogeneous population of lymphocytes than seen in (b). The larger cells resemble lymphoblasts, but are thoracic duct lymphocytes. Giemsa ×600.

having less than 25% bone marrow involvement, with more extensive marrow involvement defining leukemia. And while the cellular morphology is similar in both disorders, immunophenotyping data suggest that lymphoblastic leukemia is derived from a less differentiated cell (7). Diagnosis may be made on cytologic and immunologic evaluation of pleural effusions (Fig. 6.2(b)). Care must be taken in the interpretation of pleural fluid from young children. Thoracic surgery, such as corrective procedures for congenital heart disease frequently result in the presence of thoracic duct lymphocytes in the pleural fluid (Fig. 6.2(c)). These thoracic duct lymphocytes resemble lymphoblasts and must be interpreted with the clinical situation in mind. Lymphoblastic lymphoma may be differentiated from other T cell lymphomas by its TdT positivity and immature immunophenotype (CD1a positive, CD4 and CD8 double positive or double negative).

Large cell lymphomas represent a number of specific clinicopathologic diseases with distinctive histopathology. Diffuse large cell lymphomas may be composed of large cleaved or noncleaved cells or those with immunoblastic features. These cells have moderate to large amounts of cytoplasm which may be clear or amphophilic, with round to oval nuclei, vesicular chromatin and one to several nucleoli (Fig. 6.3(a)). Large noncleaved lymphomas must be differentiated from Burkitt lymphoma. This is generally possible using the histiocyte nucleus as a size guide, but on occasions may be difficult due to technical artifact. Large cell lymphomas have more abundant cytoplasm than Burkitt cells in both cytologic and histologic preparations. A high mitotic rate with a starry sky pattern may be seen in both lesions. While the distinction between diffuse large cell lymphoma and immunoblastic lymphoma is an issue in the Working Formulation, this distinction is extremely subjective and is not a feature of the newer classification systems.

Immunoblastic features include prominent condensation of the chromatin around the nuclear membrane, single prominent nucleolus, and eccentric position of

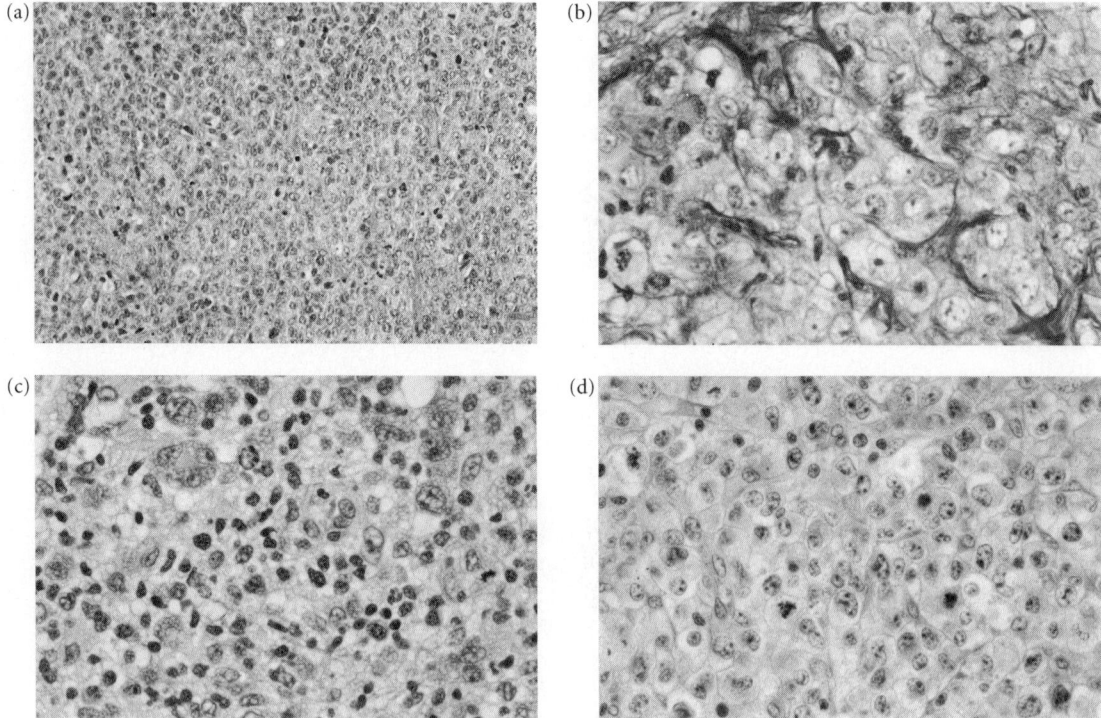

Fig. 6.3 (a) Diffuse large cell lymphoma, B cell type, high power. There is a diffuse proliferation of large lymphocytic cells with abundant cytoplasm, round nuclei, and vesicular chromatin. H&E ×600. (b) Primary mediastinal large B cell lymphoma, high power. Thin bands of fibrosis surround small clusters of large lymphoid cells. Some of these cells have prominent nucleoli. PAS ×600. (c) Anaplastic large cell lymphoma, high power. There is a pleomorphic proliferation of lymphocytic cells with many large atypical and multinucleated cells. H&E ×600. (d) Peripheral T cell lymphoma, high power. There is a diffuse infiltrate of large cells with abundant pale cytoplasm. Nuclear chromatin is fine with multiple small nucleoli. H&E ×600.

the nucleus. Large cells with abundant clear cytoplasm tend to be T cells and are classified as PTCLs because of their mature T cell phenotype (CD3, 5, 7 positive, CD4 or 8 positive).

Large cell lymphoma and occasionally Burkitt lymphoma may closely resemble granulocytic sarcoma. While some cases of granulocytic sarcoma may show evidence of granulocytic differentiation in the form of eosinophilic myelocytes, many are extremely undifferentiated morphologically. Immunophenotyping will demonstrate myeloid markers—CD13, 14, 33—and cytochemistry or immunohistochemistry will demonstrate specific esterase (alpha naphthyl ASD chloroacetate esterase) or muramidase (lysozyme) positivity in granulocytic sarcoma.

Primary mediastinal large B cell lymphoma is characterized by large lymphoid cells with abundant cytoplasm which may be amphophilic or clear, and round or irregular nuclear contours. The chromatin pattern is vesicular with prominent nucleoli. Sclerosis is a very characteristic feature of this lesion. The sclerosis may vary from thick bands of collagen to fine spider-like sclerosis surrounding small groups of cells (Fig. 6.3(b)). The major differential diagnosis involves nodular sclerosing HL and ALCL. The broad bands of collagen and nodules of lymphoid cells seen in NSHL are not seen in mediastinal large B cell lymphoma, the sclerosis while it may be dense generally surrounds single and small groups of cells. The characteristic lacunar variants of the Reed Sternberg cell are not seen in this lesion, and the background is not typical of HL. While bi- and multinucleated immunoblastic cells, resembling classic RSCs may be seen in mediastinal large B cell lymphoma, the population of atypical cells is more homogeneous than that seen in HL. ALCL does not exhibit the characteristic sclerotic pattern of mediastinal large B cell lymphoma and is generally of T cell type.

Anaplastic large cell lymphoma is characterized by a diffuse proliferation of large immunoblastic appearing cells with abundant cytoplasm and pleomorphic, often lobulated nuclei (Fig. 6.3(c)). Cells resembling RSCs may be seen. The cells tend to grow in a cohesive pattern often with a sinusoidal distribution. A number of histologic patterns have been described including a common type (24), pleomorphic and monomorphic (25), sarcomatoid (26), lymphohistiocytic (27), neutrophil rich (28), and a small cell variant (29). This lymphoma is most often of T cell type and is positive for CD30. Epithelial membrane antigen (EMA) is generally positive, but other markers are variable. Most of the common types of ALCL are positive with the ALK1 monoclonal antibody.

The differential diagnosis includes HL, metastatic carcinoma, melanoma, and sarcoma, and malignant histiocytic disorders. Immunohistochemistry is helpful in this differential. Metastatic tumors will be negative for T cell markers and CD30 and positive for cytokeratin, HMB45, or markers of muscle or other types of differentiation. ALCL does not usually express histiocytic markers. Differentiation from HL may be difficult at times, and some forms of HL (syncytial variant of NSHL and reticular LDHL) may actually represent this type of lymphoma.

Peripheral T cell lymphomas are a heterogeneous group of lymphomas similar only in their mature T cell phenotype. PTCLs are characterized by a heterogeneous cell population, ranging from small to large lymphocytes. The smaller lymphocytes may have irregular nuclear contours and coarse, clumped chromatin. Medium and larger sized cells have abundant pale or clear cytoplasm, vesicular chromatin and small nucleoli (Fig. 6.3(d)). The cytoplasmic borders between these large cells are prominent and may be accentuated with a Periodic Acid Schiff (PAS) stain. In some types of PTCL, the nuclear contour is folded or multilobated with cells resembling Reed Sternberg Cell (RSC). Eosinophils and histiocytes may be present. High endothelial venules are often prominent in these lesion (30). Differential diagnosis includes mixed and large cell lymphomas of B cell type, histiocytic malignancies, carcinoma, melanoma, and germ cell tumors. A number of these lymphomas are classified in the REAL classification or listed as provisional entities. With the exception of ALCL, all are rare in the pediatric population. Those that have been seen in children are cited in the recent review of PTCL by Agnarsson and Kadin (9).

Hodgkin lymphoma in children is similar to that seen in adults. Nodular sclerosing HL is the most common subtype seen in most institutions. Classically, NSHL presents little problem in diagnosis with its thickened capsule and collagen bands which extend into the nodal parenchyma encircling nodules of lymphoid tissue (Fig. 6.4(a)). Lacunar cells, a distinct type of RSC, are characteristic of this entity. Lacunar cells represent an artifact of formalin fixation with retraction of the cytoplasm leaving the lobulated nucleus in an empty space (lacuna) (Fig. 6.4(b)). Lacunar cells when fixed in mercury containing fixatives do not display this "lacunar" artifact, and have abundant pale cytoplasm with a low nuclear:cytoplasmic ratio and a lobulated nucleus at the periphery of the cell. The cellular composition of the nodules in NSHL varies greatly in individual cases with variable numbers of eosinophils, histiocytes, plasma cells, and lymphocytes. Necrosis may be seen in this type of HL. A type of NSHL termed the syncytial variant has been described (31) in which lacunar cells are present in large cohesive sheets and clusters. Some authors have suggested a more aggressive course for this type of NSHL (32).

Controversy exists over the prognostic implication of the cellular make-up of the nodules in NSHL. Studies conducted by the British National Lymphoma Investigation (BNLI) showed a worse response to initial therapy, increased relapse rate and decreased overall survival in patients with Grade II nodules (33). They defined Grade II nodules as those with large numbers of RSCs or pleomorphic RSCs (including the syncytial variant), and Grade I nodules as those with a predominance of lymphocytes, a mixed cell background, and a minority of RSCs. A study from the Massachusetts General Hospital also showed a longer survival and more successful salvage therapy in relapsed patients with Grade I morphology (34). Other studies have failed to show any difference in prognosis related to the cellular composition of the nodules in NSHL (35, 36).

While differential diagnosis of NSHL is generally not a problem, small biopsies or biopsies of peripheral lymph nodes may not reveal the classic features of lacunar cells and sclerosing bands. Because of the dense fibrosis associated with it, primary mediastinal large B cell lymphoma may be confused with NHL. The cells present in the large cell lymphoma are generally more homogeneous than the cellular proliferation seen in HL. The syncytial variant of NHL presents problems in differentiation from metastatic cancer, melanoma, or ALCL. Immunohistochemical stains can help differentiate the first two entities, but since ALCL cells and RSCs are both CD30 positive, this distinction may be difficult. Reed Sternberg cells are frequently CD15 positive and CD45 negative and may help in this distinction. It is likely, however, that many cases of syncytial variant NHL actually represent ALCL. Probes are now available to detect the ALK1 product of the t(2;5) translocation characteristic of ALCL.

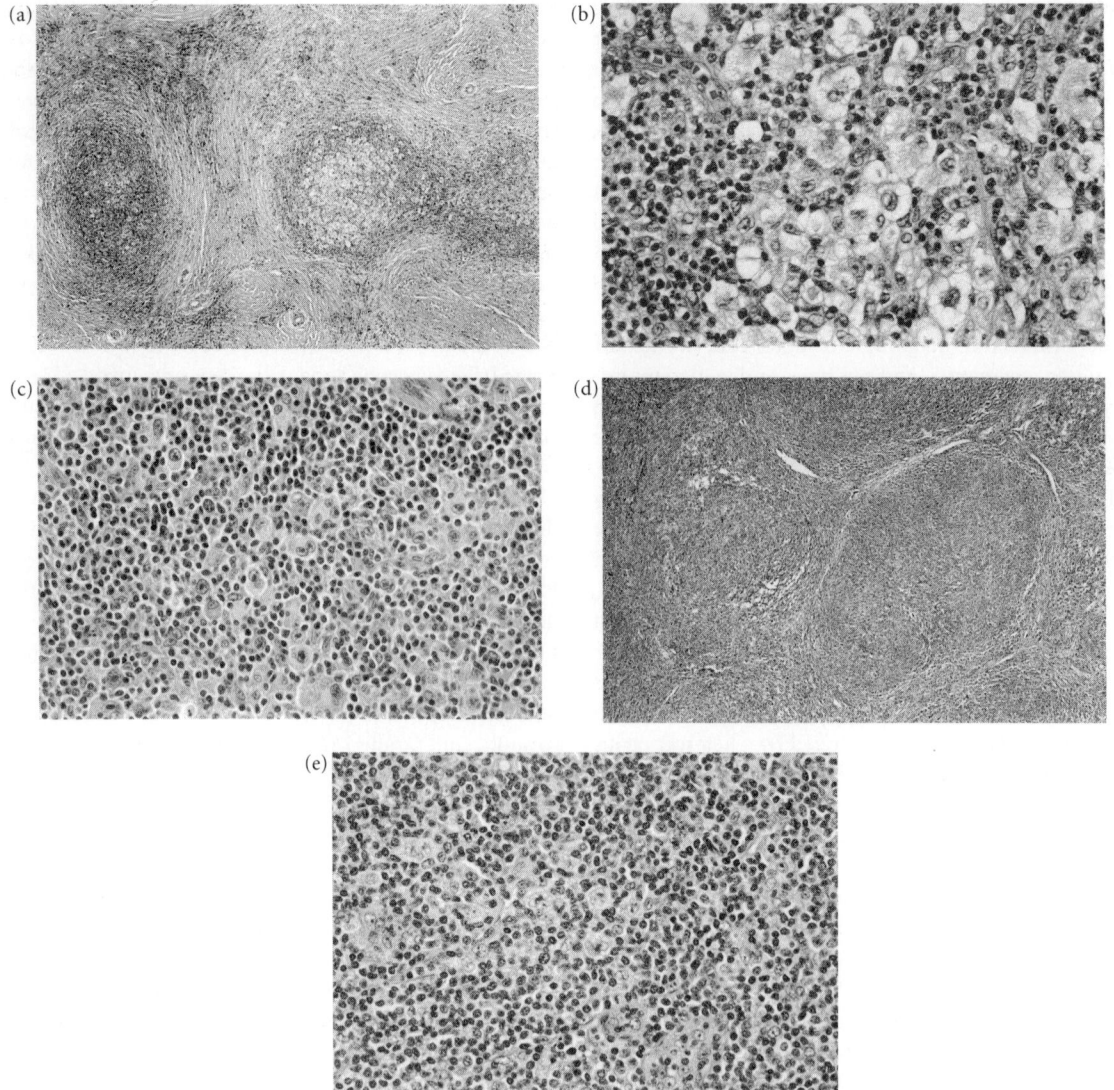

Fig. 6.4 (a) NSHL, low power. Thick bands of collagen surround nodules of lymphocytic cells. H&E ×50. (b) NSHL, high power. Lacunar cells show single and lobated nuclei and abundant clear cytoplasm. H&E ×400. (c) MCHL, high power. There is a heterogeneous population of small lymphocytes, histiocytes, eosinophils, plasma cells, and abundant Reed Sternberg cells. Both classic (binucleate) and mononuclear Hodgkins cell are present. H&E ×400. (d) LPHL, low power. A vaguely nodular pattern is seen on low power. H&E ×50. (e) LPHL, high power. The population consists of small lymphocytes with scattered L&H "popcorn" cells. H&E ×400.

Mixed cellularity HL is seen often in the pediatric population, as it is in adults. MCHL is characterized not only by a mixed population of eosinophils, histiocytes, plasma cells, and lymphocytes, but more importantly by large numbers of RSCs, both the classic binucleated, binucleolated type, and the mononuclear variant or Hodgkin cell (Fig. 6.4(c)).

Immunohistochemistry is generally not necessary to identify the numerous RSCs in MCHL, but CD15 and CD30 are positive in both the classic and mononuclear RSCs. In addition to the mixed cellular background and the number of RSCs, mixed cellularity is the subtype used to classify cases of HL that do not fit into LP, LD, or NS types, and also includes nodes partially involved by HL (37). Diagnosis of early nodal involvement by nodular sclerosis may present a problem in classification, although this distinction may not have major clinical implications. Many would classify a node with lacunar cells and minimal sclerosis as mixed cellularity, while others would call it cellular phase of NHL (38). Differential diagnosis is generally not a problem with lymph nodes totally effaced by MCHL, however, partial involvement may be difficult to detect. The interfollicular areas of reactive lymph nodes should be inspected carefully for RSCs and the appropriate cellular background. These areas often have a "moth-eaten" appearance on low power. The diagnosis of interfollicular HL, however, should be made with caution. Reactive lymph nodes with immunoblasts in the interfollicular areas may suggest focal HL. These immunoblasts have a staining pattern with CD30 that mimics RSC. CD15 is negative in these cells (39).

Cytologic preparations from FNAs or touch preparations in HL nodes may fail to show RSCs and may be confused with a benign reactive process. It is important to note as well, that the presence of RSCs in the correct background of cells is necessary to make the diagnosis of HL. Reed Sternberg cells may be seen in viral infections, such as infectious mononucleosis or in large cell lymphomas. In both these disorders, the background cells are considerably more monomorphic than the mixed background of HL. The presence of immunoblasts is helpful, since immunoblasts are seldom seen in HL.

Lymphocyte predominant HL is an uncommon type of HL in both adults and children. Lymph nodes involved by LPHL are generally large (>3 cm) and have a vaguely nodular appearance on low power examination (Fig. 6.4(d)). The architecture is effaced completely in most cases with only rare residual germinal centers present. The cells present include small lymphocytes, variable numbers of histiocytes, either singly or in small clusters, and L and H or "popcorn" cells. L and H cells are large with a high nuclear:cytoplasmic ratio and highly convoluted nucleus (Fig. 6.4(e)). Nucleoli generally are not prominent. Classic RSCs are seldom seen. The L and H cells mark as B lymphocytes, are frequently EMA positive, and do not express CD15 or 30, suggesting that this disease has features intermediate between classical HL and low grade B cell lymphoma (40). The major differential diagnosis includes progressive transformation of germinal centers (PTGC), other forms of HL, Lennert's lymphoma, and on occasion granulomatous processes. Differentiation from PTGC will be discussed below. If classic RSCs or Hodgkin cells are readily visible, the process more closely resembles MCHL and probably will behave in a more aggressive fashion than LPHL. If lacunar cells or any degree of capsular thickening and collagen bands are present, the lesion should be classified as NSHL. Lennert's lymphoma is a PTCL with numerous epithelioid histiocytes. No L and H cells should be seen in Lennert's lymphoma and the small lymphocytes in the background are atypical in appearance. Granulomatous processes such as toxoplasmosis generally have large numbers of reactive germinal centers and larger histiocytic aggregates, while the histiocytic clusters in LPHL are usually small.

Other types of lymphoma, more common in adult patients have been reported rarely in pediatric patients. These include: T cell rich B cell lymphoma (41, 42), follicular lymphoma (43), and neoplasms of reticulum cells in lymph nodes (44).

Lymphoproliferative disorders and other lesions mimicking lymphoma

In addition to the above-described lymphomas, a number of benign entities or those of questionable malignant potential may present in the pediatric patient. Acute EBV infection with the clinical features of the mononucleosis syndrome may present with lymphadenopathy and tonsillar enlargement. On occasion these lesions are biopsied and may pose a diagnostic dilemma if the complete clinical presentation, age of the patient, and EBV status are not considered. Lymph nodes or lymphoid tissue from the oropharynx in patients with mononucleosis show effacement of the normal follicular architecture by a diffuse proliferation of transformed lymphocytes or immunoblasts (Fig. 6.5). This appearance is suggestive of large cell lymphoma. Identification of EBV either serologically or in the proliferating lymphocytes as well as demonstration of their polyclonal nature of the infiltrate differentiates this lesion from large cell lymphoma.

A similar EBV-driven proliferation may be seen in patients who are transplant recipients, or immunocompromised for other reasons. These post-transplant lymphoproliferative lesions are difficult to classify and there may be little correlation between the morphologic appearance of the lesion and its biologic behavior (45). These lesions may be polymorphous or monomorphous in appearance and may be polyclonal or monoclonal. Polymorphous, polyclonal lesions tend to be less aggressive and may respond to a decrease in immunosuppression, while monomorphic, monoclonal lesions most probably represent malignant neoplasia, and generally do not respond to immune modulation.

A recently described lesion termed PTGC may be seen in children as well as adults and may be confused with LPHL. Lymph nodes involved by PTGC are frequently large (>3 cm) and often occur in the cervical region. Microscopically the node exhibits prominent follicular hyperplasia with one to several large nodular collections of lymphocytes with features different from the normal reactive germinal centers (Fig. 6.6(a)). The progressively transformed nodules are composed of small lymphocytes with round to slightly irregular nuclear contours and scattered larger transformed lymphocytes similar to those in the normal germinal centers (Fig. 6.6(b)). Histiocytes may be seen ringing the periphery of these nodules. While there is some resemblance to LPHL, PTGC is seen in the setting of a node with prominent follicular hyperplasia, and the L and H cells of LPHL are not seen in this lesion. The significance of this lesion and its relationship to LPHL are controversial. A number of studies have shown an association between the two conditions, and some authors suggest that PTGC represents a precursor lesion to LPHL (46–49). It is important to recognize this lesion and not dismiss the lymph node as reactive hyperplasia, as the patients require careful follow-up because of the reported association with HL. Likewise it is important not to confuse this benign lesion with LPHL, initiating a staging work-up and therapy for the patient.

Another recently described entity of undetermined biology termed Autoimmune Lymphoproliferative Syndrome may present in children and enter into the differential of both B and T cell lymphomas. Children with this syndrome have *FAS* gene mutations resulting in abnormal lymphocyte apoptosis. Clinical features include massive splenomegaly and lymphadenopathy with associate autoimmune disorders such as glomerulonephritis, autoimmune hemolytic anemias, immune thrombocytopenic purpura and a Guillian–Barre-like syndrome. Lymph nodes in these patients show florid follicular hyperplasia and expansion of the interfollicular regions by immunoblasts and plasma cells. There is conspicuous absence of histiocytes containing apoptotic material "tingible body macrophages." Flow cytometry shows T cells negative for both CD4 and CD8 which may suggest a diagnosis of PTCL. *FAS* gene mutations can be demonstrated in these nodes (50–52).

A number of other reactive lesions mimicking lymphoma may be seen in children. If the clinical situation

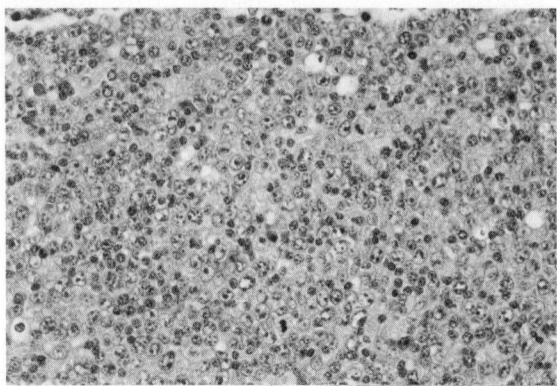

Fig. 6.5 Lymphoproliferative disease, high power. Although there are some small lymphocytes present, there is a prominent population of large lymphocytes mimicking diffuse large cell lymphoma. H&E ×400.

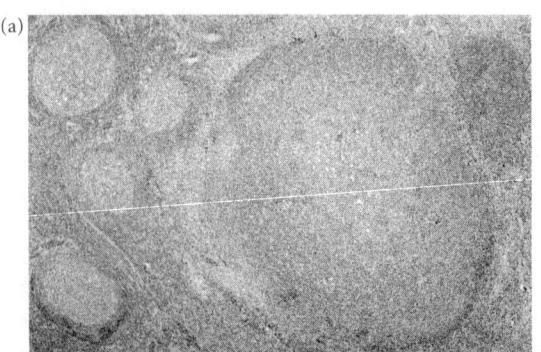
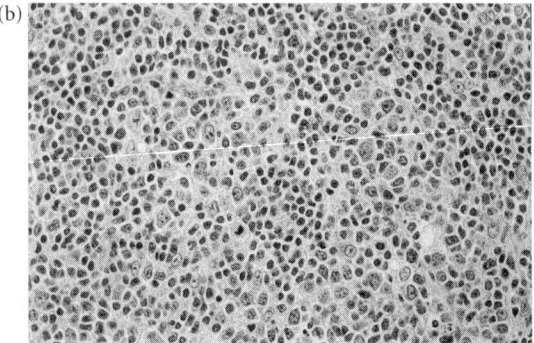

Fig. 6.6 (a) Progressive transformation of germinal centers, low power. A large lymphocytic nodule is present, surrounded by reactive germinal centers. H&E ×50. (b) Progressive transformation of germinal centers, high power. The cells of the nodule seen in (a) consist of a mixture of small and large follicular center cells. No Reed Sternberg cells are present. H&E ×400.

is not considered, lesions such as postvaccination lymphadenitis or drug-induced adenopathy may cause considerable confusion with malignancy.

Tumor markers

The availability of monoclonal antibodies has greatly enhanced our ability to characterize lymphoid proliferations. A large number of antibodies with fluorescent tags are available for use in flow cytometry, and increasing numbers of antibodies suitable for use with fixed, paraffin embedded tissue are commercially available. Flow cytometry may be used to characterize the cells in lymph nodes and other tissue biopsies, FNAs or effusions from body cavities. Consistent characteristic patterns are seen for the most common pediatric lymphomas. Burkitt lymphoma cells are positive for: CD10, 19, 20, 22 and show light chain restriction. They are TdT negative. Lymphoblastic lymphoma cells generally express pan T cell markers (CD2, 3, 5 and 7) as well as the early thymocyte marker CD1a. Lymphoblastic lymphomas are TdT positive. Large cell lymphomas may be of B cell or T cell type. Large B cell lymphomas express pan B cell markers and show light chain restriction. Large T cell lymphomas may be CD30 positive (ALCL) or may be a type of PTCL. PTCLs often show an aberrant phenotype with the loss of one or more pan T antigens, coexpression of CD4 and CD8, or loss of both CD4 and CD8. Large cell lymphomas are TdT negative. Flow cytometry is not useful in the diagnosis of HL, as the majority of the cells in the tumor are reactive host T cells.

Immunohistochemistry on fixed tissue is a useful technique and may be used when material is not available for flow cytometry. Immunohistochemistry is extremely helpful in focal lymphomas where flow cytometry may give misleading results. The use of antibodies to CD15 and CD30 to mark Reed Sternberg cells may assist in the diagnosis of HL. In LPHL, the L&H cells exhibit B cell markers.

A variety of antigen retrieval methods enhance the ability to identify surface antigens on fixed, embedded tissues (53, 54). Surface antigens as well as protein products of normal and abnormal genes may be detected in tissue sections. As more antibodies become available for use on fixed tissue sections, immunohistochemistry becomes an increasingly useful tool for the immunophenotyping of lymphomas. The most commonly used antibodies to characterize NHL and HL are listed in Table 6.6.

Table 6.6 Antibodies useful in characterization of pediatric lymphomas

	Reactivity
T cell markers	
CD1a	Common thymocytes
	Langerhans cells
CD3	Pan T cell
CD4	Helper T cells
CD5	Pan T cell
CD7	Pan T cell
CD8	Suppressor/cytotoxic T cells
CD45RO(UCHL1)	Pan T cell
CD99(O13)	Precursor T cells
TdT	Thymocytes
B cell markers	
CD19	Pan B cell
CD20(L26)	Pan B cell
CD21	Pan B cell
CD22	Pan B cell
CD79a	Pan B cell
Other markers	
CD10(CALLA)	Precursor B cells
	Follicular center B cells
CD15(LeuM1)	Myelomonocytic cells
	Reed Sternberg cells
CD30(Ki-1,BerH2)	Anaplastic large cell lymphoma
	Reed Sternberg cells
CD45RB(LCA)	Leukocytes
CD68(KP-1)	Macrophages
CD13	Myeloid cells
CD33	Myeloid cells
EMA	Anaplastic large cell lymphoma
	L and H cells

Molecular biology and cytogenetics

The application of conventional cytogenetic studies to lymphomas has led to the demonstration of the characteristic translocations seen in Burkitt lymphoma—t(8;14) (q24;q32), and less commonly t(2:8) (p11;q24) and t(8;22) (q24;q11); the t(14;18) seen most commonly in adult follicular lymphomas; and the t(2;5) (p23;q35) seen in ALCL. A number of translocations have been seen in lymphoblastic lymphoma, involving chromosomes 7 and 14, sites of the T cell receptor (TCR) gene. The most common of these translocations is t(11;14) (p13;q11). The t(14;18) and t(8;14) have been described in a few large cell lymphomas, but no consistent translocation has been described in this type of lymphoma. The most common translocations and other chromosomal abnormalities seen in pediatric lymphomas are listed in Table 6.7.

The use of newer molecular techniques such as Southern blot analysis, polymerase chain reaction (PCR), and fluorescent *in situ* hybridization (FISH) have allowed greater understanding of these genetic abnormalities seen in lymphomas. The translocations seen in most lymphomas result in the dysregulation of proto-oncogenes involved in cell proliferation and differentiation, or the creation of a novel fusion product that has effects on cell proliferation. The loss of a tumor suppressor gene, a mechanism common in many solid tumors may be seen in some patients with T cell leukemia/lymphoma and HL.

The most common molecular alterations in NHL are rearrangements in immunoglobulin and TCR genes. Normal immune function requires rearrangement of immunoglobulin heavy and light chains and all four chains of the TCR in response to antigenic stimuli. In their unstimulated germline configuration both B and T cells have numerous variable, diversity, joining and constant regions which with rearrangement can produce an almost infinite variety of molecules. In B cells heavy chain rearrangement occurs before light chains, and kappa before lambda light chains. In T cells the gamma and delta genes rearrange before the alpha and beta. DNA-PCR methods are used to identify these immunoglobulin and TCR gene rearrangements and thereby establish clonality. Most malignancies, including lymphomas are thought to be clonal proliferations of genetically altered cells, and should demonstrate a single abnormal population. Application of molecular studies to a variety of lymphocytic and histiocytic lesions, however, has demonstrated clonality in a number of disorders, which if not definitely benign, are of uncertain malignant potential. Diseases such as Langerhans cell histiocytosis, monoclonal gammopathy of unknown significance, lymphomatoid papulosis, and salivary gland lesions in Sjogrens syndrome all show clonal populations (53).

While *p53* and *BCL2* mutations have not been found in most pediatric NHL, there is some evidence that they may be involved in the pathogenesis of HL. p53 regulates a G1 checkpoint allowing only cells with intact DNA to enter S phase. Cells with DNA damage initiate DNA repair or undergo apoptosis. Bcl-2 and other proteins in this family regulate this apoptotic pathway. Proteins which inhibit apoptosis include Bcl-2, Bcl-xl, Bcl-w, Bfl-1, Mcl-1, and A1. Promoters of apoptosis include Bax, Bak, Bad, Bcl-xs, Bik, and Hrk. These proteins are located in the mitochondria. The proteins dimerize with each other, the balance of which determines if a cell will undergo apoptosis or not. Overexpression of *BCL2*, preventing apoptosis has been suggested as a mechanism in the pathogenesis of HL. *BCL2* over-expression is seen in follicular lymphomas with the t(14;18) and a few cases of HL with this translocation have been reported (54). Other mechanisms,

Table 6.7 Common chromosomal abnormalities in pediatric lymphomas

Lymphoma type	Chromosome abnormality	Genes involved
Burkitt	t(8;14) (q24;q32)	CMYC, IgH
	t(2;8) (p11;q24)	IgKappa, CMYC
	t(8;22) (q24;q11)	CMYC, IgLambda
Lymphoblastic	t(11;14) (p13;q11)	LMO2, TCRαδ
	t(11;14) (p15;q11)	LMO1, TCRαδ
	t(10;14) (q24;q11)	HOX11, TCRαδ
	t(1;14) (p34;q11)	TAL1, TCRαδ
	t(7;9) (q34;q32)	TCRβ, TAL2
	t(7;9) (q34;q34)	TCRβ, TAN1
	t(1;7) (q34;p13)	TAL1, TCRβ
	t(1;7) (p32;q34)	LCK, TCRβ
	del	TAL1
		TAL1
	p16ink4a	MTS1/MTS1
Large cell	t(2;5) (p23;q35)	ALK, NMP
T	t(8;14) (q24;q32)	CMYC, IgH
B	T(2;5) (p23;q35)	ALK, NMP

however, are also capable of causing *BCL2* over-expression. EBV, shown to up regulate *BCL2* expression, has been demonstrated in a large number of HL cases (54).

The translocation seen in Burkitt lymphoma results in the movement of the *CMYC* proto-oncogene at (8q24) to the site of the immunoglobulin heavy chain gene (14q32), kappa light chain (2p11) or lambda light chain (22q11) locus where it is abnormally expressed. The *CMYC* proto-oncogene is part of the *MYC* family which includes *CMYC*, *LMYC*, and *NMYC*. These genes are involved in cell proliferation, differentiation, and apoptosis. The proteins produced by these genes are characterized as basic helix-loop-helix (bHLH) leucine zipper nuclear phosphoproteins which act as transcription factors. Myc proteins form hetero dimers with another family of HLH leucine zipper proteins called Max. The Myc–Max hetero dimers bind to DNA in "E box" elements downstream of genes involved in cell cycle regulation. The Myc–Max complex increases transcription of the target gene. Another hetero dimer Mad–Max results in repression of gene transcription. In addition to its role in regulation of cell cycle genes in combination with Max, Myc may also repress the transcription of tumor suppressor genes (55).

It is of interest that while the t(8;14) is common to both sporadic Burkitt lymphoma and the endemic form seen in African children, the breakpoints are different in these two diseases (Fig. 6.7). In sporadic Burkitt lymphoma, the breakpoint on chromosome 8 is usually within the first exon or intron 1 of the *CMYC* gene, resulting in loss of regulation, while in endemic Burkitt it is usually upstream to the first exon of *CMYC* with loss of a normal transcriptional control point. Both mutations result in uncontrolled expression of the cMyc protein. The breakpoint on chromosome 14 is usually within a switch region in the heavy chain gene in sporadic Burkitt and within the joining (J) region in that gene in the endemic form. This implies derivation of the sporadic type of Burkitt lymphoma from a more mature B cell, which has already rearranged its immunoglobulin genes, and is undergoing secondary rearrangement with a switch in production of IgM to IgG. The endemic form is derived from a pre-B cell undergoing primary immunoglobulin gene rearrangement (55).

Consistent recognizable chromosomal abnormalities are less common in lymphoblastic lymphomas. Most of these translocations involve the T cell receptor genes on chromosome 14 ($\alpha \delta$ locus) or less commonly chromosome 7 (β locus). Many of the common abnormalities in T cell leukemia/lymphoma involve the *TAL1* gene. The molecular mechanism is similar to the Burkitt translocation—the translocation results in movement of a proto-oncogene *TAL1* to a site under the control of the TCR regulatory domain with resultant aberrant expression of the proto-oncogene. Other mutations result in

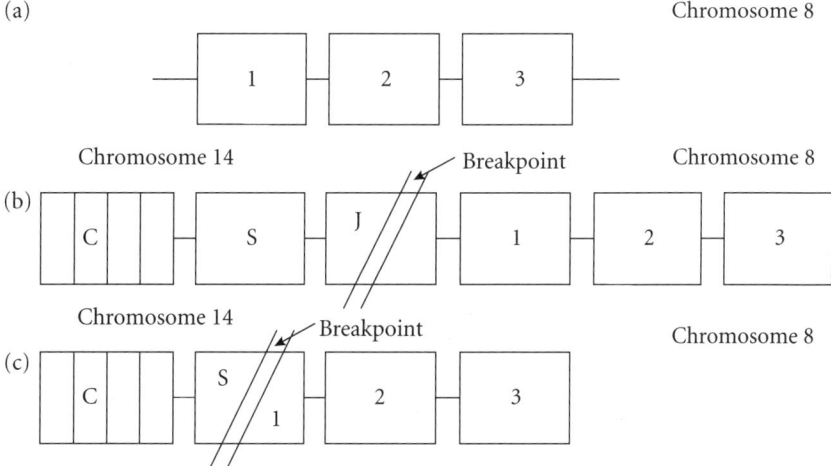

Fig. 6.7 Molecular alterations in Burkitt lymphoma. (a) The normal *CMYC* gene has three exons. (b) In endemic Burkitt lymphoma, the breakpoint is in the joining region, leaving the *CMYC* exons intact, however, mutations in the first exon lead to dysregulation of *CMYC* transcription. (c) In sporadic Burkitt lymphoma, the breakpoint occurs in the first exon in *CMYC* and the switching region of *IgH*. C: constant region *IgH*; S: switching region *IgH*; J: joining region *IgH*.

deletion of *TAL1* regulatory regions, placing *TAL1* next to the promotor of the *SIL* gene, which is active in T lymphocytes.

The *TAL* family, like *MYC*, are bHLH proteins. They are normally expressed in hematopoietic cells, but not in thymocytes. Abnormal expression of *TAL* in thymocytes may result in aberrant expression of other genes not normally expressed in these cells. The Tal proteins complex with E proteins and bind to DNA in E box regions and regulate transcription of target genes. It is also thought that normal E protein function may be suppressed by over-expression of *TAL1*. E protein homodimers have been shown to be powerful transcriptional activators, and it may be that *TAL1* over-expression, with increased Tal1-E protein hetero dimers, may be a negative regulator of transcription, thus preventing the normal function of E proteins (56). Tal1 also interacts with DRG, a GTP binding protein involved in growth control by regulation of *MYC* or *RAS* genes, and with Lim domain proteins. Other members of the *TAL* family include *TAL2* and *LYL1*. These proteins have similar functions to Tal1, but are less often involved in lymphoma translocations. Another group of proteins—the Lim proteins interact with the Tal family and may modulate the activity of Tal proteins. The genes *LMO1* and *LMO2* encode for Lim proteins and may be translocated to a region near the *TCR* in a small subset of t(11;14) mutations. Abnormal expression of both Tal and Lim proteins may have a significant role in the development of lymphomas. Studies in transgenic mouse models have shown enhanced development of tumors in mice transgenic for both *TAL1* and *LMO2* (57, 58).

Over-expression of other proto-oncogenes, not involving *TAL* expression have also been seen in a small number of T cell leukemia/lymphomas. These include: *CMYC*; *HOX11*, a developmental control gene; *LCK*, a Src family protein tyrosine kinase; and *TAN1*, a Notch protein gene (59). Another mechanism, the loss of a tumor suppressor gene *MTS1*, may also be implicated in the etiology of T cell leukemia/lymphomas. The products of *MTS1* are cycle kinase inhibitors which prevent the phosphorylation of the retinoblastoma gene protein (Rb). Rb regulates entry into the cell cycle at the G1/S checkpoint. Unphosphorylated Rb binds to E2F transcription factors and prevents cells from entering S phase from G1. Phosphorylated Rb is unable to bind E2F and allows cells to proceed from G1 to S phase and hence replicate. Loss of *MTS* may allow uncontrolled phosphorylated Rb to promote cell replication. A significant number of T cell leukemia/lymphomas have mutations in the region of chromosome 9 p21, the site of *MTS1* (60).

Large cell lymphomas are a heterogeneous group both histologically and at the molecular level. The t(14;18) is seen in many adult large B cell lymphomas. This translocation results in dysregulation of *BCL2* leading to increased cell survival by inhibition of apoptosis. This translocation has not been reported in pediatric large cell lymphomas. Also described in large cell lymphomas are t(8;14) identical to that seen in Burkitt lymphoma, and abnormalities of *BCL6*, a zinc finger-encoding gene located at 3q27. *BCL6* is normally expressed in follicular center B cells, but is downregulated as cells mature and exit the follicular center. *BCL6* rearrangements may result in over-expression of the gene and proliferation of B lymphocytes leading to large B cell lymphoma (61–64).

The best characterized of the large cell lymphomas is ALCL in which the t(2;5) (p23;q35) is seen. This translocation relocates a promoter sequence of nucleolar phosphoprotein (*NPM*) on 5q35 or other signals that cause active translation of *ALK*. NPM is thought to be involved in ribosome assembly. *ALK* is a member of the insulin receptor family and its expression is usually confined to cells of the nervous system. Over-expression of *ALK*, not normally expressed in lymphoid cells, may contribute to malignant change by inappropriate phosphorylation of intercellular growth regulators.

The primary cutaneous form of ALCL has not been shown to express *ALK* (65) although recent reports have identified *ALK* expression in these lesions (66). A monoclonal antibody to the ALK1 protein is available for use on fixed tissue. Studies using this antibody have demonstrated that some lymphomas positive for ALK1 do not have the t(2;5). It has been suggested that other chromosomal rearrangements such as inv 2 (p23;q35) (67, 68) and t(1;2) (q25;p23) (69) may also result in *ALK* expression. There is some controversy as to the occurrence of the t(2 : 5) in lesions other than ALCL as well as the significance of *ALK* expression in the absence of t(2;5) (70–73).

The receptor for the proto-oncogene *CKIT* has been identified in ALCL as well as HL (nodular sclerosis, mixed cellularity, and lymphocyte depletion). The *CKIT* product is a member of the transmembrane tyrosine kinase receptor family (74). The ligand for the cKit receptor (stem cell factor) has a putative role in the control of hematopoietic development (75). Studies using flow cytometry and immunohistochemistry have demonstrated cKit receptor expression in a number of hematologic and nonhematologic malignancies (74).

Pinto et al. (76) studied a number of lymphomas and found expression of cKit receptor protein restricted to ALCL and HL, suggesting a possible relationship between these two entities.

Prognostic factors

Many studies have been published on prognostic factors in NHL and HL. Few of these are exclusively pediatric studies. The reports on diffuse large cell lymphoma include few if any children and may not be applicable to pediatric cases. An excellent review of prognostic factors in aggressive NHL appeared in Blood (76).

Clinical factors

Tumor burden as reflected by tumor size and stage of disease and serum levels of tumor-related products has always been felt to be of prognostic significance (77, 78). Serum markers such as lactic dehydrogenase, IL2R, beta 2 microglobulin, uric acid, lactic acid, and polyamines have been studied and reflect tumor burden or rate of cell turnover (79, 80). Soluble interleukin 2 receptor has been shown to be of prognostic significance in children with Burkitt and lymphoblastic lymphomas. Levels of $sIL-2R > 1000$ were associated with a worse prognosis (81, 83).

In adult patients with aggressive NHL an International index has been shown to be predictive of overall and relapse free survival (76). Factors used in determining this index included: age, LDH level, performance status, stage and number of extranodal sites involved. Other clinical factors such as ability to tolerate chemotherapy or radiation therapy, and time to complete remission (CR) have been suggested as being significant in determining prognosis. Other clinical/hematologic parameters such as cytopenias or a leukoerythroblastic peripheral smear may reflect bone marrow involvement and patients with these peripheral blood abnormalities tend to have shorter survival times (82).

While stage remains the major prognostic indicator in HL, a number of favorable and unfavorable risk factors also have been identified. Favorable features include: absence of "B" symptoms, ESR < 20, lymphocyte predominant, or nodular sclerosis subtypes, normal spleen size and single peripheral site of involvement. Unfavorable features are: presence of "B" symptoms, ESR > 70, >4 sites of involvement, mixed cellularity histology, and splenic enlargement (14, 84).

Wasielewski et al. from the German Hodgkin Disease study group reported a worse prognosis in patients whose Reed Sternberg cells were CD15 negative (85). A multicenter study of patients with advanced stage HL demonstrated a number of factors predictive of poor outcome. These included: low serum albumin (<4 g/dl), hemoglobin <10.5 g/dl, male sex, older age (>45 years), stage IV, leukocytosis (>15,000/cc), and lymphopenia (<600/cc) (86). The youngest patients in this study were 15 years of age.

Histologic features

The histologic features of NHL are not generally of prognostic significance. In the Working Formulation classification, diffuse large cell lymphoma with immunoblastic morphology was considered a high grade lymphoma as compared with intermediate grade for diffuse large cell lymphoma without these features. Newer classifications have not continued to separate immunoblastic large cell lymphomas from other morphologic variants. Using the Kiel classification, Englehard et al. reported a better prognosis in diffuse large cell lymphoma with centroblastic morphology as compared with immunoblastic morphology (87).

Distinction between Burkitt and non-Burkitt morphology has not been shown to be of prognostic importance in POG studies (18). Likewise lymphoblastic lymphoma with or without nuclear convolutions appears to have the same prognosis (19).

Immunophenotype

The immunophenotype of lymphoma cells has been suggested as a prognostic factor. While data is controversial, some studies have shown decreased disease-free survival in large cell lymphoma with a T cell pheno-type (86, 87, 88). Mediastinal lymphomas with an immature T cell phenotype (CD2+, 7 or 5+, 3−, 4−, 8−) was shown to have a worse prognosis in one study and required more intensive therapy (89, 90).

Cytogenetics

Not surprisingly chromosomal abnormalities have been investigated for their prognostic significance. Although the data is somewhat controversial, early reports of patients with diffuse large cell lymphoma with aneuploidy seemed to have a poor prognosis (91).

Increased proliferative activity as demonstrated by increased Ki67 nuclear staining conferred a poor prognosis (92).

Adhesion molecules

CD44, the lymphocyte homing receptor which enables lymphocytes to bind to high endothelial venules has been studied as a prognostic marker. The presence of CD44 has been associated with disseminated, advanced stage disease (93). Loss of other cell adhesion molecules such as LFA-1 (CD11a) and ICAM-1 (CD54) have been suggested to confer a worse prognosis as well (94).

Molecular factors

Proteins involved in apoptosis and cell cycle regulation have been investigated in lymphoma patients. Bcl-2 is one of a family of proteins regulating apoptosis. Increased expression on Bcl-2 inhibits apoptosis in lymphoma cells treated with chemotherapy or radiation. Bax, another protein in this family enhances apoptosis and promotes tumor cell death. Studies of these proteins have shown conflicting results on overall and disease-free survival. An increase in Bcl-2 expression and high ratios of Bcl-2:Bax are seen in low grade lymphomas which are more resistant to standard chemotherapy. High grade lymphoma with lower Bcl-2 expression and Bcl-2:Bax ratios are more responsive to therapy-induced apoptosis and are potentially curable (95, 96). Other investigators have reported no difference in survival with Bcl-2 expression (95).

The role of p53 expression in NHL is also controversial. p53 is also involved in cell cycle regulation and apoptosis. Cells with DNA damage are directed into the apoptotic pathway and intact cells are allowed to enter the cell cycle. While the detection of p53 by immunohistochemical methods is generally thought to correspond to mutated p53, this has not been demonstrated in a number of studies where both immunohistochemistry and p53 mutation analysis have been performed (86). In some studies however, p53 staining has been associated with a poor prognosis (97).

Expression of *BCL6*, a proto-oncogene which encodes a cellular transcription factor has been demonstrated in approximately 30% of diffuse large cell lymphomas, many in extranodal locations (98). Translocation of *BCL6*, which resides on the long arm of chromosome 3 at 3q27, to sites of immunoglobulin genes on chromosomes 14, 22, and 2 result in overexpression of this protein. In some studies expression of *BCL6* has been associated with a better prognosis (99).

Current and future research

Much of the current research in lymphomas is focused on new therapeutic modalities: new combinations and classes of drugs, cytotoxic T cell therapy, mechanisms of drug action, monoclonal antibodies, and immuno conjugates which deliver cytotoxic drugs, toxins and radio nucleotides to targeted malignant cells, hopefully sparing normal cells. A recent review of these drug trials is reported by Liu and Press in Hematology/Oncology Clinics of North America (100). Another therapeutic technique involves targeting lymphoma cells with idiotype-specific peptides. Some of these peptides are capable of inducing apoptosis. These studies are reviewed by Lam and Zhao (101).

Work in the area of acquired drug resistance holds promise for more effective therapy for lymphoma patients. In addition to the multidrug resistance gene product (p-glycoprotein) there are additional methods to overcome the drug efflux pump. Other proteins which act in this manner such as Lung resistance-related protein (LRP) and glutathione have been studied (102). Drugs that target DNA topoisomerases, drugs that inhibit the development of DNA repair mechanism in target cells, and drugs that activate intracellular apoptosis pathways are being investigated (100).

In addition to new therapeutic strategies there is great interest in improved diagnosis and classification of lymphomas using molecular techniques. Detection of multidrug resistance gene and other mechanisms of drug resistance holds promise for salvage therapy in relapsed patients. As in pediatric leukemia and solid tumor patients, the search for good prognostic factors that would allow less therapy, and decrease therapy-related complications is a major area of research in cooperative group studies.

References

1. Murphy SB. Classification, staging and end results of treatment of childhood non-Hodgkin's lymphomas: dissimilarities from lymphomas in adults. Semin Oncol 1980, 7, 332–8.
2. Sandlund JT, Downing JR, Crist WM. Non-Hodgkin's lymphoma in childhood. New Engl J Med 1996, 334, 1238–47.

3. Gurney JG, Severson RK, Davis S, Robison LL. Incidence of cancer in children in the United States. Cancer 1995, 75, 2186–95.
4. Parkin DM, Stiller CA, Draper GJ, Bieber CA. The international incidence of childhood cancer. Int J Cancer 1988, 42, 511–20.
5. Ziegler JL. Burkitt's lymphoma. J Natl Cancer Inst 1981, 305, 735–45.
6. Perkins SL, Segal GH, Kjeldsberg CR. Classification of non-Hodgkin's lymphomas in children. Semin Diagn Pathol 1995, 12(4), 303–13.
7. Weiss LM, Bindl JM, Picozzi VJ, Link MP, Warnke RA. Lymphoblastic lymphoma: an immunophenotype study of 26 cases with comparison to T cell acute lymphoblastic leukemia. Blood 1986, 67(2), 474–8.
8. Soslow RA, Baergen RN, Warnke RA. B-lineage lymphoblastic lymphoma is a clinicopathologic entity distinct from other histologically similar aggressive lymphomas with blastic morphology. Cancer 1999, 85, 2648–54.
9. Agnarsson BA, Kadin ME. Peripheral T-cell lymphomas in children. Semin Diagn Pathol 1995, 12(4), 314–24.
10. Jacobson JO, Aisenberg AC, Lamarre L, Willett CG, et al. Mediastinal large cell lymphoma: an uncommon subset of adult lymphoma curable with combined modality therapy. Cancer 1988, 62, 1893–8.
11. Leventhal BG, Donaldson SS. Hodgkin's disease. In: Principles and practices of pediatric oncology (ed. PA Pizzo, DG Poplack). J.B. Lippincott Company, Philadelphia, 1989, 457–76.
12. Mahoney DH, Schreuders LC, Gresik MV, McClain KL. Role of staging bone marrow examination in children with Hodgkin disease. Med Pediatr Oncol 1998, 30, 175–7.
13. Meadows AT, Obringer AC, Marrero O, et al. Second malignant neoplasms following childhood Hodgkin's disease: treatment and splenectomy as risk factors. Med Pediatr Oncol 1989, 17, 477–84.
14. Raney RB. Hodgkin's disease in childhood: a review. J Pediatr Hematol/Oncol 1997, 19(6), 502–9.
15. Magrath IT. Malignant non-Hodgkin's lymphoma. In: Principles and practices of pediatric oncology (ed. PA Pizzo, DG Poplack). J.B. Lippincott Company, Philadelphia, 1989, 415–55.
16. Harris NL, Jaffe ES, Stein H, Banks PM, Chan JKC, et al. A revised European–American classification of lymphoid neoplasms: a proposal from the international lymphoma study group. Blood 1994, 84(5), 1361–92.
17. Jaffe ES, Harris NL, Diebold J, Muller-Hermelink HK. World Health Organization classification of neoplastic diseases of the hematopoietic and lymphoid tissues: a progress report. Am J Clin Pathol 1999, 111(Suppl. 1), S8–12.
18. Kelly DR, Nathwani BN, Rogers DG, Shuster JJ, Sullivan MP, et al. A morphologic study of childhood lymphoma of the undifferentiated type: the pediatric oncology group experience. Cancer 1987, 59, 1132–7.
19. Griffith RC, Kelly DR, Nathwani BN, Shuster JJ, Murphy SB, et al. A morphologic study of childhood lymphoma of the lymphoblastic type: the pediatric oncology group experience. Cancer 1987, 59, 1126–31.
20. Nathwani BN, Kim H, Rappaport H. Malignant lymphoma. Lymphoblastic. Cancer 1976, 38, 1964–83.
21. Perkins SL, Segal GH, Kjeldsberg CR. Work-up of lymphadenopathy in children. Semin Diagn Pathol 1995, 12(4), 284–87.
22. Buchino JJ, Hsiang-Kuang L. Specimen collection and preparation in fine-needle aspirations in children. Am J Clin Pathol 1998, 109(Suppl. 1), S4–8.
23. Tao Q, Robertson AM, Hildesheim A, Ambinder RF. Epstein–Barr virus (EBV) in endemic Burkitt's lymphoma: molecular analysis of primary tumor tissue. Blood 1998, 91(4), 1373–81.
24. Chan JKC, Ng CS, Hui PK, Leungs TW, et al. Anaplastic large cell Ki-1 lymphoma: delineation of two morphological types. Histopathology 1989, 15, 11–34.
25. Chott A, Kaserer K, Augustin I, Vesely M, Heinz R, et al. Ki-1 positive large cell lymphoma: a clinicopathologic study of 41 cases. Am J Surg Pathol 1990, 14, 439–48.
26. Chan JKC, Buchanan R, Fletcher CDM. Sarcomatoid variant of anaplastic large-cell Ki-1 lymphoma. Am J Surg Pathol 1990, 14(10), 983–8.
27. Pileri S, Falini B, Delsol G, Stein H, Baglioni P, Poggi S, Martelli MF, et al. Lymphohistiocytic T-cell lymphoma (anaplastic large cell lymphoma CD30+/Ki-1+ with a high content of reactive histiocytes). Histopathology 1990, 16, 383–91.
28. Mann KP, Hall B, Kamino H, Borowitz MJ, Ratech H. Neutrophil-rich, Ki-1-positive anaplastic large-cell malignant lymphoma. Am J Surg Pathol 1995, 19(4), 407–16.
29. Kinney MC, Collins RD, Greer JP, Whitlock JA, Sioutos N, Kadin ME. A small-cell-predominant variant of primary Ki-1 (CD30)+ T-cell lymphoma. Am J Surg Pathol 1993, 17(9), 859–68.
30. Waldron JA, Leech JH, Glick AD, Flexner JM, Collins RD. Malignant lymphoma of peripheral T-lymphocyte origin: immunologic, pathologic, and clinical features in six patients. Cancer 1977, 40, 1604–17.
31. Strickler JG, Michie SA, Warnke RA, Dorfman RF. The "syncytial variant" of nodular sclerosing Hodgkin's disease. Am J Surg Pathol 1986, 10(7), 470–7.
32. Ben-Yehuda-Salz D, Ben-Yehuda A, Polliack A, Ron N, Okon E. Syncytial variant of nodular sclerosing Hodgkin's disease: a new clinicopathologic entity. Cancer 1990, 65, 1167–72.
33. MacLennan KA, Bennett MH, Tu A, Hudson BV, Easterling MJ, et al. Relationship of histopathologic features to survival and relapse in nodular sclerosing Hodgkin's disease. Cancer 1989, 64, 1686–93.
34. Ferry JA, Linggood RM, Convery KM, Efird JT, Eliseo R, Harris NL. Hodgkin disease, nodular sclerosis type: implications of histologic subclassification. Cancer 1993, 71, 457–63.
35. Masih AS, Weisenberger DD, Vose JM, Bast MA, Armitage JO. Histologic grade does not predict prognosis in optimally treated, advanced-stage nodular sclerosing Hodgkin's disease. Cancer 1992, 69, 228–32.
36. Hess JL, Bodis S, Pinkus G, Silver B, Mauch P. Histopathologic grading of nodular sclerosis Hodgkin's disease: lack of prognostic significance in 254 surgically staged patients. Cancer 1994, 74, 708–14.
37. Butler JJ. The histologic diagnosis of Hodgkin's disease. Semin Diagn Pathol 1992, 9(4), 252–6.
38. Lukes RJ, Butler JJ, Hicks EB. Natural history of Hodgkin's disease as related to its pathologic picture. Cancer 1966, 19, 317–44.
39. Segal GH, Kjeldsberg CR, Smith GP, Perkins SL. CD30 antigen expression in florid immunoblastic proliferations: a

clinicopathologic study or 14 cases. Am J Clin Pathol 1994, **102**, 292–8.
40. Mason DY, Banks PM, Chan J, Cleary ML, Delsol G, deWolf-Peeters C, Falini B, et al. Am J Surg Pathol 1994, **18**(5), 526–30.
41. Ng CS, Chan JKC, Hui PK, Lau WH. Large B-cell lymphomas with a high content of reactive T cells. Human Pathol 1989, **20**, 1145–54.
42. Krishnan J, Wallberg K, Frizzera G. T-cell-rich large B-cell lymphoma: a study of 30 cases, supporting its histologic heterogeneity and lack of clinical distinctiveness. Am J Surg Pathol 1994, **18**(5), 455–65.
43. Winberg CD, Nathwani BN, Bearmann RB, et al. Follicular (nodular) lymphoma during the first two decades of life: a clinicopathologic study of 12 patients. Cancer 1981, **48**, 2223–35.
44. Koo CH, Reifel J, Kogut N, Cove JK, Rappaport H. True histiocytic malignancy associated with a malignant teratoma in a patients with 46XY gonadal dysgenesis. Am J Surg Pathol 1992, **16**(2) 175–83.
45. Craig FE, Gulley ML, Banks PM. Posttransplantation lymphoproliferative disorders. Am J Clin Pathol 1993, **99**, 265–76.
46. Poppema S, Kaiserling E, Lennert K. Hodgkin's disease with lymphocytic predominance, nodular type (nodular paragranuloma) and progressively transformed germinal centres—a cytohistological study. Histopathology 1979, **3**, 295–308.
47. Osborne BM, Butler JJ. Clinical implications of progressive transformation of germinal centers. Am J Surg Pathol 1984, **8**(10), 725–33.
48. Hansmann M-L, Fellbaum C, Hui PK, Moubayed P. Progressive transformation of germinal centers with and without association to Hodgkin's disease. Am J Clin Pathol 1990, **93**, 219–26.
49. Osborne BM, Butler JJ, Gresik V. Progressive transformation of germinal centers: comparison of 23 pediatric patients to the adult population. Mod Pathol 1997, **5**, 135–40.
50. Drappa J, Vaishnaw AK, Sullivan KE, Chu J-L, Elkon KB. Fas gene mutations in the Canale–Smith syndrome, an inherited lymphoproliferative disorder associated with autoimmunity. New Eng J Med 1996, **335**, 1643–9.
51. Sneller MC, Wang J, Dales JK, Strober W, Middelton LA, Youngnim C, et al. Clinical, immunologic, and genetic features of an autoimmune lymphproliferative syndrome associated with abnormal lymphocyte apoptosis. Blood 1997, **89**(4), 1341–8.
52. Lim MS, Straus SE, Dale JK, Fleisher TA, Stetler-Stevenson M, Strober W, Sneller MC, Puck JM, Lenardo MJ, Elenitoba-Johnson KSJ, et al. Pathological findings in human autoimmune lymphoproliferative syndrome. Am J Pathol 1998, **153**, 1541–50.
53. Shi S-R, Key ME, Kalra KL. Antigen retrieval in formalin-fixed, paraffin-embedded tissues: an enhancement method of immunohistochemical staining based on microwave oven heating of tissue sections. J Histochem Cytochem 1991, **39**, 741–8.
54. Taylor CR, Shi S-R, Chaiwun B, Young L, Imam SA, Cote RJ. Strategies for improving the immunohistochemical staining of various intranuclear prognostic markers in formalin-paraffin section: androgen receptor, estrogen receptor, progesterone receptor, p53 protein, proliferating cell nuclear antigen, and Ki-67 antigen revealed by antigen retrieval techniques. Human Pathol 1994, **25**, 263–70.
55. Collins RD. Is clonality equivalent to malignancy: specifically, is immunoglobulin gene rearrangement diagnostic of malignant lymphoma? Human Pathol 1997, **28**, 757–9.
56. Bhagat SKM, Medeiros LJ, Weiss LM, Wang J, Raffeld M, Stetler-Stevenson M. bcl-2 expression in Hodgkin's disease: correlation with the t(14;18) translocation and Epstein–Barr virus. Am J Clin Pathol 1993, **99**, 604–8.
57. Goldsby RE, Carroll WL. The molecular biology of pediatric lymphomas. J Pediatr Hematol/Oncol 1998, **20**(4), 282–96.
58. Bain G, Engel I, Robanus-Maandag EC, et al. E2A deficiency leads to abnormalities in alphabeta T-cell development and to rapid development of T-cell lymphomas. Mol Cell Biol 1997, **14**, 1256–65.
59. Robb L, Begley CG. The SCL/TAL1 gene: roles in normal and malignant hematopoiesis. Bioessays 1997, **19**, 607–13.
60. Larson RC, Larvenir I, Larson TA, et al. Protein dimerization between Lmo2 (Rbtn2) and Tall alters thymocyte development and potentiates T cell tumorigenesis in transgenic mice. Eur J Microbiol Oncol 1996, **15**, 1021–7.
61. Hwang LY, Baer RJ. The role of chromosome translocations in T cell acute leukemia. Curr Opin Immunol 1995, **7**, 659–64.
62. Cayuela J-M, Madani A, Sanhes L, et al. Multiple tumor-suppressor gene 1 inactivation is the most frequent genetic alteration in T-cell acute lymphoblastic leukemia. Blood 1996, **87**, 2180–6.
63. Ye BH, et al. Alterations of a zinc-finger encoding gene, BCL-6, in diffuse large-cell lymphoma. Science 1993, **262**, 747–50.
64. Onizuka T, Masatsugu M, Yamochi T, Toshihiko K, Kazama A, et al. BCL-6 gene product, a 92- to 98-kD nuclear phosphoprotein, is highly expressed in germinal center B cells and their neoplastic counterparts. Blood 1995, **86**(1), 28–37.
65. Cattoretti G, Chih-Chao C, Cechova K, Zhang J, Ye BH, Falini B, et al. BCL-6 protein is expressed in germinal-center B cells. Blood 1995, **86**(1), 45–53.
66. Ye BH, Cattoretti G, Shen Q, Zhang J, Hawe N, deWaard R, Leung C, et al. The BCL-6 proto-oncogene controls germinal-centre formation in the Th2-type inflammation. Nature Genet 1997, **16**, 161–70.
67. Wood G, Hardman D, Boni R, et al. Lack of the t(2;5) or other mutations resulting in expression of anaplastic lymphoma kinase catalytic domain in CD30+ primary cutaneous lymphoproliferative disorders and Hodgkin's disease. Blood 1996, **88**, 1765–70.
68. Beylot-Barry M, Groppi V, Vergier B, Pulford K, Merlio JP. Characterization of t(2;5) reciprocal transcripts and genomic breakpoints in CD30+ cutaneous lymphoproliferations. Blood 1998, **91**(12), 4668–76.
69. Benharroch D, Meguerian-Bedoyan Z, Lamant L, Amin C, et al. ALK-positive lymphoma: a single disease with a broad spectrum morphology. Blood 1998, **91**(6), 2076–84.
70. Wlodarska I, deWolf-Peeters C, Falini B, Verhoef G, Morris SW, et al. The cryptic inv(2)(p23q35) defines a new molecular genetic subtype of ALK-positive anaplastic large-cell lymphoma. Blood 1998, **92**(8), 2688–95.
71. Lamant L, Dastugue N, Pulford K, Delsol G, Mariame B. A new fusion gene TPM3-ALK in anaplastic large cell lymphoma created by a (1;2)(q25;p23) translocation. Blood 1999, **93**(9), 3088–95.

72. Chan JKC. CD30+ (Ki-1) lymphoma: t(2;5) translocation, the implicated genes and more (commentary). Adv Anat Pathol 1995, **2**(2), 99–104.
73. Arber DA, Sun L-H, Weiss LM. Detection of the t(2;5)(p23;q35) chromosomal translocation in large B-cell lymphomas other than anaplastic large cell lymphoma. Human Pathol 1996, **27**, 590–4.
74. Delsol G, Lamant L, Mariame B, Pulford K, Dastugue N, Brousset P, Rigal-Huguet F, Saati TA, Cerretti DP, Morris SW, et al. A new subtype of large b-cell lymphoma expressing the ALK kinase and lacking the 2;5 translocation. Blood 1997, **89**(5),1483–90.
75. Falini B, Bigerna B, Fizzotti M, Pulford K, Pileri SA, Delsol G, Carbone A, et al. ALK expression defines a distinct group of T/Null lymphomas ("ALK lymphomas") with a wide morphological spectrum. Am J Pathol 1998, **153**(3), 875–86.
76. Pinto A, Gloghini A, Gattei V, Aldinucci D, Zagonel V, Carbone A. Expression of the c-kit receptor in human lymphomas is restrcited to Hodgkin's disease and DC30+ anaplastic large cell lymphomas. Blood 1994, **83**(3), 785–92.
77. Broxmeyer HE, Maze R, Miyazawa K, Carow C, Hendrie PC, Cooper S, et al. The kit receptor and its ligand, steel factor, as regulators of hemopoiesis. Cancer Cells 1991, **3**, 480–7.
78. Shipp MA. Prognostic factors in aggressive non-Hodgkin's lymphoma: who has "high risk" disease? Blood 1994, **83**(5), 1165–73.
79. Magrath IT, Lee YJ, Anderson T, Henle W, Ziegler J, Simon R, Schein P. Prognostic factors in Burkitt's lymphoma: importance of total tumor burden. Cancer 1980, **45**, 1507–15.
80. Magrath IT, Janus C, Edwards B, et al. An effective therapy for both undifferentiated (including Burkitt's) lymphoma and lymphoblastic lymphomas in children and young adults. Blood 1984, **63**, 1102.
81. Gordon LI, Andersen J, Colgan J, Glick J, Resnick GD, et al. Advanced diffuse non-Hodgkin's lymphoma: analysis of prognostic factors by the international index and by lactic dehydrogenase in an intergroup study. Cancer 1995, **75**, 865–73.
82. Swan F, Jr, Velasquez WS, Tucker S, Redman JR, Rodriguez MA, McLaughlin P, et al. A new serologic staging system for large-cell lymphomas based on initial β2-micro-globulin and lactage dehydrogenase levels. J Clin Oncol 1989, **7**, 1518.
83. Wagner DD, Kiwanuka J, Edwards BK, et al. Soluble interleukin II receptor levels in patients with undifferentiated and lymphoblastic lymphomas. J Clin Oncol 1987, **5**, 1262–74.
84. Conlan MG, Armitage JO, Bast M, Weisenberger DD. Clinical significance of hematologic parameters in non-Hodgkin's lymphoma at diagnosis. Cancer 1991, **67**, 1389–95.
85. von Wasielewski R, Mengel M, Fischer R, Hansmann M-L, Huebner K, Franklin J, Tesch H, et al. Classical Hodgkin's disease: clinical impact of the immunophenotype. Am J Pathol 1997, **151**, 1123–30.
86. Hasenclever D, Diehl V. A prognostic score for advanced Hodgkin's disease. New Eng J Med 1998, **339**, 1506–14.
87. Engelhard M, Brittinger G, Huhn D, Gerhartz HH, Meusers P, Siegert W, Thiel E, et al. Subclassification of diffuse large B-Cell lymphomas according to the Kiel Classification: distinction of centroblastic and immunoblastic lymphomas is a significant prognostic risk factor. Blood 1997, **87**(7), 2291–7.
88. Gascoyne RD. Pathologic prognostic factors in diffuse aggressive non-Hodgkin's lymphoma. Hematol/Oncol Clin North Am 1997, **11**(5), 847–62.
89. Gisselbrecht C, Gaulard P, Lepage E, Coiffier B, Briere J, Haioun C, Cazals-Hatem D, et al. Prognostic significance of T-cell phenotype in aggressive non-Hodgkin's lymphomas. Blood 1998, **92**(1), 76–82.
90. Yumura-Yagi K, Ishihara S, Hara J, Mitsunori M, Izumi Y, Tawa A, Sato A, et al. Poor prognosis of mediastinal non-Hodgkin's lymphoma with an immature phenotype of CD2+, CD7 (or CD5)+, CD3−, CD4−. And CD8−. Cancer 1989, **63**, 671–4.
91. Salmon I, Swan F, dargent J-L, Pasteels J-L, Kiss R, Katz R. Relationship between DNA ploidy level, nuclear size, and survival in large cell lymphoma. Am J Clin Pathol 1995, **103**, 568–73.
92. Grogan TM, Lippmann SM, Spier CM, Slymen DJ, Ryski JA, Rangel CS, et al. Independent prognostic significance of a nuclear proliferation antigen in diffuse large cell lymphomas as determined be the monoclonal antibody Ki-67. Blood 1988, **71**(4), 1157–60.
93. Horst E, Meijer CJLM, Radaszkiewicz R, Ossekoppele GJ, vanKrieken JHJM, Pals ST Adhesion molecules in the prognosis of diffuse large-cell lymphoma: expression of a lymphocyte homing receptor (CD44), LFA-1 (CD11a/18), and ICAM-1 (CD54). Leukemia 1990, **4**, 595.
94. Grogan TM. A philosophical perspective: the biologic principles underlying poor prognosis and therapy failure. Am J Surg Pathol 1996, **20**(3), 376–9.
95. Wheaton S, Netser J, Guinee D, Rahn M, Perkins S. Bcl-2 and Bax protein expression in indolent versus aggressive B-cell non-Hodgkins's lymphomas. Human Pathol 1998, **29**, 820–5.
96. Gascoyne R, Adomat S, Krajewski S, et al. Prognostic significance of bcl-2 protein expression and Bcl-2 gene rearrangement in diffuse aggressive non-Hodgkin's lymphoma. Blood 1997, **90**, 244–51.
97. Piris MA, Pezella F, Martinez-Montero JC, Orradre JL, Villuendas R, Sanchez-Beato M. P53 and bcl-2 expression in high-grade B-cell lymphomas: correlation with survival time. Cancer 1994, **69**, 337–41.
98. Ye BH, Lista F, LoCoco F, et al. Alterations of a zinc finger-encoding gene, BCL-6, in diffuse large-cell lymphoma. Science 1993, **262**, 747–50.
99. Offit K, LoCoco F, Louie DC, Parsa NZ, Leung D, Portlock C, Ye BH, et al. Rearrangement of the bcl-6 gene as a prognostic marker in diffuse large-cell lymphoma. New Eng J Med 1994, **331**, 74–80.
100. Lui SY, Press OW. The potential for immunoconjugates in lymphoma therapy. Hematol/Oncol Clin North Am 1997, **11**(5), 987–1006.
101. Lam KS, Zhao Z-G. Targeted therapy for lymphoma with peptides. Hematol/Oncol Clin North Am 1997, **11**(5), 1007–19.
102. Dalton WS. Alternative (non-p-glycoprotein) mechanisms of drug resistance in non-Hodgkin's lymphoma. Hematol/Oncol Clin North Am 1997, **11**(5), 975–86.

7 | Tumors of the central nervous system and eye

Venita Jay, Jeremy A. Squire, and Maria Zielenska

Primary brain tumors represent the most common solid neoplasms in children (1). They contrast significantly in location, type, and natural history from brain tumors occurring in adults. While the mainstay of morphologic diagnosis rests on recognition of cytologic characteristics using conventional light microscopic and ultrastructural techniques, recent advances in immunohistochemistry, tumor kinetics, and molecular genetics have widened the spectrum of diagnostic modalities. This monograph is intended merely as a brief overview of how different laboratory techniques of today have enabled us to recognize common tumors, their important variants, and new tumor entities. The need for brevity precludes an exhaustive review of pediatric brain and eye tumors, which may be found in several excellent texts (2–7).

Classification of pediatric brain tumors

Pediatric neuropathologists are becoming increasingly aware that many "tumors" are not readily classifiable by conventional classification schemes (8). Some low-grade neoplasms may coexist with malformative or hamartomatous elements. Classification criteria for brain tumors are being continually refined and supplemented, especially with recent advances in immunohistochemistry and molecular diagnostic tools. With respect to tumor grading, sampling error remains a significant factor in brain tumors, which may show significant regional heterogeneity. This is particularly true of situations when the pathologist is confronted with small samples from stereotactic biopsies.

In children, infratentorial tumors (those below the tentorium, most commonly involving the cerebellum and brainstem) are more frequent, and about 75% involve the cerebellum (9). Astrocytoma is the most common type among both supratentorial and infratentorial locations. Of the infratentorial tumors, about 50% are astrocytomas, 20% medulloblastomas, 15% ependymomas, and 15% other types; of the supratentorial tumors, 65% are astrocytomas, 15% primitive neuroectodermal tumors (PNETs), 15% ependymomas, and 5% other types. The most common suprasellar tumors are the craniopharyngioma (85%) and germ cell tumor (15%). Tumors in the pineal region include germ cell tumors, astrocytomas and rarely, pineocytomas and pineoblastomas.

Brain tumor sampling

At the Neuropathology laboratory at The Hospital for Sick Children, we receive up to 100 new cases of brain tumors each year. At the time of frozen section analysis, lesional tissue is sampled for electron microscopy (EM), molecular genetic studies, and cytogenetic analysis.

For frozen section analysis, tumor imprints and smear preparations are of great value providing excellent cytologic detail. While each pathologist develops a personal preference for either smears or frozen sections, we favor doing both, as architectural patterns such as perivascular rosettes of ependymoma are better appreciated on tissue sections rather than smears. Smear preparations quite elegantly highlight various cytologic features such as the fibrillary processes of tumor cells in astrocytoma (Fig. 7.1(a)), the dense cellularity and high nuclear cytoplasmic ratio of PNET, the two cell populations of germinoma, the psammoma bodies in a meningioma, and the papillary nature of choroid plexus papilloma.

In the ensuing paragraphs, an overview of cell kinetic and molecular genetic studies and important immunohistochemical markers will be presented, followed by a discussion of individual tumors.

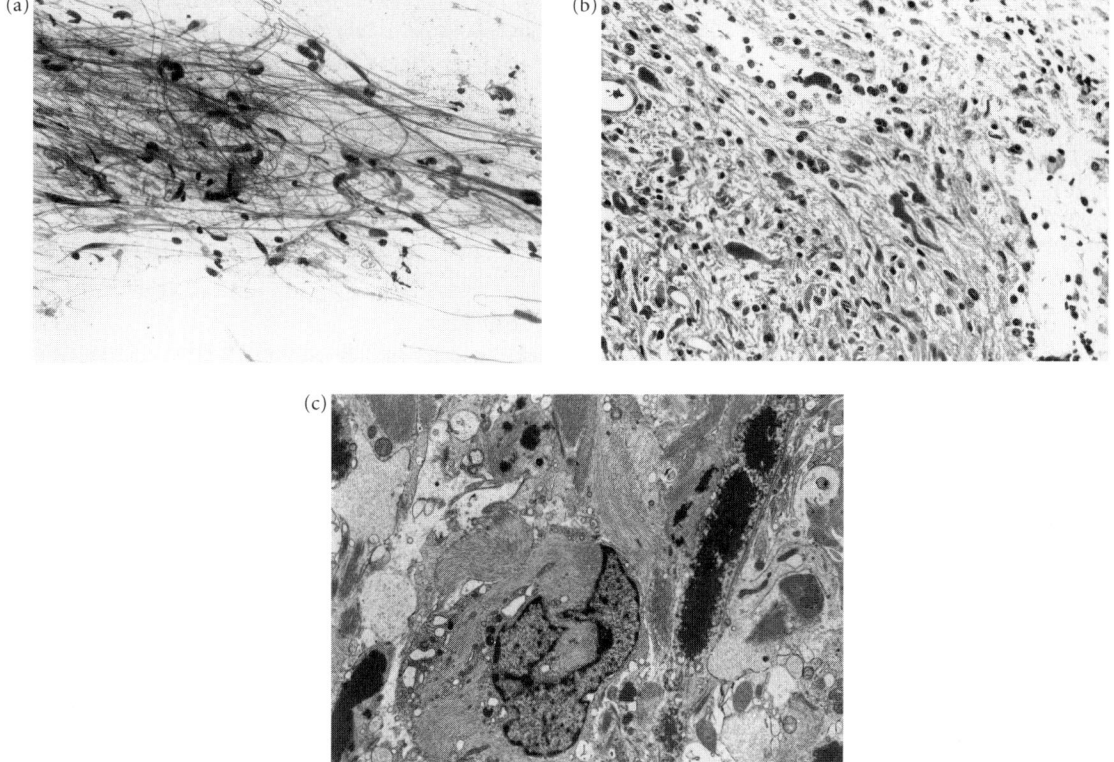

Fig. 7.1 Pilocytic astrocytoma. (a) Smear preparation in a cerebellar pilocytic astrocytoma reveals elongated hair like processes of tumor cells (hematoxylin and eosin (HE), × 225). (b) Medium power micrograph reveals compact and cystic areas, with the former containing many Rosenthal fibers. HE stain, × 225. (c) Low power electron micrograph reveals tumor cells filled with bundles of intermediate filaments and Rosenthal fibers, which appear as dense osmiophilic condensations, Uranyl acetate with lead citrate stain, ×18, 240.

Cell kinetic and molecular genetic studies

Cell kinetic indices provide an objective means of assessing the growth potential of brain tumors (10). Relying on traditional histological parameters such as necrosis, cellular atypia, mitoses, hypercellularity, and endothelial hyperplasia does not always provide consistent prediction of biologic outcome for every tumor. For example, in pilocytic astrocytomas of the cerebellum, presence of endothelial hyperplasia and some degree of cellular atypia is not correlated with an adverse outcome. Recently, one of the authors encountered a cerebellar ganglioglioma, which showed very marked atypia, but had a MIB-1 labeling index of 1.5%, attesting to a very low growth potential (11). On the other hand, tumors such as PNETs may reveal a MIB-1 labeling index as high as 20% or more (10).

In the past, proliferative indices were obtained by autoradiographic analysis of tissue exposed to tritiated thymidine. Now, easier and safer alternatives are available with *in vitro* methods such as Ki-67/MIB-1 immunohistochemistry (10, 12). The MIB-1 antibody recognizes nuclei of proliferating cells and identifies all phases of the cell cycle except G0. Being applicable to paraffin embedded material, MIB-1 remains a useful adjunct in tumor grading and can be used with archival material. Measurement of the amount of DNA with automated flow cytometry has also been widely applied to brain tumors.

In addition to conventional karyotype analysis, brain tumor samples can be assessed by polymerase chain reaction (PCR), fluorescence *in situ* hybridization (FISH), and comparative genomic hybridization (CGH) for the presence of chromosomal gains and losses and oncogene amplification. Brain tumor cytogenetics is often frustrating as tumors often fail to grow in culture.

Recently, techniques such as differential PCR (13–15) have provided an useful alternative to Southern blotting for evaluation of oncogene amplification. Differential PCR has several advantages over Southern blot analysis, which requires about 100 times more DNA and takes longer time (1–2 weeks for Southern blotting, 1–2 days for differential PCR). Furthermore, the results of PCR can be read from ethidium bromide-stained agarose gels thus obviating the need for radioisotopes.

The technique of FISH has the extraordinary advantage over conventional cytogenetic analysis in its applicability to interphase cells. FISH provides information about translocations, gene amplifications, and other chromosomal alterations (16). Powerful screening methods based on FISH analysis include the multiplex FISH and spectral karyotyping (SKY), which apply labeled painting probes to visualize each chromosome within a metaphase in different colors (17). Chromosome classification is based on the unique spectral information for each chromosome in SKY analysis.

While karyotype analysis and FISH require interphase nuclei or metaphase spreads, CGH in contrast, uses DNA extracted from the tumor sample. CGH measures the relative DNA sequence copy number of the tumor without the need for cultures, by cohybridizing with differentially labeled tumor DNA and reference normal DNA to normal metaphase chromosomes (18, 19). Recognition of previously unknown abnormalities is thus possible by CGH, which is based on competitive binding of tumor and control DNA to normal metaphase chromosomes. Gains or losses of whole chromosomes or segments of chromosomes are visualized as intensity differences in the fluorescence, which can be quantified. Thus CGH is applicable to both frozen and paraffin embedded material and is a genome wide test that assesses changes in the entire genome in a single step, without prior knowledge of which gene or chromosome is involved.

Commonly used immunohistochemical markers

Glial fibrillary acidic protein (GFAP)

It is a 48–50-kDa protein recognized as the chemical subunit of the intermediate filaments of astrocytes (20, 21). It is present in immature, normal, and reactive astrocytes. Thus, GFAP positivity is seen in both neoplastic and non-neoplastic astrocytic proliferation. It is not exclusive to astrocytes (22), and can be found in ependymal cells, pituicytes, as well as in non-glial cells such as satellite cells of sensory ganglia. In spite of this, GFAP remains an excellent immunohistochemical marker of astrocytic differentiation and is perhaps the most frequently utilized tumor marker in diagnostic neuropathology (23, 24). Use of this antiserum has helped to define and recognize entities such as pleomorphic xanthoastrocytoma (PXA) and desmoplastic tumors of childhood (25–28).

Vimentin

This 57-kDa protein is seen in a wide range of normal, reactive, and neoplastic cells of varied histogenesis. Immunoreactivity to vimentin can be seen in sarcomas, meningiomas, schwannomas, astrocytomas, and other tumors. Vimentin positivity is a consistent feature of the malignant rhabdoid tumor (MRT) (29, 30), which demonstrates intracytoplasmic whorls of intermediate filaments, which are both vimentin and cytokeratin positive.

S100 protein

This 21-kDa protein is found in the nucleus and cytoplasm of a variety of glial and nonglial cell types. S100 positivity is encountered in a variety of glial tumors, choroid plexus tumors, and nerve sheath tumors. This broad distribution limits its specificity as a diagnostic marker, although they are commonly used as a marker for Schwann cells.

Neurofilaments

Neurofilaments (NFs) are the intermediate filaments of neurons and their processes, and are composed of protein triplets with three major subunits of 68, 150, and 200 kDa (31). Use of anti-NF antibodies reveals immunoreactivity in neoplastic ganglion cells as well as in other tumors exhibiting neuronal differentiation (ganglioglioma, PNETs, and neuronal components of teratomas) (31, 32). Antibodies to both phosphorylated and nonphosphorylated NFs are available. Due to NF protein heterogeneity, failure to detect immunopositivity with antibodies to phosphorylated NF may reflect methodological variations rather than actual absence of these antigens; microwave antigen retrieval may be useful (33).

Synaptophysin

This is a specific and sensitive marker of neuronal differentiation (34, 35). Synaptophysin is an integral membrane glycoprotein of presynaptic vesicles. Synaptophysin positivity is found in PNETs and other tumors with neuronal differentiation, such as ganglioglioma and dysembryoplastic neuroepithelial tumor.

Neuron specific enolase

Initially thought to be restricted to neurons, NSE has subsequently been found in a variety of non-neural tissues, thus it cannot be used as a specific marker of neuronal differentiation.

Epithelial markers

In primary brain tumors, positivity for epithelial markers such as cytokeratin and epithelial membrane antigen (EMA) may be seen in choroid plexus tumors, meningiomas, some ependymomas, craniopharyngiomas, epithelial elements of teratomas, and MRT. Positivity for these markers has been described in epithelial-like areas in glioblastomas and gliosarcomas. Chordomas are also positive for these markers, but are rare in childhood. EMA positivity is seen in perineurial cells and their reactive and neoplastic proliferations (36–38). Perineurial cells are EMA-positive and S-100-negative in contrast to Schwann cells which are S-100 positive and EMA-negative (37).

p53 immunohistochemistry

Mutations of the p53 gene located on the short arm of chromosome 17 represent the most common genetic alterations in human cancer. In recent years, voluminous literature has appeared on abnormalities of the p53 gene in primary brain tumors (39–43). While it was generally assumed that immunohistochemistry detects the mutant p53 protein, which is said to be more stable than wild type protein, it is now evident that, in many instances, the observed p53 positivity may reflect wild type p53 accumulation and p53 accumulation that can result from a number of different underlying mechanisms. Despite possible discrepancies between findings at the DNA level, on the one hand and the protein level, a number of immunohistochemical studies have been undertaken on brain tumors, in almost all of which, higher grade astrocytomas have been more frequently immunopositive than lower grade tumors, but a consistent relationship between number of positive cells and tumor grade has not emerged. Lang et al. (43) reported a high frequency of p53 protein accumulation without gene mutation in juvenile pilocytic astrocytomas. In a recent immunohistochemical study of p53 expression in choroid plexus tumors, we (44) observed consistent p53 positivity in choroid plexus carcinomas (six out of six cases) while three out of four papillomas were negative. Of the carcinomas, three cases showed a labeling index of over 70% (44).

In the subsequent paragraphs, individual tumors will be discussed with examples highlighting the role of various laboratory techniques in diagnostic neuropathology.

Astrocytoma and variants

The most common pediatric brain tumor is the low-grade astrocytoma, particularly of the pilocytic type (Fig. 7.1(a)–(c)). The cerebellar pilocytic astrocytoma is often cystic and may contain a mural nodule. The tumor displays a characteristic histologic pattern, with compact and cystic areas. Individual tumor cells especially in smear preparations reveal hair like elongated cytoplasmic processes ("pilocytes") (Fig. 7.1(a)). There are prominent accumulations of Rosenthal fibers (Fig. 7.1(c)), which are ubiquitin positive and are composed of alpha B-crystallin. Generally, the center of the Rosenthal fiber is GFAP negative. Ultrastructurally, Rosenthal fibers show dense osmiophilic cores surrounded by intermediate filaments (GFAP) (Fig. 7.1(c)). Eosinophilic granular bodies (aggregates of eosinophilic globules) are frequent. They are immunoreactive for alpha-1-antitrypsin and alpha-1-chymotrypsin.

The pilocytic astrocytoma may also occur in the hypothalamus, brainstem, and optic pathways (3, 5, 6). This tumor, particularly in the cerebellum, is associated with an excellent outcome after surgical resection, which is the mainstay of therapy. Local extension into the subarachnoid space is common. In other sites such as the hypothalamus or brainstem, even low-grade astrocytomas may be associated with poor outcome by virtue of the strategic location of the tumor. Optic nerve gliomas are slow growing tumors, but extension posteriorly into the hypothalamic region will affect the prognosis, despite the low histologic grade.

Pilocytic astrocytomas of the optic nerve are the principal tumors encountered in neurofibromatosis 1 (NF1) and may be bilateral. Stern et al. (45) reported that a circumferential perineural growth pattern with proliferation in the subarachnoid space correlated with presence of NF1, while optic nerve gliomas not associated with NF1 showed an expansile intraneural mass.

Pilocytic astrocytoma versus other astrocytic tumors

Typically, the pilocytic astrocytoma is associated with an excellent prognosis and has to be distinguished from other types of gliomas (5, 6). The *fibrillary astrocytoma* is a histologic variant of the low-grade diffuse astrocytoma that is predominantly composed of fibrillary astrocytes with scanty cytoplasm, creating the appearance of naked nuclei (5, 6). Some lesions may have a loose fibrillary stroma and contain microcysts. The *gemistiocytic astrocytoma* reveals plump gemistiocytic astrocytes with glassy cytoplasm and eccentric nuclei. This variant is particularly prone to progression to anaplasia (5, 6). The *protoplasmic astrocytoma* is a rare, poorly defined variant composed of neoplastic astrocytes with few processes and low content of glial filaments. High-grade astrocytomas may be found in the cerebrum and brainstem, but are less frequent in children compared to adults.

The two critical issues with respect to astrocytoma are histologic subtyping and grading. Traditionally, higher grade tumors (anaplastic astrocytoma and gliblastoma) have increased cellularity, greater cytologic atypia, mitoses, necrosis, and endothelial hyperplasia (5, 6). Necrotic foci may be rimmed by viable tumor, a pattern referred to as "pseudopalisading necrosis," which is commonly seen in glioblastoma. In pilocytic astrocytomas of the cerebellum in children, there may frequently be prominent endothelial hyperplasia. Such tufts of hyperplastic endothelium may mistakenly lead to a diagnosis of a high-grade astrocytoma, but in cerebellar pilocytic astrocytomas, this finding does not have ominous implications as in gliomas in adults.

Rarely, some cerebellar gliomas in children may be associated with very marked atypia, leading to a mistaken diagnosis of anaplastic astrocytoma. One of the authors (11) recently encountered such a situation with a cerebellar ganglioglioma, which had tremendous cytologic atypia, but less than 1 mitosis/50 high power fields and a MIB-1 labeling index of 1.5%. This case underscores the value of MIB-1 staining, which confirmed low growth potential of this tumor. This was reaffirmed clinically with no evidence of tumor recurrence or neurological deterioration 21 years after surgery. This case reinforces the need for careful evaluation and grading of cerebellar gliomas in children, which show extreme nuclear pleomorphism and yet demonstrate no other features of malignancy. This is particularly significant in view of the fact that cerebellar astrocytomas in children carry an excellent prognosis after surgical resection and high-grade astrocytomas (anaplastic astrocytoma and glioblastoma) are exceptionally rare in this age group in this location.

Pleomorphic xanthoastrocytoma and desmoplastic cerebral tumors of childhood

GFAP immunohistochemistry has been invaluable in identifying unusual astrocytic variants such as the PXA and desmoplastic cerebral gliomas (25–28). The PXA was described in 1979 by Kepes *et al.* (26) as a variant of the supratentorial astrocytoma in young patients. The lipidized tumor cells in PXA exhibit GFAP positivity and often show marked pleomorphism and nuclear atypia, but mitoses and necrosis are generally absent. Neuronal elements are infrequent in the PXA, but have been reported. Although prognosis is generally favorable, malignant transformation has been infrequently reported in PXA (46), and increased mitotic activity is a negative prognostic indicator, which may herald subsequent anaplastic transformation. There may be extensive reticulin deposition in the tumor. By EM, the tumor cells display a basal lamina, which is considered to be a feature of subpial astrocytes.

In recent years, there is greater awareness amongst pediatric pathologists of a group of central nervous system (CNS) tumors, which display prominent desmoplasia and a neoplastic component of glial and/or neuronal elements (25–28). CNS tumors with a prominent desmoplastic stroma include the *gliofibroma*, *desmoplastic infantile ganglioglioma* (DIG), *desmoplastic cerebral astrocytoma* (also referred to as superficial cerebral astrocytoma) and *PXA*. Taratuto *et al.* (28) described tumors of a similar appearance attached to the convexity dura in infants and referred to them as *"superficial cerebral astrocytomas."* In 1987, VandenBerg *et al.* (47) described large supratentorial tumors in infants, which had in addition to the mature collagen and astrocytes, an added feature of ganglion cells. These authors advocated the terminology of *desmoplastic infantile ganglioglioma* for this lesion. In VandenBerg's original report, 11 cases were described, all under 18 months of age. The tumors usually presented in the first 4 months of life and most often involved the frontal and parietal regions. Grossly, they were invariably cystic and the cysts often accounted for a significant fraction of the tumor volume. There was variable dural attachment.

The desmoplastic cerebral tumors are rich in reticulin and at surgery, the firm rubbery texture and consistency may mimic a tumor of meningeal origin. Thus immunohistochemistry, particularly for GFAP is an important diagnostic tool in delineating the glial component, which is invariably seen in all desmoplastic cerebral tumors of childhood. Application of neuronal markers such as synaptophysin and NF highlights the neuronal elements, which may be less pronounced compared to the prominent glial component. Thus immunohistochemistry plays an important role in distinction of these desmoplastic glial tumors from fibroblastic meningiomas, which occur in a similar location, have a similar gross appearance, and at superficial glance, even similar histology. The desmoplastic cerebral tumors appear to be associated with a more favorable outcome despite the massive size and presence of foci of undifferentiated cells (47).

Cell kinetic and molecular genetic analysis of astrocytomas

In a study of cell kinetic analysis of 117 brain tumors, Jay et al. (10) evaluated 29 low-grade astrocytomas, 5 anaplastic astrocytomas, 4 glioblastomas and 1 gliosarcoma by flow cytometry and Ki-67 quantitation. The Ki-67 labeling index in the low-grade astrocytomas ranged from 0% to 2.76% (10). This contrasts with the higher labeling index in high-grade astrocytomas. In this regard, the inherent problem of regional variability and presence or absence of necrosis is particularly significant in astrocytic tumors in the interpretation of labeling indices. Thus, a low labeling index in a glioblastoma may reflect a large area of necrosis rather than viable tumor. When performing quantitative analysis of positively labeled nuclei (Ki-67/MIB-1), one should also be cognizant of labeling in nuclei of endothelial cells in foci of endothelial hyperplasia; if these are included in the quantitation, there would be a spurious increase in the "labeling" index in some pilocytic astrocytomas. Ploidy abnormalities, higher S phase fractions, and differences in DNA index values have been more consistently associated with higher grade astrocytomas compared with low-grade tumors.

Deletions of chromosomal material and the loss or inactivation of tumor suppressor genes appear to be involved in the development of many pediatric tumors. Specific chromosomal and molecular genetic abnormalities have been recognized in low- and high-grade astrocytomas and glioblastomas (17, 48–61). These involve structural or numerical abnormalities of chromosomes 1, 6, 7, 9, 10, 19, 22, and the sex chromosome. Malignant gliomas show a pattern of nonrandom abnormalities involving chromosomes 7 (gains), 10 (losses), and rearrangements (primarily deletions) of 9p as well as other rearrangements and losses of chromosome 22. Low-grade astrocytomas on the other hand have mainly shown either normal karyotypes or loss of one sex chromosome, but when clonal abnormalities occur, they are similar to those found in the malignant variety. Thus, polysomy of 7 and monosomy of 10 and 22 as well as loss of sex chromosomes have been described also in low-grade gliomas. Besides karyotype analysis, chromosome aberrations have also been detected in metaphase and interphase tumor cells by *in situ* hybridization using chromosome specific library probes (49, 50). In gliomas, interphase cytogenetics has revealed an over-representation of chromosome 7 and under-representation of chromosome 10, in keeping with observations from conventional karyotypic analysis.

We previously reported an aggressive malignant glioma in a child with MYCN amplification and double minutes (62). Double minutes in glioblastomas usually correlate with amplification of epidermal growth factor receptor (EGFR) and less commonly of MYCN, gli, or c-MYC. Loss of 9p usually reflects homozygous deletion of the CDKN2 gene. In the study of Barker et al. (63), homozygous p16 deletions were significantly more common in high-grade gliomas compared with low-grade gliomas. The majority of glioblastomas also have homozygous deletions of the CDKN2 (p16/MTS1) gene (60) and CDKN2 deletions occur twice as commonly in glioblastomas with EGFR amplification. Glioblastoma multiforme can be divided into two genetic subsets: one-third of cases (primarily in older adults) have EGFR amplification, while another one-third (primarily in younger adults) have p53 mutation (60).

Recently, there has been much interest in assessing telomerase activity in human neoplasms. Telomerase is a ribonucleoprotein containing an RNA template that synthesizes telomeric DNA. Somatic cells do not normally have telomerase activated. In a study of 41 brain tumors, Nakatani et al. (64) found telomerase activity in 12/20 glioblastomas, 2/2 oligodendrogliomas, and 3/3 metastases, while the anaplastic astrocytomas, low-grade astrocytomas, and meningiomas exhibited no activity. Based on these results, these authors suggested that telomerase activity may be an important marker of brain tumor malignancy (64). Patients with telomerase activity had a worse prognosis compared to those with undetectable activity, suggesting that telomerase activity may be a useful prognosticator for brain tumors.

Primitive neuroectodermal tumors

Nosology

In the last decade, there has been an emergence and greater acceptance of the diagnostic term, primitive neuroectodermal tumor (PNET) to designate tumors such as the medulloblastoma (8). The conceptual basis for this nomenclature is the assumption that PNETs share a common progenitor cell population, which may undergo anaplastic transformation at a number of sites in the CNS, leading to tumors with similar morphology. Some neuropathologists propose use of the term PNET for all embryonal tumors of the CNS, while others prefer to use specific designations, for example, medulloblastoma for such tumors in the cerebellum. In the revised WHO classification of brain tumors proposed in 1993 (8), the majority of participants supported the inclusion of the term PNET. However, the WHO classification voted also to use PNET selectively, rather than applying to all small cell embryonal childhood tumors, thus retaining the use of terminology such as pineoblastoma, medulloepithelioma, medulloblastoma, and ependymoblastoma (8). Notwithstanding this controversy in precise terminology and nosology and differences in tumor biology, at a morphological level, there are unifying features, which are characteristic of this group of CNS embryonal tumors. Immunohistochemistry and EM play an integral role in the diagnosis of this group of tumors and are invaluable in distinguishing them from other entities such as MRT.

Cerebral and cerebellar PNET (medulloblastoma) and variants

Since the initial description of medulloblastoma (PNET of the cerebellum) by Bailey and Cushing (65), this tumor has been extensively studied from pathological and molecular biologic persectives. While medulloblastomas comprise 7–8% of all intracranial tumors of neuroepithelial origin, they account for up to 25% of intracranial tumors in children being second in frequency only to the cerebellar astrocytomas. Medulloblastoma is the most common malignant brain tumor in childhood. About 50% occur in the first decade. Tumors can also be seen in young adults and even congenital medulloblastomas are recognized. Medulloblastoma may be associated with certain hereditary or familial syndromes such as nevoid basal cell carcinoma syndrome and Turcot syndrome (66).

In childhood examples of medulloblastoma, a midline location is common. The tumor is soft, friable, and moderately well demarcated from the adjacent cerebellar tissue. Other tumors may show necrosis; cyst formation and calcification are not prominent. The tumor may extend into the cavity of the fourth ventricle. The laterally situated tumors present as usually well-demarcated masses.

The "undifferentiated" medulloblastoma forms the largest subgroup of medulloblastoma and conforms closely to the original descriptions of the tumor. These are cellular tumors with no specific architectural arrangement of tumor cells with round, oval, or carrot shaped hyperchromatic nuclei and relatively scanty cytoplasm. Number of mitoses varies and individual cell necrosis is prominent. A high MIB-1 labeling index and apoptotic cells are common in this tumor type. Large geographic areas of tumor necrosis are uncommon. There may be tumor involvement of the leptomeninges with positive cerebrospinal fluid cytology (67).

In most medulloblastomas, some degree of neuronal differentiation is usually apparent, especially with application of immunocytochemical markers. Homer Wright rosettes, when encountered (Fig. 7.2(a)) are considered the hallmark of neuroblastic differentiation. Here, the cytoplasm of tumor cells form tapering processes converging into a central core. Advanced neuronal differentiation occurs only in a small percentage of cases (15, 68), where immature or even fully mature ganglion cells may be apparent.

A well-recognized variant of medulloblastoma is the *desmoplastic medulloblastoma*, which most frequently but not exclusively arises in the lateral lobes of adolescents and young adults (66). This distinctive variant is often demarcated and firm in texture and shows pale islands of cells (follicles) surrounded by dense mantles of small dark cells. These tumors show a lightly stained reticulin-free islands or follicles contiguous to more compact reticulin rich stroma, and these tumors frequently invade the leptomeninges. Relationship to prognosis has been controversial, with reportedly worse prognosis in children (69) and better prognosis in adults. The reticulin-free islands show prominent neuronal and glial differentiation (70).

In recent years, another variant of medulloblastoma with an aggressive clinical course has been reported (71). In 1992, Giangaspero *et al.* (71) described a distinct variant of medulloblastoma in four infants, associated with highly aggressive clinical behavior and proposed the designation of "*large cell medulloblastoma.*" In contrast to the classic medulloblastoma which exhibits a relatively monotonous population of tumor cells with hyperchromatic oval or carrot-shaped nuclei

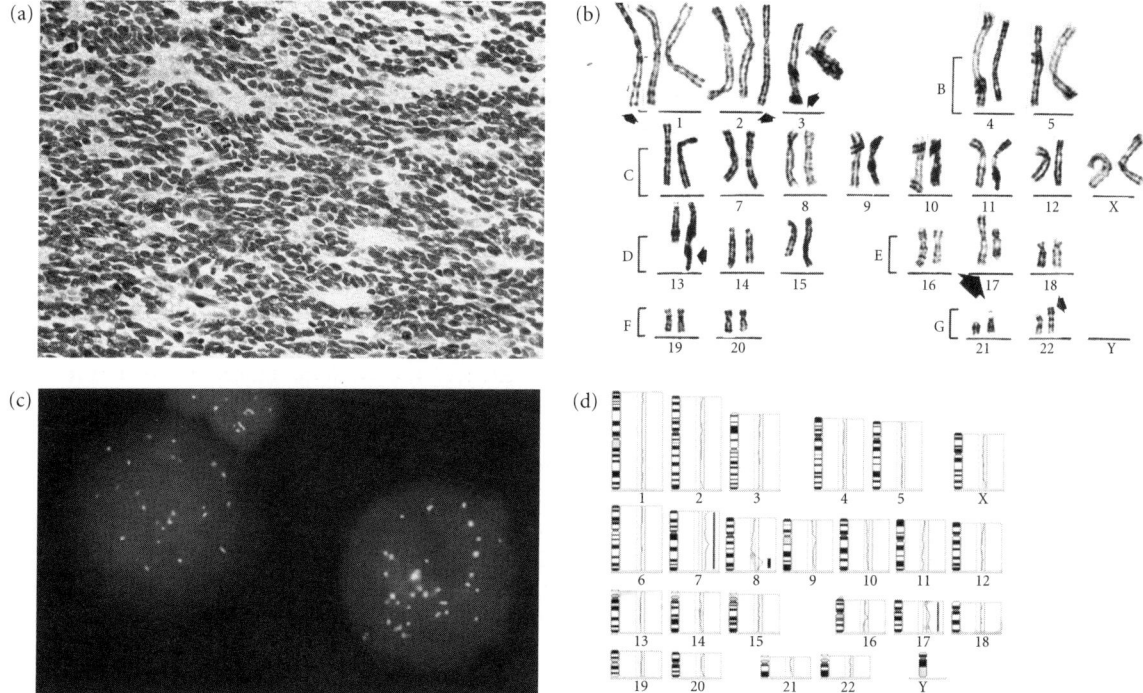

Fig. 7.2 PNET/medulloblastoma. (a) Medium power micrograph of a cerebellar medulloblastoma reveals Homer Wright rosettes where tumor cell processes converge into a central core. Tumor cells exhibit hyperchromatic nuclei. HE stain, ×225. (b) Abnormal karyotype in a supratentorial PNET: 48, XX, +i(1q), +2, 3q+, 13q+, i(17q), 22p+ (arrows). (c) FISH analysis reveals MYCN amplification in the 20–30-fold range in a medulloblastoma. (d) Ideogram summarizing the results of CGH analysis of large cell medulloblastoma: gains are represented by vertical lines to the right of schematic chromosomes. CGH diagram shows increased copy number of chromosome 7, amplification corresponding to MYCC gene locus on chromosome 8 and gain of long arm of chromosome 17 corresponding to i(17q).

and scanty cytoplasm, these tumors were associated with large vesicular nuclei and prominent nucleoli. In a recent case of large cell medulloblastoma encountered in our laboratory, the MIB-1 index was 56%. Spinal drop metastases were observed early in the clinical course and this tumor remained unresponsive to chemotherapy and total neuraxis irradiation and the patient died of disseminated subarachnoid and intraventricular tumor spread, within 8 months of initial presentation.

Rarely, medulloblastomas exhibit myogenic differentiation ("medullomyoblastoma") or reveal melanin pigment within tumor cells. Some authors regard "ependymoblastoma" as distinct entity, while others view it as a medulloblastoma with prominent ependymal differentiation.

With application of immunocytochemical markers, focal glial and neuronal differentiation is well documented in medulloblastoma. Positivity for a number of neuronal markers including NF proteins, beta 3 tubulin, MAP-2 and Tau (microtubule associated proteins), and synaptophysin is well documented in medulloblastoma (34, 70). The relationship between prognosis and differentiation in medulloblastomas remains controversial with some advocating worse outcome and others advocating better survival (72, 73).

By EM, typically, even in the so-called "undifferentiated" medulloblastoma, there is invariably evidence of some degree of neuronal differentiation, with cell processes containing microtubules and short profiles of rough endoplasmic reticulum, neurosecretory granules, and poorly developed junctions. Evidence of glial differentiation in medulloblastoma is indicated by bundles of glial filaments in a tumor cell. Less commonly there may be prominent ependymal differentiation, with very well developed cell junctions and intracytoplasmic lumina with microvilli. Skeletal muscle differentiation is rare with thick and thin myofilaments and Z bands within tumor cells. PNETs of the pineal (pineoblastoma) have distinctive ultrastructural features including intercellular junctions, dense core granules, 9 + 0 pattern cilia, microtubules, intermediate filaments, and synaptic junctions. Medulloepitheliomas (5) are exceedingly rare tumors which are considered to be the most primitive of neuroepithelial tumors and show a morphologic appearance reminiscent of primitive medullary plate and neural tube epithelium; these tumors reveal tubules and cords with a pseudostratified primitive neuroepithelium with inner (luminal) and outer (true) membranes. Heterotopic tissues such as cartilage and skeletal muscle may be present.

Cell kinetic and molecular genetic analysis of medulloblastoma and cerebral PNETs

Abnormalities of ploidy are recognized in medulloblastoma by flow cytometry (10). But in contrast to the neuroblastoma, where there is a significant correlation between prognosis and tumor ploidy, the relevance of ploidy to outcome is less well established in medulloblastomas although some authors advocate a better outcome for aneuploid tumors (74).

Isochromosome 17q has been recognized as the most common specific abnormality in the CNS PNETs (Fig. 7.2(b)), most of which have been cerebellar medulloblastomas (75, 76). Trisomy of 1q and monosomy for 17p are common in these tumors. Although the p53 gene is located on 17p, it is infrequently mutated in medulloblastomas. In contrast to peripheral PNETs (those occuring outside the CNS), which consistently demonstrate a primary chromosomal abnormality (77), characterized by a reciprocal translocation t(11;22)(q24;q12), PNETs of the CNS are typically not associated with this translocation (78). Using RT-PCR, we (78) demonstrated absence of t(11;22) in PNETs of the CNS.

The frequency of oncogene amplification is greater in medulloblastoma cell lines than in primary tumor samples (14, 15, 68, 79–82). In medulloblastomas, amplification of MYCC and less commonly of MYCN is described. Using differential PCR and FISH, we previously reported MYCN amplification in medulloblastomas with prominent neuronal differentiation (14, 15). Figure 7.2(c) shows MYCN amplification detected by FISH analysis in a medulloblastoma.

In a CGH study of 27 cases of medulloblastoma, Reardon et al. (83) found a number of genomic abnormalities including, nonrandom losses in regions on chromosomes 10q, 11, 16q, 17p, and 8p, gains of chromosomes 17q and 7, and amplifications of chromosome bands 5p15.3 and 11q22.3. In a study of 18 primitive neuroectodermal tumors (PNETs) Schütz et al. (84) found loss of 17p, gain of 17q, amplification of 2p24 corresponding to MYCN, and amplification of 8q24 corresponding to MYCC. We (85) previously reported 2p24 amplification in a medulloblastoma by CGH, corresponding to the MYCN locus. In a recent case of large cell medulloblastoma in our laboratory, CGH revealed gains of chromosome 7, 8q24, and long arm of chromosome 17 suggesting the presence of i(17q) (Fig. 7.2(d)). There was no evidence of MYCN amplification or 1p deletion in this tumor. Southern blotting confirmed that the oncogene amplified was MYCC.

With respect to MYCC, Bigner et al. (80) reported amplification of this oncogene in three cell lines and four xenografts derived from four primary medulloblastomas with double minutes and suggested that the MYCC gene provides a growth advantage to the tumor cells *in vitro* and in nude mice. In a large series of 27 medulloblastomas, Badiali and colleagues (79) found a single case with an aggressive course and 27-fold MYCC amplification. Tomlinson et al. (86) reported MYCN amplification as well as a rearranged MYCC gene in an aggressive medulloblastoma in a 27-year-old man.

In the report of Schütz et al. (84), none of the three patients with high copy number amplifications of MYCN responded to therapy. On the other hand, we recently encountered two medulloblastomas with exceptionally prominent neuronal differentiation and MYCN amplification associated with a relatively indolent course (15). Thus, the exact prognostic significance of MYCN and MYCC amplification and prognosis in medulloblastoma remains to be fully defined.

Ependymoma

In children, ependymomas are the third most common intracranial neoplasm, with two-thirds of cases being located in the infratentorial region. Variants such as the myxopapillary ependymoma occur in the region of the filum terminale (5). About 15% of ependymomas are anaplastic, with presence of increased cellularity, mitoses, cellular pleomorphism, and necrosis.

Ependymomas express both glial and epithelial characteristics. An important diagnostic feature, particularly valuable for diagnosis of frozen sections is the "perivascular pseudorosette." These are perivascular nuclear-free zones and are comprised of elongated tumor cell processes abutting on a vessel. In choroid plexus papillomas, tumor cells lie around a vessel, but there is a fibrovascular core. The perivascular processes in

(10). One hypodiploid tumor showed consistent monosomies of chromosomes 2, 10, and 22 by karyotypic analysis (Fig. 7.3(b)). Losses of chromosome 22 is common in ependymomas. Other inconsistent chromosomal abnormalities are also reported in this tumor.

Oligodendroglioma

This tumor is uncommon in childhood. It is recognized histologically by the presence of small cells with dark nuclei and perinuclear haloes, the so-called "fried egg" appearance. The cells are separated by a delicate vascular meshwork and there are variable degrees of microcystic change and calcification. Since a satisfactory immunohistochemical marker for oligodendroglioma remains to be developed, reliance is placed on the characteristic light microscopic and ultrastructural features. By EM, the tumor cells show microtubules and closely packed cells with condensation of nuclear heterochromatin. The most frequent genetic alteration in oligodendrogliomas is loss of heterozygosity (LOH) in 1p and 19q and is detectable in both low- and high-grade tumors (87). Inactivation of tumor suppressor genes at 1p and 19q may represent cooperative alterations occurring in early stages of oncogenesis for oligodendrogliomas (87).

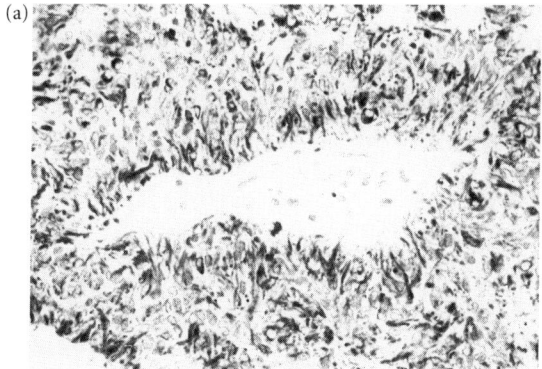

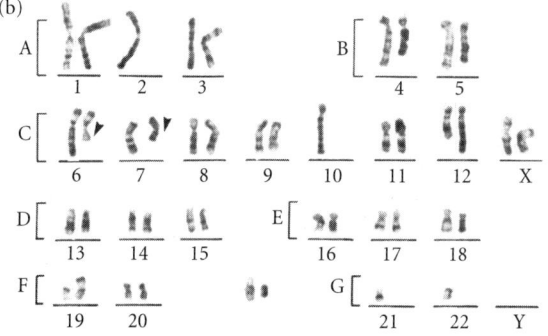

Fig. 7.3 Ependymoma. (a) Immunoperoxidase stain for GFAP reveals positivity in the perivascular processes of tumor cells (perivascular pseudorosettes), ×225. (b) Karyotype analysis in an ependymoma revealed hypodiploidy with consistent monosomies of chromosomes 2, 10, and 22 and two inconsistent abnormalities (6q− and 7q−), with markers.

ependymoma are GFAP-positive (Fig. 7.3(a)). There may also be cytokeratin positivity in this tumor.

Another finding, not universally present, is the true ependymal rosette, where tumor cells lie around a central lumen. EM is valuable in confirming ependymal lineage and shows cell junctions, cilia, basal bodies, and microvilli.

The problem of regional heterogeneity is significant in ependymomas, which may show well differentiated foci of low cellularity and other areas of higher cellularity associated with increased mitoses in the same tumor. Such tumors, which do not display frank anaplastic features, but contain focal hypercellular foci with occasional mitoses, may show abnormalities by flow cytometry with abnormal ploidy or increased G2M values (10). In a series of eight ependymomas (10), we found diploidy in four cases, diploidy with increased G2M in two cases, and aneuploidy in two cases by flow cytometric analysis. Four of seven anaplastic ependymomas showed ploidy abnormalities including hypodiploidy and polyhypertetraploidy

Neurocytoma

An important tumor in the differential diagnosis of oligodendroglioma is the neurocytoma (88–90). These tumors are quite rare, and characteristically occur in an intraventricular location. Histologically, this tumor is composed of small uniform cells, which have regular round nuclei and perinuclear haloes. Immunostaining and EM help to confirm the diagnosis. Immunostaining reveals prominent neuronal differentiation with positivity for synaptophysin and by EM, one sees evidence of neuronal differentiation with microtubules, NFs and dense core neurosecretory granules.

In an intraventricular neurocytoma in an 11-year-old boy, we found no evidence of MYCN amplification or 1p deletion (88). This tumor had a complex karyotype with counts in the near diploid range (45–48), with additional copies of 1q present in rearrangements with 4 and 7 (88). Although the literature on molecular genetic abnormalities in this tumor are limited, its karyotypic profile appears to be different from that of neuroblastoma and PNET.

Mixed gliomas and other malformative lesions

Ganglioglioma is a mixed glioma, composed of both neoplastic glial and neuronal elements. These tumors are slow-growing and have a predilection for the third ventricle and temporal lobe. Histologically, there is a low-grade astrocytoma as well as varying degrees of neuronal differentiation. The neoplastic neurons are distinguished from normal trapped cortical neurons by the marked variability in morphology including variable size, shape, and Nissl pattern and presence of binucleate or multinucleate forms. An interesting variant is the DIG (47), which has been included under the rubric of desmoplastic cerebral tumors.

Anaplastic transformation in a ganglioglioma is extremely rare. While such anaplasia is usually restricted to the glial component, we (91) encountered an unusual example of malignant transformation, a ganglioglioma with anaplastic neuronal and glial components; this anaplastic tumor emerged 3 years post-irradiation and showed a complex karyotype with clonal abnormalities.

Gangliogliomas are common in surgical resections done for medically refractory seizure disorder (92). Another common tumor in this patient population is the relatively recently described entity, the *Dysembryoplastic neuroepithelial tumor* (DNET) (93, 94). These tumors are most common in the temporal lobe and are characterized by a multinodular appearance. There is a heterogeneous population of astrocytes and oligodendroglial-like small cells, which appear to be small neurons based on the immunohistochemical and ultrastructural profile. Areas of calcification and small microcysts may be present. An interesting abnormality involves the cortex, which shows disorganized neuronal layering consistent with cortical dysplasia. The MIB1 labeling index is low and generally the tumor is associated with a good prognosis. Ganglioglioma and DNET are of particular interest to neuropathologists, as they represent examples of lesions where there is transition from malformative to neoplastic elements.

Subependymal giant cell tumor

These intriguing tumors are associated with tuberous sclerosis (95). Typically, they occur in a subependymal location near the foramen of Monro. In patients with tuberous sclerosis, the precursors of these tumors are seen as "candle gutterings," which are nodular protuberances

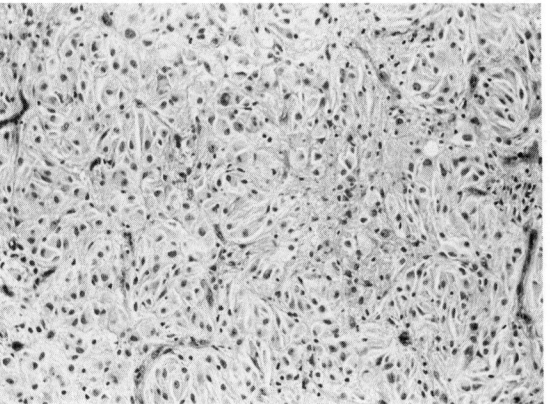

Fig. 7.4 Subependymal giant cell tumor. Plump cells with glassy cytoplasm in a fascicular arrangement typical of SEGT, HE stain, ×225.

composed of cells, which give rise to the subependymal giant cell tumor. While frequently referred to as the "subependymal giant cell astrocytoma," the tumor cells are not truly astrocytic in origin; rather, they seem to be composed of unique cells capable of both neuronal and glial differentiation (92, 95). Histologically, they present a characteristic pattern with a fascicular arrangement of cells with abundant eosinophilic glassy cytoplasm (Fig. 7.4) and may be calcified. Although giant cells with nuclear pleomorphism may be present, these are very slow growing tumors, which generally tend to be diploid and have very low proliferative index. Patients with tuberous sclerosis also reveal retinal astrocytic hamartomas, which are generally asymptomatic unlike the intracranial lesions.

In our experience, the Subependymal giant cell tumors are usually vimentin positive and exhibit variable positivity for GFAP, Neuron specific enolase, and synaptophysin. Ultrastructurally, they show prominent "lysosomal" inclusions, which are a characteristic feature. Other findings include prominent Golgi complexes, well-developed rough and smooth endoplasmic reticulum, cytoplasmic intermediate filaments, and rarely, even neurosecretory granules, microvilli, and even synapses may be found. Jay *et al.* previously reported on the finding of crystalline rhomboidal or rectanglular inclusions in a subependymal giant cell tumor (95). These may be quite prominent even by light microsopy and may be found not only in tumor cells, but also in nontumorous cells in the cortical tubers.

In tuberous sclerosis, molecular genetic studies have implicated two chromosomal loci, TSC1 on chromosome 9q and TSC2 on chromosome 16p (96, 97).

The exact function of the protein encoded by the TSC2 gene, tuberin, remains speculative.

There is no consistent pattern of cytogenetic abnormality in the SEGT. In a SEGT in a 15-year-old boy with tuberous sclerosis, we found an abnormal karyotype, which was pseudodiploid, hypodiploid, and hypotetraploid with fragments, dicentric and marker chromosomes, multiple structural rearrangements, and random losses and gains of whole chromosomes. Reports of karyotypic and molecular genetic analyses of the SEGT are limited. Ye et al. (98) found no evidence of LOH for chromosome 10 in one case of SEGT. A normal karyotype was described by Chadduck et al. (54) in one case. Vagner-Capodano et al. (99) reported normal karotype in one and 47,XY,+mar in another case of SEGT. These changes are distinct from those in low-grade gliomas.

Choroid plexus tumors

Choroid plexus tumors account for less than 1% of all intracranial tumors, but account for 2–5% of primary pediatric brain tumors. The benign choroid plexus papilloma is far more common. These tumors mimic the architecture of the normal choroid plexus (Fig. 7.5) and may be associated with overproduction of the cerebrospinal fluid. Choroid plexus carcinoma is invariably a disease of childhood. Although rare, it may account for over 25% of all choroid plexus tumors in children.

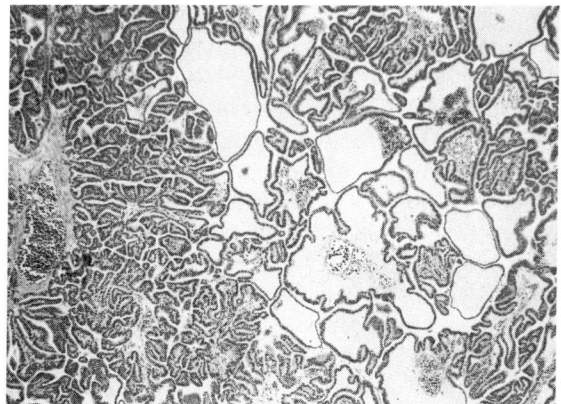

Fig. 7.5 Choroid plexus papilloma. The architecture of the tumor mimics that of normal choroid plexus. Tumor cells lie around a fibrovascular core. Choroid plexus papillomas can lead to an overproduction of cerebrospinal fluid. HE stain, ×125.

Choroid plexus papillomas show a prominent papillary pattern, with a fibrovascular core. By EM, unlike an ependymoma, these cells rest on a basal lamina. Junctions, microvilli, and cilia are present. Choroid plexus tumors can display S100, keratin, and EMA positivity as well as focal GFAP positivity. Our experience suggests that the choroid plexus carcinomas consistently show p53 immunopositivity while the papillomas appear to be negative (44).

Karyotype analysis in choroid plexus tumors in our laboratory revealed interesting abnormalities. In one choroid plexus papilloma, we found hypodiploidy, diploidy, and hypertriploidy, while a second case revealed hyperdiploidy with miscellaneous trisomies and a consistent −22. In a 5-month-old girl with choroid plexus carcinoma, all cells examined showed monosomy 22 with a karyotype, 45,XX,−22. In another case of choroid plexus carcinoma, a highly complex karyotype was evident: 76,XXX,+1,−3,+8, +8,+9,+12,+14,−16,+20,+21,+22. Five of six cells examined were hyperdiploid with 75–78 chromosomes. The karyotypic abnormalities correlated well with assessment of ploidy by flow cytometry, which revealed hyperdiploidy with increased S phase. Thus chromosome 22 abnormalities may be encountered also in choroid plexus tumors, but this is not a consistent finding.

We (10) previously reported ploidy abnormalities in six choroid plexus tumors studied by flow cytometry. An adverse outcome was reported for aneuploid tumors by Qualman et al. (100) while Coons et al. (101) reported that aneuploidy is common in choroid plexus tumors and in itself is not related to a poor outcome. In a study of 10 choroid plexus tumors including 4 carcinomas, Coons et al. (101) reported that the mean S phase fraction for choroid plexus papillomas was 1.1 ± 0.82% SD, which was significantly different from that of the choroid plexus carcinoma group (7 ± 1.25% SD) and concluded that lower S phase fractions were correlated with favorable outcome.

Monosomy 22 characterizes several neurogenic tumors. Using restriction fragment length polymorphism (RFLP) analysis, Seizinger et al. (102–104) demonstrated partial deletions of 22q in neurofibromas, meningiomas, and acoustic neuromas of patients with bilateral acoustic neurofibromatosis as well as in sporadic meningiomas and unilateral acoustic neuromas. The defective gene responsible for bilateral acoustic neurofibromatosis is located on chromosome 22. These findings suggest that sporadic neurogenic tumors with losses or deletions of chromosome 22 including unilateral acoustic neuromas, meningiomas, and gliomas have lost through somatic mutation the gene which is defective in bilateral acoustic neurofibromatosis patients.

Meningioma

Meningiomas are not common in childhood. Several histological patterns are identified, including meningothelial (Fig. 7.6(a)), psammomatous, transitional, and fibroblastic areas. But these are of no prognostic significance. The papillary meningioma is associated with a poorer prognosis as are the meningeal hemangiopericytomas (105).

The charateristic histological pattern is that of whorls of cells without distinct cytoplasmic borders. This syncytial pattern is due to close interdigitation of tumor cell cytoplasm, well seen by EM. By EM, desmosomal junctions are also seen. Meningiomas show vimentin, EMA, and keratin positivity as well as positivity for laminin and fibronectin.

Meningiomas can show interesting abnormalities by flow cytometry and cytogenetic analysis. Monosomy for chromosome 22 is a consistent cytogenetic abnormality (Fig. 7.6(b)). Meningiomas are also frequently aneuploid (10), but the prognostic significance of ploidy is not definitely established.

Malignant rhabdoid tumor

It is an extremely aggressive malignant tumor, with as yet, undetermined histogenesis. The rhabdoid tumor of the kidney was reported by Beckwith and Palmer (106) and subsequently extrarenal MRT have been found in a number of sites including the CNS (30, 107–112). These tumors show cytoplasmic perinuclear filamentous whorls, which appear as globular inclusions, which are immunopositive for vimentin and cytokeratin, and composed of a mass of intermediate filaments by EM. Classically, the tumors exhibit a polyphenotypic profile, with consistent immunopositivity for EMA, cytokeratin, and vimentin.

The proportion of cells with such "rhabdoid" features is variable from case to case and the more undifferentiated element may resemble a PNET. The term "atypical teratoid rhabdoid tumor" has been used to designate anaplastic tumors in young children, which show a variety of histological patterns including rhabdoid cells in combination with foci of PNET (6, 108). Other morphological patterns including clear cells and cells with mesenchymal/epithelial features may also be present. The immunocytochemical profile of these tumors is complex including positivity for a wide range of markers. EM characteristics vary depending on the area sampled, but cells with typical rhabdoid features are also identified. These tumors may thus exhibit an array of findings including prominent junctions, cytoplasmic intermediate filaments, and evidence of neuronal differentiation with microtubules and neurosecretory granules.

Both MRTs and atypical teratoid rhabdoid tumors carry a dismal prognosis and their distinction from PNETs, which are associated with a far more favorable outcome is of paramount importance. Olson *et al.* (110) reported survival in three patients with no evidence of disease at 5 years, 2 years, and 9 months from diagnosis after surgical resection, chemotherapy, radiotherapy, and triple intrathecal chemotherapy.

The exact histogenesis of CNS MRTs remains speculative. Some authors favor a neural differentiation (107), but the pattern of cytogenetic abnormalities in CNS MRTs is quite different from that of CNS PNETs,

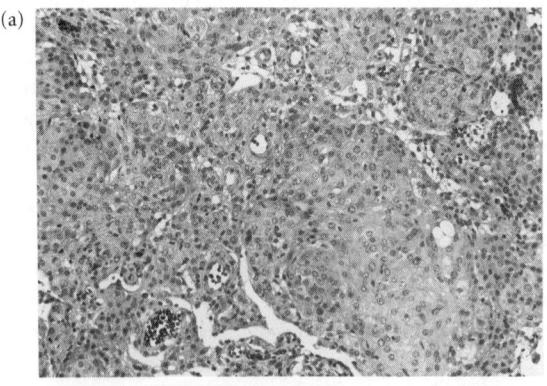

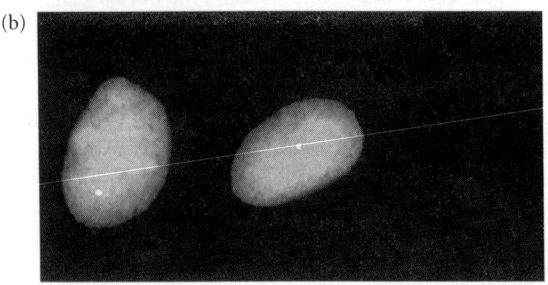

Fig. 7.6 Meningioma. (a) Meningothelial nests in a meningioma with the characteristic syncytial whorling pattern, where individual cell borders are indistinct. HE stain, ×225. (b) FISH analysis reveals monosomy 22 in this tumor.

which are commonly associated with an isochromosome 17q. Monosomy 22 has been reported in CNS MRTs (61).

Other lesions

Other lesions that a pediatric neuropathologist might encounter include germ cell neoplasms, craniopharyngioma, and intracranial cysts. Pituitary adenomas, acoustic neuromas, hemangioblastomas, and chordomas are relatively uncommon in children.

Intraocular neoplasms

Retinoblastoma

Retinoblastoma is the most common intraocular neoplasm in children with no significant sex or race predilection; a third of cases are bilateral (resulting from germline mutations). The average age at diagnosis is between 12 and 24 months, with an average age of 18 months (113). Typically, children with heritable disease present at an earlier age than those with unilateral disease.

Children with retinoblastoma may have other congenital abnormalities such as 13q− deletion syndrome, other trisomies, PHPV, and congenital cataracts. Bilateral retinoblastoma in association with pineoblastoma has been referred to as trilateral retinoblastoma (114). Retinoblastoma behaves as an autosomal dominant trait with 90–95% penetrance and represents a prototype for human cancers characterized by loss of tumor suppressor genes at the constitutional or tumor level (115). The Knudson's two hit hypothesis (116) states that retinoblastoma arises as a result of two mutational events (Fig. 7.7(a)). If both chromosomal 13q14 regions are normal, no retinoblastoma develops; if one of the two 13q14 regions is abnormal, no retinoblastoma results. If both chromosomes 13 have a 13q14 deletion, retinoblastoma results. When both mutations occur in the same somatic postzygotic cell, a single unilateral retinoblastoma results. Since the mutations occur in a somatic cell, this condition is therefore not inherited. In the hereditary form, the first mutation occurs in a germinal prezygotic cell, which means that this mutation is present in all resulting somatic cells and a second mutation occurs in the somatic postzygotic cells, resulting in multiple retinal tumors as well as tumors in other sites such as sarcomas. The RB gene (locus name RB1) was cloned by isolating and sequencing genomic DNA fragments from band 13q14 (117). It appears to be transcribed in all cells, and it is not clear why the mutant allele predisposes retinal or osteoid cells, in particular, to malignancy. Some individuals with breast, bladder, or lung cancer have structural abnormalities of the RB gene suggesting that it may play a role in the carcinogenesis of different types of cancer.

The RB gene product (pRB), a 110 kDa protein is is 928 amino acids long and found in cell nuclei; it has a fundamental role in regulating cell proliferation and exists in both phosphorylated and dephosphorylated forms (117). Phosphorylation of pRB is at a low level at the beginning of the cell cycle (G1) and increases as the cycle progresses (S and G2). Recently, it has been shown that pRB binds to and potentially inactivates the E2F transcription complex, which is involved in cell cycle regulation.

Early presentation in retinoblastoma may include visual difficulties or strabismus. More prominent lesions may present as leukocoria (white pupillary reflex), or a picture of psedoinflammation simulating uveitis, endophthalmitis, or panophthalmitis. In terms of growth patterns, retinoblastomas may be endophytic (toward the vitreous), exophytic (toward the subretinal space), or mixed. The diffuse infiltrating retinoblastoma is uncommon and presents the greatest difficulty in clinical diagnosis, simulating a pseudohypopyon and intraocular inflammation (113). Another uncommon presentation of retinoblastoma is complete spontaneous tumor necrosis (spontaneous regression), which is accompanied by a severe inflammatory reaction followed by pthisis bulbi (113).

There is extensive mitotic activity and necrosis and frequent calcification in the tumor. Basophilic staining of blood vessels and lens capsule represents DNA deposition from tumor necrosis. The *Flexner Wintersteiner* rosettes are the characteristic rosettes of retinoblastoma, where cells with basal nuclei form an irregular apical limiting membrane surrounding a lumen, which contains hyaluronidase-resistant acid mucopolysacharide (Fig. 7.7(b)). By EM, these cells exhibit a 9 + 0 pattern of cilia and show photoreceptor differentiation. *Fleurettes* are flower like arrangements of tumor cells, which represents marked photoreceptor differentiation (Fig. 7.7(c)). In the fully differentiated tumor, the retinocytoma, fleurettes are prominent.

The mode of spread for retinoblastoma includes local extension, extension into the optic nerve and intracranial spread, and distant metastases. In terms of prognostic factors, besides tumor size and location, a

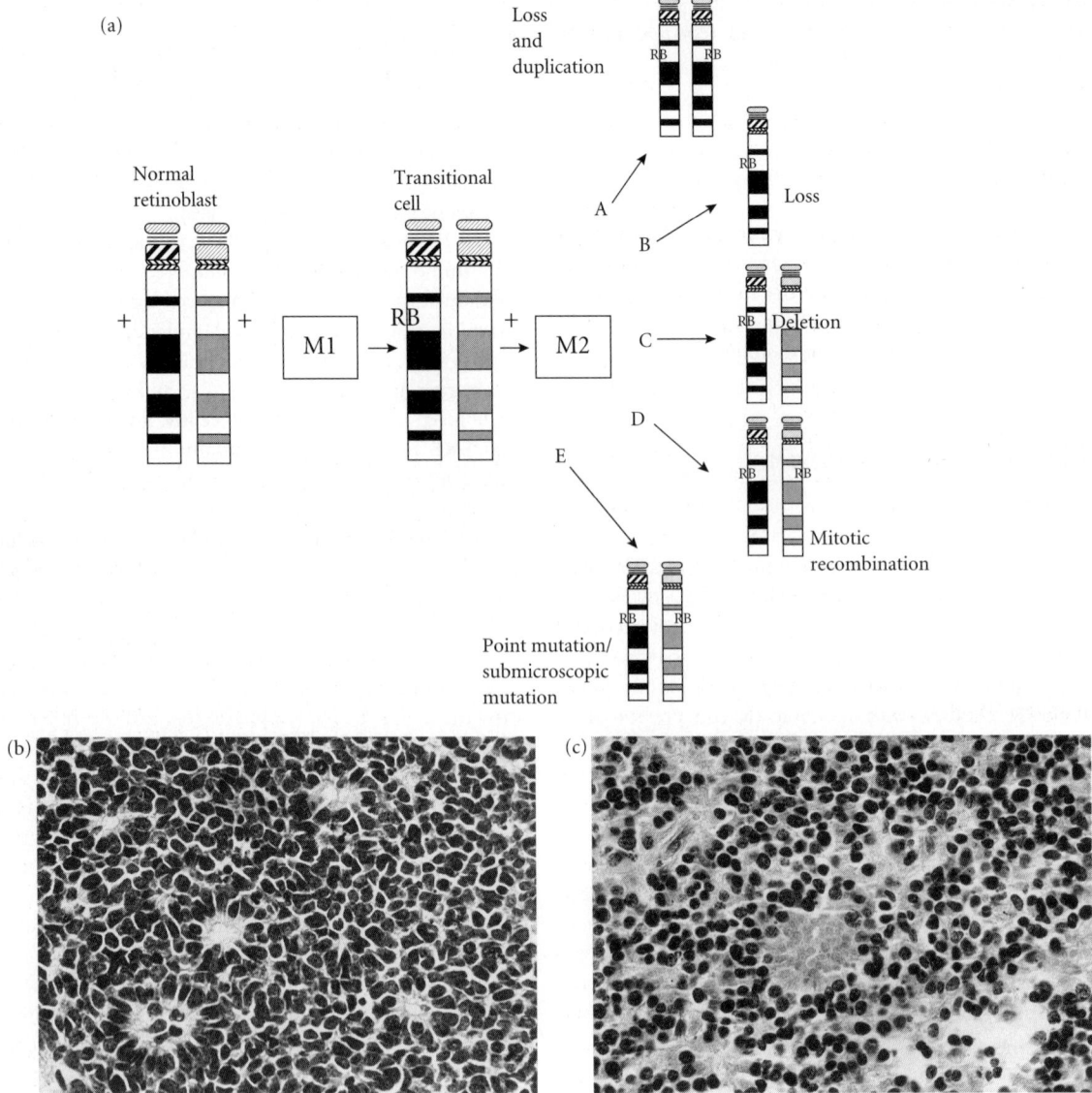

Fig. 7.7 Retinoblastoma. (a) Mechanisms of mutational inactivation of a tumor suppressor gene (RB1). Retinoblastoma occurs when two independent mutations M1 and M2 inactivate both normal alleles at the RB1 (RB) locus on chromosome 13 at band 13q14. The most frequent mechanism (A) results in the chromosome carrying the normal gene being lost completely and chromosomes carrying the mutant RB1 allele being duplicated. In mechanism B, the normal chromosome is lost with one mutant chromosome. Occasionally, a small deletion at band 13q14 is identified as shown in mechanism C. Mitotic recombination is also possible as shown in mechanism D. In some patients, no gross chromosomal mechanism is involved; rather such patients have two independent mutations in each RB1 allele as shown in mechanism E. (b) Photomicrograph reveals Flexner Wintersteiner rosettes in a retinoblastoma. HE stain, ×300. (c) More advanced differentiation is evident in this retinoblastoma with formation of fleurettes. HE stain, ×300.

differentiated tumor with abundant Flexner Wintersteiner rosettes or fleurettes has a much better prognosis (118); the extent of invasion is important with extension into the optic nerve and ocular coats being the two most important predictors of outcome (4, 119) and extraocular invasion being the most important predictor of death. Massive choroidal invasion and extension into the sclera are associated with high incidence of systemic metastases. With respect to assessing extraglobal extension, it is important to note that isolated episcleral "free floating" tumor cells may sometimes represent artifactually dislodged tumor cells during opening of the globe. Subretinal pigment epithelial or superficial choroidal extension is frequent and is not very significant (113). With respect to invasion of the optic nerve, invasion up to but not beyond the lamina cribrosa has relatively little prognostic significance, but invasion up to the line of transection carries a poor prognosis. Tumor beyond the lamina cribrosa and involving the pia arachnoid also is associated with a poor prognosis (113).

Important considerations in the differential diagnosis of leukocoria (2, 7) include Coats' disease, persistent hyperplastic primary vitreous, Toxocara infection, retinopathy of prematurity, and retinal dysplasia.

Medulloepithelioma (diktyoma) is a rare congenital tumor arising almost exclusively in the ciliary body (4, 120, 121). It may achieve massive proportions and may be low grade or anaplastic. These tumors consist of cords and sheets of primitive neuroepithelium, often interlaced with spaces rich in hyaluronic acid. Heterotopic tissues such as hyaline cartilage, skeletal muscle, or neural elements may be present (teratoid medulloepitheliomas).

Conclusion

Pediatric brain tumors are unique in several respects. Few are completely amenable to total surgical resection and despite recent advances in surgery, radiotherapy, and chemotherapy, many children with malignant brain gliomas or medulloblastoma die of their tumors. In the near future, analysis of gene rearrangements and amplifications should allow in a manner complementary to histopathological analysis, identification of biological differences between brain tumors. Also, new biotherapeutic strategies may be developed to reduce tumor cell proliferation by blocking specific cell cycle proteins or by enhancing the function of cyclin dependent kinase inhibitors. An understanding of basic tumor kinetics and tumor biology will contribute greatly to more accurate prognostication, advancement in targeting cells with gene therapy and newer, safer therapeutic strategies.

References

1. Young JLJ, Miller RW. Incidence of malignant tumors in U.S. children. J Pediatr 1975, 86, 254–8.
2. Yanoff M, Fine BS. Ocular pathology. A text and atlas, 3rd edn. Philadelphia, JB Lippincott, 1989.
3. Russell DS, Rubinstein LJ. Pathology of tumours of the nervous system, 5th edn. Williams & Wilkins, Baltimore, 1989.
4. McLean IW, Burnier MN, Zimmerman LE, Jakobiec FA. Tumors of the eye and ocular adnexa, Fascicle 12, 3rd series vol. Armed Forces Institute of Pathology, Washington, DC, 1994.
5. Kleihues P, Cavenee WK. Pathology and genetics of tumours of the central nervous system. International Agency for Research on Cancer, Lyon, 1997.
6. Burger PC, Scheithauer BW. Atlas of tumor pathology. Tumors of the central nervous system, 10, 3rd series vol. Armed Forces Institute of Pathology, Washington, DC, 1993.
7. Apple DJ, Rabb MF. Ocular pathology. Clinical applications and self assessment, 4th edn. Mosby Year Book, St Louis, 1991.
8. Kleihues P, Burger PC, Scheithauer BW. Histological typing of tumours of the central nervous system, 2nd edn. Springer-Verlag, New York, 1993.
9. Becker LE, Jay V. Tumors of the central nervous system in children. Martinus Nijhoff Company, The Hague, Netherlands, 1990.
10. Jay V, Parkinson D, Becker L, Chan F-W. Cell kinetic analysis in pediatric brain and spinal tumors: a study of 117 cases with Ki-67 quantitation and flow cytometry. Pediatr Pathol 1994, 14, 253–76.
11. Jay V, Greenberg M. Unusual cerebellar ganglioglioma with marked atypia. Pediatr Pathol 1997, 17, 105–14.
12. McCormick D, Chong H, Hobbs C, Datta C, Hall PA. Detection of the Ki-67 antigen in fixed and wax-embedded sections with the monoclonal antibody MIB1. Histopathology 1993, 22, 355–60.
13. Boerner S, Squire J, Thorner P, McKenna G, Zielenska M. Assessment of MYCN amplification in neuroblastoma biopsies by differential polymerase chain reaction. Pediatr Pathol 1994, 14, 823–32.
14. Jay V, MacNeill S, Zielenska M. MYCN amplfication in pediatric brain tumors. J Histotechnol 1997, 20, 115–18.
15. Jay V, Marrano P, Zielenska M. MYCN amplification in medulloblastoma. Ped Pathol Mol Med 1999, 18, 127–42.
16. Gray JW, Pinkel D, Brown JM. Fluorescence in situ hybridization in cancer and radiation biology. Radiation Res 1994, 137, 275–89.
17. Bigner SH, Schrock E. Molecular cytogenetics of brain tumors. J Neuropathol Exp Neurol 1997, 56, 1173–81.
18. Kallioniemi A, Kallioniemi O-P, Sudar D, et al. Comparative genomic hybridization for molecular cytogenetic analysis of solid tumors. Science 1992, 258, 818–21.
19. Kallioniemi OP, Kallioniemi A, Sudar D, et al. Comparative genomic hybridization: a rapid new method for detecting and mapping DNA amplification in tumors. Semin Cancer Biol 1993, 4, 41.
20. Bignami A, Eng LF, Dahl D, Uyeda CT. Localization of glial fibrillary acidic protein in astrocytes by immunofluorescence. Brain Res 1972, 43, 429–35.
21. Eng LF, Vanderhaeghen JJ, Bignami A, Gerstl B. An acidic protein isolated from fibrous astrocytes. Brain Res 1971, 28, 351–4.

22. Budka H. Non-glial specificities of immunocytochemistry for the glial fibrillary acidic protein (GFAP). Triple expression of GFAP, vimentin and cytokeratins in papillary meningioma and metastasizing renal carcinoma. Acta Neuropathol 1986, 72, 43–54.
23. Jay V, Becker LE. Brain tumors. Curr Opin Neurol Neurosurg 1990, 3, 934–42.
24. Perentes E, Rubinstein LJ. Recent applications of immunoperoxidase histochemistry in human neuro-oncology. Arch Pathol Lab Med 1987, 111, 796–812.
25. Louis DN, von Deimling A, Dickersin GR, Dooling EC, Seizinger BR. Desmoplastic cerebral astrocytomas of infancy: a histopathologic, immunohistochemical, ultra-structural, and molecular genetic study. Hum Pathol 1992, 23, 1402–9.
26. Kepes JJ, Rubinstein LJ, Eng LF. Pleomorphic xanthoastrocytoma: a distinctive meningocerebral glioma of young subjects with relatively favorable prognosis. A study of 12 cases. Cancer 1979, 44, 1839–52.
27. Rushing EJ, Rorke LB, Sutton L. Problems in nosology of desmoplastic tumors of childhood. Pediatr Neurosurg 1993, 19, 57–62.
28. Taratuto AL, Monges J, Lylyk P, Leiguardia R. Superficial cerebral astrocytoma attached to dura. Report of six cases in infants. Cancer 1984, 54, 2505–12.
29. Tsokos M, Kouraklis G, Chandra RS, Bhagavan BS, Triche TJ. Malignant rhabdoid tumor of the kidney and soft tissues. Evidence for a diverse morphological and immunocytochemical phenotype. Arch Pathol Lab Med 1989, 113, 115–20.
30. Chou SM, Anderson JS. Primary CNS malignant rhabdoid tumor (MRT): report of two cases and review of the literature. Clin Neuropathol 1991, 10, 1–10.
31. Trojanowski JQ. Immunohistochemistry of neurofilament proteins and their diagnostic applications. In: Advances in immunohistochemistry (ed. RA DeLellis). Raven Press, New York, 1988, 237–60.
32. Molenaar WM, Jansson DS, Gould VE, et al. Molecular markers of primitive neuroectodermal tumors and other pediatric central nervous system tumors. Monoclonal antibodies to neuronal and glial antigens distinguish subsets of primitive neuroectodermal tumors. Lab Invest 1989, 61, 635–43.
33. Yachnis AT, Trojanowski JQ. Studies of childhood brain tumors using immunohistochemistry and microwave technology: methodological considerations. J Neurol Sci 1994, 55, 191–200.
34. Gould VE, Rorke LB, Jansson DS, et al. Primitive neuroectodermal tumors of the central nervous system express neuroendocrine markers and may express all classes of intermediate filaments. Hum Pathol 1990, 21, 245–52.
35. Miller DC, Koslow M, Budzilovich GN, Burstein DE. Synaptophysin: a sensitive and specific marker for ganglion cells in central nervous system neoplasms. Hum Pathol 1990, 21, 93–8.
36. Bilbao JM, Khoury NJS, Hudson AR, Briggs SJ. Perineurioma (localized hypertrophic neuropathy). Arch Pathol Lab Med 1984, 108, 557–60.
37. Jay V, Vasjar J, Haslam RHA. Axonal neuropathy with perineurial hyperplasia: report of a case with multifocal involvement. J Child Neurol, in press.
38. Theaker JM, Fletcher CDM. Epithelial membrane antigen expression by the perineurial cell: further studies of peripheral nerve lesions. Histopathol 1989, 14, 581–92.
39. Barbareschi M, Iuzzolino P, Pennella A, et al. p53 protein expression in central nervous system neoplasms. J Clin Pathol 1992, 45, 583–6.
40. Louis DN. The p53 gene and protein in human brain tumors. J Neuropathol Exp Neurol 1994, 53, 11–21.
41. Louis DN, Rubio M-P, Correa KM, Gusella JF, von Deimling A. Molecular genetics of pediatric brain stem gliomas. Application of PCR techniques to small and archival brain tumor specimens. J Neuropathol Exp Neurol 1993, 52, 507–15.
42. Ng HK, Lo SY, Huang DP, Poon WS. Paraffin section p53 protein immunohistochemistry in neuroectodermal tumors. Pathology 1994, 26, 1–5.
43. Lang FF, Miller DC, Pisharody S, Koslow M, Newcomb EW. High frequency of p53 protein accumulation without p53 gene mutation in human juvenile pilocytic, low grade and anaplastic astrocytomas. Oncogene 1994, 9, 949–54.
44. Jay V, Ho M, Chan F, Malkin D. p53 expression in choroid plexus neoplasms: an immunohistochemical study. Arch Pathol Lab Med 1996, 120, 1061–5.
45. Stern J, Jakobiec FA, Housepian EM. The architecture of optic nerve gliomas with and without neurofibromatosis. Arch Ophthalmol 1980, 98, 505–11.
46. Macaulay RJB, Jay V, Hoffman HJ, Becker LE. Increased mitotic activity as a negative prognostic indicator in pleomorphic xanthoastrocytoma. J Neurosurg 1993, 79, 761–8.
47. VandenBerg SR, May EE, Rubinstein LJ, et al. Desmoplastic supratentorial neuroepithelial tumors of infancy with divergent differentiation potential ("desmoplastic infantile gangliogliomas"). J Neurosurg 1987, 66, 58–71.
48. Agamanolis DP, Malone JM. Chromosomal abnormalities in 47 pediatric brain tumors. Cancer Genet Cytogenet 1995, 81, 125–34.
49. Arnoldus EP, Noordermeer IA, Peters AC, et al. Interphase cytogenetics of brain tumors. Genes Chromosomes Cancer 1991, 3, 101–7.
50. Arnoldus EPJ, Wolters LBT, Voormolen JHC, et al. Interphase cytogenetics: a new tool for the study of genetic changes in brain tumors. J Neurosurg 1992, 76, 997–1003.
51. Bigner SH, Mark J, Burger PC, et al. Specific chromosomal abnormalities in malignant human gliomas. Cancer Res 1988, 88, 405–11.
52. Bigner SH, Mark J, Bigner DD. Cytogenetics of human brain tumors. Cancer Genet Cytogenet 1990, 47, 141–54.
53. Bigner SH, Vogelstein B. Cytogenetics and molecular genetics of malignant gliomas and medulloblastomas. Brain Pathol 1990, 1, 12–18.
54. Chadduck WM, Boop FA, Sawyer JR. Cytogenetic studies of pediatric brain and spinal cord tumors. Pediatr Neurosurg 1991–92, 17, 57–65.
55. Griffin CA, Hawkins AL, Packer RJ, Rorke LB, Emanuel BS. Chromosome abnormalities in pediatric brain tumors. Cancer Res 1988, 48, 175–80.
56. James CD, He J, Carlbom E, et al. Loss of genetic information in central nervous system tumors common to children and young adults. Genes Chromosomes Cancer 1990, 2, 94–102.

57. Karnes PS, Tran TN, Cui MY, et al. Cytogenetic analysis of 39 pediatric central nervous system tumors. Cancer Genet Cytogenet 1992, 59, 12–19.
58. Jenkins RB, Kimmel DE, Moertel CA, et al. A cytogenetic study of 53 human gliomas. Cancer Genet Cytogenet 1989, 39, 253–79.
59. Rey JA, Bello MJ, deCampos JM, Kusak ME, Moreno S. Chromosomal composition of a series of 22 human low-grade gliomas. Cancer Genet Cytogenet 1987, 29, 223–7.
60. Hayashi Y, Ueki K, Waha A, Wiestler OD, Louis DN, von Deimling A. Association of EGFR gene amplification and CDKN2 (p16/MTS1) gene deletion in glioblastoma multiforme. Brain Pathol 1997, 7, 871–5.
61. Bhattacharjee M, Armstrong D, Vogel H, Cooley LD. Cytogenetic analysis of 120 primary pediatric brain tumors and literature review. Cancer Genet Cytogenet 1997, 97, 39–53.
62. Jay V, Rutka J, Becker LE, Squire J. Pediatric malignant glioma with tuboloreticular inclusions and MYCN amplification. Cancer 1994, 73, 1987–93.
63. Barker FG, Chen P, Furman F, Aldape KD, Edwards MS, Israel MA. p16 deletion and mutation analysis in human brain tumors. J Neuro-Oncol 1997, 31, 17–23.
64. Nakatani K, Yoshimi N, Mori H, et al. The significant role of telomerase activity in human brain tumors. Cancer 1997, 80, 471–6.
65. Bailey P, Cushing H. Medulloblastoma cerebelli: a common type of midcerebellar glioma of childhood. Arch Neurol Psychiatr 1925, 14, 192–224.
66. Russell DS, Rubinstein LJ. Tumours of central neuroepithelial origin: cerebellar medulloblastomas, 5th edn. Williams & Wilkins, Baltimore, 1989, 261–3.
67. Murakami M, Jay V, Al-Shail E, Rutka JT. Brain tumors that disseminate along cerebrospinal fluid pathways and beyond. In: Brain tumor invasion: Biological, clinical, and therapeutic considerations (ed. T Mikkelsen, R Bjerkving, OD Laerum, ML Rosenblum). Wiley-Liss, Inc., 1998, 111–32.
68. Jay V, Squire J, Zielenska M, Gerrie B, Humphreys R. Molecular and cytogenetic analysis of a cerebellar primitive neuroectodermal tumor with prominent neuronal differentiation: detection of MYCN amplification by differential polymerase chain reaction and Southern blot analysis. Pediatr Pathol 1995, 15, 733–744.
69. Park TS, Hoffman HJ, Hendrick EB, Humphreys RP, Becker LE. Medulloblastoma: clinical presentation and management. Experience at The Hospital for Sick Children, Toronto, 1950–1980. J Neurosurg 1983, 58, 543–52.
70. Katsetos CD, Herman MM, Frankfurter A, et al. Cerebellar desmoplastic medulloblastomas. A further immunohistochemical characterization of the reticulin-free pale islands. Arch Pathol Lab Med 1989, 113, 1019–29.
71. Giangaspero F, Rigobello L, Badiali M, et al. Large-cell medulloblastomas. A distinct variant with highly aggressive behavior. Am J Surg Pathol 1992, 16, 687–93.
72. Caputy AJ, McCullough DC, Manz HJ, Patterson HJ, Hammock MK. A review of factors influencing the prognosis of medulloblastoma. J Neurosurg 1987, 66, 80–7.
73. Packer RJ, Sutton LN, Rorke LB, et al. Prognostic importance of cellular differentiation in medulloblastoma of childhood. J Neurosurg 1984, 61, 296–301.
74. Tomita T, Das L, Radkowski MA. Bone metastases of medulloblastoma in childhood: correlation with flow cytometric DNA analysis. J Neuro-Oncol 1990, 8, 113–20.
75. Bigner SH, Mark J, Friedman HS, Biegel JA, Bigner DD. Structural chromosomal abnormalities in human medulloblastoma. Cancer Genet Cytogenet 1988, 30, 91–101.
76. Biegel JA, Rorke LB, Packer RJ, et al. Isochromosome 17q in primitive neuroectodermal tumors of the central nervous system. Genes Chromosomes Cancer 1989, 1, 139–47.
77. Whang-Peng J, Triche TJ, Knutsen T, Miser J, Douglass EC, Israel MA. Chromosome translocation in peripheral neuroepithelioma. New Engl J Med 1984, 311, 584–5.
78. Jay V, Pienkowska M, Becker LE, Zielenska M. Primitive neuroectodermal tumors of the cerebrum and cerebellum: absence of t(11;22) translocation by RT-PCR analysis. Modern Pathol 1995, 8, 488–91.
79. Badiali M, Pession A, Basso G, et al. N-myc and c-myc oncogenes amplification in medulloblastomas. Evidence of particularly aggressive behavior in a tumor with c-myc amplification. Tumori 1991, 77, 118–21.
80. Bigner SH, Friedman HS, Vogelstein B, Oakes WJ, Bigner DD. Amplification of the c-myc gene in human medulloblastoma cell lines and xenografts. Cancer Res. 1990, 50, 2347–50.
81. Friedman HS, Burger PC, Bigner SH, Trojanowski JQ, Brodeur GMea. Phenotypic and genotypic analysis of human medulloblastoma cell line and transplantable xenograft (D 341 Med) demonstrating amplification of c-myc. Am J Pathol 1988, 130, 472–84.
82. Fujimoto M, Sheridan PJ, Sharp ZD, Weaker FJ, Kagan-Hallet KS, Story JL. Proto-oncogene analyses in brain tumors. J Neurosurg 1989, 70, 910–15.
83. Reardon DA, Michalkiewicz E, Boyett JM, et al. Extensive genomic abnormalities in childhood medulloblastoma by comparative genomic hybridization. Cancer Res 1997, 57, 4042–7.
84. Schütz BR, Scheurlen W, Krauss J, et al. Mapping of chromosomal gains and losses in primitive neuroectodermal tumors by comparative genomic hybridization. Genes Chromosomes Cancer 1996, 196–203.
85. Bayani J, Thorner P, Zielenska M, Pandita A, Beatty B, Squire JA. Application of a simplified comparative genomic hybridization technique to screen for gene amplification in pediatric solid tumors. Ped Pathol Lab Med 1995, 15, 831–44.
86. Tomlinson FH, Jenkins RB, Scheithauer BW, et al. Aggressive medulloblastoma with high-level N-myc amplification. Mayo Clin Proc 1994, 69, 359–65.
87. Bello MJ, Leone PE, Vaquero J, et al. Allelic loss of 19 and 19q frequently occurs in association and may represent early oncogenenic events in oligodendroglial tumors. Intl J Cancer 1995, 64, 207–10.
88. Jay V, Edwards V, Hoving E, et al. Central neurocytoma: morphological, flow cytometric, polymerase chain reaction, fluorescence in situ hybridization, and karyotypic analysis. J Neurosurg 1999, 90, 348–54.
89. Hassoun J, Soylemezoglu F, Gambarelli D, Figarella-Branger D, von Ammon K, Kleihues P. Central neurocytoma: a synopsis of clinical and histological features (Review). Brain Pathology 1993, 3, 297–306.

90. Hassoun J, Gambrelli D, Grisoli F, et al. Central neurocytoma. An electron-microscopic study of two cases. Acta Neuropathol 1982, 56, 151–6.
91. Jay V, Squire J, Becker LE, Humphreys R. Malignant transformation in a ganglioglioma with anaplastic neuronal and astrocytic components. Cancer 1994, 73, 2862–8.
92. Jay V, Becker LE. Surgical pathology of epilepsy: a review. Pediatr Pathol 1994, 14, 731–50.
93. Daumas-Duport C, Scheithauer BW, Chodkiewicz JP, Laws ERJ, Vedrenne C. Dysembryoplastic neuroepithelial tumor: a surgically curable tumor of young patients with intractable partial seizures. Neurosurgery 1988, 23, 537–44.
94. Hirose T, Scheithauer BW, Lopes MB, VandenBerg SR. Dysembryoplastic neuroepithelial tumor (DNT): an immunohistochemical and ultrastructural study. J Neuropathol Exp Neurol 1994, 53, 184–95.
95. Jay V, Edwards V, Rutka JT. Crystalline inclusions in a subependymal giant cell tumor in a patient with tuberous sclerosis. Ultrastructural Pathol 1993, 17, 503–13.
96. Kerfoot C, Wienecke R, Menchine M, et al. Localization of tuberous sclerosis 2 mRNA and its protein product tuberin in normal human brain and in cerebral lesion of patients with tuberous sclerosis. Brain Pathol 1996, 6, 367–77.
97. Short MP, Richardson EPJ, Haines JL, Kwiatkowski DJ. Clinical, neuropathological and genetic aspects of the tuberous sclerosis complex. Brain Pathol 1995, 5, 173–9.
98. Ye Z, Qu JK, Darras BT. Loss of heterozygosity for alleles on chromosome 10 in human brain tumours. Neurol Res 1993, 15, 59–62.
99. Vagner-Capodano AM, Gentet JC, Gambarelli D, et al. Cytogenetic studies in 45 pediatric brain tumors. Pediatr Hematol Oncol 1992, 9, 223–35.
100. Qualman SJ, Shannon BT, Boesel CP, Jacobs D, Jinkens C, Hayes J. Ploidy analysis and cerebrospinal fluid nephelometry as measures of clinical outcome in childhood choroid plexus neoplasia. Pathol Annual 1992, 305–20.
101. Coons SW, Johnson PC, Haskett D, Rider R. Flow cytometric analysis of deoxyribonucleic acid ploidy and proliferation in choroid plexus tumors. Neurosurgery 1992, 31, 850–6.
102. Seizinger BR, Martuza RL, Gusella JF. Loss of genes on chromosome 22 in tumorigenesis of human acoustic neuroma. Nature 1986, 322, 644–7.
103. Seizinger BR, delaMonte S, Atkins L, Gusella JF, Martuza RL. Molecular genetic approach to human meningioma: loss of genes on chromosome 22. Proc Natl Acad Sci USA 1987, 84, 5419–23.
104. Seizinger BR, Rouleau G, Ozelius LJ, et al. Common pathogenetic mechanism for three tumor types in bilateral acoustic neurofibromatosis. Science 1987, 236, 317–19.
105. Guthrie BL, Ebersold MJ, Scheithauer BW, Shaw EG. Meningeal hemangiopericytoma: histopathological features, treatment, and long-term follow-up of 44 cases. Neurosurgery 1989, 25, 514–22.
106. Beckwith JB, Palmer NF. Histopathology and prognosis of Wilms' tumor. Cancer 1978, 41, 1937–48.
107. Behring B, Bruck W, Goebel H, et al. Immunohistochemistry of primary central nervous system malignant rhaboid tumors: report of five cases and review of the literature. Acta Neuropathol 1996, 91, 578–86.
108. Bhattacharjee M, Hicks J, Langford L, et al. Central nervous system atypical teratoid/rhabdoid tumors of infancy and childhood. Ultrastruct Pathol 1997, 21, 369–78.
109. Bhattacharjee M, Hicks J, Dauser R, et al. Primary malignant rhabdoid tumor of the central nervous system. Ultrastruct Pathol 1997, 21, 361–8.
110. Olson TA, Bayar E, Kosnik E, et al. Successful treatment of disseminated central nervous system malignant rhabdoid tumor. [Review]. J Ped Hem/Oncol 1995, 17, 71–75.
111. Parham DM, Weeks DA, Beckwith JB. The clinicopathologic spectrum of putative extrarenal rhabdoid tumors. An analysis of 42 cases studied with immunohistochemistry or electron microscopy. Am J Surg Pathol 1994, 18, 1010–29.
112. Satoh H, Goishi J, Sogabe T, Uozumi T, Kiya K, Migita K. Primary malignant rhabdoid tumor of the central nervous system: case report and review of the literature. Surg Neurol 1993, 40, 429–34.
113. Rootman J, Carruthers JD, Miller RR. Retinoblastoma. Perspectives Ped Pathol 1987, 10, 208–58.
114. Brownstein S, De Chadarevian JP, Little JM. Trilateral retinoblastoma. Report of two cases. Arch Ophthalmol 1984, 102, 257–62.
115. Smith BJ, O'Brien JM. The genetics of retinoblastoma and current diagnostic testing. J Ped Ophthalmol Strab 1996, 33, 120–3.
116. Knudson AG. Hereditary cancer: two hits revisited. J Cancer Res Clin Oncol 1996, 122, 135–40.
117. Squire JA, Whitmore GF, Phillips RA. Genetic basis of cancer. In: The basic science of oncology (ed. I Tannock, R Hill). McGraw Hill, New York, 1998, 48–78.
118. Margo C, Hidayat A, Kopelman J, Zimmerman LE. Retinocytoma. A benign variant of retinoblastoma. Arch Ophthalmol 1983, 101, 1519–31.
119. McLean IW. Retinoblastomas, retinocytomas, and pseudoretinoblastomas. In: Ophthalmic pathology, vol. 2 (ed. W Spencer). W.B. Saunders Company; Philadelphia, 1996, 1332–438.
120. Brownstein S, Barsoum-Homsy M, Conway VH, Sales C, Condon G. Nonteratoid medulloepithelioma of the ciliary body. Ophthalmology 1984, 91, 1118–22.
121. Zimmerman LE, Font RL, Andersen SR. Rhabdomyosarcomatous differentiation in malignant intraocular medulloepitheliomas. Cancer 1972, 30, 817–35.

8 | Neuroblastoma

Sadick Variend and Susan A. Burchill

Neuroblastoma is the third most common solid malignant tumour of infancy and childhood, being surpassed only by neoplasms of the lymphoid tissue and cerebral tumours (1, 2). Its incidence is about 1 per 10,000 live births in the United States (3), and constitutes some 8–10% of all cancers seen in children up to the age of 15 years. It is rarely reported in Africa. Ninety per cent of neuroblastomas occur in children less than 10 years old, usually between birth and 5 years (4). The median age at diagnosis is 22 months. The tumour is slightly more common in white children than black children, and shows a higher incidence in boys than girls (5).

The cumulative incidence of neuroblastoma during childhood in Britain increased by 23% between 1971–75 and 1986–90 (6), while age-standardized mortality fell by 27% between 1971–73 and 1981–85. There was an accompanying marked decrease in recorded diagnosis of neuroblastoma in children aged 10–14 years. These changes may reflect improved methods for diagnosis, which ultimately result in more appropriate and successful therapeutic intervention.

At diagnosis, the majority of children have advanced stage disease (7). Spontaneous regression or maturation can occur, but usually only in those children under the age of 1 (stage 4s, see below) for whom prognosis is usually good. However, for most children who are older and present with high stage disease, the disease is generally lethal.

Most cases of neuroblastoma are sporadic, but a subset of patients exhibit an autosomal dominant predisposition (8, 9). The median age at diagnosis for familial neuroblastoma is 9 months, compared to 22 months for the general population. There is evidence that parental exposure to environmental agents may increase the risk of neuroblastoma, for example, foetal alcohol syndrome (10), maternal use of hair colouring products (11), exposure to electromagnetic fields (12, 13), though it seems unlikely that environmental factors have a major role in the aetiology.

Neuroblastoma arises in cells of the neural crest, and can occur at any point along the migratory pathway of the sympathetic nervous system (7). Intra-abdominal tumours are the most common, arising in the adrenal medulla or paraspinal autonomic ganglia. Extra-abdominal locations, in the order of decreasing frequency, are the posterior mediastinum (14) and cervical region (15). Large adrenal tumours may be difficult to distinguish from those arising from the paraspinal autonomic chain. Paraspinal tumours may insinuate through the intervertebral foramina and cause spinal cord compressions (16). Calcification within the tumour is often demonstrated on x-ray, but is more often seen histologically (17, 18). Neuroblastic tumours exist in three forms: neuroblastoma, ganglioneuroblastoma, and ganglioneuroma (19).

Diagnostic considerations

The second International Neuroblastoma Staging System conference recommended the following criteria for the clinical diagnosis of neuroblastoma (20):

1. the demonstration of tumour tissue by light microscopy (with or without immunohistology or electron microscopy), increased urine or serum catecholamines or their metabolites; or
2. bone marrow aspirate or trephine biopsy containing unequivocal tumour cells (e.g. syncytial or immunocytologically positive clumps of cells) and increased urine or serum catecholamines or their metabolites.

A bone marrow biopsy by itself can be used for diagnosis but would not be suitable for subtyping or prognostic evaluation (21). On the other hand, a fresh sample of bone marrow can be used to assess prognostic molecular markers such as amplification of *MYCN*.

Microscopy

Neuroblastoma shows a spectrum of histology ranging from undifferentiated, poorly differentiated to differentiating tumours that vary in behaviour, morphology, and molecular genetic profile. It is typically composed of nests of small hyperchromatic cells (neuroblasts) in a neurofibrillary stroma (neuropil), surrounded by fibrovascular septa. Homer–Wright rosettes with neuroblasts around a central tangle of neuropil are characteristic but not essential for diagnosis (17, 18). Undifferentiated neuroblastoma is characterized by sheets of small round-to-oval cells frequently compartmentalized by strands of vascular fibrous connective tissue. Nuclei reveal a coarse chromatin pattern with variable mitotic activity. Homer–Wright rosettes and patches of pink fibrillary material (neuropil) indicate early differentiation ('poorly differentiated neuroblastoma'). Early neuronal differentiation is also accompanied by cellular enlargement, nuclear vesiculation, and the emergence of prominent nucleoli. Necrosis and calcification are common, the latter sometimes associated with a foreign body-type giant cell reaction. Calcification may be found in areas of viable or necrotic tumour. A small number of neuroblastomas include occasional foci of ganglioneuromatous tissue at the periphery, or within septa between tumour lobules. Tumour may occasionally show intracytoplasmic glycogen detected using periodic acid schiff stain (PAS), but *en bloc* or punctate PAS positivity commonly seen in rhabdomyosarcoma, Ewing's sarcoma, neuroepithelioma, and common acute lymphoblastic leukaemia (ALL) is not described. Cytological preparations may show clumping of small groups of tumour cells with tapering cytoplasmic extensions directed radially or linking adjacent individual tumour cells.

Schwannian stromal development may or may not be present in differentiating neuroblastoma. Other tumours expressing neural rosettes listed in Table 8.1 should be considered in their differential diagnosis.

Ganglioneuroblastoma shows a predominant ganglioneuromatous component of ganglion cells and Schwann cells, with less than 50% neuroblastomatous elements, and is subdivided into nodular and intermixed types (according to the recent INC classification (22), see later).

Ganglioneuromas are benign, generally circumscribed, often encapsulated tumours (23). Microscopically, mature or maturing neoplastic ganglionic cells are seen either singly or clustered in a matrix which is predominantly composed of Schwannian stroma. The Schwannian stroma is a reactive and not a neoplastic part of the tumour (24). The ganglion cells may or may not be surrounded by satellite cells and may show some degree of multinuclearity. Mitoses are uniformly absent. Foci of cystic degeneration, haemorrhage, or calcification are encountered occasionally. Multiple sections should be examined in order to exclude the presence of residual malignant neuroblasts, though care must be taken not to confuse focal lymphocytic infiltration (which is fairly frequent) for neuroblasts. Immunohistochemistry for leucocyte common antigen (CD45) facilitates the distinction between lymphocytes and neuroblasts. Children with ganglioneuroma are generally older at diagnosis than those with neuroblastoma, the mean age at diagnosis being 10 years. There is usually no prior history of neuroblastoma, supporting the hypothesis that these tumours are a different tumour entity rather than the differentiated counterpart of neuroblastoma. Metabolites of catecholamines are rarely secreted into the urine of children with ganglioneuroma. These neoplasms have an anatomical distribution similar to that of neuroblastoma and they may attain an enormous size (23).

Table 8.1 Tumours to be considered in the differential diagnosis of neuroblastoma

Small round cell tumours of childhood	Tumours capable of expressing neural rosettes
Neuroblastoma	Neuroblastoma
Rhabdomyosarcoma	Malignant ectomesenchymoma
Tumours of the Ewing's sarcoma family	Neuroepithelioma/pPNET
Lymphoma	Neural Ewing's sarcoma
	Retinal anlage tumour*

* Retinal anlage tumour is also known as melanotic neuroectodermal tumour of infancy.

Immunohistochemistry

It is important to distinguish undifferentiated neuroblastoma from other small round cell tumours of similar microscopic appearance (Table 8.1). This is in part achieved by immunohistochemistry. Commonly used antibodies include those directed at neuron-specific enolase, synaptophysin, chromogranin A, and protein-gene product 9.5 (25, 26). These immunomarkers vary in their specificity and sensitivity, and an immunoprofile

Table 8.2 Recommended immunohistochemistry for distinguishing neuroblastoma from other small round cell tumours of childhood

Antibody/target	Expression in neuroblastoma	
	Positive	Negative
NB84/neuroblastoma antigen	+	
P30/32^{MIC2}/cell surface glycoprotein		+
Actin		+
Myogenic proteins (MyoD1, myogenin)		+

using several different antibodies is usually recommended (25) (Table 8.2). A positive reaction for neural markers alone is insufficient for diagnosis, and interpretation should be carried out in conjunction with a negative reaction for other markers (e.g. desmin, myoglobin, vimentin, and CD99) (21). Neuroblastomas are uniformly negative for the CD99 (p30/32^{MIC2}; MIC2), helping to distinguish them from tumours of the Ewing's sarcoma family (27). Ninety per cent of neuroblastomas stain for NB84 (28), an antibody produced using human neuroblastoma as the source of antigen. This antibody works reliably on paraffin sections. However, about 60% of Ewing's sarcomas are also found to react positively with NB84 (28) though other small round cell tumours (rhabdomyosarcoma, Wilms' tumour, and lymphomas) do not stain with NB84 (29). Antibodies to S100 protein have successfully been used to identify cells of the supporting stroma in poorly differentiated and differentiating neuroblastoma, and may indicate early tumour differentiation (30).

Electron microscopy

Ultrastructurally, the cytoplasm is scant and contains abundant free ribosomes, rough endoplasmic reticulum, some mitochondria, microfilaments, and occasional Golgi complexes (31, 32). The tumour cell nuclei are large with dispersed chromatin and occasionally prominent nucleoli.

Catecholamine granules (neurosecretory or electron-dense granules) measuring 50–200 nm in diameter, and a compact meshwork of inter-digitating neurites (Fig. 8.1(a)) are the principal features of neuroblastoma (26, 30–32). The secretory granules, whilst present in the cell body, are more frequently found in the cytoplasmic extensions (Fig. 8.1(b)) (31), and should be distinguished from lysosomes which are normally found close to the Golgi regions.

Neurotubules (about 25 nm in diameter) are usually found in the cytoplasmic processes. The intertwining cytoplasmic processes correspond to the eosinophilic fibrillar material (neuropil) seen in routine sections of 'poorly differentiated' or 'differentiating neuroblastoma'. Schwann cells may be observed (33). Clear vesicles approximately the size of catecholamine granules may be present, probably containing cholinergic enzymes (31, 32). Increased differentiation and neurite extension are associated with a greater number of catecholamine granules (32, 33). The neurite extensions contain longitudinally orientated neurofilaments and neurotubules (31), and their number and length increase with increasing tumour differentiation. These are particularly pronounced in ganglioneuroma (32).

Junctional complexes are often present between plasma membranes of adjacent tumour cells or their processes. Synaptic structures have been reported, but true desmosomes are rare. Undifferentiated neuroblastomas often contain scattered Schwann cells that may indicate early tumour differentiation.

Electron microscopy can be especially useful in undifferentiated neuroblastoma where its differential diagnosis from other small round cell tumours is essential, and immunohistochemistry has produced equivocal results.

Prognostic parameters

Neuroblastoma is known for its broad spectrum of clinical behaviour (34), varying from aggressive malignant disease to spontaneous maturation and even regression. The biological mechanisms responsible for this variable behaviour are unclear. A number of parameters are considered useful in predicting outcome and may influence the choice of optimal therapy. These prognostic markers may usefully be divided into four groups: clinical, morphological, biochemical, or genetic.

Clinical

At diagnosis, important clinical determinants of prognosis are the age of the child at diagnosis, stage of disease, and anatomical location of tumour (35). Children under

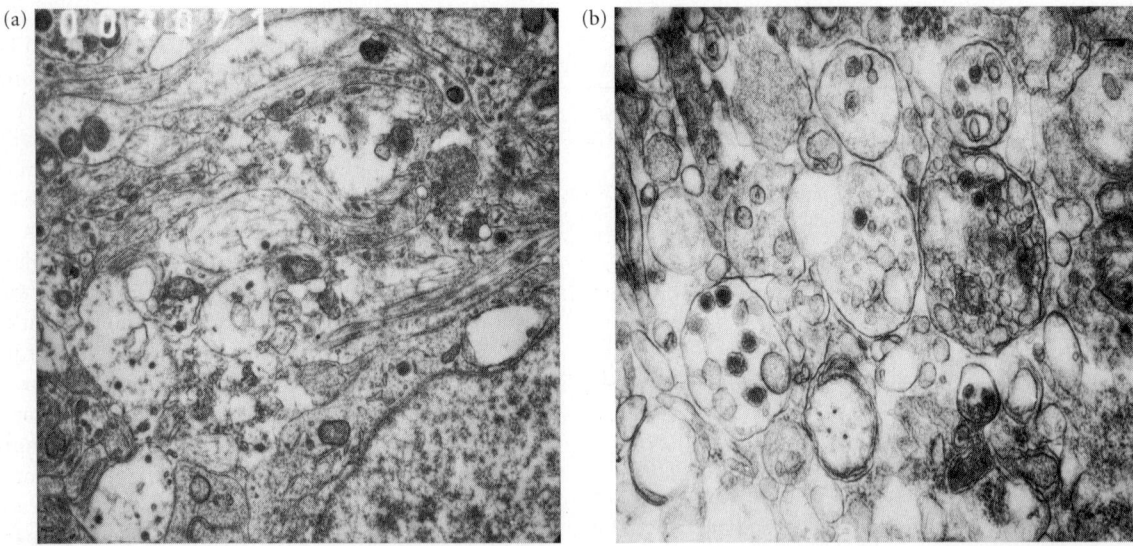

Fig. 8.1 Ultrastructure of poorly differentiated neuroblastoma showing (a) a tight network of intertwining neurites corresponding to neuropil, readily visible by conventional light microscopy and (b) numerous electron-dense neurosecretory granules.

1 year of age with neuroblastoma tend to have less aggressive disease and a correspondingly better clinical outcome (36). It is usually a highly lethal neoplasm when diagnosed in children over the age of 2 years. The most common site for neuroblastoma is the adrenal. These tumours tend to be poorly differentiated and are associated with a poor outcome. A revised International Neuroblastoma Staging System (INSS) is shown in Table 8.3 (20). Clinical stage 1 and 2 neuroblastoma (localized disease) generally have a good overall prognosis, whereas metastatic disease (stage 4) is frequently associated with a fatal outcome despite aggressive therapy. Children with stage 3 disease (regional disease) appear to constitute a heterogeneous group with characteristics of non-metastatic (stages 1 and 2) and metastatic disease (stage 4). Stages 1, 2, and 4s neuroblastoma, are associated with a favourable histology (37).

In children under the age of 1 year with metastatic disease the outlook is not necessarily as gloomy as might be expected, as the disease often undergoes spontaneous regression. This is largely attributed to infants with stage 4s disease (38), in whom metastases are found in the liver, skin, and bone marrow but without osseous involvement. In stage 4s disease, the adrenal is the primary tumour site in the majority of cases (39). Maturation of stage 4s neuroblastoma to ganglioneuroma to fibrosis has been documented, but progression does not necessarily precede regression (40). As a group, children with stage 4s disease have an excellent prospect for survival regardless of treatment, more than 80% becoming long-term survivors (7). However, those less than 2 months old without skin involvement seem to do much worse than the rest of this group (41); death possibly resulting from the mechanical effect of massive hepatomegaly, chemotherapy, or late disease progression/recurrence (39).

It is clear that the presence of disseminated disease detected by light microscopy and/or immunocytology in children with neuroblastoma is a poor prognostic indicator, with the usual exception of children with 4s disease as discussed above (42–44). More recently the sensitive detection of small numbers of circulating tumour cells using reverse transcriptase polymerase chain reaction (RT-PCR) has been shown to identify clinically significant disease in bone marrow and peripheral blood (45–49). The molecular detection of clinically significant small numbers of circulating tumour cells by RT-PCR may ultimately lead to a redefinition of metastatic disease and disease-free status, resulting in a change in therapeutic strategy. This may also be an important method to monitor disease status in patients with neuroblastoma (48, 50). Of the different targets that have been used for the detection of low level disease in neuroblastoma tyrosine hydroxylase

Table 8.3 Staging system for neuroblastoma

Stage 1	Localized tumour with complete gross excision, with or without microscopic residual disease; representative ipsilateral lymph nodes negative for tumour microscopically (nodes attached to and removed with the primary tumour may be positive).
Stage 2A	Localized tumour with incomplete gross excision: representative ipsilateral non-adherent lymph nodes negative for tumour microscopically.
Stage 2B	Localized tumour with or without complete gross excision; with ipsilateral non-adherent lymph nodes positive for tumour. Enlarged contralateral lymph nodes must be negative microscopically.
Stage 3	Unresectable unilateral tumour, infiltrating across the midline,* with or without regional lymph node involvement; or localized unilateral tumour with contralateral regional lymph node involvement; or midline tumour with bilateral extension by infiltration or lymph node involvement.
Stage 4	Any primary tumour with dissemination to distant lymph nodes, bone, bone marrow, liver, and/or other organs (except as defined for stage 4s).
Stage 4s	Localized primary tumour (as defined for stage 1 or 2A or 2B), with dissemination limited to liver, skin, and/or bone marrow (limited to infants <1 year of age).

Note: Stage 1 and 2 (A and B) disease is regarded as localized disease, while stage 3 is accepted as regional disease.
* The midline is the lateral border of the vertebral column on the side opposite to the origin of the primary tumour.

appears to be the most useful (45, 50–52). The biology of these circulating tumour cells may be evaluated using a computer assisted scanning system for automatic cell search and gene analysis (53).

Morphological parameters

Evidence suggests that children with histologically differentiated neuroblastoma have a more favourable outcome than those with poorly differentiated tumours (54). This has formed the basis for an age-linked classification that includes several histologically determined prognostic variables (55). The key features of the classification included assessment of the amount of Schwannian stroma, proliferation and supporting elements, the degree of tumour differentiation, and nuclear morphology, determined by the mitosis-karyorrhexis index (MKI) in multiple microscopic fields. Karyorrhectic cells are characterized by nuclear condensation and fragmentation, with condensed eosinophilic cytoplasm; care must be taken not to confuse this with pyknotic cells characterized by nuclear shrinkage and hyperchromasia without fragmentation. Karyorrhexis is an expression of apoptosis in which endonuclease-induced DNA fragmentation is a fundamental feature (21). MYCN is reported to promote both mitoses and karyorrhexis, depending on the expression of growth factors (21). In the presence of growth factors, MYCN induces proliferation and in their absence induces apoptosis. A high MKI probably reflects rapid cell turnover in neuroblastoma (Fig. 8.2(a)). Areas showing necrosis, crush artefact, discrete foci of haemorrhage and poor fixation or preservation should be avoided when assessing the MKI. Cells with mixed-histological features are not included in the assessment.

The time taken to assess the MKI, and the increasing reliance on small biopsy samples or aspiration cytology for diagnosis, are limitations. Furthermore, MKI assessment is not valid in post-treatment samples, since increased karyorrhexis, differentiation and/or maturation may occur secondary to radiotherapy or chemotherapy. Various schemes have been suggested to facilitate the assessment of the MKI (17, 18). Joshi *et al.* (17, 18) proposed that where the cell density is uniform, the degree of density and the average number of tumour cells per high-power microscopy field should be determined. This method has the advantage of accuracy, but is time consuming and complex. Alternatively, the procedure may be facilitated by using a micrometer fitted to an eye-piece. A 100 squares (10×10) grid is superimposed on the microscopic field of neuroblastoma so that 5–10 tumour cell nuclei (depending on cellularity) are framed in each square (Fig. 8.2(b)). This allows rapid identification of 500–1000 cells and the number of cells with mitoses and karyorrhexis can be counted within the group with relative ease. Three grades of MKI are recognized: low MKI $\leq 2\%$ of mitotic/karyorrhectic cells: intermediate MKI = 2–4% of mitotic/karyorrhectic cells; high MKI $\geq 4\%$ of such cells (21).

Stroma-rich tumours are additionally subcategorized into (a) well-differentiated, (b) intermixed, and

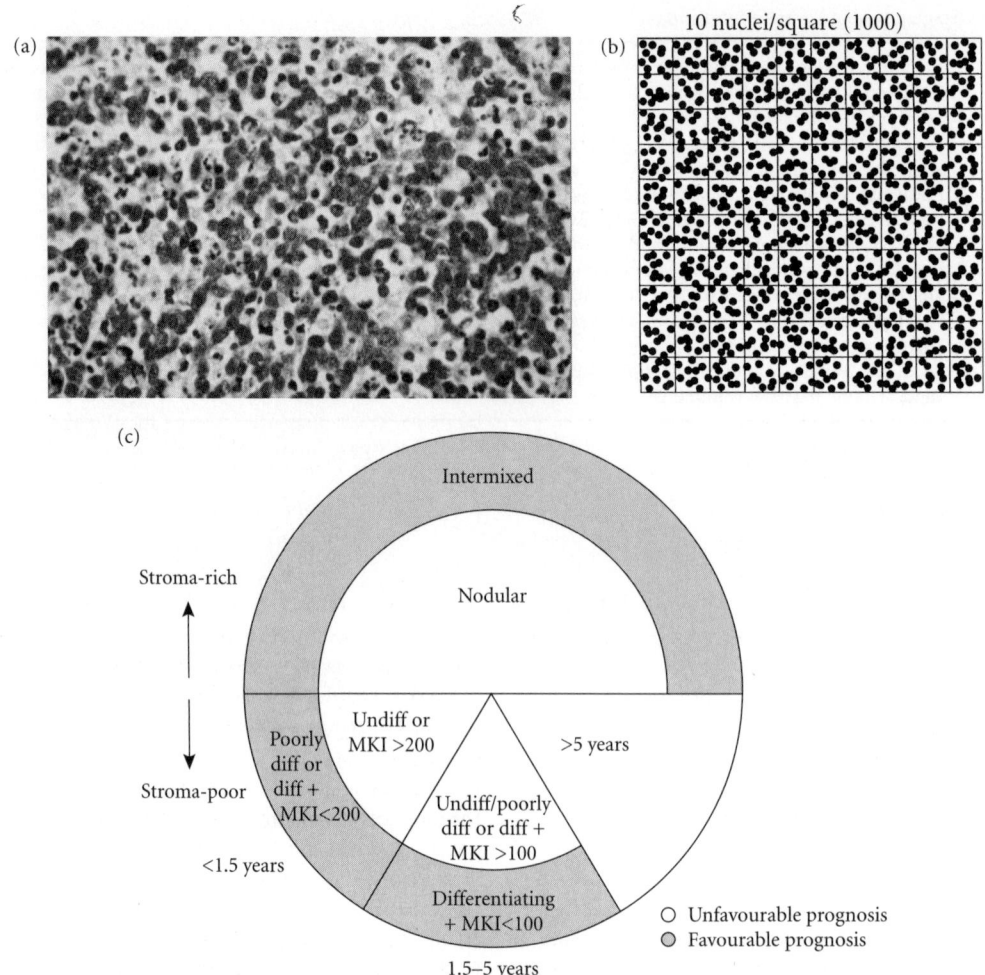

Fig. 8.2 (a) Microscopy of undifferentiated neuroblastoma displaying a high MKI. (b) Diagrammatic representation of a grid (10 × 10) which can be used to ring-fence a finite number of nuclei to facilitate assessment of the MKI. If each of the squares is shown to contain roughly 10 nuclei, the entire grid will delimit around 1000 cells. (c) Different prognostic groups employing histological features such as degree of stroma differentiation, MKI, and age (after Tsokos 1992) and employing new INPC data. (Abbr: undiff = undifferentiated; diff = differentiating.)

(c) nodular. Nodular tumours (i.e. those tumours with macroscopically identifiable nodules of neuroblastoma) are regarded as unfavourable, whereas the other two subtypes are considered favourable. The MKI is not normally assessed in stroma-rich tumours (ganglioneuroblastomas and ganglioneuromas).

Stroma-poor tumours are viewed as prognostically favourable or unfavourable depending on the MKI, degree of differentiation, and the age of the child (Fig. 8.2(c)). For children aged 1.5–5 years with stroma-poor tumours, MKI values greater than 100 per 5000 viable tumour cells or lack of differentiation are considered unfavourable. In children over 5 years old, stroma-poor tumours are considered unfavourable. MKI values over 200 in children younger than 1.5 years are unfavourable. Neuroblastomas with favourable histology are almost always found in clinical stages 1, 2, and 4s (56). However, a small proportion (6%) of stage 4s tumours can have unfavourable histology with a corresponding poor survival rate (37).

The presence of S100 protein in the septal component of the supporting stroma correlates with early Schwannian differentiation, and has been associated with a favourable clinical outlook. The cells expressing S100 protein are probably immature or precursors of Schwann cells. However, the great majority of neuroblastomas seen by the histopathologist are stroma poor (56), and most of these are poorly differentiated making staining for S100 of limited value. Differentiated tumours are usually associated with a low MKI and none, according to Shimada et al. (56), exhibit amplification of MYCN. Of the undifferentiated tumours, 30% showed amplification of MYCN. Neuroblastomas with amplification of MYCN are nearly always stroma poor and undifferentiated, with a high MKI (see below).

Nuclear anaplasia has been described in neuroblastoma, but unlike some of the other childhood tumours this does not necessarily indicate a potential for aggressive behaviour (17, 18). A small proportion of neuroblastomas have a distinct organoid pattern, characterized by a large number of S100-protein positive spindle cells, which has been associated with favourable prognosis in young children with neuroblastoma (57).

Biochemical parameters

Neuroblastoma and its congeners are frequently biologically active, produce catecholamines, and secrete their metabolites in urine (58). The catecholamine metabolites vanillylmandelic acid (VMA), homovanillic acid (HVA), or both are secreted in the urine of over 95% of children with neuroblastoma (36), and are often used as biochemical markers to assist in diagnosis and to monitor the effectiveness of therapy. Although one might expect this to be associated with hypertension in children with neuroblastoma (59), this is actually very rare. Compression of the renal pedicle by retroperitoneal tumours is an alternative explanation for hypertension (59). The secretion of catecholamine metabolites reflects the neurotransmitter function of the normal cells in which these tumours arise.

The ratio of VMA:HVA has been employed as a prognostic index (25), ratios greater than one being predictive of a more favourable outcome. Since HVA is a precursor of VMA, tumours that elaborate more HVA were thought to be biochemically immature and therefore potentially more aggressive. However, this is rarely informative. The real power of detecting catecholamine metabolites in the urine is to aid differential diagnosis of neuroblastoma from other small round cell tumours, and monitor response to therapy (a change in metabolites reflecting a decrease or increase in tumour bulk).

Raised serum neuron specific enolase (>100 ng/ml) has been reported to correlate with large tumour burden and advance stage disease (35), all of which are associated with a poor prognosis. Similarly, high serum levels of ferritin (>150 ng/ml; 60, 61) and lactate dehydrogenase ($\geq 1\,500$ IU/l) (62) have been associated with large tumour burden and an unfavourable outcome. Tumours occasionally produce vasoactive intestinal peptide and patients may present with intractable diarrhoea (63).

Biology

The cellular and molecular characterization of neuroblastoma is becoming increasingly important for improved diagnosis, predicting clinical behaviour and monitoring disease activity in children. In addition these studies have given insight into the mechanisms of malignant transformation and progression in neuroblastoma, identifying potential targets for novel therapeutic strategies.

As neuroblastomas are derived from postganglionic sympathetic neuroblasts they sometimes exhibit features of neuronal differentiation, which are of prognostic significance (see above). The mechanisms involved in the induction of this differentiated phenotype are not well understood, but several growth factor-receptor pathways are most likely involved. In particular, the neurotrophin nerve growth factor (NGF) and its high affinity receptor TrkA appear to be of biological and clinical significance. High expression of TrkA (64) is associated with clinically favourable tumours, such as those in children under the age of 1 year and stage 1, 2, or 4s disease. Furthermore, since primary neuroblastoma cells in culture with high levels of TrkA differentiate when treated with NGF, but die in the absence of NGF (64, 65), the NGF-TrkA pathway may explain the propensity for some neuroblastomas to differentiate or regress spontaneously.

Two neurosecretory proteins that are associated with differentiation of neuroblastomas are chromogranin A and neuropeptide Y. Both have been used to characterize the differentiation status of neuroblastomas, or monitor disease activity and response to therapy in children with this disease (66–68). Similarly, the peptide hormone somatostatin and expression of its receptors are associated with differentiation in neuroblastoma, and consequently a good prognosis (69).

Cytogenetically, neuroblastomas are characterized by DNA index, deletion of the short arm of chromosome 1, gain of chromosome 17, double-minute chromatin bodies (DMs) and homogenously staining regions (HSRs) (Fig. 8.3).

DNA ploidy is linked with prognosis in children less than 2 years old, with poor outcome in patients with diploid and tetraploid tumours and favourable outcome in hyperdiploid and triploid tumours (70). The DNA index of neuroblastomas from infants can also provide important information on the response of disease to therapy: infants with tumours that are hyperdiploid are most likely to have low stage disease that responds well to therapy, unlike those with diploid DNA content who

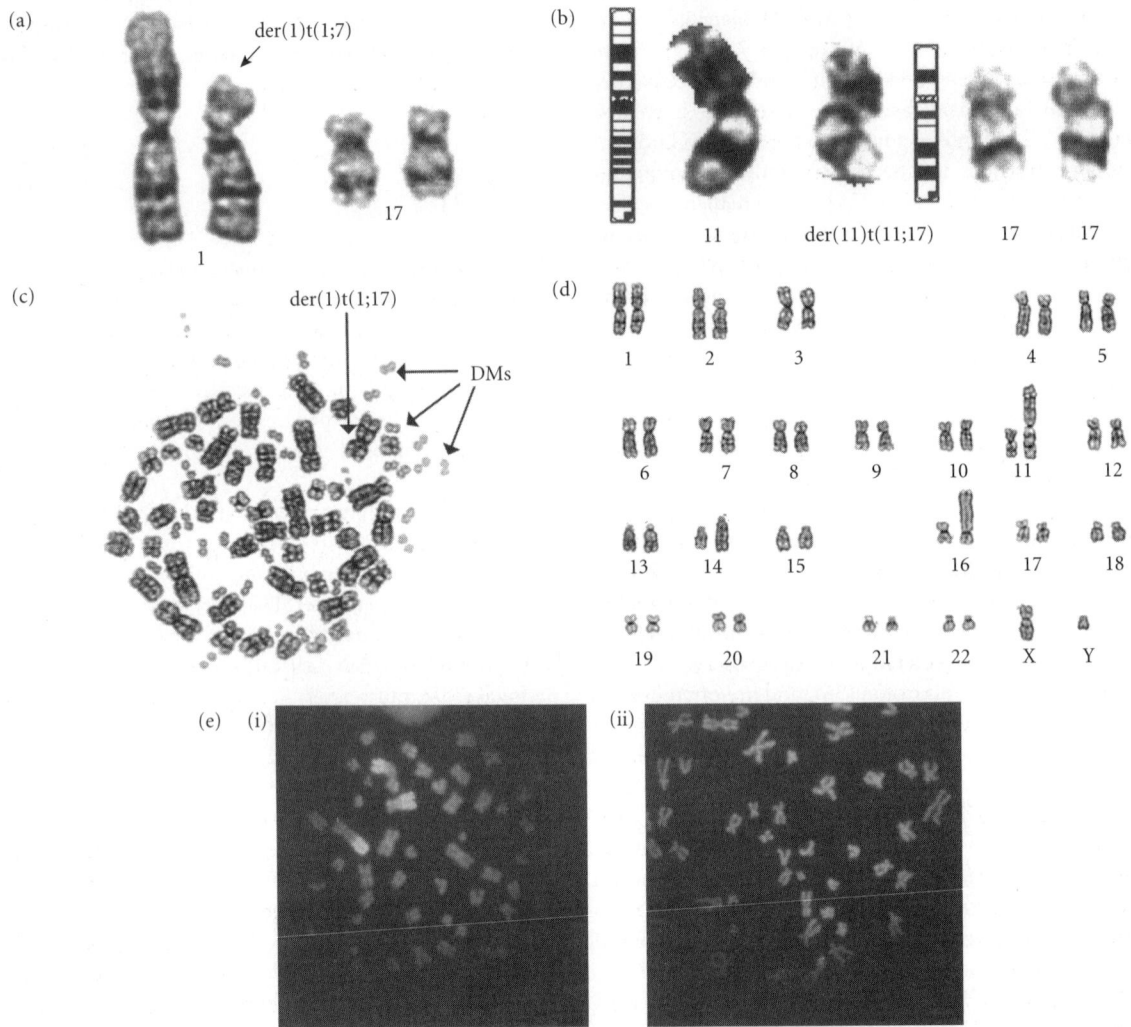

Fig. 8.3 Common cytogenetic abnormalities in neuroblastoma. Cytogenetically neuroblastomas are characterized by deletion of the short arm of chromosome 1, gain of chromosome 17, and DMs and HSRs predominantly resulting from amplification of MYCN. (a) deletion of short arm of chromosome 1, which has formed an unbalanced translocation with 17; (b) unbalanced t(11;17) translocation, resulting in loss of 11q and gain of chromosome 17q; (c) DMs: this tumour also has an unbalanced t(1;17); (d) HSRs inserted into 16p; (e) amplification of MYCN demonstrated by FISH using a digoxogenin labelled probe. Amplification of MYCN is shown in (i) as a concentration of fluorescent spots on chromosome 2p, but not in the single copy cells (ii).

are more likely to have aggressive disease that does not respond to chemotherapy (71). Flow cytometric analysis of DNA content is a simple and semi-automated way of measuring total cell DNA content, which correlates with chromosome number. Although this method cannot detect specific chromosome rearrangements, the simplicity of the test and its correlation with outcome in this age group make it attractive.

Cytogenetic aberrations of 1p are reported in at least 70% of the near-diploid neuroblastomas (72), the most consistent site of deletion being 1p36.3-p36.2 (73). Abnormalities of 1p in neuroblastoma are associated with poor prognosis (74, 75) and most frequently identified by conventional G-banding (Fig. 8.3(a)) or fluorescent *in situ* hybridization (FISH). Loss of 1p frequently correlates with amplification of MYCN (76). Although the tumour suppressor gene on 1p has not been identified, several possible candidate genes have been mapped (70); currently the most compelling candidate is p73, a gene showing high homology to p53 and mapping to 1p36.33 (77). Familial neuroblastoma however, does not map to chromosome 1p36 (9).

Gain of chromosome 17, either the whole chromosome or 17q21 to 17pter, has recently been shown by FISH and comparative genomic hybridization (CGH) to be the most powerful cytogenetic prognostic indicator in neuroblastoma, partial 17q gain being an indicator of poor prognosis (78) (Fig. 8.3(b)). The biological explanation for this association is currently unknown.

DMs and HSRs are manifestations of gene amplification. In neuroblastoma the amplified gene is usually derived from the short arm of chromosome 2, which contains the *MYCN* proto-oncogene. Amplification of the *MYCN* gene (>10 copies) is found in approximately 25% of primary neuroblastomas, and up to 40% of high stage tumours (Fig. 8.3(e)). It is usually seen in tumours from children over the age of 1 year, and associated with rapid progression of disease and poor prognosis (79, 80). The amplification status of *MYCN* is usually analyzed by Southern blot or FISH. The function of the *MYCN* gene, located on chromosome 2p24 and normally expressed in developing neural tissue, is unclear (70). It has been suggested *MYCN* may regulate expression of multi-drug resistance-associated protein (MRP) expression (81) or the DEAD box protein gene, DDX1 (82). Histopathological assessment of *MYCN* amplified tumours has shown a predominance of undifferentiated neuroblastoma with high MKI (56).

Less-well established indicators of poor prognosis include deletion of chromosome 14q (83), high telomerase activity (84, 85), and elevated expression of MRP (81). Although mutations of the tumour suppressor gene p53 are not common in neuroblastoma (86, 87), the novel p53-related gene p73 has been proposed as a putative tumour suppressor with prognostic significance in neuroblastoma (88). Indicators of good prognosis include increased expression of H-*ras* (89, 90) and cell surface CD44+ (91). Markers of poor prognosis tend to be associated with each other, and are inversely correlated with markers of good prognosis (92–94).

Combining clinical and molecular genetic features, Brodeur *et al.* (94) defined three prognostically significant groups of neuroblastomas:

1. *favourable prognosis*: hyperdiploidy, high TrkA expression, low stage, usually found in infants, that is, under 1 year of age.
2. *intermediate prognosis*: near-diploidy, 1p deletion, no MYCN amplification, low TrkA expression, high stage, usually in older children.
3. *poor prognosis*: MYCN amplification, 1p deletion, diploidy, no expression of TrkA, high stage with rapid progression, usually in children aged 1–5 years.

These groups have been refined and incorporated into a new classification for neuroblastoma that incorporates pathological and biological features.

International Neuroblastoma Pathology Committee (INPC) terminology

The INPC reported a classification grading system for neuroblastoma, with important prognostic implications and biological relevance (22). The advantages of this classification are: (a) high inter-observer concordance, (b) high statistical significance between survival and histological categories, and (c) biological significance (21). The INPC classification is a modified version of the Shimada scheme, and has retained the traditional staging nomenclature. Table 8.4 shows the relationship with previously reported classifications. The classification uses histological, biochemical, and biological features to classify tumours into favourable and

Table 8.4 Comparison of neuroblastoma terminology

Previous	Shimada	Joshi	INPC
Classic NB	SP—NB	Undifferentiated NB Poorly differentiated NB	Undifferentiated NB Poorly differentiated NB
NB or GNB	SP—NB (differentiating sub-type)	Differentiating NB	Differentiating NB
Composite GNB	SR—NB (nodular)	GNB—nodular	GNB—nodular
Composite GNB	SR—NB (intermixed)	GNB—intermixed	GNB—intermixed
GNB	SR—NB (well-differentiated)	GNB—borderline	GN—maturing subtype

Note: Intermixed and nodular stroma-rich neuroblastomas correspond to the composite type of ganglioneuroblastoma. The diffuse type ganglioneuroblastoma corresponds to the 'differentiating' category referred to by Joshi.
NB = neuroblastoma   GNB = ganglioneuroblastoma   GN = ganglioneuroma   SP = schwannian stroma-pool

unfavourable prognostic groups. This is summarized below.

Neuroblastoma (Schwannian stroma-poor)

Undifferentiated subtype

The tumour cells are undifferentiated; neuropil is inconspicuous or absent (Fig. 8.4(a)). Nucleoli may or may not be present. Histological differential diagnosis includes other small round cell tumours (primitive rhabdomyosarcoma, lymphoma, or peripheral primitive neuroectodermal tumour/Ewing's sarcoma) and a definitive diagnosis calls for ancillary methods such as immunohistochemistry and electron microscopy. The tumour is associated with a poor prognosis.

Poorly differentiated subtype

Five per cent or less of tumour cells show cellular differentiation towards ganglion cells. Differentiation towards ganglion cells should be synchronously expressed in nuclei (enlargement with nucleolar formation and increased vesicular pattern) and cytoplasm (increased volume and eosinophilia). S100 protein positive cells are commonly demonstrated in the separating fibrovascular septa. A variable amount of neuropil is present and rosettes may be seen (Fig. 8.4(b)). The proportion of neuropil may vary between microscopic fields and between different tumours.

Differentiating subtype

Five per cent or more of tumour cells show synchronous differentiation towards ganglion cells (Fig. 8.4(c)). Neuropil is easily recognizable. Such tumours also often show substantial amounts of Schwannian stroma, but by definition should not exceed 50% of tumour volume assessed in representative sections.

Ganglioneuroblastoma

According to the INPC classification, ganglioneuroblastoma is limited to two components: mature stroma-rich tissue, which includes differentiated ganglion cells, and stroma-poor neuroblastoma. Nodular and intermixed subtypes represent the two histological categories of ganglioneuroblastoma (Fig. 8.5(a)).

Nodular (composite Schwannian stroma-rich/stroma-dominant and stroma-poor)

One or more grossly visible discrete nodules of neuroblastoma are present in a mature or maturing Schwannian stroma. The nodules may be encapsulated and are often haemorrhagic (Fig. 8.5(b)). The two components are clearly demarcated by compressed stroma,

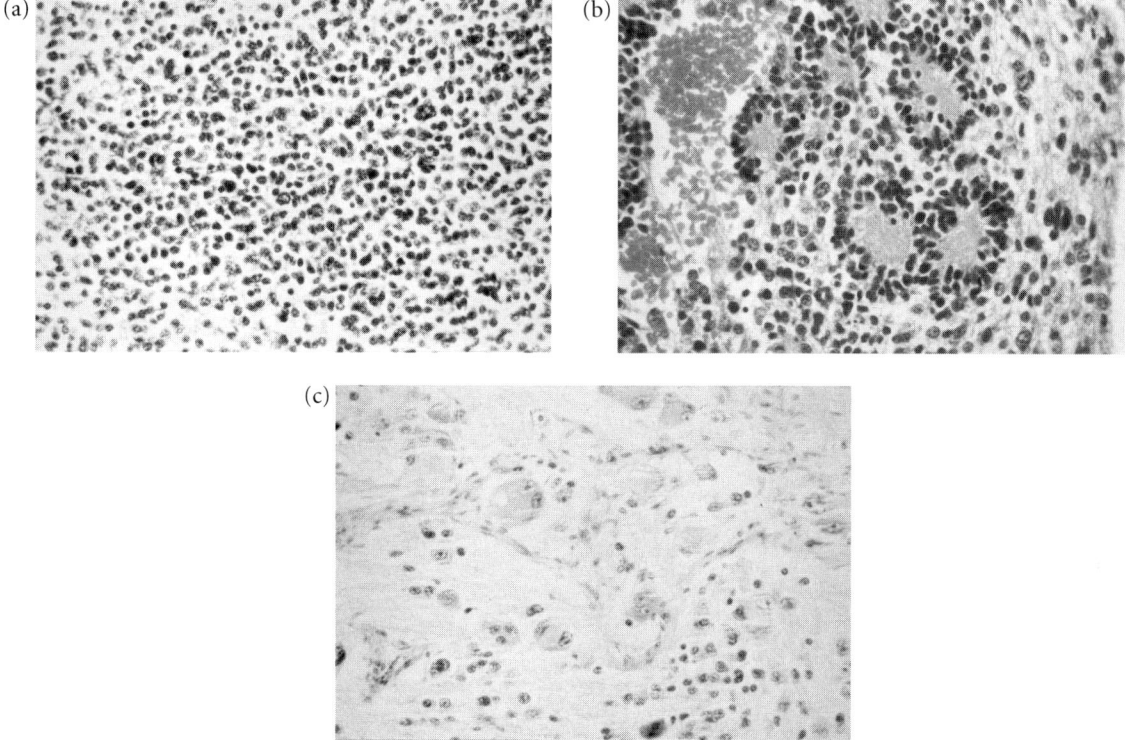

Fig. 8.4 Neuroblastoma subtypes. (a) Undifferentiated neuroblastoma showing essentially a small round cell tumour with no differentiation. These tumours must be distinguished from other small round cell tumours. (b) Poorly differentiated neuroblastoma showing variable amounts of neuropil and rosette formation. (c) Differentiating neuroblastoma displaying prominent ganglionic differentiation in association with abundant neuropil.

microscopy representing a pushing border and indicative of an expansile process (Fig. 8.5(c)). The nodules are thought to indicate the emergence of new malignant clones. The ganglioneuromatous tissue can appear as variable thickness septa separating the nodules, or remain as a thin rim at the periphery of the tumour. The distinction between reactive fibrosis and Schwannian stroma is important, and deeper sections or immunostaining for S100 protein may be helpful in making the distinction. Equally important is the distinction between Schwannian stroma and an entrapped normal ganglion. Regional lymph nodes may show neuroblastomatous tissue alongside an intermixed ganglioneuroblastoma or ganglioneuroma of mature or maturing type; these tumours should be categorized as nodular subtype (Fig. 8.5(d)) ganglioneuroblastoma. For this reason, the surgeon carrying out the biopsy or resection should be encouraged to sample regional lymph nodes adequately. Only a small biopsy showing neuroblastoma may conceivably originate from a nodule of such a tumour. Conversely, a biopsy that only features ganglioneuromatous or ganglioneuroblastomatous (intermixed) tissue may equally not be representative. Imaging studies of the original tumour may be valuable in these circumstances as they may demonstrate the nodules of nodular ganglioneuroblastoma (21).

Intermixed (Schwannian stroma-rich)

The neuroblastomatous component is present as variable-sized, well-defined nests of neuroblasts and neuropil scattered within a predominant Schwannian (stroma-rich) background. The proportion of Schwannian stroma should exceed 50% of tumour volume in representative sections. The nests of neuroblasts, which show variable differentiation, can only be diagnosed on microscopic examination (Fig. 8.5(e)). This pattern can also be seen in lymph nodes.

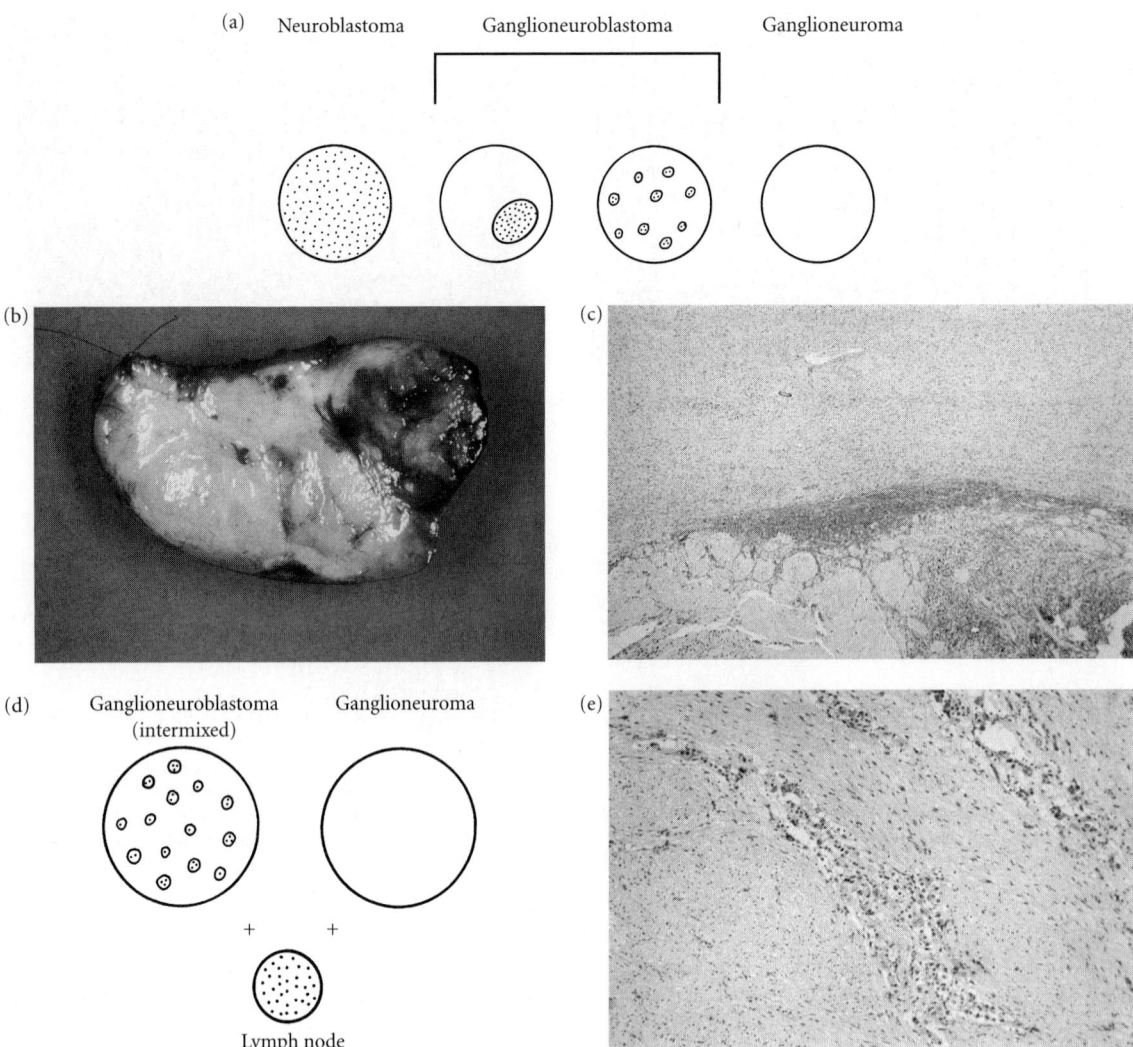

Fig. 8.5 (a) Diagrammatic representation to show intermixed and nodular subtypes of ganglioneuroblastoma. (b) Cut surface of a tumour demonstrating a variable appearance with relatively homogenous stroma in association with a large haemorrhagic nodule (upper right hand corner). (c) Microscopic view to show expansile border of a nodule in a nodular ganglioneuroblastoma. The edge of the nodule is partially haemorrhagic. (d) Diagrammatic representation showing atypical forms of nodular ganglioneuroblastoma. (e) Intermixed type (Schwannian stroma-rich) subtype of ganglioneuroblastoma showing microscopic foci of variably differentiated neuroblastoma against a background of ganglioneuroma. The ganglioneuromatous component must represent more than 50% of the tumour as assessed in representative sections. The ganglioneuromatous component of a nodular ganglioneuroblastoma may be compressed along the periphery of the tumour and may not be grossly visible. It is thus important to sample tumours along the edge for histology.

Ganglioneuroma (Schwannian stroma-dominant)

In the new classification this is referred to as ganglioneuroma (Schwannian stroma-dominant) and may be subtyped into 'maturing' and 'mature'. The 'maturing' subtype is characterized by a few scattered moderately to well-differentiated neuroblasts and neuropil, merging with the predominant ganglioneuromatous component (Fig. 8.6(a)). There are no discrete foci of neuroblastomatous tissue. Ganglioneuroma-mature subtype is composed of ganglion cells and mature Schwannian stroma. Mature ganglion cells are normally rimmed by satellite cells and a neuroblastomatous component is

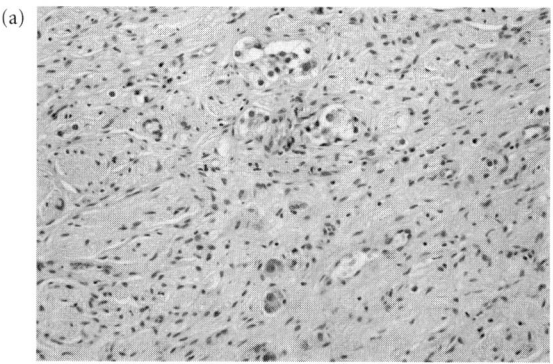 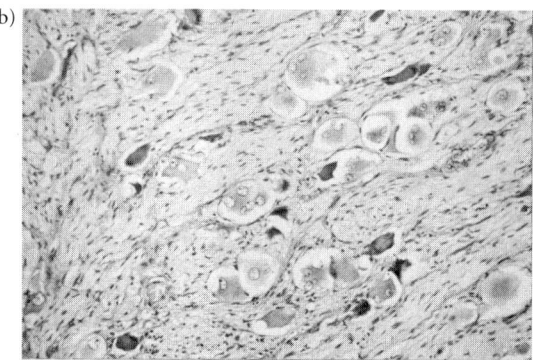

Fig. 8.6 (a) Mature ganglion cells with a few scattered neuroblasts against a neurocollagenous background is the hallmark of a maturing subtype of ganglioneuroma. (b) The presence of mature ganglion cells frequently surrounded by satellite cells characterize a mature ganglioneuroma.

typically absent (Fig. 8.6(b)). The 'maturing' subtype is included in favourable histology category, while ganglioneuroma-mature subtype is an entirely benign tumour.

Despite advances in therapy, the overall survival rate for children diagnosed with neuroblastoma remains poor. Improved methods for diagnosis, staging, and assessment of response to therapy appears to be improving outcome for some children, though for others this has had little impact. In this chapter we have reviewed current diagnostic criteria and prognostic markers for children with neuroblastoma. Increased knowledge of the correlation between morphological and non-morphological markers may more usefully define children with neuroblastoma as low, intermediate, or high-risk subgroups, ultimately directing appropriate therapeutic strategies to specific risk groups. The current challenge remains the correlation of these markers to design an algorithm for risk-specific therapy, though this knowledge may also be helpful in understanding the pathogenesis of neuroblastoma and lead to the identification of targets for novel therapeutic strategies.

Acknowledgement

Thank you to Mr Paul Roberts, Department of Cytogenetics, St James's University Hospital for allowing us to reproduce Figs 8.3(a)–(e).

References

1. Marsden HB, Steward JB (ed.). Tumours in children, vol. 1. Springer, Berlin, Heidelberg, New York, 1976.
2. Young JL, Miller RW. Incidence of malignant tumors in children. J Pediatr 1975, **86**, 254–8.
3. Bolande RP. The spontaneous regression of neuroblastoma. Experimental evidence for a natural host immunity. Pathol Ann 1991, **26**(part 2), 187–99.
4. Kinnier Wilson LM. Neuroblastoma, its natural history and prognosis: a study of 487 cases. Br Med J 1974, **3**, 301–7.
5. Young JL, Jr, Ries LG, Silverberg E, Horm JW, Miller RW. Cancer incidence, survival, and mortality for children younger than age 15 years. Cancer 1986, **15**, 598–602.
6. Stiller CA. Trends in neuroblastoma in Great Britain: indicence and mortality 1971–1990. Eur J Cancer 1993, **29A**, 1000–12.
7. Seeger RC, Siegal SE, Sidell N. Neuroblastoma clinical perspectives, monoclonal antibodies, and retinoic acid. Ann Intern Med 1982, **97**, 873–4.
8. Kushner BH, Gilbert F, Helson L. Familial neuroblastoma. Case reports, literature review, and etiologic considerations. Cancer 1986, **57**, 1887–93.
9. Maris JM, Kyemba SM, Rebbeck TR, White PS, Sulman EP, Jensen SJ, *et al*. Familial predisposition to neuroblastoma does not map to chromosome band 1p36. Cancer Res 1996, **56**, 3421–5.
10. Kinney H, Faix R, Brazy J. The fetal alcohol syndrome and neuroblastoma. Pediatrics 1980, **66**, 130–2.
11. Kramer S, Ward E, Meadows AT, Malone KE. Medical and drug risk factors associated with neuroblastoma: a case–control study. J Nat Cancer Inst 1987, **78**, 797–804.
12. Spitz MR, Johnson CC. Neuroblastoma and paternal occupation. A case–control analysis. Am J Epidemiol 1985, **121**, 924–9.
13. Wilkins JR 3rd., Hundley VD. Paternal occupational exposure to electromagnetic fields and neuroblastoma in offspring. Am J Epidemiol 1990, **131**, 995–1008.
14. Adam A, Hocholzer L. Ganglioneuroblastoma of the posterior mediastinum: a clinicopathologic review of 80 cases. Cancer 1981, **47**, 373–81.
15. Brown RJ, Szymula NJ, Lore JM. Neuroblastoma of the head and neck. Arch Otolaryngol 1978, **104**, 395–8.

16. Punt J, Pritchard J, Pincott JR, Till K. Neuroblastoma: a review of 21 cases presenting with spinal cord compression. Cancer 1980, 45, 3095–4001.
17. Joshi VV, Cantor AB, Altshuler G, Larkin EW, Neill JS, Shuster JJ, et al. Recommendations for modification of terminology of neuroblastic tumors and prognostic significance of Shimada classification: A clinicopathologic study of 213 cases from the Pediatric Oncology Group. Cancer 1992, 69(8), 2183–96.
18. Joshi VV, Cantor AB, Altshuler G, Larkin EW, Neill JS, Shuster JJ, et al. Age-linked prognostic categorization based on a new histologic grading system of neuroblastomas: A clinicopathologic study of 211 cases from the Pediatric Oncology Group. Cancer 1992, 69(8), 2197–2211.
19. Joshi VV, Silverman JF. Pathology of neuroblastic tumors. Semin Diagn Pathol 1994, 11, 107–17.
20. Brodeur GM, Pritchard J, Berthold F, Carisen NL, Castel V, Castelberry RP, et al. Revisions of the International Criteria etc. J Clin Oncol 1993, 11, 1466–77.
21. Joshi VV. Peripheral neuroblastic tumors: pathologic classification based on recommendations of international neuroblastoma pathology committee (modification of Shimada classification). Pediatr Dev Pathol 2000, 3, 184–99.
22. Shimada H, Ambros IM, Dehner LP, Hata J-i, Joshi VV, Roald B. Terminology and morphologic criteria of neuroblastic tumors. Cancer 1999, 86(2), 349–63.
23. Stout AP. Ganglioneuroma of the sympathetic nervous system. Surg Gynecol Obstet 1947, 84, 101–9.
24. Ambros IM, Ambros PF. Schwann cells in neuroblastoma. Eur J Cancer 1995, 31a, 429–34.
25. Triche TJ. Neuroblastoma and other childhood neural tumors: review. Pediatric Pathol 1990, 10, 175–93.
26. Carter RL, Al-Sam SZ, Corbett RP, Clinton S. A comparative study of immunohistochemical staining for neuron-specific enolase protein gene product 9.5 and S100 protein in neuroblastoma, Ewing's sarcoma and other round cell tumours in children. Histopathology 1990, 16, 461–7.
27. Perlman EJ, Dickman PS, Askin FB, Grier HE, Miser JS, Link MP. Ewing's sarcoma—routine diagnostic utilization of MIC2 analysis: a Pediatric Oncology Group/Children's Cancer group Intergroup Study. Human Pathol 1994, 3, 304–7.
28. Thomas JO, Nijjar J, Turley H, Micklem K, Gatter KC. NB84: a new monoclonal antibody for the recognition of neuroblastoma in routinely processed material. J Pathol 1991, 163, 69–75.
29. Miettinen M, Chatten J, Paetau A, Stevenson A. Monoclonal antibody NB84 in the differential diagnosis of neuroblastoma and other small round cell tumors. Am J Surg Pathol 1998, 22(3), 327–32.
30. Shimada H, Aoyama C, Chiba R, Newton WA. Prognostic subgroups for undifferentiated neuroblastoma: immunohistochemical study with anti-S100 protein antibody. Human Pathol 1985, 16, 471–6.
31. Misugi K, Misugi N, Newton WA. Fine structural study of neuroblastoma, ganglioneuroblastoma and phaechromocytoma. Arch Pathol Lab Med 1968, 86, 160–9.
32. Yokoyama M, Okada K, Tolue A, Takayasu H, Yamada R. Ultrastructural and biochemical study of neuroblastoma and ganglioneuroblastoma. Invest Urol 1971, 9, 156–63.
33. Taxy JB. Electron microscopy in the diagnosis of neuroblastoma. Arch Pathol Lab Med 1980, 104, 355–60.
34. Bill AH. The regression of neuroblastoma. J Pediatr Surg 1968, 3, 103–6.
35. Oppedal BR, Storm-Mathisen I, Lie SO, Brandtzaeg P. Prognostic factors in neuroblastoma. Clinical, histopathological, and immunohistochemical features and DNA ploidy in relation to prognosis. Cancer 1988, 62, 772–80.
36. Evans AE. Staging and treatment of neuroblastoma. Cancer 1980, 45, 1799–802.
37. Katzenstein HM, Bowman LC, Brodeur GM, Thorner PS, Joshi VV, Smith EL, et al. Prognostic significance of age, MYCN oncogene amplification, tumor cell ploidy, and histology in 110 infants with stage D(S) neuroblastoma: The Pediatric Oncology Group experience—A Pediatric Oncology Group Study 1998, 16(6), 2007–17.
38. D'Angio GJ, Evans AE, Koop CE. Special pattern of widespread neuroblastoma with a favourable prognosis. Lancet 1971, 1, 1046–9.
39. Wilson PC, Coppes MJ, Solh H, Chan HS, Jenkin D, Greenberg ML, et al. Neuroblastoma stage IV-S: a heterogeneous disease. Med Pediatr Oncol 1991, 19, 467–72.
40. Haas D, Ablin AR, Miller C, Zoger S, Matthay KK. Complete pathologic maturation and regression of stage IVS neuroblastoma without treatment. Cancer 1988, 62, 818–25.
41. Stephenson SR, Cook BA, Mease AD, Ruymann FB. The prognostic significance of age and pattern of metastases in stage IV-S neuroblastoma. Cancer 1986, 58, 372–5.
42. Rogers DW, Treleaven JG, Kemshead JT, Pritchard J. Monoclonal antibodies for detecting bone marrow invasion by neuroblastoma. J Clin Pathol 1989, 42, 422–6.
43. Moss TJ, Sanders DG. Detection of neuroblastoma cells in blood. J Clin Oncol 1990, 8, 736–40.
44. Moss TJ, Reynolds CP, Sather HN, Romansky SG, Hammond GD, Seeger RC. Prognostic value of immunocytological detection of bone marrow metastases in neuroblastoma. New Engl J Med 1991, 324, 219–26.
45. Burchill SA, Bradbury FM, Smith B, Lewis IJ, Selby P. Neuroblastoma cell detection by reverse transcriptase-polymerase chain reaction (RT-PCR) for tyrosine hydroxylase mRNA. Int J Cancer 1994, 57, 671–5.
46. Miyajima Y, Horibe K, Fukuda M, Matsumoto K, Numata S, Mori H, et al. Sequential detection of tumour cells in the peripheral blood and bone marrow of patients with stage IV neuroblastoma by the reverse transcription-polymerase chain reaction for TH mRNA. Cancer 1996, 77, 1214–19.
47. Kuroda T, Saeki M, Nakano M, Mizutani SJ. Clinical application of minimal residual neuroblastoma cell detection by reverse transcriptase-polymerase chain reaction. J Pediatr Surg 1997, 32, 69–72.
48. Burchill SA, Lewis IJ, Abrams K, Riley R, Imeson J, Pearson ADJ, Pinkerton R, Selby P. Circulating neuroblastoma cells detected by reverse transcriptase polymerase chain reaction for tyrosine hydroxylase mRNA are an independent poor prognostic indicator in stage 4 neuroblastoma in children over 1 year. J Clin Oncol 2001, 19, 1795–801.
49. Seeger RC, Reynolds CP, Gallego R, Stram DO, Gerbing RB, Matthay KK. Quantitative tumor cell content of bone marrow and blood as a predictor of outcome in stage IV

neuroblastoma: a Children's Cancer Group Study. J Clin Oncol 2000, 18, 4067–76.
50. Burchill SA, Bradbury FM, Selby P, Lewis IJ. Early clinical evaluation of neuroblastoma cell detection by reverse transcriptase-polymerase chain reaction (RT-PCR) for tyrosine hydroxylase mRNA. Eur J Cancer 1994, 31, 553–6.
51. Gilbert J, Norris MD, Marshall GM, Haber M. Low specificity of PGP9.5 expression for detection of micrometastatic neuroblastoma. Br J Cancer 1997, 75, 1779–81.
52. Mattano LA, Jr, Moss TJ, Emerson SG. Sensitive detection of rare circulating neuroblastoma cells by the reverse transcriptase-polymerase chain reaction. Cancer Res 1992, 52, 4701–5.
53. Mehes G, Luegmayr A, Hattinger CM, Lorch T, Ambros IM, Gadner H, Ambros PF. Automatic detection and genetic profiling of disseminated neuroblastoma cells. Med Pediatr Oncol 2001, 36, 205–9.
54. Beckwith JB, Martin RF. Observations on the histopathology of neuroblastoma. J Pediatr Surg 1968, 3, 106–10.
55. Shimada H, Chatten J, Newton WA, Jr, Sachs N, Hamoudi AB, Chiba T, et al. Histopathologic prognostic factors in neuroblastic tumors: definition of subtypes of ganglioneuroblastoma and age linked classification of neuroblastomas. J Nat Cancer Inst 1984, 73, 405–16.
56. Shimada H, Stram DO, Chatten J, Joshi VV, Hachitanda Y, Brodeur GM, et al. Identification of subsets of neuroblastomas by combined histopathologic and N-myc analysis. J Nat Cancer Inst 1995, 87(19), 1470–6.
57. Hachitanda Y, Tsuneyoshi M. Neuroblastoma with a distinct organoid pattern: a clinicopathologic, immunohistochemical and ultrastructural study. Human Pathol 1994, 25(1), 67–72.
58. Schweisguth O. Excretion of catecholamine metabolites in the urine of neuroblastoma patients. J Pediatr Surg 1968, 3, 118–20.
59. Kogut MD, Kaplan SA. Systemic manifestations of neurogenic tumors. J Pediatr 1962, 60, 694–704.
60. Hann HW, Evans AE, Siegel SE, Wong KY, Sather H, Dalton A. Prognostic importance of serum ferritin in patients with stage III and IV neuroblastoma: The Children's Cancer Study Group experience. Cancer Res 1985, 45, 2843–8.
61. Evans AE, D'Angio GJ, Propert K, Anderson J, Hann HW. Prognostic factors in neuroblastoma. Cancer 1987, 59, 1853–9.
62. Shuster JJ, McWilliams NB, Castleberry R, Nitschke R, Smith EI, Altshuler G, Kun L, Brodeur G, Joshi V, Vietti T, et al. Serum lactate dehydrogenase in childhood neuroblastoma. A Pediatric Oncology Group recursive partitioning study. Am J Clin Oncol 1992, 15, 295–303.
63. Mendelsohn G, Eggleston JC, Olson JL, Said SL, Baylin SB. Vasoactive intestinal peptide and its relation to ganglion cell differentiation in neuroblastic tumors. Lab Invest 1979, 41, 144–9.
64. Nakagawara A, Arima-Nakagawara M, Scavarda NJ, Azar CG, Cantor AB, Brodeur GM. Association between high levels of expression of the TRK gene and favorable outcome in human neuroblastoma. New Engl J Med 1993, 328, 847–54.
65. Buckley SL. The role of nerve growth factor and its receptors in paediatric neurally derived tumours. PhD Thesis, 1999.
66. Qualman SJ, O'Dorisio MS, Fleshman DJ, Shimada H, O'Dorisio TM. Neuroblastoma. Correlation of neuropeptide expression in tumor tissue with other prognostic factors. Cancer 1992, 70, 2005–12.
67. Kogner P, Bjork O, Theodorsson E. Neuropeptide Y in neuroblastoma: increased concentration in metastasis, release during surgery, and characterization of plasma and tumor extracts. Med Pediatr Oncol 1993, 21, 317–22.
68. Rascher W, Kremens B, Wagner S, Feth F, Hunneman DH, Lang RE. Serial measurements of neuropeptide Y in plasma for monitoring neuroblastoma in children. J Pediatr 1993, 122, 914–16.
69. Kogner P, Borgstrom P, Bjellerup P, Schilling FH, Refai E, Jonsson C, et al. Somatostatin in neuroblastoma and ganglioneuroma. Eur J Cancer 1997, 33, 2084–9.
70. Thorner PS, Squire JA. Molecular genetics in the diagnosis and prognosis of solid pediatric tumors. Pediatr Dev Pathol 1998, 1, 337–65.
71. Look AT, Hayes FA, Nitschke R, McWilliams NB, Green AA. Cellular DNA content as a predictor of response to chemotherapy in infants with unresectable neuroblastoma. New Engl J Med 1984, 311, 231–5.
72. Weith A, Martinsson T, Cziepluch C, Bruderlein S, Amler LC, Berthold F, Schwab M. Neuroblastoma consensus deletion maps to 1p36.1-2. Genes Chromosomes Cancer 1989, 1, 159–66.
73. White PS, Maris JM, Sulman EP, Jensen SJ, Kyemba SM, Beltinger CP, et al. Molecular analysis of the region of distal 1p commonly deleted in neuroblastoma. Eur J Cancer 1997, 33, 1957–61.
74. Caron H, van Sluis P, Buschman R, Pereira do Tanque R, Maes P, Beks L, et al. Allelic loss of chromosome 1p as a predictor of unfavourable outcome in patients with neuroblastoma. New Engl J Med 1996, 334, 225–30.
75. Ambros IM, Zellner A, Roald B, Amann G, Ladenstein R, Printz D, et al. Role of ploidy, chromosome 1p, and Schwann cells in the maturation of neuroblastoma. New Engl J Med 1996, 334, 1505–11.
76. Fong CT, Dracopoli NC, White PS, Merrill PT, Griffith RC, Housman DE, et al. Loss of heterozygosity for the short arm of chromosome 1 in human neuroblastomas: correlation with N-myc amplification. Proc Natl Acad Sci, USA 1989, 86, 3753–7.
77. Matos P, Isidro G, Vieira E, Lacerda AF, Martins AG, Boavida MG. P73 expression in neuroblastoma: a role in the biology of advanced tumors? Pediatr Hematol Oncol 2001, 18, 37–46.
78. Lastowska M, Cotterill S, Pearson AD, Roberts P, McGuckin A, Lewis I, et al. Gain of chromosome arm 17q predicts unfavourable outcome in neuroblastoma patients. U.K. Children's Cancer Study Group and the U.K. Cancer Cytogenetics Group. Eur J Cancer 1997, 33, 1627–33.
79. Brodeur GM, Seeger RC, Schwab M, Varmus HE, Bishop JM. Amplification of N-myc in untreated human neuroblastomas correlates with advanced disease stage. Science 1984, 224, 1121–4.
80. Bordow SB, Norris MD, Haber PS, Marshall GM, Haber M. Prognostic significance of MYCN oncogene expression in

childhood neuroblastoma. J Clin Oncol 1998, 16, 3286–94.
81. Norris MD, Bordow SB, Marshall GM, Haber PS, Cohn SL, Haber M. Expression of the gene for multi-drug-resistance-associated protein and outcome in patients with neuroblastoma. New Engl J Med 1996, 334, 231–8.
82. George RE, Kenyon RM, McGuckin AG, Malcolm AJ, Pearson AD, Lunec J. Investigation of co-amplification of the candidate genes ornithine decarboxylase, ribonucleotide reductase, syndecan-1 and a DEAD box gene, DDX1, with N-myc in neuroblastoma. United Kingdom Children's Cancer Study Group. Oncogene 1996, 12, 1583–7.
83. Fong CT, White PS, Peterson K, Sapienza C, Cavenee WK, Kern SE. Loss of heterozygosity for chromosomes 1 or 14 defines subsets of advanced neuroblastomas. Cancer Res 1992, 52, 1780–5.
84. Hiyama E, Hiyama K, Yokoyama T, Matsuura Y, Piatyszek MA, Shay JW. Correlating telomerase activity levels with human neuroblastoma outcomes. Nat Med 1995, 1, 249–55.
85. Hiyama E, Hiyama K, Ohtsu K, Yamaoka H, Ichikawa T, Shay JW. Telomerase activity in neuroblastoma: is it a prognostic indicator of clinical behaviour? Eur J Cancer 1997, 33, 1932–6.
86. Kusafuka T, Fukuzawa M, Oue T, Komoto Y, Yoneda A, Okada A. Mutation analysis of p53 gene in childhood malignant solid tumors. J Pediatr Surg 1997, 32(8), 1175–80.
87. Hosoi G, Hara J, Okamura T, Osugi Y, Ishihara S, Fukuzawa M, et al. Low frequency of the p53 gene mutations in neuroblastoma. Cancer 1994, 73(12), 3087–93.
88. Kaghad M, Bonnet H, Yang A, Creancier L, Biscan JC, Valent A, et al. Monoallelically expressed gene related to p53 at 1p36, a region frequently deleted in neuroblastoma and other human cancers. Cell 1997, 90(4), 809–19.
89. Tanaka T, Hiyama E, Sugimoto T, Sawada T, Tanabe M, Ida N. Trk A gene expression in neuroblastoma: the clinical significance of an immunohistochemical study. Cancer 1995, 76, 1086–95.
90. Tanaka T, Slamon DJ, Shimada H, Shimoda H, Fujisawa T, Ida N, Seeger RC. A significant association of Ha-ras p21 in neuroblastoma cells with patient prognosis. A retrospective study of 103 cases. Cancer 1991, 68 1296–1302.
91. Combaret V, Gross N, Lasset C, Frappaz D, Peruisseau G, Philip T, et al. Clinical relevance of CD_{44} cell surface expression and N-myc gene amplification in a multivariate analysis of 121 pediatric neuroblastomas. J Clin Oncol 1996, 14, 25–34.
92. George RE, Variend S, Cullinane C, Cotterill SJ, McGuckin AG, Ellershaw C, Lunec J, Pearson AD; United Kingdom Children Cancer Study Group. George Med. Relationship between histopathological features, MYCN amplification, and prognosis: a UKCCSG study. United Kingdom Children Cancer Study Group. Pediatr Oncol 2001, 36, 169–76.
93. Lastowska M, Cullinane C, Variend S, Cotterill S, Bown N, O'Neill S, Mazzocco K, Roberts P, Nicholson J, Ellershaw C, Pearson AD, Jackson MS; United Kingdom Children Cancer Study Group and the United Kingdom Cancer Cytogenetics Group. Comprehensive genetic and histopathologic study reveals three types of neuroblastoma tumors. J Clin Oncol 2001, 19, 3080–90.
94. Brodeur GM, Maris JM, Yamashiro DJ, Hogarty MD, White PS. Biology and genetics of human neuroblastomas. J Pediatr Hematol Oncol 1997, 19, 93–101.

9 | Primitive neuroectodermal tumours

Catherine J. Cullinane and Susan A. Burchill

Primitive neuroectodermal tumours (PNET)

Primitive neuroectodermal tumours are a group of small round cell tumours, which share morphological, immunohistochemical, and ultrastructural features of neural differentiation. They have been classified into two main groups, central or peripheral, depending on the localization of the primary tumour at diagnosis (1). The central PNET (cPNET) arises in the brain; medulloblastoma is the prototype. Those arising from the peripheral nervous system include neuroblastoma, peripheral PNET (pPNET; sometimes known as neuroepithelioma), and Ewing's sarcoma (ES), as well as a number of rare entities (1, 2). Their cell of origin remains speculative, though it is postulated to be a pluripotent neural crest cell or a mesenchymal stem cell that differentiates along neural lines (3). The cPNET and neuroblastomas can readily be distinguished from pPNET and ES by their clinical, biological, and genetic features. The cPNETs and neuroblastoma are discussed elsewhere in this text.

The Ewing's sarcoma family of tumours (ESFT)

The ESFT, including ES and pPNET are aggressive malignant tumours of children and young adults, which may arise in bone or soft tissues (4). ES is predominantly of skeletal origin, and pPNET usually presents in soft tissues. In recent years it has become apparent that they share not only similar morphological and biological features but also specific chromosomal rearrangements between the *EWS* gene on chromosome 22 and various members of the *ETS* gene family (1, 4, 5). These common, non-random gene rearrangements provide strong evidence for the common histogenesis of these tumours, and provide a valuable tool for their differential diagnosis from other small round cell tumours.

The second most common malignant tumour of bone is the ES accounting for 10–15% of all primary bone tumours (6). It affects 13 per million 0–24 year olds per year in the United Kingdom (7), and is slightly more common in males than females (ratio 1.5:1). It has been described in siblings (8, 9), although this is rare and the disease does not appear to be implicated in familial cancer syndromes. Genetic influences may play some role in its aetiology as Black Afro-Caribbean and Chinese populations are less frequently affected than the White population (9, 10). It may affect any bone but the most common sites are lower extremity (45%), followed by pelvis (20%), upper extremity (13%), axial skeleton and ribs (13%), and face (2%) (11). The femur is the most frequently affected bone, the tumour usually arising in the mid-shaft; on X-ray an osteolytic mass with characteristic 'onion-skinning' appearance due to concentric periosteal new bone deposition is apparent.

The second most common soft tissue malignancy in childhood is the pPNET accounting for 20% of sarcomas (12). It shows a predilection for the chest wall (Askin tumour), followed by paraspinal tissues, abdominal wall, head and neck, and extremities (12, 13). It may also arise in bone and rarely in kidney (14), skin (15, 16), pancreas (17), and lung (18). Soft tissue extension is common in osseous ESFT, and infiltration of adjacent bone is frequent in soft tissue ESFT, which can make it difficult to determine the primary site of tumour origin.

The ESFTs are typically aggressive with an overall 7.5-year disease-free survival of 45–60% (19). Approximately 30% of patients with ESFT have metastases at presentation (20), for these patients' overall survival is 10–20% (21, 22). Overall survival for patients with localized disease is reported to be about 60% (23). Relapse is very common, even occurring in up to 50%

of patients with apparently localized disease at diagnosis (20). This suggests these patients have low-level metastatic disease that is not detected by current routine methods such as imaging and histological examination of bone marrow at diagnosis. For these patients reverse transcriptase polymerase chain reaction (RT-PCR) for EWS–ETS fusion transcripts may identify low levels of clinically significant disease with improved sensitivity and specificity (24–26) (see below).

Pain and swelling in the affected area are the usual presenting symptoms. ESFT is often associated with systemic symptoms, especially in patients with metastatic disease, which may include weight loss, fever, and fatigue (11, 20). Patients with ESFT arising in or adjacent to the ribs within the pleural cavity may present with pleural effusion and respiratory symptoms. Osteomyelitis may be suspected when fever and leucocytosis are found in association with a bony lesion, and thus may result in delayed diagnosis of ESFT. Paraspinal tumours may infiltrate the cord, leading to neurological symptoms and signs. Delayed diagnosis may also be a feature of pelvic primaries, as the tumour may attain a large size before the patient presents. ESFT metastasise to lungs, bones, liver, and brain, but rarely to the lymph nodes or bone marrow which are the usual sites of metastases in neuroblastomas (11, 27). Raised serum lactate dehydrogenase (LDH) (28, 29) and erythrocyte sedimentation rate (ESR) (30) are common features of ESFT, reflecting tumour mass and anaemia, respectively. There is no consensus staging system for ESFT.

Ewing's sarcoma family of tumours are thought to be of neural origin, largely based on the presence of limited neuronal differentiation characterized by immunohistochemical analysis for neuronal antigens and electron microscopy for the presence of neurosecretory granules or primitive neurites (19, 31). Further evidence for a neural histogenesis is illustrated by the capacity of ESFT cell lines to undergo neuronal differentiation *in vitro* (32, 33). These tumours are predominantly cholinergic, synthesizing acetylcholine transferase essential for the production of acetylcholine (34–36). This suggests that they are derived from postganglionic parasympathetic primordial cells, located throughout the parasympathetic autonomic nervous system. The wide distribution of these pluripotent stem cells may explain the variety of soft tissue and bony locations in which ESFT are found. Although some tumours express adrenergic neurotransmitters and their precursors, they do not secrete catecholamines or their metabolites in urine. This feature is useful in distinguishing ESFT from neuroblastoma.

Diagnosis

Accurate diagnosis of ESFT is critical for the most appropriate clinical management of patients. This is based on radiological investigations, haematological and biochemical assessment, bone marrow and tumour biopsy. Adequate clinical information, recognition of morphological, immunohistochemical, ultrastructural, and cytogenetic features of ESFT are all required for differential diagnosis from other small round cell tumours of childhood (Tables 9.1 and 9.2).

Pathology

The macroscopic appearance of the excised primary tumour, rarely seen today, is grey–white and fleshy with foci of necrosis, haemorrhage, and cystic degeneration. By light microscopy, ESFT are small round cell tumours. All are regarded as high-grade malignancies. Accurate diagnosis is facilitated by the application of a panel of immunohistochemical antibodies and electron microscopy. Ultrastructural analysis is used less frequently as a routine diagnostic technique today, this being superseded by immunohistochemistry and molecular diagnostic techniques.

A range of appearances, depending on the extent of neural differentiation, are apparent in ESFT, from an undifferentiated (ES) to neural differentiation (pPNET). All consist of closely packed primitive cells, divided into lobules by fibrous tissue bands. A trabecular or filigree pattern may also be present. There is scant if any stroma between the cells, usually no neuropil, and very rarely reticulin fibres in the cellular component. A positive periodic acid-Schiff (PAS) stain, with and without diastase, demonstrating abundant cytoplasmic glycogen is also of value in the diagnosis of this tumour. The presence of glycogen is best demonstrated on imprints and frozen sections, as formalin fixation may lead to a variable result. However, glycogen is absent in about one-third of cases and has occasionally been reported in other small round cell tumours such as rhabdomyosarcoma and neuroblastoma. Focal or more extensive geographic necrosis may be evident, with peri-vascular preservation of tumour cells. ESFT has a fine capillary framework and haemorrhage is common.

The histological definition of ES and pPNET has varied in the past (1, 3, 19). Currently ES is defined morphologically by the absence of neural differentiation whereas pPNET shows neural differentiation either by light microscopy, immunohistochemistry, or electron microscopy. Typical ES has small cells with round,

Table 9.1 Immunohistochemistry and ultrastructure of pPNET, ES, and other common small cell tumours of childhood

IHC	pPNET	ES	NBL	RMS	NHL
Vimentin	+	+	−	+	− (+)
NSE	+	−	+	− (+)	−
PGP 9.5	+	−	+	−	−
S100	+	−	− (+)	−	−
Chromogranin	− (+)	−	+	−	−
GFAP	− (+)	−	−	−	−
Leu 7	+	−	−	−	− (+)
MIC2	+	+	−	− (+)	+ (−)
NB84	−	−	+	−	−
Desmin	− (+)	− (+)	−	+	−
MyoD1	−	−	−	+	−
Myogenin	−	−	−	+	−
Actin	−	−	−	+	−
CD45	−	−	−	−	+
Cytokeratin	− (+)	− (+)	−	− (+)	−
EM	G++	G+++	G+	G+	G+
	Occasional cell processes, neurosecretory granules	Primitive cells, few organelles	Abundant cell processes and neurosecretory granules	Myofilaments Z-band material	Few organelles scanty cell junctions

Abbreviations: IHC = Immunohistochemistry; EM = Electron microscopy; pPNET = peripheral primitive neuroectodermal tumour (neuroepithelioma); ES = Ewing's sarcoma; ESFT = Ewing's sarcoma family of tumours; NBL = Neuroblastoma; RMS = Rhabdomyosarcoma; NHL = Non-Hodgkin's lymphoma, G = glycogen.
Markers in **bold** are useful to aid diagnosis in the tumour types indicated.

Table 9.2 Different EWS fusion types described in ESFT and other sarcomas

Translocation	Gene fusion	Tumour type (EWS–ETS gene rearrangement as a % in ESFT)
t(11;22)(q24;q12)	EWS–FLI1	ESFT (85%)
t(21;22)(q22;q12)	EWS–ERG	ESFT (10%)
t(7;22)(p22;q12)	EWS–ETV1	ESFT (rare)
t(17;22)(q12;q12)	EWS–E1AF	ESFT (rare)
t(2;22)(q33;q12)	EWS–FEV	ESFT (rare)
t(12;22)(q13;q12)	*EWS–AFT1*	*Clear cell sarcoma*
t(11;22)(q13;q12)	*EWS–WT1*	*Desmoplastic small round cell tumour*
t(9;22)(q22;q12)	*EWS–CHN*	*Myxoid chondrosarcoma*
t(12;22)(q13;q12)	*EWS–CHOP*	*Myxoid liposarcoma*

Note: The presence of *EWS–ETS* gene rearrangements is increasingly used to define ESFT. The breakpoint on chromosome 22q at the location of the *EWS* gene is consistent; this can partner with a number of different *ETS* gene family members from various chromosomes. Rearrangements of the *EWS* gene on chromosome 22q12 with other chromosomes have also been described in other less common sarcoma types (shown in italics and bold).

monotonous nuclei, finely dispersed chromatin and inconspicuous nucleoli and a narrow rim of clear or pale cytoplasm with abundant glycogen (Fig. 9.1(a)). Mitoses are often infrequent (1, 31). Ultrastructurally, ES contains primitive cells with a smooth nuclear surface, scanty organelles, and cytoplasmic glycogen in pools or aggregates (Fig. 9.1(b)). A mixture of pale viable and dark shrunken necrotic tumour cells imparts a characteristic light and dark appearance though this is a non-specific feature often reported in other tumour types. The atypical (large cell) ES shows variation in nuclear size, indented nuclei, coarse chromatin, large nucleoli, low levels of glycogen, and more mitoses. Ultrastructural findings in atypical ES are similar to those in pPNET.

Peripheral PNET is defined by the presence of neural differentiation, although this is rare and often difficult to identify. Poorly formed rosettes may be present, less frequently Homer–Wright rosettes and/or peri-vascular rosettes, and rarely ganglion cells and neurofibrillary stroma (neuropil) (19, 27). Generally pPNET shows increased cell and nuclear size, pleomorphism, increased mitoses, and less glycogen (Fig. 9.2(a)). Occasionally an alveolar pattern, due to dissolution of cells, may suggest a diagnosis of alveolar rhabdomyosarcoma (Fig. 9.2(b)). Also, if the tumour is deep within soft tissues, entrapment of muscle or regenerating myofibres may cause diagnostic confusion with rhabdomyosarcoma. Divergent differentiation along neuroglial, epithelial, and myogenic lines has been described in subsets of these tumours (37, 38). Electron microscopy reveals primitive cells with larger nuclei, nuclear indentation and coarse chromatin, and neural features including cytoplasmic filaments, microtubules, cell processes, and neurosecretory granules, although the latter are much less common than in neuroblastoma. Glycogen is also present, in pools or aggregates, even though it may not always be obvious by light microscopy (39).

Immunohistochemistry

The immunohistochemical reactions in ESFT also reflect the continuum of neural differentiation and aid

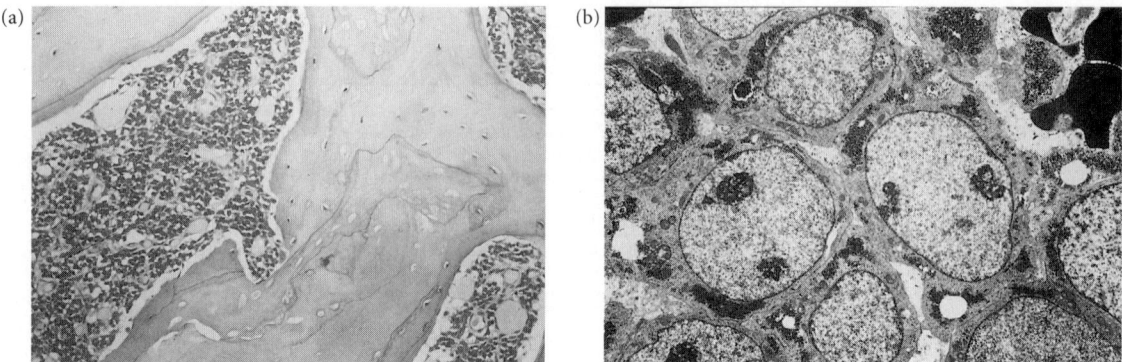

Fig. 9.1 (a) ES of bone showing undifferentiated small cells filling the marrow spaces (H&E). (b) Ultrastructurally the primitive cells of ES have scanty cytoplasm containing particulate glycogen, few organelles, and oval or round nuclei with smooth nuclear membranes.

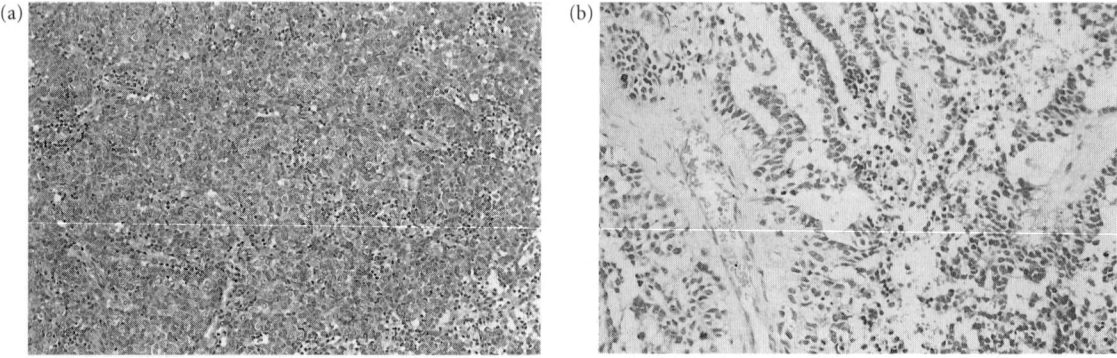

Fig. 9.2 (a) pPNET (neuroepithelioma) has larger more pleomorphic oval nuclei and scanty pale or clear cytoplasm. Focally the cells form pseudorosettes (H&E). (b) The alveolar pattern in this tumour with cells clinging to the fibrous septa suggests alveolar rhabomyosarcoma. However, the immunoprofile and cytogenetic analysis t(11;22) were typical of pPNET (H&E).

classification from other small round cell tumours of childhood (Table 9.1). Typical ES is positive for vimentin, and negative for neural markers. Rarely focal desmin and/or cytokeratin positivity is noted. Atypical ES usually shows vimentin and focal neural marker positivity. pPNETs are positive for vimentin, and variably positive for one or more neural markers such as neuron specific enolase (NSE), protein gene product 9.5 (PGP 9.5), leucocyte antigen 7 (Leu-7), synaptophysin, S100 and neurofilaments, and less frequently cells focally positive for desmin and cytokeratin.

Of particular value in the differential diagnosis of ESFT from other small round cell tumours of childhood is the antibody CD99, which recognizes the cell surface glycoprotein p30/32^{MIC2} (4, 40–44) (Fig. 9.3). The MIC2 gene, a pseudoautosomal gene, is present on chromosomes Xp and Y and is usually over-expressed in ESFT (45). It is also expressed by normal cortical thymocytes, pancreatic Islet of Langerhans cells, and sertoli cells (43), and has been described in mesenchymal chondrosarcoma (46), rhabdoid tumour (47), synovial sarcoma (48), sex cord stromal tumours (49), lymphomas, leukaemia, and rhabdomyosarcoma (41, 43). In lymphoid lesions expression is diffuse whereas in rhabdomyosarcoma the positive reaction tends to be focal (43). Rhabdomyosarcoma is further defined by immunohistochemical staining with myogenic antibodies including Myo-D1 and myogenin. Furthermore, a proportion of rhabdomyosarcomas (alveolar sub-type), have translocations involving *PAX-FKHR* gene rearrangements that can be identified by G-banding, RT-PCR, or fluorescent *in situ* hybridization (FISH).

Ewing's sarcoma family of tumours is very rare in children younger than 5 years of age. In this age group the main differential diagnosis for ESFT is from neuroblastoma. Neuroblastomas (98%) produce and secrete elevated levels of catecholamine metabolites, that can be readily detected in the urine. These tumours are also positive by immunohistochemistry for neural antibodies such as NSE, S100 and NB84, which can be used to distinguish neuroblastoma from classic ES. However, some ESFT share some of the same histological

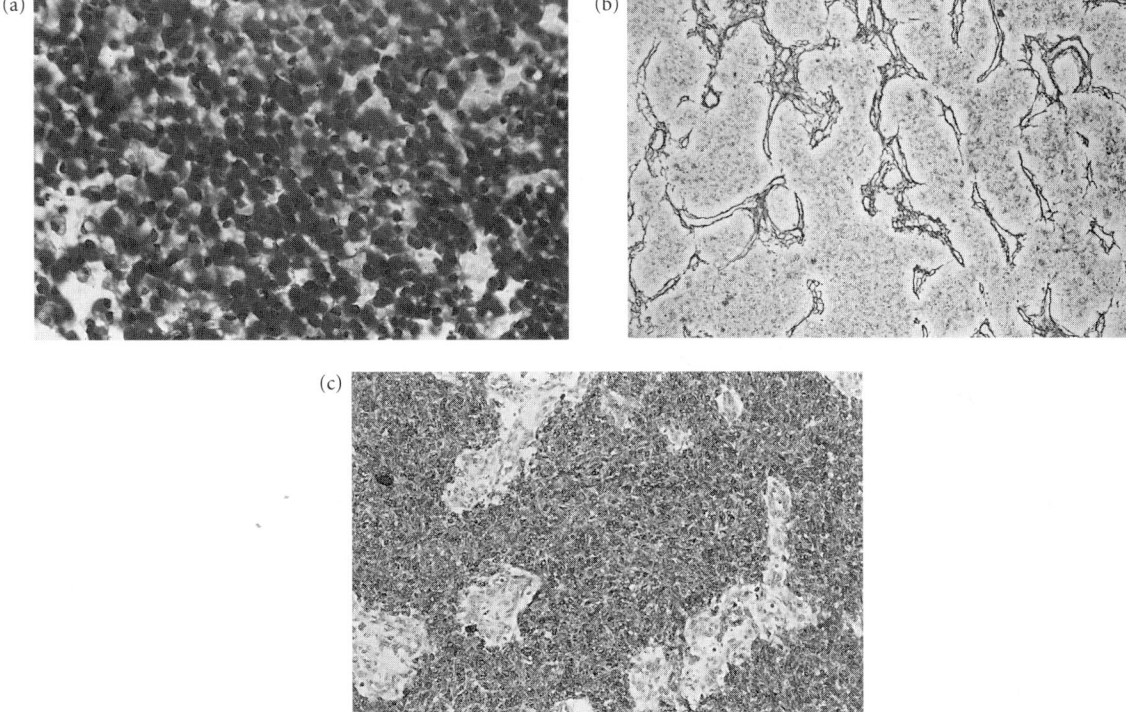

Fig. 9.3 Special stains (PAS and reticulin) and immunohistochemistry, especially for CD99, are particularly helpful in the diagnosis of ESFT. (a) The presence of glycogen in the cytoplasm is demonstrated by the Periodic Acid Schiff stain (PAS). (b) Typically there are scanty reticulin fibres in the cellular component compared to the septa (Reticulin). (c) Positive CD99 immunostaining of the cell membranes (CD99 antibody).

characteristics as neuroblastoma; in these cases cytogenetic differences are particularly important.

Cytogenetics

Increasingly ESFT are characterized by rearrangements between the *EWS* gene on 22q12, with various members of the *ETS* gene family (Table 9.2). The most frequent gene rearrangement is the t(11;22)(q24;q12) translocation, found in about 85% of these tumours (Fig. 9.4). Fusion of the amino-terminal of the *EWS* gene on 22q12 with the carboxy-terminal of the *FLI1* gene on 11q24, results in a chimeric fusion transcript EWS–FLI1 (Fig. 9.5(a)). Other *EWS–ETS* gene family rearrangements have been identified in the remaining 15% of tumours, the t(21;22)(q22;12) resulting in fusion of *EWS* with the *ERG* gene on 21q22 being the second most common (50) (Table 9.2). The fusion protein derived from EWS–ERG is similar to that of the *EWS–FLI1* gene product. Other variant translocations have been described where *EWS* is fused with *ETV1* t(7;22)(p22;q12), (50); *E1AF* t(17;22)(q21;q12), (51); and *FEV* t(2;22)(q33;q22), (52); in addition to more complex translocations involving multiple chromosomes such as t(11;14;22)(q24;q11;q12) and t(10;11;22.) (p11.2;q24;q12). The biological significance of these more complex gene-rearrangements is not clear.

The presence of these non-random *EWS–ETS* gene rearrangements in ES and pPNET is strong evidence for their common histogenesis, and provides a valuable characteristic for the differential diagnosis of ESFT from other small round cell tumours of childhood. Two molecular techniques have successfully been used to detect these EWS–ETS fusion transcripts, RT-PCR and FISH (Fig. 9.5(b) and 9.6). RT-PCR requires the conversion of tumour derived RNA to cDNA, which is subsequently amplified by PCR for the chimeric fusion transcripts. Primers designed to the gene for each fusion transcript type ensure sensitive and specific detection of fusion transcripts. Using this approach, EWS–FLI1 or EWS–ERG fusion transcripts have been detected in over 95% of ESFT. The presence of EWS–ETS fusion products detected by RT-PCR correlates well with conventional G-banding studies, but perhaps more interestingly RT-PCR can be used to identify *EWS–ETS* gene fusions in tumours where conventional G-banding

KARYOTYPE:
47,XX,+8, del(11)(q23),t(11;22)(q24;q12),+12,add(14)(p11),–16, add(17)(p13),der(19)t(17;19)(q21;q13),add(21)(q22)

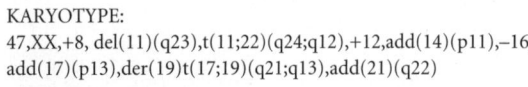

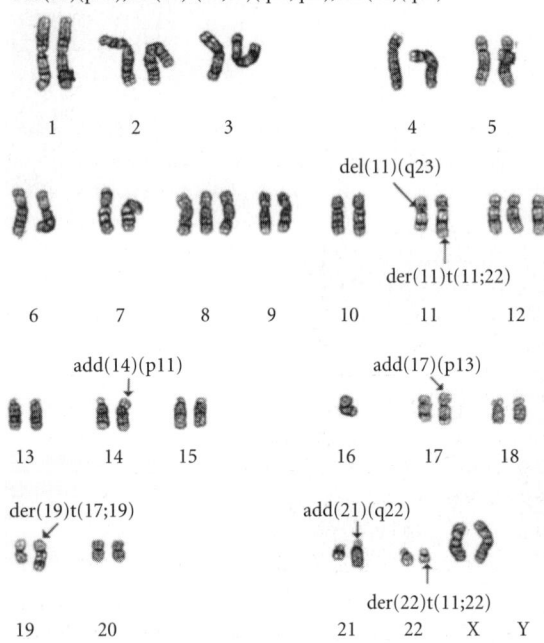

Fig. 9.4 G-banding of chromosomes from an ES showing the t(11.22)(q12.24). This tumour also has trisomy of chromosome 8 and 12, and loss of 16, all common features of ESFT.

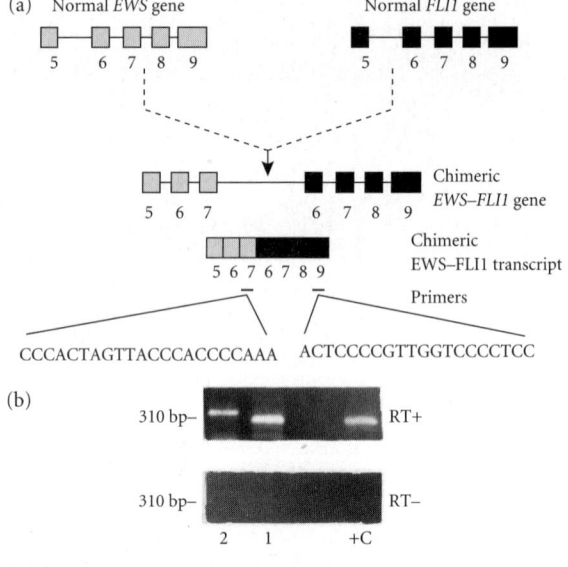

Fig. 9.5 RT-PCR for EWS–FLI1 fusion transcripts. (a) Diagrammatic representation of the EWS–FLI1 type 1 fusion transcript. Primer sequences for the amplification of the EWS–FLI1 fusion transcript are shown. (b) RT-PCR for EWS–FLI1 gene rearrangements in two tumours showing type 1 (1) and type 2 (2) fusion transcripts. +c = amplification of RNA from the TC-32 cell line demonstrating the type 1 EWS–FLI1 fusion transcript; RT+ contains reverse transcriptase enzyme and the negative control RT– does not.

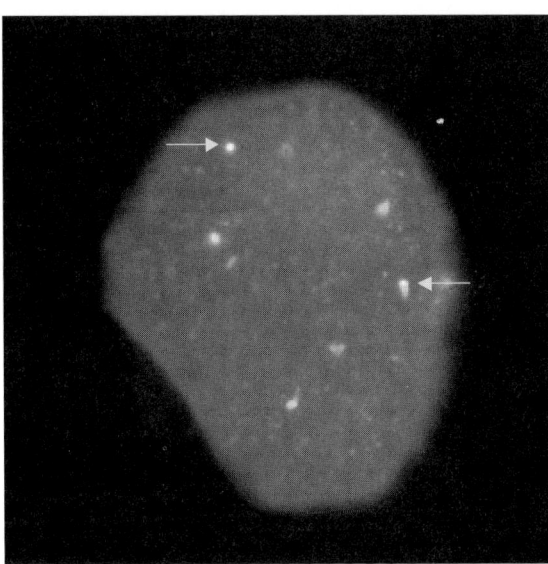

Fig. 9.6 FISH on tetraploid interphase of an ESFT showing 2 copies of t(11.22)(q24.q12). Arrows denote *EWS–FLI 1* fusion on the der(22). EWS. BAC (222M10) labelled green; FLI-1 BAC (428J4) labelled red. Note the der(11) exhibits a green signal generated by translocated EWS sequences. See Plate 10.

has been uninformative, either due to a very complex gene rearrangement or lack of mitotic cells. Indeed the ability of RT-PCR to detect fusion transcripts in small pieces of tumour, even in fine-needle biopsies or bone marrow aspirations, makes this a very attractive tool to aid in the diagnosis of ESFT. It has also been used to detect small numbers of tumour cells in cytologically normal bone marrow aspirates and peripheral blood. The molecular detection of these small numbers of circulating tumour cells may ultimately lead to a redefinition of the terms metastatic disease and disease-free. FISH has also been successfully used to identify these gene rearrangements in ESFT. FISH uses fluorescent-tagged probes for two involved loci to label tumour cells. The fusion of the *EWS* and *ETS* gene members is visualized by microscopy of the fluorescent-labelling in inter-phase cells; a translocation has occurred if the two fluorescent probes are adjacent to each other on the same chromosome (Fig. 9.6). Like RT-PCR, FISH can often be particularly valuable to identify *EWS–ETS* gene rearrangements when conventional G-banding studies are uninformative.

Using RT-PCR many alternative forms of EWS–FLI1 transcripts have been described, reflecting variations in the breakpoint in *EWS* and *FLI1*. The most common type, designated type 1, consists of the first seven exons of *EWS* joined to exons 6–9 of *FLI1* and accounts for approximately 60% of cases. The type 2 EWS–FLI1 fusion also includes FLI1 exon 5 and is present in a further 25% (53). Recent studies have shown these different fusion transcript types to be of prognostic significance (see below).

The *EWS–ETS* gene arrangements have been detected in bi-phenotypic sarcomas with muscle and neural differentiation (38), and rarely in rhabdomyosarcomas (54), neuroblastomas (55), rhabdoid tumour (56), and extraskeletal mesenchymal chondrosarcoma (57). Whether these examples represent extremes of the ESFT or rare pathological entities themselves is not clear.

The *EWS* gene is also rearranged in several other tumours, which are clinically and morphologically distinct from ESFT (Table 9.2). In desmoplastic small round cell tumour (DSRCT) the recurrent chromosomal translocation t(11;22)(p13;q12) results in a fusion transcript of the *EWS* gene at 22q12 and the Wilm's tumour gene *WT1* at 11p13, while in clear cell sarcoma, the recurrent translocation t(9;22)(q22;q12) fuses the *AFT1* gene at 9q22 to the *EWS* gene (50). In extraskeletal myxoid chondrosarcoma, the recurrent translocation t(9;22)(q22;q12) leads to the formation of a chimeric transcript of *CHN* gene at 9q22 and *EWS* (58). A multiplex RT-PCR to detect EWS fusion transcripts in small pieces of tumour, even in fine-needle biopsies or bone marrow aspirations, makes an attractive tool to aid in the diagnosis of ESFT (59).

Prognostic factors

Evaluation of tumour status occurs at the time of diagnosis, and subsequently to assess treatment response or for assessment on follow-up. Initial findings or changes in radiology or tumour marker status provide important information to aid the process of risk stratification and patient management. A number of prognostic factors have been described in ESFT (Table 9.3); a recent systematic review has reported on the statistical power of 23 different markers (NHS Health and Technology Assessment (HTA) programme; grant number 97/15/03; for further details of these results see http://www.prw.le.ac.uk/epidemio/personal/rdr3/paed.html). These can be grouped into clinical, pathological, and genetic factors. The most frequently used prognostic markers in clinical practice are those that belong to the clinical group.

Clinical

Metastatic disease at the time of diagnosis, determined by standard imaging methods and histological examination

Table 9.3 Prognostic factors in ESFT

	Adverse	Favourable
Clinical	Metastatic disease at diagnosis	Localized disease at diagnosis
	Pelvic, axial primary	Peripheral primary
	Age >12 years	Age <12 years
	Male sex	Female sex
	High serum LDH at diagnosis	Low serum LDH at diagnosis
	Anaemia and fever	Lack of systemic symptoms
	Tumour volume >100 ml	Tumour volume <100 ml
Pathological	Post-chemotherapy necrosis <90%	Post-chemotherapy necrosis >90%
	Neural differentiation (controversial)	Absence of neural differentiation
Genetic		Type 1 EWS–FLI1 transcript
	Chromosome 1p deletion	Trisomy 8
	Aneuploidy	Diploidy
	p53 expression present	p53 expression absent

of bone marrow, is the most powerful predictor of adverse prognosis in patients with ESFT (60, 61). Since a number of patients without detectable metastasis at diagnosis subsequently develop secondary disease, this suggests there may be a patient population with clinically unidentified small volume disease. The EWS–ETS fusion transcripts have been successfully used as targets for RT-PCR to detect such low-level disease (24–26). Disease detected in the peripheral blood by RT-PCR appears not to be clinically informative, although in bone marrow may predict a poor clinical outcome (24, 25, 62–65). This suggests that RT-PCR for EWS–ETS fusion transcript type in bone marrow may be useful to improve stratification of patients for therapy and result in a redefinition of the term disease-free.

In patients with non-metastatic localized ESFT, a large tumour volume (>100 ml) (66) and pelvic primary (67) at presentation are associated with a worse prognosis than for patients with tumours of <100 ml or disease localized to the distal bones and ribs. Diagnosis in boys and young men over 12 years of age is also thought to predict a poor outcome in non-metastatic ES of the bone (68). Response to therapy has been reported as being of prognostic value, although treatment intensification may make this less important and also change the power of specific tumour volumes (23).

Pathological

Classification of ESFT into typical ES, atypical ES, and pPNET has been reported as an independent prognostic indicator in patients with localized primary tumours of the distal extremities (69); patients with typical ES having an improved survival compared to those with atypical ES or pPNET. However, more recent studies have found no difference in the outlook between typical and atypical ES (1, 31). Early studies suggested that the degree of differentiation, defined by either morphological or immunohistochemical criteria, was predictive of a worse outcome in ESFT (1, 3, 19, 70), although several recent studies have shown no such correlation (31, 71, 72).

Although much effort has been made to define the differences between ES and pPNET, the identification of EWS–ETS gene rearrangements in both these tumour types is consistent with the hypothesis these tumours are of a common histogenesis and share key cytogenetic abnormalities. This supports the theory that the processes of development and progression of these two tumour types are likely to be similar, and consequently suggests they will respond to the same therapeutic strategies. This is substantiated in current clinical studies, in which the outcome for patients with ES or pPNET is comparable after modern chemotherapy (73). Currently the most important molecular factor in ES and pPNETs is the presence of the EWS–ETS gene rearrangements (see below), although the identification of new molecular markers that define behaviour in ESFT is needed.

The histological response to initial chemotherapy, defined as the development of necrosis, is currently the most powerful histopathological feature of prognostic value (60, 61, 66, 68, 74). A 5-year disease-free survival of 95% is reported in patients with total tumour necrosis post-treatment, compared to 35% in those with little or no necrosis (61). Less than 90% necrosis is reported to be an adverse prognostic factor (61, 75).

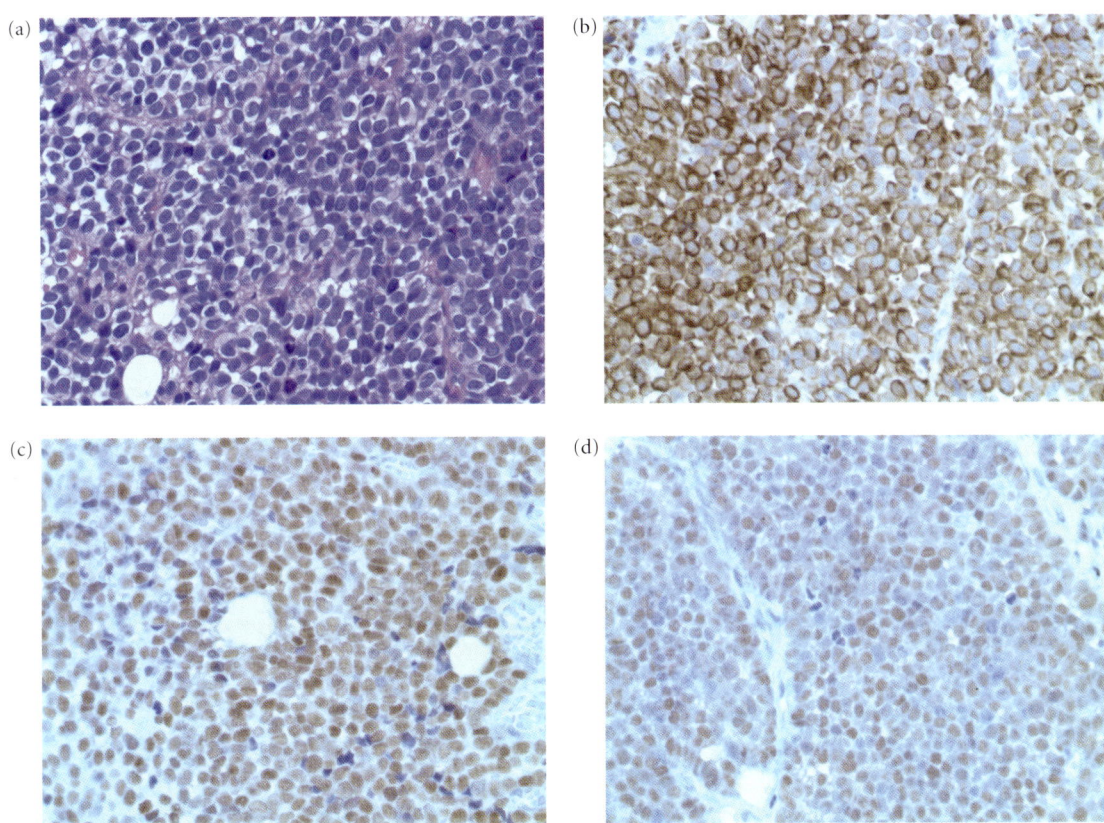

Plate 1. Use of desmin, myogenin, and MYOD1 to distinguish rhabdomyosarcoma from other small RCT.

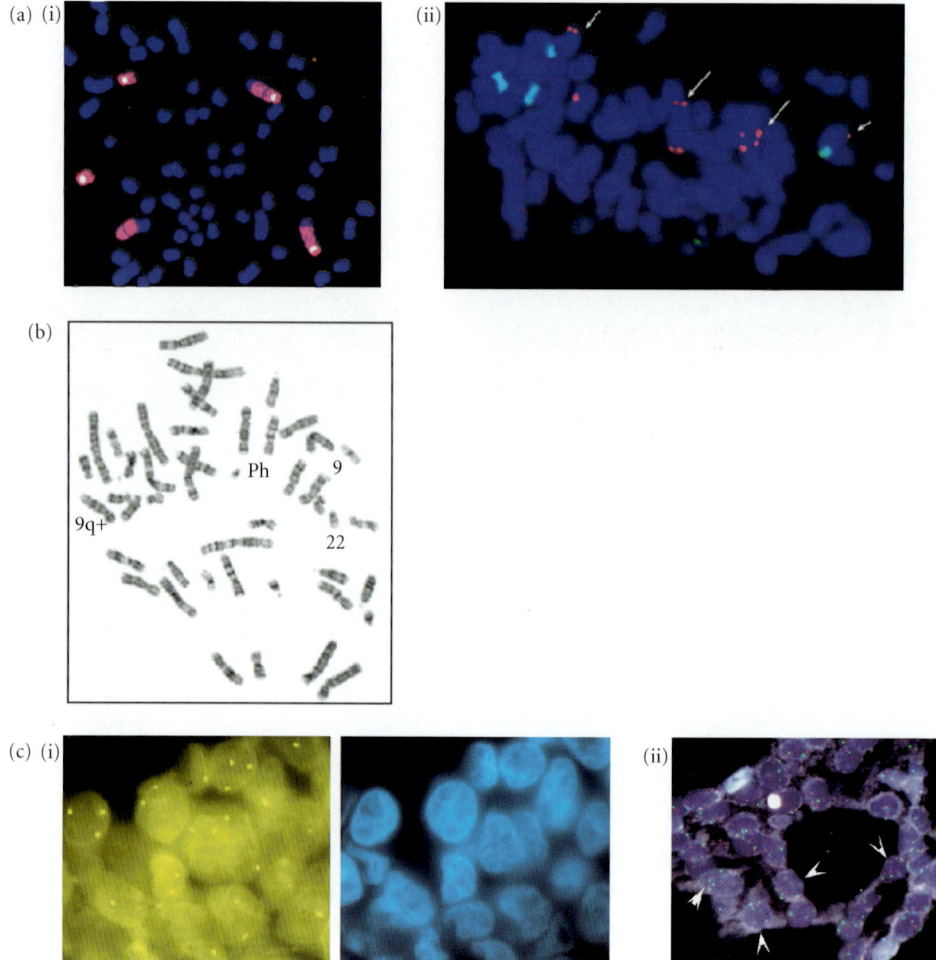

Plate 2. Examples of FISH on metaphase and interphase cells.

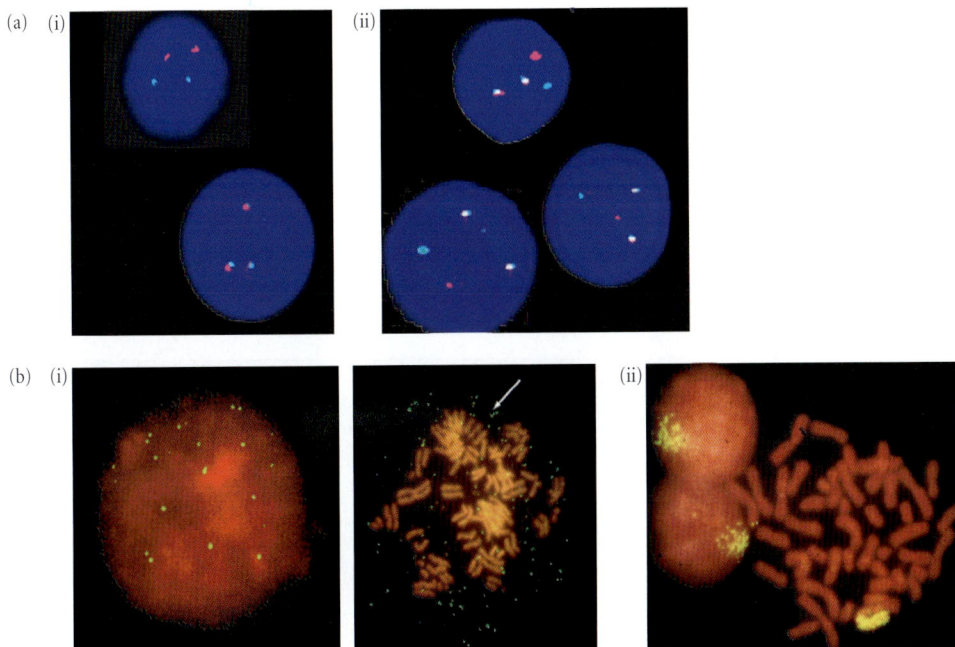

Plate 3. FISH analysis for the detection of translocations and gene amplification.

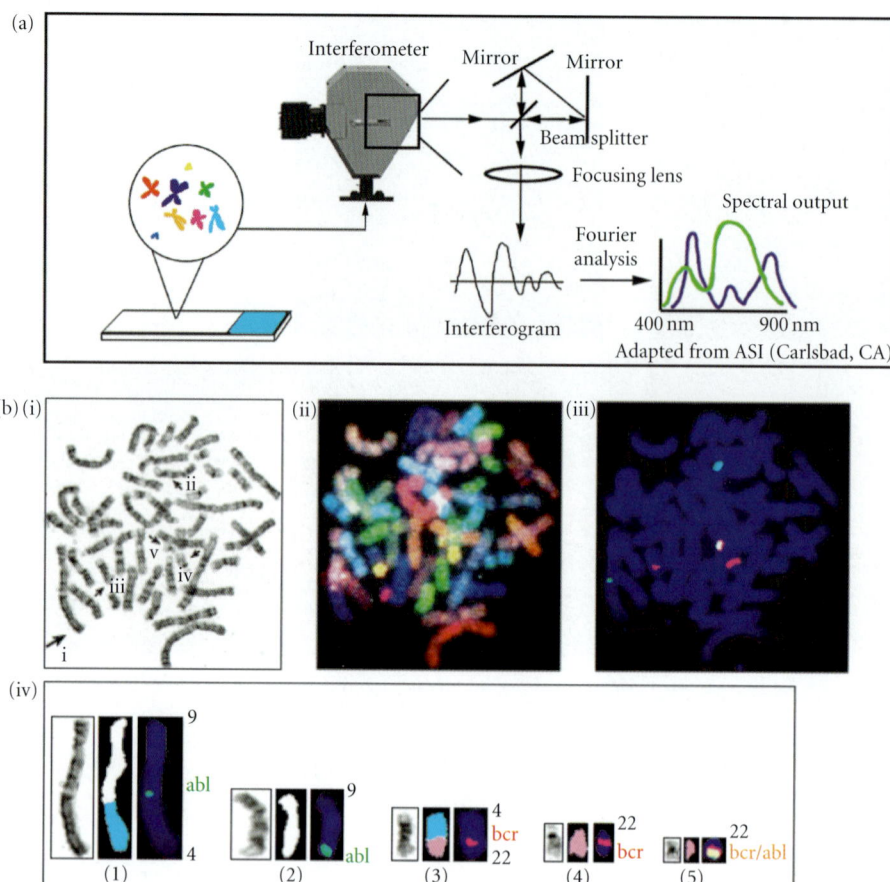

Plate 4. Spectral karyotyping.

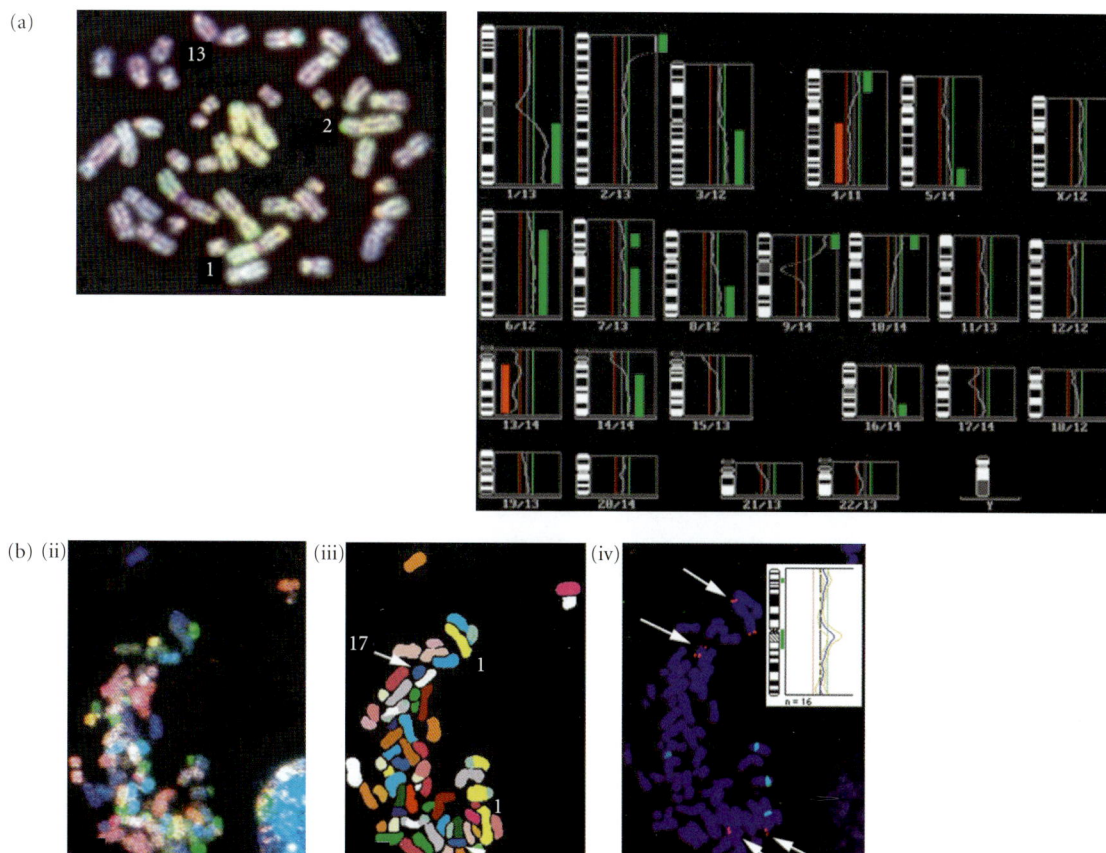

Plate 5. CGH analysis and combined molecular cytogenetic techniques.

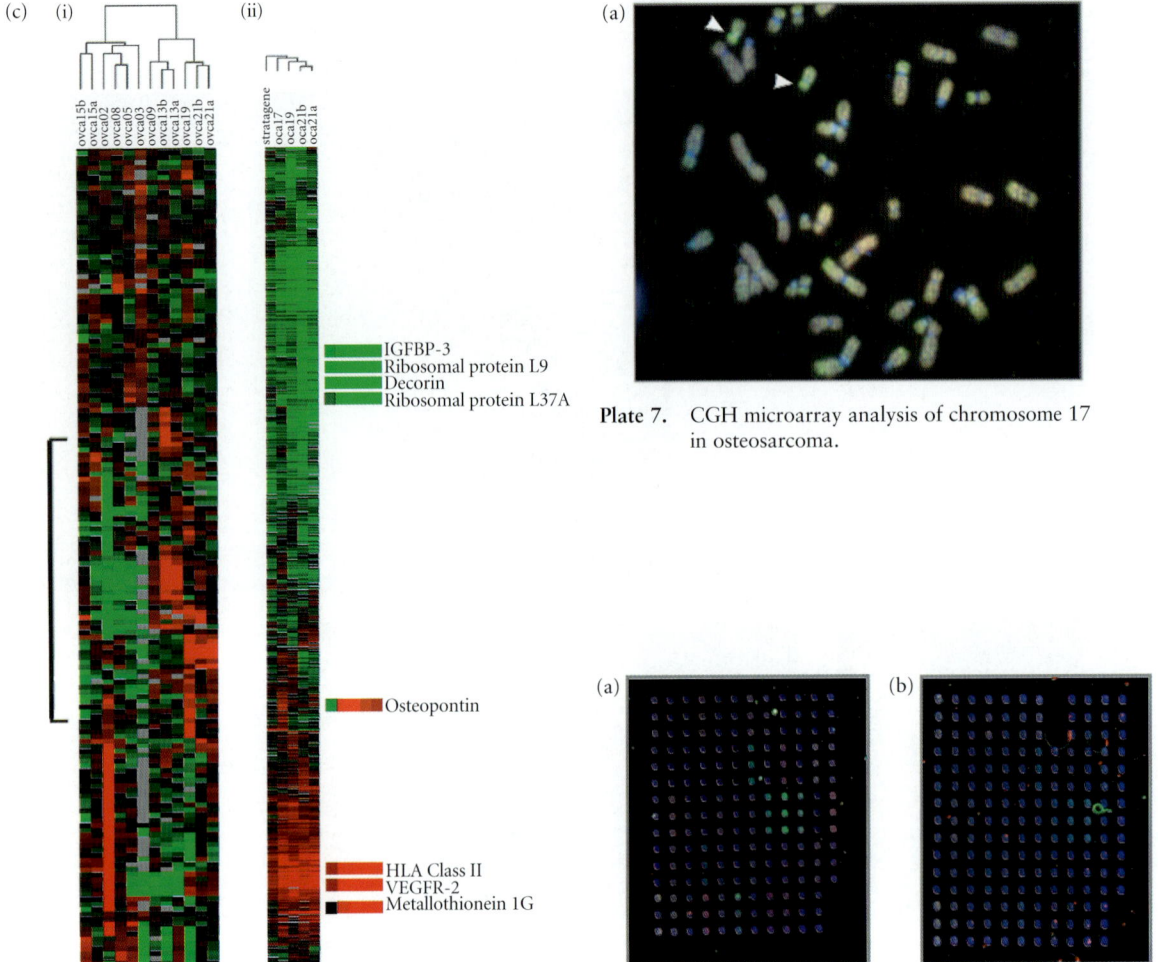

Plate 6. Expression microarray technology.

Plate 7. CGH microarray analysis of chromosome 17 in osteosarcoma.

Plate 8. CGH array using nick translated PCR products.

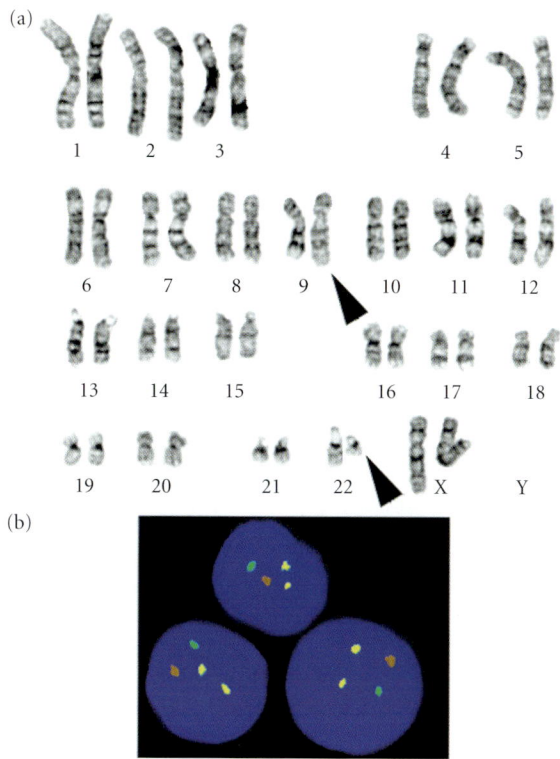

Plate 9. G-banded and interphase FISH analyses of CML.

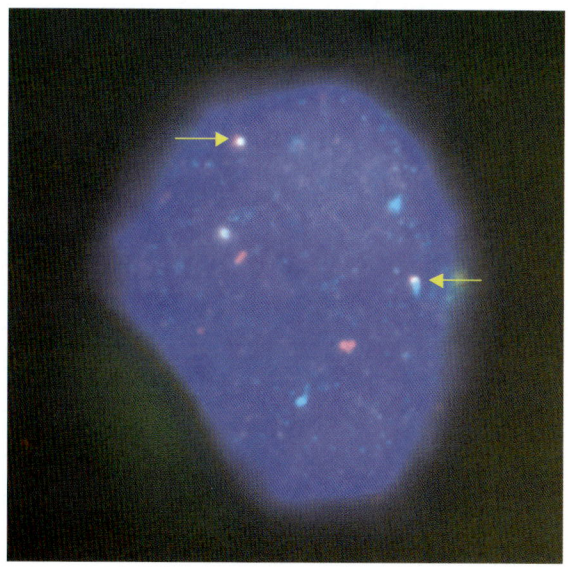

Plate 10. FISH on tetraploid interphase of an ESFT showing 2 copies of t(11.22)(q24.q12).

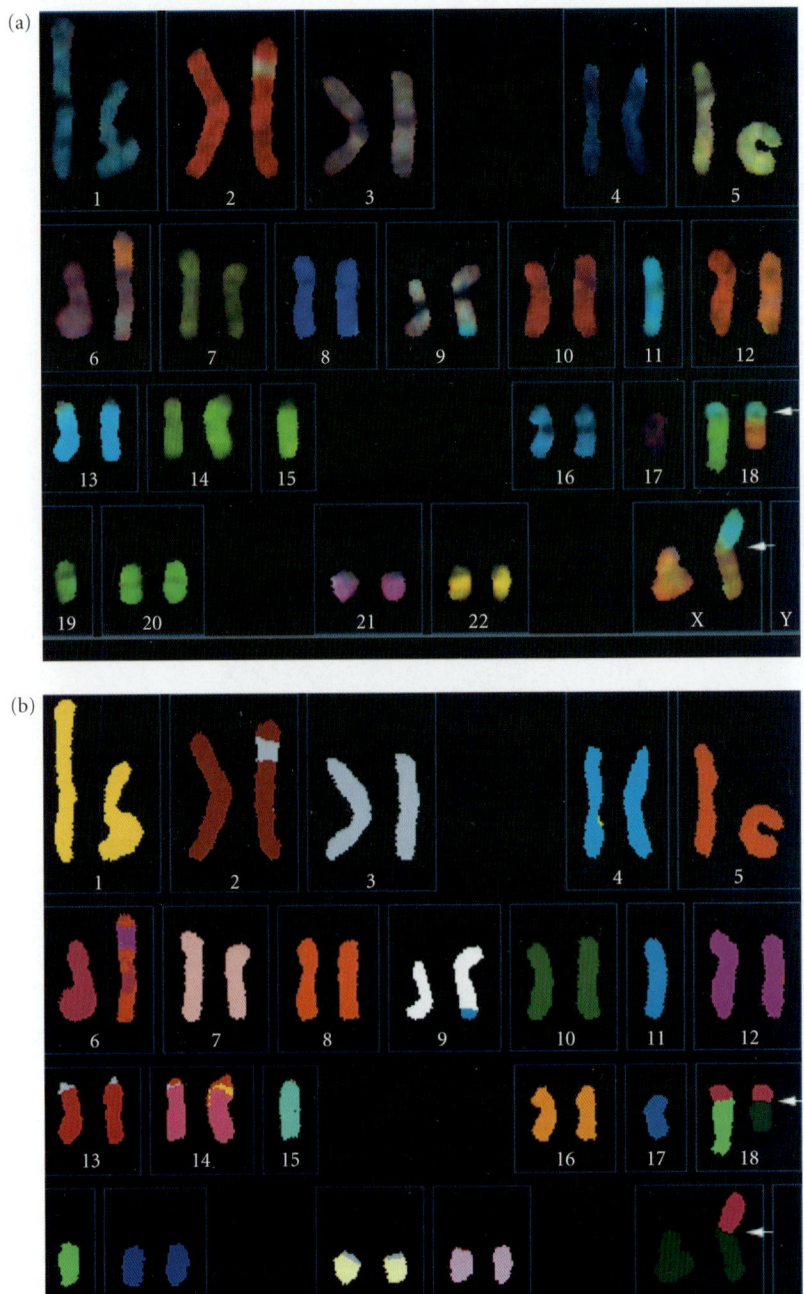

Plate 11. Spectral karyotype of a synovial sarcoma showing primary and secondary aberrations.

However, in the recent CESS 86 report, the prognostic significance of histological response to therapy was lost, probably reflecting adaptation of treatment intensity to initial tumour volume (23). This emphasizes the need to re-evaluate the value of prognostic markers with improved multi-modal therapy.

Genetic

The alternative forms of the EWS–ETS fusion transcripts are reported to be of prognostic significance, either in patients with localized (53) or metastatic disease (26). Tumours with the most common EWS–FLI1 fusion product type 1 (see above) appear to predict a better outcome for patients than those with an EWS–FLI1 type 2 fusion, or indeed any other EWS–ETS fusion transcript type. The type 1 EWS–FLI1 fusion appears to encode a less active chimeric transcription factor than the other fusion transcript types, which may provide the molecular basis for such clinical heterogeneity (76). However, other studies have shown that the two gene fusion products EWS–FLI1 and EWS–ERG do not define distinct clinical phenotypes, suggesting that differences in the c-terminal partner of EWS gene fusions are not associated with significant phenotypic differences (77).

Less frequent secondary chromosomal abnormalities have also been described in ESFT, including trisomy of chromosome 8 (78–82) and 12 (79–81), the unbalanced translocation t(1;16) (78, 82–84), and deletions at the short arm of chromosome 1 (82, 84). The frequency and clinical significance of these secondary chromosome rearrangements is not clear, although initial studies suggest individuals with gain of chromosome 8 may have a poor clinical outcome (79, 81) although this has recently been disputed (84). Deletion of chromosome 1 is reported to be associated with an unfavourable outcome in individuals with localized disease (84). DNA ploidy and proliferation studies of ESFT are limited. Although the number of patients studied is small ($n = 37$), those with diploid tumours are reported to have a good prognosis (58% survival at 7.5 years) compared to those with aneuploid tumours (all patients died of disease) (85). However, a separate flow cytometric study of childhood soft tissue sarcomas suggested 77% of ESFTs were diploid or near diploid, compared to aneuploidy in 23% (86). If both these observations were true for all ESFT, one would predict that the long-term survival for patients with ESFT would be around 77%, which it clearly is not. More complex karyotypes and multiple chromosomal aberrations in ESFT appear to be associated with poor outcome (82, 87).

In ESFT abrogation of the G1 checkpoint appears to be important in the progression and development of clinical phenotype (88–90), consistent with the hypothesis of unchecked cell division. Frequent aberrations include homozygous deletions and/or mutations of the INK4a gene on chromosome 9p21 (88, 91), and mutation of the $p21^{WAF}$ gene and/or down-regulation of its nuclear expression (90, 92). However, loss of pRb expression (88, 90), and mutations of p53 (89, 92–94) are rare events. Amplification of the MDM2 gene which inactivates p53 protein is also rare in ESFTs (89, 95), consistent with the hypothesis that p53 and regulators of its activity may not play a dominant role in ESFT's transformation and progression. However, one study has suggested that expression of p53 (<15% of cases) correlates with a poor prognosis (96). Unlike neuroblastoma, ESFTs do not demonstrate MYCN amplification but do express high levels of MYCC (97–99).

Expression of the proliferation antigens Ki 67 (61, 100, 101) and PCNA (100) are relatively high in ESFT, although the clinical significance of the proliferation index in ESFT at diagnosis is not clear. This uncertainty most likely reflects the variability in reported proliferation index and the small number of patients studied. However, a correlation between proliferation index and necrosis with disease-free overall survival suggests this may be a useful prognostic marker (61). This is supported by our own studies showing a relationship between proliferation index, apoptosis, and prognosis (Burchill, unpublished observation). Proliferation index is also reported to correlate with expression of the proto-oncogene MYCC (101) and EWS–FLI1 fusion transcript type (102), both of which are thought to play a role in the ESFT phenotype. However, unlike EWS–FLI1 fusion transcript type, expression of MYCC appears not to be of prognostic significance (97–99). Further studies have suggested the relationship between EWS–FLI1 fusion transcript type and proliferation may reflect differential regulation of the insulin growth factor receptor 1 pathway (102), which is thought to be important in the biology of ESFT (103–105).

Rare primitive neuroectodermal tumours

Malignant ectomesenchymoma is a very rare malignant tumour with neoplastic mesenchymal and neuroblastic components (1). The name is derived from ectomesenchyme, the embryonic migratory pluripotential cells of the neural crest. The majority present in young children usually before age 3 years, with a third of cases arising in infancy (106). The abdomen is the commonest site followed by perineum, head, and neck, and rarely extremity (106) and kidney (107). Typically in children these tumours consists of a rhabomyosarcoma (embryonal or alveolar) and ganglion cells, with less frequent foci of primitive neuroblastic elements. Cartilaginous foci may be present (106, 107). MIC2 is reported to be negative and a normal karyotype detected in the small number of cases examined (106). It has been suggested, however, that a subset of the tumours may be related to ESFT; biphenotypic tumours with features of neural and myogenic differentiation and the t(11;22)(q24;q12) may represent 'primitive' malignant ectomesenchymomas and account for up to 10% of primitive sarcomas with myogenic differentiation (38, 108). Malignant ectomesenchymoma may be a heterogenous group of neoplasms with different genotypes and origins (107). The outcome is similar to that expected for rhabdomyosarcoma. Older age, large tumour size, alveolar rhabdomyosarcoma component, and lymph node dissemination appear to be adverse prognostic features (106).

Esthesioneuroblastoma (Olfactory neuroblastoma) (ENB) is a very uncommon locally aggressive tumour of the nasal cavity and presents usually in adulthood in the 5th decade and rarely in children in the 2nd decade (1). Histologically it typically consists of nests of small round hyperchromatic cells in a fibrillary background (109). It is positive for neuroendocrine markers and negative for MIC2 antigen. It appears to arise from neuronal or neuroendocrine cells of the olfactory mucosa. The histology overlaps with neuroblastoma and ESFT. Clinical presentation differs from neuroblastoma and absence of expression of the enzyme tyrosine hydroxylase, which is widely expressed in neuroblastoma, and absence of *MYCN* amplification suggests that these tumours are not neuroblastomas (110). A relationship with ESFT was suggested by the presence of the reciprocal translocation t(11;22)(q24;q12) (111) as well as expression of EWS–FLI1 transcripts (110). Subsequent studies however have not found any *EWS* rearrangements in ENB (109, 112, 113) indicating that they are unrelated to ESFT. Trisomy 8 has also been identified and although also noted in ESFT it is not a tumour specific feature, being reported in a variety of small cell tumours (113, 114).

Melanotic neuroectodermal tumour of infancy (MNETI) is a rare distinctive neoplasm that occurs almost exclusively in children, usually in infancy (115, 116). It is also called retinal anlage tumour. The vast majority arise in the maxilla, and infrequently in brain, mediastinum, and genital tract (115, 116). Serum and urinary catecholamine metabolites and serum alpha-fetoprotein levels may be raised (117, 118). It is characterized histologically by a biphasic population of cells; neuroblasts in a neurofibrillary stroma, and larger epithelial cells with abundant cytoplasm containing melanin pigment. Focal desmin positivity and rhabdomyoblastic differentiation may also be present (119, 120).

Because they are so rare little information is available regarding their molecular profile. A study of three cases demonstrated absence of neuroblastoma features such as 1p deletion and MYCN amplification. In addition *EWS* gene rearrangements, characteristic of ESFT and DSRCT, were not detected by RT-PCR (121).

The majority follow a benign course but local recurrence occurs in 15–45% of cases and an aggressive malignant course is pursued in fewer than 7% of cases (116, 119).

In summary, improved diagnostic and staging methodologies leading to better risk group analysis are essential so that treatment and clinical management of children and young adults with ESFT can be tailored appropriately. The identification and characterization of the *EWS* gene rearrangements in ESFT has been the most important advance made in these tumours in the last decade, leading to improvements in diagnosis and potentially prognosis. Current biological investigations of these gene fusions will define targets for much needed novel therapeutic approaches. The elucidation of specific pathogenetic phenotypes will provide insight into the development and progression of the primitive neuroectodermal family of tumours that may ultimately be of benefit to individuals afflicted with these diseases.

Acknowledgements

Thank you to Mr Paul Roberts, Department of Cytogenetics, St James's University Hospital for allowing us to reproduce Figs 9.4 and 9.6.

References

1. Tsokos M. Peripheral primitive neuroectodermal tumors. Diagnosis, classification, and prognosis. Perspect Pediatr Pathol 1992, 16, 27–98. In: Molecular pathology: quantitation and applications (ed. Garvin AJ, O'Leary TJ, Bernstein J, Rosenberg HS). Karger, Basel.

2. Schmidt D. Malignant peripheral neuroectodermal tumor. In: Current topics in pathology, Vol. 89 (ed. Harms D, Schmidt D). Springer-Verlag, Berlin, Heidelberg, 1995.
3. Dehner LP. Primitive neuroectodermal tumor and Ewing's sarcoma. Am J Surg Pathol 1993, 17, 1–13.
4. Ambros IM, Ambros PF, Strehl S, Kovar H, Gadner H, Salzer-Kuntschik. MIC2 is a specific marker for Ewing's sarcoma and peripheral primitive neuroectodermal tumors. Evidence of a common histogenesis of Ewing's sarcoma and peripheral primitive neuroectodermal tumors from MIC2 expression and specific chromosome aberration. Cancer 1991, 67, 1886–93.
5. Dehner LP. Neuroepithelioma (primitive neuroectodermal tumor) and Ewing's sarcoma. At least a partial consensus. Arch Pathol Lab Med 1994, 118, 606–7.
6. Huvos AG. Ewings sarcoma. In: Bone tumors: diagnosis, treatment and prognosis, 2nd edn (ed. Huvos AG). PA Sanders, Philadelphia, 1991, 523–52.
7. Cotterill SJ, Parker L, Malcolm AJ, Reid M, More L, Craft AW. Incidence and survival for cancer in children and young adults in the North of England, 1968–1995: a report from the Northern Region Young Persons' Malignant Disease Registry. Br J Cancer 2000, 83, 397–403.
8. Hutter RVP, Francis KC, Foote FW. Ewing's sarcoma in siblings. Am J Surg 1964, 107, 598.
9. Zamora P, Garcia de Paredes ML, Gonzalez Baron M, Diaz MA, Escobar Y, Ordonez A, Lopez Barea F, Gonzalez JM. Ewing's tumor in brothers. An unusual observation. Am J Clin Oncol 1986, 9, 358–60.
10. Joyce MJ, Harmon DC, Mankin HJ, Suit HD, Schiller AL, Truman JT. Ewing's sarcoma in female siblings: a clinical report and review of the literature. Cancer 1984, 53, 1959–62.
11. Grier HE. The Ewing family of tumors. Ewing's sarcoma and primitive neuroectodermal tumors. Pediatr Clin North Am 1997, 44, 991–1004.
12. Harms D. Soft tissue sarcoma in the Kiel Pediatric Registry. Curr Top Pathol 1995, 89, 31–45.
13. Kimber C, Michalski A, Spitz L, Pierro A. Primitive neuroectodermal tumours: anatomic location, extent of surgery, and outcome. J Pediatr Surg 1998, 33, 39–41.
14. Marley ER, Liapis H, Humphrey PA, Nadler RB, Siegel CL, Zhu X, Brand JM, Dehner LP. Primitive neuroectodermal tumor of the kidney-another enigma: pathologic, immunohistochemical, and molecular diagnostic study. Am J Surg Pathol 1997, 21, 354–9.
15. Smith LM, Adams RH, Brothman AR, Vanderhooft SL, Coffin CM. Peripheral primitive neuroectodermal tumor presenting with diffuse cutaneous involvement and 7; 22 translocation. Med Pediatr Oncol 1998, 30, 357–63.
16. Hasegawa SL, Davison JM, Rutten A, Fletcher CDM. Primary cutaneous Ewing's sarcoma. Immunophenotypic and molecular cytogenetic evaluation of 5 cases. Am J Surg Pathol 1998, 22, 300–8.
17. Danner DB, Hiruban RH, Pitt HA, Hayashi R, Griffin CA, Perlman EJ. Primitive neuroectodermal tumor arising in the pancreas. Mod Pathol 1994, 7, 200–4.
18. Tsuji S, Hisoaka M, Morimitsu Hashimoto H, Jimi A, Watanabe J, Eguchi H, Kaneko Y. Peripheral primitive neuroectodermal tumour of the lung: report of two cases. Histopathology 1998, 33, 369–74.
19. Schmidt D, Hermann C, Jurgens H, Harms D. Malignant peripheral neuroectodermal tumor and its necessary distinction from Ewing's sarcoma: a report from the Kiel Pediatric Tumor Registry. Cancer 1991, 68, 2251–9.
20. Granowetter L. Ewing's sarcoma and extracranial primitive neuroectodermal tumors. Curr Opin Oncol 1992, 4, 696–703.
21. Kinsella TJ, Miser JS, Waller B, Venzon D, Glatstein E, Weaver-McClure L, Horowitz ME. Long-term follow-up of Ewing's sarcoma of bone treated with combined modality therapy. Int J Radiat Oncol Biol Phys 1991, 20, 389–95.
22. Sandoval C, Meyer WH, Parham DM, Kun LE, Hustu HO, Luo X, Pratt CB. Outcome of 43 children presenting with metastatic Ewing sarcoma: the St. Jude Children's Research Hospital experience, 1962 to 1992. Med Pediatr Oncol 1996, 26, 180–5.
23. Arhens S, Hoffman C, Jabar S, Braun-Munzinger G, Paulussen M, Dunst J, Rube C, Winkelman W, Heinecke A, Gobel U, Winkler K, Harms D, Treuner J, Jurgens H. Evaluation of prognostic factors in a tumor volume-adapted treatment strategy for localised Ewing's sarcoma of bone: the CESS 86 experience. Cooperative Ewing Sarcoma Study. Med Ped Oncol 1999, 32930, 186–95.
24. Peter M, Magdelenat H, Michon J, Melot T, Oberlin O, Zucker JM, Thomas G, Delattre O. Sensitive detection of occult Ewing's cells by the reverse transcriptase-polymerase chain reaction. Br J Cancer 1995, 72, 96–100.
25. West DC, Grier HE, Swallow MM, Demetri GD, Granowetter L, Sklar J. Detection of circulating tumor cells in patients with Ewing's sarcoma and peripheral primitive neuroectodermal tumor. J Clin Oncol 1997, 15, 583–8.
26. de Alava E, Lozano MD, Patino A, Sierrasesumaga L, Pardo-Mindan FJ. Ewing family tumours: potential prognostic value of reverse-transcriptase polymerase chain reaction detection of minimal residual disease in peripheral blood samples. Diagn Mol Pathol 1998, 7, 152–7.
27. Williams S, Parham DM, Jenkins JJ 3rd. Peripheral neuroepithelioma with ganglion cells: report of two cases and review of the literature. Pediatr Dev Pathol 1999, 2, 42–9.
28. Huijgen HJ, Sanders GT, Koster RW, Vreeken J, Bossuyt PM. The clinical value of lactate dehydrogenase in serum: a quantitative review. Eur J Clin Chem Clin Biochem 1997, 35, 569–79.
29. Bacci G, Ferrari S, Longhi A, Rimondini S, Versari M, Zanone A, Forni C. Prognostic significance of serum LDH in Ewing's sarcoma of bone. Oncol Rep 1999, 6, 807–11.
30. Hannisdal E, Solheim OP, Theodorsen L, Host H. Alterations of blood analyses at relapse of osteosarcoma and Ewing's sarcoma. Acta Oncol 1990, 29, 585–7.
31. Parham DM, Hijazi Y, Steinberg SM, Meyer WH, Horowitz M, Tzen CY, Wexler LH, Tsokos M. Neuroectodermal differentiation in Ewing's sarcoma family of tumors does not predict tumor behaviour. Hum Pathol 1999, 30, 911–18.
32. Cavazzana AO, Miser JS, Jefferson J, Triche TJ. Experimental evidence for a neural origin of Ewing's sarcoma of bone. Am J Pathol 1987, 127, 507–18.
33. Sugimoto T, Umezawa A, Hata J. Neurogenic potential of Ewing's sarcoma cells. Virchows Arch 1997, 430, 41–6.
34. Thiele CJ. Pediatric peripheral neuroectodermal tumors, oncogenes, and differentiation. Cancer Invest 1990, 8, 629–39.

35. Thiele CJ. Biology of pediatric peripheral neuroectodermal tumors. Cancer Metastasis Rev 1991, 10, 311–19.
36. O'Regan S, Diebler MF, Meunier FM, Vyas SA. Ewing's sarcoma cell line showing some, but not all, of the traits of a cholinergic neuron. J Neurochem 1995, 64, 69–76.
37. Hachitanda Y, Tsuneyoshi M, Enjoji M, Nakagawara A, Ikeda K. Congenital primitive neuroectodermal tumor with epithelial and glial differentiation. An ultrastructural and immunohistochemical study. Arch Pathol Lab Med 1990, 114, 101–5.
38. Sorensen PHB, Shimada H, Liu XF, Lim JF, Thomas G, Triche TJ. Biphenotypic sarcomas with myogenic and neural differentiation express the Ewing's sarcoma *EWS/FLI1* fusion gene. Cancer Res 1995, 55, 1385–92.
39. Mierau GW, Weeks DA, Hicks MJ. Role of electron microscopy and other special techniques in the diagnosis of childhood round cell tumors. Hum Pathol 1998, 29, 1347–55.
40. Fellinger EJ, Garin-Chesa P, Glasser DB, Huvos AG, Rettig WJ. Comparison of cell surface antigen HBA71 (p30/32MIC2), neuron-specific enolase, and vimentin in the immunohistochemical analysis of Ewing's sarcoma of bone. Am J Surg Pathol 1992, 16, 746–55.
41. Ramani P, Rampling D, Link M. Immunocytochemical study of 12E7 in small round-cell tumours in childhood: an assessment of its sensitivity and specificity. Histopathology 1993, 23, 557–61.
42. Weidner N, Tjoe J. Immunohistochemical profile of monoclonal antibody 013: antibody that recognises glycoprotein p30/32 MIC2 and is useful in diagnosing Ewing's sarcoma and peripheral neuroepithelioma. Am J Surg Pathol 1994, 18, 486–94.
43. Perlman EJ, Dickman PS, Askin FB, Grier HE, Miser JS, Link MP. Ewing's sarcoma—routine diagnostic utilization of MIC2 analysis: a pediatric oncology group/children's cancer group intergroup study. Hum Path 1994, 25, 304–7.
44. Lee CS, Southey MC, Waters K, Kannourakis G, Georgiou T, Armes JE, Chow CW, Venter DJ. EWS/FLI1 fusion transcript and MIC2 immunohistochemical staining in the diagnosis of Ewing's sarcoma. Pediatr Pathol Lab Med 1996, 16, 379–92.
45. Smith MJ, Goodfellow PJ, Goodfellow PN. The genomic organisation of the human pseudoautosomal gene MIC2 and the detection of a related locus. Hum Mol Genet 1993, 2, 417–22.
46. Granter SR, Renshaw AA, Fletcher CD, Bhan AK, Rosenberg AE. CD99 reactivity in mesenchymal chondrosarcoma. Hum Pathol 1996, 27, 1273–6.
47. Fanburg-Smith, JC, Hengge M, Hengge UR, Smith JS, Jr, Miettinen M. Extrarenal rhabdoid tumors of soft tissue: a clinicopathologic and immunohistochemical study of 18 cases. Ann Diagn Pathol 1998, 2, 351–62.
48. Fisher C. Synovial sarcoma. Ann Diagn Pathol 1998, 2, 401–21.
49. Gordon MD, Corless C, Renshaw AA, Beckstead J. CD99, keratin and vimentin staining in sex cord-stromal tumors, normal ovary and testis. Mod Pathol 1998, 11, 769–73.
50. Sorensen PH, Triche TJ. Gene fusions encoding chimaeric transcription factors in solid tumours. Semin Cancer Biol 1996, 7, 3–14.
51. Urano F, Umezawa A, Hong W, Kikuchi H, Hata J. A novel chimera gene between EWS and EIA-F, encoding the adenovirus enhancing-binding protein, in extraosseous Ewing's sarcoma. Biochem Biophys Res Commun 1996, 219, 608–12.
52. Peter M, Couturier J, Pacquement H, Michon J, Thomas G, Magdelenat H, Delattre O. A new member of the ETS family fused to EWS in Ewing's tumors. Oncogene 1997, 14, 1159–64.
53. Zoubek A, Dockhorn-Dworniczak B, Delattre O, Christiansen H, Niggli F, Gatterer-Menz I, Smith TL, Jurgens H, Gadner H, Kovar H. Does expression of different EWS chimeric transcripts define clinically distinct risk groups of Ewing tumor patients? J Clin Oncol 1996, 14, 1245–51.
54. Thorner P, Squire J, Chilton-MacNeil S, Marrano P, Bayani J, Malkin D, Greenberg M, Lorenzana A, Zielenska M. Is the EWS–FLI-1 fusion transcript specific for Ewing sarcoma and peripheral primitive neuroectodermal tumor? A report of four cases showing this transcript in a wider range of tumor types. Am J Pathol 1996, 148, 1125–38.
55. Burchill SA, Wheeldon J, Cullinane C, Lewis IJ. EWS–FLI1 fusion transcripts identified in patients with typical neuroblastoma. Eur J Cancer 1997, 33, 239–43.
56. Mastik MF, Molenaar WM, Boudewijn E, de Graaf, SSN, Hogendoorn PCW, Van Der Hout AH, Van Den Berg E. Translocation (11;22)(Q24;q120) in a small cell tumor of the thigh in a two-year-old boy: immunohistology, cytogenetics, molecular genetics, and review of the literature. Human Pathol 1999, 30, 352–5.
57. Sainati L, Scapinello A, Montaldi A, Bolcato S, Ninfo V, Carli M, Basso G. A mesenchymal chondrosarcoma of a child with the reciprocal translocation (11; 22)(q24;q12). Cancer Genet Cytogenet 1993, 71, 144–7.
58. Clark J, Benjamin H, Gill S, Sidhar S, Goodwin G, Crew J, Gusterson BA, Shipley J, Cooper CS. Fusion of the EWS gene to CHN, a member of the steroid/thyroid receptor gene superfamily, in a human myxoid chondrosarcoma. Oncogene 1996, 12, 229–35.
59. Peter M, Gilbert E, Delattre O. A multiplex real-time PCR assay for the detection of gene fusions observed in solid tumors Lab Invest 2001, 81, 905–12.
60. Terrier P, Llombart-Bosch A, Contesso G. Small round blue tumors in bone: prognostic factors correlated to Ewing's sarcoma and neuroectodermal tumors. Semin Diagn Pathol 1996, 13, 250–7.
61. Picci P, Böhling T, Bacci G, Ferrari S, Sangiorgi L, Mercuri M, Ruggieri P, Manfrini M, Ferraro A, Casadei R, Benassi MS, Mancini AF, Rosito P, Cazzola A, Barbieri E, Tienghi A, Brach del Prever A, Comandon A, Bacchini P, Bertoni F. Chemotherapy-induced tumor necrosis as a prognostic factor in localized Ewing's sarcoma of the extremities. J Clin Oncol 1997, 15, 1553–9.
62. Pfleiderer C, Zoubek A, Gruber B, Kronberger M, Ambros PF, Lion T, Fink FM, Gadner H, Kovar H. Detection of tumour cells in peripheral blood and bone marrow from Ewing tumour patients by RT-PCR. Int J Cancer 1995, 64(2), 135–9.
63. Toretsky JA, Neckers L, Wexler LH. Detection of (11;22)(q24;q12) translocation-bearing cells in peripheral blood progenitor cells of patients with Ewing's sarcoma family of tumors. J Natl Cancer Inst 1995, Mar 1, 87(5), 385–6.

64. Zoubek A, Ladenstein R, Windhager R, Amann G, Fischmeister G, Kager L, Jugovic D, Ambros PF, Gadner H, Kovar H. Predictive potential of testing for bone marrow involvement in Ewing tumor patients by RT-PCR: a preliminary evaluation. Int J Cancer 1998, Feb 20, **79**(1), 56–60.
65. Fagnou C, Michon J, Peter M, Bernoux A, Oberlin O, Zucker JM, Magdelenat H, Delattre O. Presence of tumor cells in bone marrow but not in blood is associated with adverse prognosis in patients with Ewing's tumor. J Clin Oncol 1998, **16**, 1707–11.
66. Koscielniak E, Jürgens H, Winkler K, Bürger D, Herbst M, Keim M, Bernhard G, Treuner J. Treatment of soft tissue sarcoma in childhood and adolescence. Cancer 1992, **70**, 2557–67.
67. Nesbit ME, Jr, Gehan EA, Burgert EO, Jr, Vietti TJ, Cangir A, Tefft M, Evans R, Thomas P, Askin FB, Kissane JM, et al. Multimodal therapy for the management of primary, nonmetastatic Ewing's sarcoma of bone: a long-term follow-up of the First Intergroup study. J Clin Oncol 1990, **8**, 1664–74.
68. Bacci G, Ferrar, S, Bertoni F, Rimondini S, Longhi A, Bacchini P, Forni C, Manfrini M, Donati D, Picci P. Prognostic factors in nonmetastatic Ewing's sarcoma of bone treated with adjuvant chemotherapy: analysis of 359 patients at the Istituto Ortopedico Rizzoli. J Clin Oncol 2000, **18**, 4–11.
69. Hartman KR, Triche TJ, Kinsella TJ, Miser JS. Prognostic value of histopathology in Ewing's sarcoma. Long-term follow-up of distal extremity primary tumors. Cancer 1991, **67**, 163–71.
70. Brinkhuis M, Wijnaendts LC, van der Linden JC, van Unnik AJ, Voute PA, Baak JP, Meijer CJ. Peripheral primitive neuroectodermal tumour and extra-osseous Ewing's sarcoma; a histological, immunohistochemical and DNA flow cytometric study. Virchows Arch 1995, **425**, 611–16.
71. Terrier P, Henry-Amar M, Triche TJ, Horowitz ME, Terrier-Lacombe MJ, Miser JS, Kinsella TJ, Contesso G, Llombart-Bosch A. Is neuro-ectodermal differentiation of Ewing's sarcoma of bone associated with an unfavourable prognosis? Eur J Cancer 1995, **31A**, 307–14.
72. Luksch R, Sampietro G, Collini P, Boracchi P, Massimino M, Lombardi F, Gandola L, Giardini R, Fossati-Bellani F, Migliorini L, Pilotti S, Scopsi L. Prognostic value of clinicopathologic characteristics including neuroectodermal differentiation in osseous Ewing's sarcoma family of tumors in children. Tumori 1999, **85**,101–7.
73. Wexler LH, Meyer WH, Parham DM, Tsokos M. Neural differentiation and prognosis in peripheral primitive neuroectodermal tumor. J Clin Oncol 2000, **18**, 2187–8.
74. Göbel V, Jürgens H, Etspüler G, Kemperdick H, Jungblut RM, Stienen U, Göbel U. Prognostic significance of tumor volume in localized Ewing's sarcoma of bone in children and adolescents. J Cancer Res Clin Oncol 1987, **113**, 187–91.
75. Van der Woude HJ, Bloem JL, Taminiau AHM, Nooy MA, Hoogendoorn PCW. Classification of histopathologic changes following chemotherapy in Ewing's sarcoma of bone. Skeletal Radiol 1994, **23**(7), 501–7.
76. Lin PP, Brody RI, Hamelin AC, Bradner JE, Healey JH, Ladanyi M. Differential transactivation by alternative EWS–FLI1 fusion proteins correlates with clinical heterogeneity in Ewing's sarcoma. Cancer Res 1999, **59**, 1428–32.
77. Ginsberg JP, de Alava E, Ladanyi M, Wexler LH, Kovar H, Paulussen M, Zoubek A, Dockhorn-Dworniczak B, Juergens H, Wunder JS, Andrulis IL, Malik R, Sorensen PH, Womer RB, Barr FG. EWS–FLI1 and EWS–ERG gene fusions are associated with similar clinical phenotypes in Ewing's sarcoma. J Clin Oncol 1999, **17**, 1809–14.
78. Mugneret F, Lizard S, Aurias A, Turc-Carel C. Chromosomes in Ewing's sarcoma. II. Nonrandom additional changes, trisomy 8 and der(16)t(1;16). Cancer Genet Cytogenet 1988, **32**, 239–45.
79. Armengol G, Tarkkanen M, Virolainen M, Forus A, Valle J, Bohling T, Asko-Seljavaara S, Blomqvist C, Elomaa I, Karaharju E, Kivioja AH, Siimes MA, Tukiainen E, Caballin MR, Myklebost O, Knuutila S. Recurrent gains of 1q, 8 and 12 in the Ewing family of tumours by comparative genomic hybridisation. Br J Cancer 1997, **75**, 1403–9.
80. Maurici D, Perez-Atayde A, Grier HE, Baldini N, Serra M, Fletcher JA. Frequency and implications of chromosome 8 and 12 gains in Ewing sarcoma. Cancer Genet Cytogenet 1998, **100**, 106–10.
81. Tarkkanen M, Kiuru-Kuhlefelt S, Blomqvist C, Armengol G, Bohling T, Ekfors T, Virolainen M, Lindholm T, Monge O, Picci P, Knuutila S, Elomaa I. Clinical correlations of genetic changes by comparative genomic hybridization in Ewing sarcoma and related tumors. Cancer Genet Cytogenet 1999, **114**, 35–41.
82. Zielenska M, Zhang ZM, Ng K, Marrano P, Bayani J, Ramirez OC, Sorensen P, Thorner P, Greenberg M, Squire JA. Acquisition of secondary structural chromosomal changes in pediatric ewing sarcoma is a probable prognostic factor for tumor response and clinical outcome. Cancer 2001, **91**, 2156–64.
83. Douglass EC, Rowe ST, Valentine M, Parham D, Meyer WH, Thompson EI. A second nonrandom translocation, der(16)t(1;16)(q21;q13), in Ewing sarcoma and peripheral neuroectodermal tumor. Cytogenet Cell Genet 1990, **53**, 87–90.
84. Hattinger CM, Rumpler S, Strehl S, Ambros IM, Zoubek A, Pötschger U, Gadner H, Ambros PF. Prognostic impact of deletions at lp36 and numerical aberrations in Ewing tumors. Genes Chromosomes Cancer 1999, **24**, 243–54.
85. Dierick AM, Langlois M, van Oostveldt, Roels H. The prognostic significance of the DNA content in Ewing's sarcoma: a retrospective cytophotometric and flow cytometric study. Histopathology 1993, **23**, 333–9.
86. Niggli FK, Powell JE, Parkes SE, Ward K, Raafat F, Mann JR, Stevens MC. DNA ploidy and proliferative activity (S-phase) in childhood soft-tissue sarcomas: their value as prognostic indicators. Br J Cancer 1994, **69**, 1106–10.
87. Kullendorff CM, Mertens F, Donner M, Wiebe T, Akerman M, Mandahl N. Cytogenetic aberrations in Ewing sarcoma: are secondary changes associated with clinical outcome? Med Pediatr Oncol 1999, **32**, 79–83.
88. Kovar H, Jug G, Aryee DN, Zoubek A, Ambros P, Gruber B, Windhager R, Gadner H. Among genes involved in the RB dependent cell cycle regulatory cascade, the p16 tumor suppressor gene is frequently lost in the Ewing family of tumors. Oncogene 1997, **15**, 2225–32.
89. Lopez-Guerrero JA, Pellin A, Noguera R, Carda C, Llombart-Bosch A. Molecular analysis of the 9p21 locus and p53 genes in Ewing family tumors. Lab Invest 2001, **81**, 803–14.

90. Maitra A, Roberts H, Weinberg AG, Geradts J. Aberrant expression of tumor suppressor proteins in the Ewing family of tumors. Arch Pathol Lab Med 2001, 125(9), 1207–12.
91. Wei G, Antonescu CR, de Alava E, Leung D, Huvos AG, Meyers PA, Healey JH, Ladanyi M. Prognostic impact of INK4A deletion in Ewing sarcoma. Cancer 2000, 89, 793–9.
92. de Alava E, Gerald WL. Molecular biology of the Ewing's sarcoma/primitive neuroectodermal tumor family. J Clin Oncol 2000, 18, 204–13.
93. Wadayama B, Toguchida J, Yamaguchi T, Sasaki MS, Yamamuro T. P53 expression and its relationship to DNA alterations in bone and soft tissue sarcomas. Br J Cancer 1993, 68, 1134–9.
94. Radig K, Schneider-Stock R, Rose I, Mittler U, Oda Y, Roessner A. p53 and ras mutations in Ewing's sarcoma. Pathol Res Pract 1998, 194, 157–62.
95. Kovar H, Auinger A, Jug G, Aryee D, Zoubek A, Salzer-Kuntschik M, Gadner H. Narrow spectrum of infrequent p53 mutations and absence of MDM2 amplification in Ewing tumours. Oncogene 1993, 8, 2683–90.
96. Abudu A, Mangham DC, Reynolds GM, Pynsent PB, Tillman RM, Carter SR, Grimer RJ. Overexpression of the p53 protein in primary Ewing's sarcoma of bone: relationship to tumour stage, response and prognosis. Br J Cancer 1999, 79, 1185–9.
97. Thiele CJ, McKeon C, Triche TJ, Ross RA, Reynolds CP, Israel MA. Differential protooncogene expression characterises histopathologically tumors of the peripheral nervous system. J Clin Invest 1987, 80, 804–11.
98. McKeon C, Thiele J, Ross RA, Kwan M, Triche TJ, Miser JS, Israel MA. Indistinguishable patterns of protooncogene expression in two distinct but closely related tumors: Ewing's sarcoma and neuroepithelioma. Cancer Res 1988, 48, 4307–11.
99. Yeger H, Mor O, Pawlin G, Kapkinsky C, Shiloh Y. Importance of phenotypic and molecular characterisation for identification of a neuroepithelioma tumor cell line, NUB-20. Cancer Res 1990, 50, 2794–802.
100. Hicks J, Murray J, Dreyer Z, Horowitz M, Ostrowski M, Brown R, Smith B, Spjut H. Expression of proliferation-associated markers and glycoprotein p30/32^{MIC2} in Ewing's sarcoma: a clinicopathologic study. Am J Clin Pathol 1995, Abstract 104, 352.
101. Sollazzo MR, Benassi SS, Mogagnoli G, Gamberi G, Molendini L, Ragazzini P, Merli M, Ferrari C, Balladelli A, Picci P. Increased C-MYC oncogene expression in Ewing's sarcoma: correlation with Ki67 proliferation index. Tumori 1999, 85, 167–73.
102. de Alava E, Panizo A, Antonescu CR, Huvos AG, Pardo-Mindán FJ, Barr FG, Ladanyi M. Association of EWS–FLI1 type 1 fusion with lower proliferative rate in Ewing's sarcoma. Am J Pathol 2000, 156, 849–55.
103. Hofbauer S, Hamilton G, Theyer G, Wollmann K, Gabor F. Insulin-like growth factor-I-dependent growth and *in vitro* chemosensitivity of Ewing's sarcoma and peripheral primitive neuroectodermal tumour cell lines. Eur J Cancer 1993, 29, 241–5.
104. Scotlandi K, Benini S, Sarti M, Serra M, Lollini PL, Maurici D, Picci P, Manara MC, Baldini N. Insulin-like growth factor I receptor-mediated circuit in Ewing's sarcoma/peripheral neuroectodermal tumor: a possible therapeutic target. Cancer Res 1996, 56, 4570–4.
105. Xie Y, Skytting B, Nilsson G, Brodin B, Larsson O. Expression of insulin-like growth factor-1 receptor in synovial sarcoma: association with an aggressive phenotype. Cancer Res 1999, 59, 3588–91.
106. Boue DR, Parham DM, Webber B, Crist WM, Qualman SJ. Clinicopathologic study of ectomesenchymomas from Intergroup Rhabdomyosarcoma Study Groups 111 and 1V. Pediatr Dev Pathol 2000, 3, 290–300.
107. Goldsby RE, Bruggers CS, Brothman AR, Sorensen PHB, Beckwith JB, Pysher TJ. Spindle cell sarcoma of the kidney with ganglionic elements (malignant ectomesenchymoma) associated with chromosomal abnormalities and a review of the literature. J Pediatr Hematol/Oncol 1998, 20(2), 160–4.
108. Galili N, Davis RJ, Fredericks WJ, Mukhopadhyay S, Rauscher FJ 3rd, Emanuel BS, Rovera G, Barr FG. Fusion of a fork head domain gene to PAX3 in the solid tumour alveolar rhabdomyosarcoma. Nat Genet 1994, 5, 230–5 [Published erratum appears in Nat Genet, 6, 214].
109. Argani P, Perez-Ordonez B, Xiao H, Caruana SM, Huvos AG, Ladanyi M. Olfactory neuroblastoma is not related to the Ewing family of tumors: absence of EWS/FLI1 gene fusion and MIC2 expression. Am J Surg Pathol 1998, 22, 391–8.
110. Sorensen PHB, Wu JK, Berean KW, Lim JF, Donn W, Frierson HF, Reynolds CP, Lopez-Terrada D, Triche TJ. Olfactory neuroblastoma is a peripheral neuroectodermal tumor related to Ewing sarcoma. Proc Natl Acad Sci, USA, 93, 1038–43.
111. Whang-Peng J, Freter CE, Knutsen T, Nanfro JJ, Gazdar A. Translocation t(11;22) in esthesioneuroblastoma. Cancer Genet Cytogenet 1987, 29, 155–7.
112. Kumar S, Perlman E, Pack S, Davis M, Zhang H, Meltzer P, Tsokos M. Absence of EWS/FLI1 fusion in olfactory neuroblastomas indicates these tumors do not belong to the Ewing's sarcoma family. Hum Pathol 1999, 30, 1356–60.
113. Mezzelani A, Tornielli S, Minoletti F, Pierotti MA, Sozzi G, Pilotti S. Esthesioneuroblastoma is not a member of the primitive peripheral neuroectodermal tumour—Ewing's group. Br J Cancer 1999, 81, 586–91.
114. VanDevanter DR, George D, McNutt MA, Vogel A, Luthardt F. Trisomy 18 in primary esthesioneuroblastoma. Cancer Genet Cytogenet 1991, 57, 133–6.
115. Carpenter BF, Jimenez C, Robb IA. Melanotic neuroectodermal tumor of infancy. Pediatr Pathol 1985, 3, 227–44.
116. Kapadia SB, Frisman DM, Hitchcock CL, Ellis GL, Popek EJ. Melanotic neuroectodermal tumor of infancy: clinicopathological, immunohistochemical and flow cytometric study. Am J Surg Pathol 1993, 17, 566–73.
117. Dourov N, Mayer R, de Martelaere F, Godart S, Gepts W, Maurus R. Melanotic neuroectodermal tumor of infancy with high serum levels of alpha-fetoprotein. Ultrastructural study and immunological evidence of glial fibrillary protein and alpha-fetoprotein. J Oral Pathol 1987, 16, 251–5.
118. Hoshino S, Takahashi H, Shimura T, Nakazawa S, Naito Z, Asano G. Melanotic neuroectodermal tumor of infancy in the skull associated with high serum levels of

catecholamines. Case report. J Neurosurg 1994, 80(5), 919–24.
119. Pettinato G, Manivel JC, d'Amore ESG, Jaszcz W, Gorlin RJ. Melanotic neuroectodermal tumour of infancy: a re-examination of a histogenetic problem based on immunohistochemical, flow cytometric, and ultrastructural study of 10 cases. Am J Surg Pathol 1991, **15**, 233–45.
120. Roa I, Araya J, Gonzalez S, Garrido C. Peripheral pigmented neuroectodermal tumor of infancy with rhabdomyoblastic differentiation. Pathol Res Pract 1990, **186**, 404–7.
121. Khoddami M, Squire J, Zielenska M, Thorner P. Melanotic neuroectodermal tumor of infancy: a molecular genetic study. Pediatr Dev Pathol 1998, **1**, 295–9.

10 Rhabdomyosarcoma

Ivo Leuschner

Introduction

Rhabdomyosarcoma (RMS) is the most common soft tissue sarcoma in childhood and adolescence (1). The incidence decreases in relation to age, with predominance in childhood and the lowest incidence in late adolescence (2). Approximately 5% of RMS are found in children under 1 year of age. Two percent of RMS are already present at birth (3). In adults, especially over forty years of age, RMS is a rare tumor (4, 5). Two hundred and fifty new cases of RMS are diagnosed every year in the United States. Epidemiological studies have shown that a slight predominance exists in Caucasians. An incidence of 8.4 cases per million inhabitants was found in Caucasians compared to 3.9 cases in Black inhabitants in the United States (6, 7). There is a slight predominance in males (1.4 : 1) (6, 7). For certain subtypes of RMS some association between site, age, and sex is known. This will be discussed later.

Rhabdomyosarcoma is a heterogeneous group of tumors. The tumors are composed of cells that histologically resemble fetal muscle cells at 10–12 weeks of gestation (8). By the early 1950s it was realized that the rhabdomyosarcoma had at least two distinct morphological subtypes which were named embryonal and alveolar rhabdomyosarcoma. Molecular genetic studies of the last decade have shown that these different histological patterns are caused by different genetic changes. Today, the two basic subtypes of rhabdomyosarcoma are regarded as probably distinct sarcoma entities sharing myogenic differentiation. A different biological behavior of the two subtypes of rhabdomyosarcoma has been shown in large clinical oncology studies (9–11), that demonstrated that the alveolar rhabdomyosarcoma is associated with a less favorable prognosis compared to the embryonal type. This resulted in development of treatment protocols with regard to the variable aggressiveness of the different subtypes of RMS.

Prognosis of children with RMS has improved a lot during the last decades. The good response to radiotherapy of RMS was seen in the early 1950s (12). A combined complete and partial response rate of 33% was achieved using single cytotoxic drugs in the 1950s, 1960s, and early 1970s (7). In the 1970s and early 1980s large national and international paediatric oncology studies were founded to establish treatment protocols on the basis of treatment results of large numbers of patients. Today an event-free survival of about 70% for embryonal RMS and about 50% for alveolar RMS can be achieved using a combined therapy including chemotherapy, surgery, and in some cases, additional radiotherapy (13, 14).

Genetic predisposition and association with other diseases

Various epidemiological studies have investigated possible risk factors for development of RMS. Paternal cigarette smoking (15), parental cocaine and marijuana use (16), and *in utero* X-ray exposure (7) were associated with increased risk. A large study covering 555 children did not reveal a significant influence of past medical history on the development of cancer in children (17). Interestingly, the study showed a high excess number of the children studied had not been immunized. Single cases of RMS and fetal alcohol syndrome (18) or hydantoin syndrome (19) are reported in the literature. Congenital anomalies, such as malformations in central nervous system (CNS), kidneys, or heart, were found in patients with RMS in 32% of cases (20).

Rhabdomyosarcoma may be associated with syndromes, for example, Beckwith–Wiedemann syndrome (21, 22) (discussed below), Rubenstein Taybi syndrome (20), and Roberts syndrome (23). In addition RMS have been reported in association with neurofibromatosis (24, 25). There is also an increased incidence of RMS in families with Li Fraumeni syndrome (26).

Classification

Currently the rhabdomyosarcomas are classified according to the International Classification of Rhabdomyosarcomas (IRC) which was developed by an international group of soft tissue sarcoma experts (27). This classification (Table 10.1) is based on the Horn and Enterline classification (28), but also includes various aspects of the National Institutes of Health (NIH) classification (29), the SIOP classification (30), and the cytological classification (31). In general three prognostically relevant groups are distinguished. This grouping should not be confused with a grading, because all RMS are regarded as grade 3 sarcomas. The groups refer to the behavior of the different types of RMS under the current treatment protocols.

Staging

Staging of RMS is based on a combined clinical and pathological approach. In many clinical studies the Intergroup Rhabdomyosarcoma Study (IRS) staging system is used (32). The most important prognostic feature is the complete or incomplete removal of the tumor at surgery (see Table 10.2). The TNM system (33) is less informative, but can be used in addition to the IRS staging system.

Table 10.1 International classification of rhabdomyosarcoma

Favorable prognosis
    Botryoid subtype of embryonal RMS
    Spindle cell subtype of embryonal RMS

Intermediate prognosis
    "Classical" embryonal RMS
        (all embryonal rhabdomyosarcomas except the botryoid subtype and the spindle cell subtype)

Unfavorable prognosis
    Alveolar rhabdomyosarcoma including "solid variant"

Table 10.2 Modified IRS-staging system as used by the German Cooperative Soft Tissue Sarcoma Study (CWS)

IRS-stage	Definition	pT-stage
I	Localized disease, completely resected (regional lymph nodes not involved)	
IA	Confined to muscle or organ of origin	pT1
IB	Contiguous involvement with infiltration outside the muscle or organ of origin, as through fascial planes	pT2
II	Grossly resected tumor with microscopic residual disease	
IIA	Regional lymph nodes not involved	pT3a
IIB	Regional lymph nodes involved, but completely resected	
IIC	Regional lymph nodes involved, but incompletely resected	
III	Incomplete resection or biopsy with gross residual disease	pT3b
	Malignant ascites in neighbouring cavities	pT3c
IV	Distant metastatic disease present at the onset (lung, liver, bones, bone marrow, and distant muscle and nodes)	pT4

Histopathological diagnostic features

Favorable prognosis

Botryoid subtype of embryonal rhabdomyosarcoma

The botryoid subtype of embryonal RMS is found in organs that form cavities such as nasopharynx, vagina, urinary bladder, and the bile duct system. This subtype compromises about 7% of all RMS (11). The tumor shows a "grape-like" growth pattern with polypoid projections into the lumen. Microscopically the tumor shows a typical band-like hypercellular tumor cell arrangement beneath the covering epithelium called the cambium layer (Fig. 10.1). This contrasts with the hypocellular deeper portions of the tumor. The cytology of the tumor cells is basically the same as in the "classical" embryonal RMS as described later.

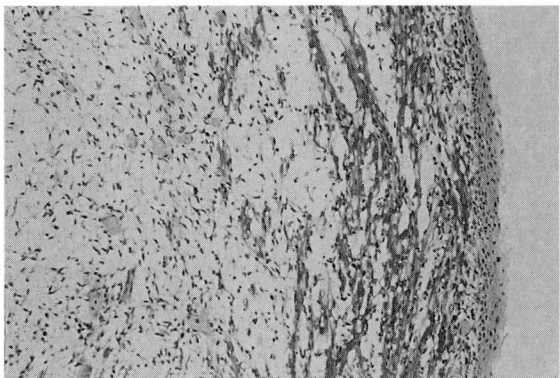

Fig. 10.1 Botryoid embryonal RMS with condensation of tumor cell beneath the surface epithelium ("cambium layer"). Desmin intermediate filaments, alkaline phosphate–anti-alkaline phosphatase (APAAP), ×20.

Spindle cell type of embryonal rhabdomyosarcoma

This rare variant of embryonal RMS occurs mostly in the paratesticular region. It represents a highly differentiated tumor composed of spindle cells in more than 75% of the tumor (Fig. 10.2). Histologically the cells resemble smooth muscle cells, but strongly express skeletal muscle proteins as myoglobin, myosin, and titin (34, 35). Often a storiforme growth pattern of whirls and bundles can be seen. A spindle cell differentiation can occur in embryonal RMS, although this is usually focal. The association with a favorable prognosis is only seen if more than 75% of the tumor is composed of spindle cells. In addition the paratesticular site seems to influence the good prognosis as well (35).

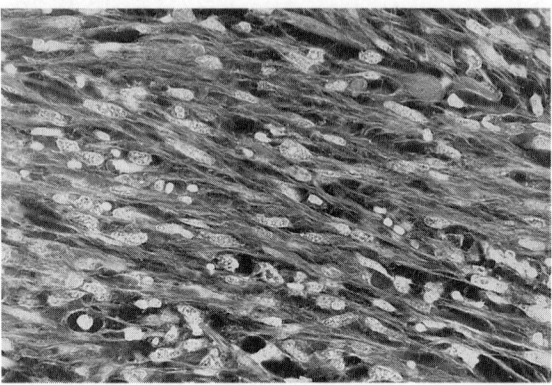

Fig. 10.2 Spindle cell embryonal RMS consisting almost entirely of well-differentiated spindle cells resembling myotubes. Hematoxylin and eosin (H&E), ×80.

Intermediate prognosis group

"Classical" embryonal rhabdomyosarcoma

All rhabdomyosarcoma not classified as one of the two favorable subtypes of embryonal RMS or alveolar RMS belong to this group. The group is rather heterogeneous and also includes the pleomorphic RMS of childhood and adolescence.

In general "classical" embryonal RMS can occur in most sites of the body, with a high prevalence in the head and neck region (about 46% of all embryonal RMS) and urogenital region (about 28%) (11). By contrast the extremities have a low incidence of embryonal RMS (about 8%). In the urinary bladder and the prostate practically all RMS are of the embryonal type (36). The age of onset is between birth and about 15 years, with a major peak incidence between the first and the fifth year of life (37). RMS of adults, which often has pleomorphic features, should be regarded as a separate group of tumors (8).

Microscopy shows spindle-shaped to ovoid tumor cells of varying cellularity. The cells can be arranged in a loose pattern or in bundles and solid areas of high cellularity. The amount of fibrous tissue and reticulin fibers is variable. PAS stain is positive if appropriate fixation of tissue is achieved. At least some of the tumor cells have a distinct eosinophilic cytoplasm, which represents the myogenesis (Fig. 10.3). Focal myoblasts with broad eosinophilic cytoplasm or "tadpole" cells can be found. "Tandem cells" with nuclei arranged in a myotube-like pattern show a higher degree of differentiation (Fig. 10.4). Cross striation is not mandatory for the diagnosis of embryonal RMS. It is most frequently associated with a better prognosis (38). The degree of differentiation varies a lot in embryonal RMS. An association between the degree of differentiation and prognosis has been discussed (39), but needs to be proven. This may be complicated by the induction of differentiation after chemotherapy.

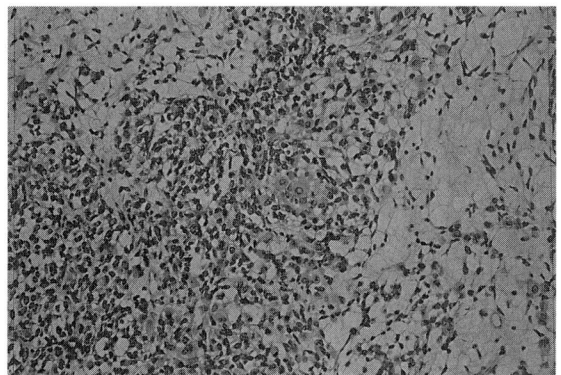

Fig. 10.3 Poorly differentiated embryonal RMS showing small to stellate-shaped tumor cells with sometimes eosinophilic cytoplasm. H&E, ×20.

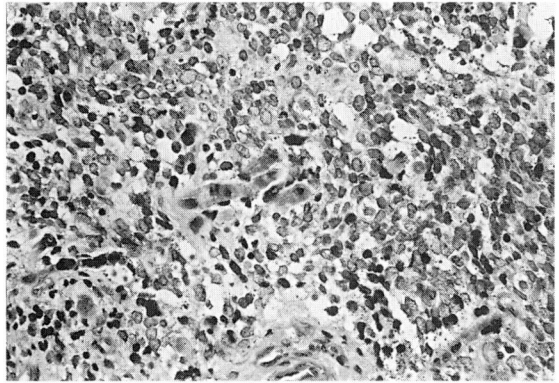

Fig. 10.4 Well differentiated tumor cells in an embryonal RMS with broad cytoplasm forming "tadpole" and "tandem" cells. Periodic Acid Schiff (PAS) stain, ×80.

Anaplastic cells, as described in Wilms' tumours, can be found in embryonal RMS. It has been shown that the occurrence of anaplastic cells (using the criteria for Wilms' tumors (40)) could also be used as an indicator of a worse prognosis, as seen in Wilms' tumors (41). This finding does not yet influence the treatment of patients.

Unfavorable prognosis group

Alveolar rhabdomyosarcoma

This group of RMS has to be considered as a distinct type of myogenic tumor and needs to be separated from the embryonal RMS. In the 1950s it was realized that these tumors seemed to be different from the rest of RMS. The typical histological pattern with alveolar-like spaces gave the name to this entity.

The age range of patients with an alveolar RMS is different from embryonal RMS. They are usually rare in children below 1 year, followed by an increase until 5 years of age. After this age there is quite an even age distribution until early adulthood (37). Boys have a slightly higher incidence of alveolar RMS than girls (37). The alveolar RMS are mostly found in the extremities (about 45% of tumors), followed by head and neck region (about 22%) and trunk (about 12%) (11). The incidence of lymph node metastasis at the time of diagnosis is much higher in patients with alveolar RMS than in patients with embryonal RMS (42).

The morphological pattern of alveolar RMS is very typical. The tumors are composed of small round cells with a quite large nucleus and scanty rim of cytoplasm. The cytology of the cells is very different from embryonal RMS. The nuclei in embryonal RMS are usually smaller and have a condensed chromatin. The typical stellate to ovoid shape of cells in embryonal RMS does not occur in alveolar RMS. The tumor cells of alveolar RMS are arranged in large solid areas which can show "alveolar"-like spaces with a single layer of tumor cells ('lining') along the fibrous septa (Fig. 10.5). These are regressive changes in the tumor and in some tumors only the solid growth pattern is seen. The latter tumors are called "solid variant" of alveolar RMS (43). The identification of the "solid variant" of alveolar RMS is very important to ensure it is not confused with embryonal RMS (due to the lack of the alveolar spaces). Nevertheless these tumors behave like alveolar RMS and need a more aggressive therapy than embryonal RMS.

The distinction between embryonal and alveolar RMS is based on the cytology of cells, the growth patterns and the reticulin fiber pattern. The different

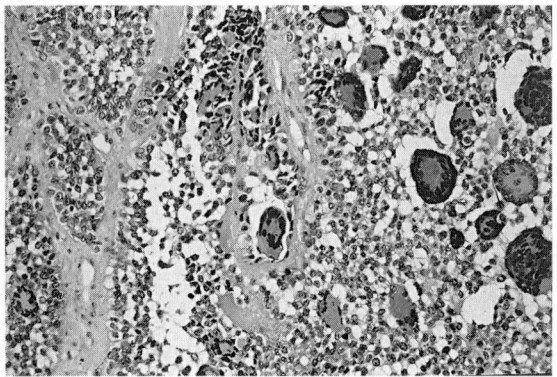

Fig. 10.5 Alveolar RMS with regressive spaces lined by layers of tumor cells and multinucleated cells in the center. H&E, ×40.

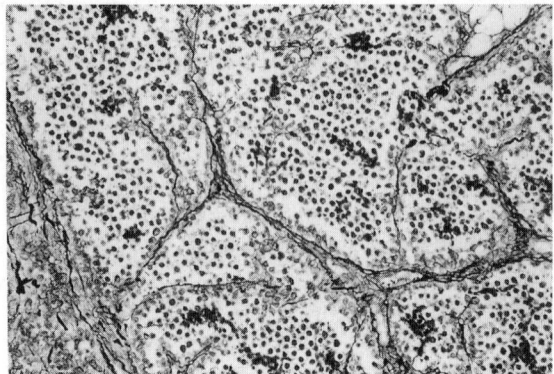

Fig. 10.6 Reticulin fiber pattern of alveolar RMS with fiber-free tumor cell nests. Bielschowski reticulin stain, ×40.

cytology and growth pattern is described above. The reticulin fiber pattern is very typical in alveolar RMS. Although the tumor cell nests are completely free of fibers, the surrounding fibrous septa show an intense amount of fiber strands (Fig. 10.6). By contrast the embryonal RMS have a diffuse network of reticulin fibers in the tumor cell nests. Using a reticulin stain the identification of a "solid variant" of alveolar RMS should be possible.

Immunohistochemistry

Using monoclonal or polyclonal antibodies various myogenic antigens can be demonstrated in RMS. The expression pattern of these antigens is not dependent on the type of RMS but is related to the degree of differentiation in these tumors. Therefore the antibodies will be discussed for all RMS.

Vimentin is a mesenchymal marker often expressed in RMS (44–46), but it is not helpful in the differential diagnosis. Desmin is more specific for a myoid differentiation and is a very sensitive marker (47–49). Nevertheless it is expressed in various mesenchymal tumors and not specific for RMS. Usually the expression of desmin in non-RMS is less intensive than in RMS. The demonstration of actin using pan-actin antibodies like HHF 35 (50, 51) shows a similar expression pattern to desmin. Proteins of skeletal muscle differentiation, for example, myoglobin (52, 53), myosin (54, 55), Troponin T (56, 57), Titin (49) are specific for skeletal muscle differentiation, but can also be found in non-RMS, e.g. Wilms' Tumor and ectomesenchymoma. The positivity of the antigens is dependent on the degree of differentiation in the RMS. Poorly differentiated RMS, especially alveolar RMS, usually do not express these antigens. Therefore expressing one of these skeletal muscle proteins is diagnostic of RMS, although quite a large number of RMS do not express these markers of differentiation. Antibodies against alpha sarcomeric actin can be helpful (58, 59), but are usually not so specific to distinguish between sarcomeric and other types of actin. Interestingly both embryonal and alveolar RMS express the fetal form of the acetylcholine receptor (60).

Other myogenic proteins as creatin kinase MM and BB (61, 62), beta-enolase (63), Z-protein (64), and some more (overview in (8)) not suitable for the use in routine diagnostics but may be helpful in research work.

The myoD family of myogenic regulatory proteins plays an important role in the development of RMS. To this group belong MyoD 1, myf-4 (myogenin), MRF-4, and myf-5. Myo D1 has been shown to convert mouse fibroblasts into determined myoblasts (65) and appears essential for the induction of myogenesis (66). It is expressed earlier than desmin in myogenesis (65), and consequently its nuclear expression may be more sensitive for the detection of myogenesis than desmin antibodies (8, 67). Nevertheless, the demonstration of MyoD1 in paraffin-embedded tissue is not as sensitive as in frozen tissue (68) and a negative or cytoplasmic staining should be interpreted with caution in routinely processed formalin-fixed tissue. Using frozen tissue or molecular techniques, MyoD1 can be used to distinguish RMS from other tumors (67, 69, 70). By contrast myf-4 (myogenin) can be demonstrated in paraffin-embedded tissue including RMS in a reliable way (71). In addition the intensity of the nuclear myogenin expression might be helpful in distinguishing embryonal from alveolar RMS because the latter usually has a much higher expression of myogenin (72).

In summary the immunhistochemical demonstration of desmin, myf-4 (myogenin) in combination with MyoD1 is useful for proving the diagnosis of RMS.

Electron microscopy

Many studies have been published describing the ultrastructure of RMS (73–77). The demonstration of thin and thick filaments or Z-bands is used as typical structures for skeletal muscle differentiation in a tumor. Nevertheless these structures can only be found if the tumor shows some degree of differentiation by conventional morphology (78). The immunohistochemical detection of myogenic proteins is much more sensitive, therefore, the ultrastructural investigation of RMS in the routine diagnostic procedure has become less important.

DNA ploidy

The estimation of DNA content in RMS seems to be less important than in other tumors of childhood. This reflects the large number of reports with contradicting results in the literature. An initial report using frozen tissue showed an association between a better prognosis and a triploid DNA content in embryonal RMS (79). This association could also been shown by subsequent reports using paraffin-embedded tumor tissue (80–83). However, other studies have not been able to confirm this association between tumor type, DNA ploidy, and prognosis (84–87). The value of the DNA content in RMS remains unclear.

Cytogenetics and molecular genetics

Genetic changes have been found for both embryonal and alveolar RMS (for review see (88)). In embryonal RMS a loss of heterozygosity (LOH) on chromosome 11p15.5 has been shown (89, 90). The involved gene or genes have not yet been clearly identified but several interesting genes are located in this area, for example, the MyoD1 gene (91), the IGF-2 gene (92, 93), the LDH (muscle subunit) gene (94), and the WT 1 gene (95). It has been considered that the involved gene could be a tumor suppressor gene ('rhabdomyosarcoma locus') (96). A possible imprinting of this gene and a mechanistic relationship to the association between Beckwith–Wiedemann syndrome has also been postulated (96, 21). Putative candidate tumor suppressor genes in this region include GOK, H19, and BWR1A. GOK expression was found to be absent in several embryonal RMS and alveolar RMS cell lines while its expression is high in normal skeletal muscle. Transfection of GOK cDNA induced cell death specifically in the embryonal RMS cell line (RD), suggesting GOK as tumor suppressor with its growth suppressive effect specific to RMS (97). Expression of H19 was also found to be significantly suppressed with respect to normal skeletal muscle in a majority of embryonal RMS (11/15) and some alveolar RMS (3/11) tumors (98). For BWR1A, a point mutation that results in an amino acid substitution was found in an embryonal RMS cell line (TE125-T) (99). Since this change was present only when homozygous it supports the idea of the loss of a tumor suppressor. Two different growth factor genes have been found on the short and long arm of chromosome 11, which seem to play a role in embryonal RMS (100). The locus of the growth factor gene on the short arm of chromosome 11 may be the same region which is involved in Wilms' tumors. This could explain why Wilms' tumors may have features of myogenesis and how both embryonal RMS and Wilms' tumors can occur in Beckwith–Wiedemann syndrome (101). A more recent report demonstrated that the region of LOH in embryonal RMS and Wilms' tumor on chromosome 11p15.5 is similar (102). Using comparative genomic hybridization a recent study has shown that several chromosomes including chromosomes 2, 7, 8, 11, 12, 13, and 20 demonstrated a gain of chromosomal material, whereas losses were most prominent on chromosomal regions 1p35–36, 6, 9q22, 14q, and 17 (103). The 1p36 region corresponds to the PAX7 gene altered in alveolar RMS (see below) and the 9q22 corresponds to the PTCH gene, a putative tumor suppressor gene, which has been shown to play a role in rhabdomyosacroma in a mouse model of Gorlin syndrome (104).

Alveolar RMS has different genetic changes, which can be shown in the majority of cases. A balanced reciprocal translocation, t(2;13)(q35;q14), involves the PAX 3 gene on chromosome 2 and the FKHR gene on chromosome 13 (105–109). The result is a PAX3-FKHR fusion protein that can be demonstrated by various molecular methods (110–113). This translocation is also found in the solid variant of alveolar RMS (114, 115). The t(2;13) translocation juxtaposes the PAX3 DNA-binding domain on chromosome 2 to the FKHR trans-activation domain on chromosome 13, resulting in a more potent transcriptional activator (116–120). The PAX gene family includes several paired homeobox-containing genes which are important for the organ development (121). The potential gain-of-function of FKHR rearrangements is thought to contribute to the more aggressive behavior of alveolar RMS through the dysregulation of downstream target genes. The t(1;13) translocation found in a subset of alveolar RMS involves rearrangement of FKHR with the PAX7 gene, which shows a high homology to PAX3, at chromosomal region 1p36 (122). Overexpression of both fusion products was noted when compared to wild type PAX3 or PAX7. The PAX7-FKHR over-expression was found to be the result of gene amplification, while the PAX3-FKHR over-expression was the result of a copy number-independent process (123). Moreover, the PAX3-FKHR and PAX7-FKHR fusion-positive RMS were found to associate with distinct clinical phenotypes. Compared to the PAX3-FKHR fusion-positive tumors, the PAX7-FKHR fusion-positive tumors tend to occur in younger individuals, present more often with extremity lesions, are more localized, metastasize only to bone and distant nodes, and have a better overall prognosis (124). Wild type PAX3 expression was elevated in some cases of embryonal RMS and alveolar RMS when compared with normal adult skeletal muscle, regardless of the presence of PAX3/7-FKHR translocations (125). Increased PAX3 expression can inhibit myogenic differentiation and thus is thought to contribute to tumorigenesis by preventing terminal differentiation. PAX3's role as a transcription factor and growth promoter was recently demonstrated by the up-regulation of the growth factor receptor c-met (126).

The role of disruption of apoptotic pathways has been implicated by the finding of increased N-myc and c-myc expression in alveolar RMS that positively correlated to growth and metastatic potential (127, 128). RMS cells also appear to increase proliferation by disrupting other apoptotic pathways. Both germ-line p53 mutations and MDM2 gene amplification (also resulting in nonfunctioning p53 protein) are known to be involved in a subset of RMS tumors, which includes both the embryonal RMS and alveolar RMS subtypes (129).

Despite all the differences in molecular changes between embryonal and alveolar RMS there seem to be some tumors with overlapping genetic abnormalities. Recent reports have shown that some alveolar RMS have alterations on chromosome 11 in the same region as seen in embryonal RMS (130, 131). Also the initial reports concerning the t(2;13) translocation in alveolar RMS included tumors classified as embryonal RMS, which showed the same translocation. The observation of molecular heterogeneity within each major subtype likely suggests more complex variations in genotypes that can lead to varied tumor behavior despite an apparent similar phenotype. Understanding of these changes will aid in the elucidation of RMS tumorigenesis.

Prognostic factors

Primary site and clinical stage are the most important prognostic factors in RMS (13, 132). The IRS-III study of the United States showed that patient outcome is related to primary site of tumor. Orbit and genitourinary non-bladder/prostate tumors represent the most prognostically favorable site, followed by genitourinary bladder/prostate, head and neck, extremities, parameningeal, and other sites. When patients were analyzed according to clinical stage, patients with stage I and II disease had a much better prognosis than those with more advanced tumors. This has also been demonstrated by other studies (133, 134).

Histology is also an important prognostic factor. In earlier studies patients with an alveolar RMS had a worse prognosis compared to those with embryonal RMS (9, 11). This was confirmed in the large German Soft Tissue Tumor Study (CWS) (135), despite a more aggressive treatment for patients with an alveolar RMS. The IRS-III study did not show this difference (13). Nevertheless, alveolar RMS is more frequently associated with advanced disease (42) than embryonal RMS. In addition the identification of the correct histological type of RMS is extremely important, because alveolar RMS requires more aggressive therapeutic intervention.

Other factors such as DNA ploidy, proliferation, chemoresistance, have not proven to be of prognostic importance.

Treatment strategies

The low incidence of RMS necessitates treatment within national or international pediatric oncology trials such as the IRS-Studies in the USA, SIOP MMT studies in some European countries, or the German

CWS studies. All these trials use a similar treatment protocol with some minor differences. Experience over the last four decades has shown that only a combined surgical and chemotherapeutic approach, sometimes with additional radiotherapy, is effective for patients with RMS. Using the German CWS protocol as an example, the patients are grouped into one of four 'risk groups' (low, standard, high risk, and stage IV disease) according to stage, site, and histological type of RMS. If a complete resection of the tumor is not possible (without mutilation) a two or three drug chemotherapy (including vincristin, actinomycin D, ifosfamide, and adriamycin) is given primarily. In some cases preoperative radiotherapy is also performed. The tumor is then resected after 9–10 weeks of chemotherapy. Response to chemotherapy of the residual tumor, estimated by CT scan or MRI, is very important in cases to define further treatment strategies. After resection of the tumor the patients receive further chemotherapy and in some cases additional radiotherapy. Overall the children receive treatment for 25 weeks or even more (14). For those with recurrences a special treatment protocol is available.

Current and future research

Current research on RMS is focused on several aspects. Looking at the molecular aspects of these tumors using modern methods such as comparative genomic hybridization and PCR in combination with microdissection techniques will allow the identification of new interesting genetic abnormalities. Genetic imprinting, for example, H19 on chromosome 11, is already under investigation. In addition the microdissection technique will allow study of the tumor heterogeneity at both a molecular and morphological level. This latter technique might be used to investigate a possible link between embryonal and alveolar RMS.

Mechanisms of chemoresistance in RMS are not well understood. Despite some initial reports the classical p170-mediated multidrug resistance does not seem to play an important role in soft tissue sarcomas of childhood and adolescence (136). Other mechanisms are not well understood. The prediction of response to chemotherapy would be of great value for treatment planning. Cell culture testing of different drug combination simulating the treatment protocol will be necessary in the future.

Clinically the treatment study designs focus on an individual treatment plan according to stage, site, and histological subtype of disease, to achieve the optimal treatment but avoiding unnecessary side-effects due to over treatment. This includes evaluation of individual tumor parameters, drug monitoring, and optimizing the radiotherapy by using acceleration and hyperfraction of doses. Future treatment studies will include immunotherapy by coupling cytotoxic agent to antibodies specific to tumor antigens.

References

1. Robinson LL. General principles of epidemiology of childhood cancer. In: Principles and practice of paediatric oncology, 2nd edn (ed. P Pizzo, DG Poplack). Lippincott, Philadelphia, 1989, 3–10.
2. Enzinger FM, Weiss SH. Rhabdomyosarcoma. In: Soft tissue tumours, 3rd edn (ed. FM Enzinger, SW Weiss). Mosby, St Louis, 1995, 539–77.
3. Ragab AH, Heyn R, Tefft M, Hays DM, Newton WA, Jr, Beltangady M. Infants younger than 1 year of age with rhabdomyosarcoma. Cancer 1986, **58**, 2606–10.
4. Miettinen M. Rhabdomyosarcoma in patients older than 40 years of age. Cancer 1988, **62**, 2060–5.
5. Seidal T, Kindblom LG, Angervall L. Rhabdomyosarcoma in middle-aged and elderly individuals. Acta Path Microbiol Immunol Scand Sect A 1989, **97**, 236–48.
6. Raney RB, Jr, Hays DM, Tefft, M, Triche TJ. Rhabdomyosarcoma and the undifferentiated sarcomas. In: Principles and practice of paediatric oncology (2nd edn) (ed. PA Pizzo, DG Poplack). Lippincott, Philadelphia, 1993, 769–94.
7. Ruymann FB, Grufferman S. Introduction and epidemiology of soft tissue sarcomas. In: Rhabdomyosarcoma and related tumours in children and adolescents (eds HM Maurer, FB Ruymann, C Pochedly). CRC Press, Boca Raton, 1991, 3–18.
8. Parham D. Rhabdomyosarcoma and related tumors. In: Pediatric neoplasia. Morphology and Biology (ed. D Parham). Lippincott-Raven, Philadelphia, 1996, 87–104.
9. Crist WM, Garnsey L, Beltangady M, Gehan E, Ruymann F, Webber B, Hays DM, Wharam M, Maurer HM, for the Intergroup Rhabdomyosarcoma Study Committee. Prognosis in children with rhabdomyosarcoma: a report of the Intergroup Rhabdomyosarcoma Studies I and II. J Clin Oncol 1990, **8**, 443–52.
10. Koscielniak E, Harms D, Henze G, Jürgens H, Gadner H, Herbst M, Klingebiel T, Schmidt BF, Morgan M, Knietig R, Treuner J. Results of treatment for soft tissue sarcoma in childhood and adolescence: a final report of the German Cooperative Soft Tissue Sarcoma Study CWS-86. J Clin Oncol 1999, **17**, 3706–19.
11. Newton WA, Jr, Soule EH, Hamoudi AB, Reiman HM, Shimada H, Beltangady M, Maurer H. Histopathology of childhood sarcomas, Intergroup Rhabdomyosarcoma Studies I and II: clinicopathologic correlation. J Clin Oncol 1988, **6**, 67–75.

12. Stobbe GD, Dargeon HW. Embryonal rhabdomyosarcoma of head a neck in children and adolescents. Cancer 1950, 3, 826–36.
13. Crist W, Gehan EA, Ragab AH, Dickman PS, Donaldson SS, Fryer C, Hammond D, Hays DM, Herrmann J, Heyn R, Jones PM, Lawrence W, Newton W, Ortega J, Raney RB, Ruymann FB, Tefft M, Webber B, Wiener E, Wharam M, Vietti TJ, Maurer HM The Third Intergroup Rhabdomyosarcoma Study. J Clin Oncol March 1995, 13, 610–30.
14. CWS-96. Study protocol of the German Cooperative Soft Tissue Sarcoma Study CWS-96. Stuttgart, Germany, 1997.
15. Grufferman S, Wane HH, DeLong ER, Kimm SY, Delzell ES, Falletta JM. Environmental factors in the etiology of rhabdomyosarcoma in childhood. J Natl Cancer Inst 1982, 68, 107–13.
16. Grufferman S, Schwartz AG, Ruymann FB, Maurer HM. Parents' use of cocaine and marijuana and increased risk of rhabdomyosarcoma in their children. Cancer Causes Control 1993, 4, 217–24.
17. Hartley AL, Birch JM, McKinney PA, Blair V, Teare MD, Carrette J, Mann JR, Stiller CA, Draper GJ, Johnston HE, et al. The Inter-Regional Epidemiological Study of Childhood Cancer (IRESCC): past medical history in children with cancer. J Epidemiol Community Health 1988, 42, 235–42.
18. Becker H, Zaunschirm A, Muntean W, Domej W. Fetales Alkohol-Syndrom und maligne Tumoren (Fetal alcohol syndrome and malignant tumours). Wien Klin Wochenschr 1982, 94, 364–5.
19. Cohen MM, Jr. Neoplasia and the fetal alcohol and hydantoin syndromes. Neurobehav Toxicol Teratol 1981, 3, 161–2.
20. Ruymann FB, Maddux HR, Ragab A, Soule EH, Palmer N, Beltangady M, Gehan EA, Newton WA, Jr. Congenital anomalies associated with rhabdomyosarcoma: an autopsy study of 115 cases. A report from the Intergroup Rhabdomyosarcoma Study Committee (representing the Chidren's Cancer Study group, the Paediatric Oncology Group, The United Kingdom Children's Cancer Study Group, and the Paediatric Intergroup Statistical Center). Med Pediatr Oncol 1988, 16, 33–9.
21. Steenman M, Westerveld A, Mannens M. Genetics of Beckwith–Wiedemann syndrome-associated tumors: common genetic pathways. Genes Chromosomes Cancer 2000, 28, 1–13.
22. Smith AC, Squire JA, Thorner P, Zielenska M, Shuman C, Grant R, Chitayat D, Nishikawa JL, Weksberg R. Association of alveolar rhabdomyosarcoma with the Beckwith–Wiedemann syndrome. Pediatr Dev Pathol 2001, 4, 550–8.
23. Wenger SL, Blatt J, Steele MW, Lloyd DA, Bellinger M, Phebus CK, Horn M, Jaffe R. Rhabdomyosarcoma in Roberts syndrome. Cancer Genet Cytogenet 1988, 31, 285–9.
24. McKeen EA, Bodurtha J, Meadows AT, Douglass EC, Mulvihill JJ. Rhabdomyosarcoma complicating multiple neurofibromatosis. J Pediatr 1978, 93, 992–3.
25. Warrier RP, Kini KR, Shumaker B, Schwartz G, Raju U, Raman BS. Neurofibromatosis, factor IX deficiency, and rhabdomyosarcoma. Urology 1986, 28, 295–6.
26. Li FP, Fraumeni JF, Jr. Prospective study of a family cancer syndrome. JAMA 1982, 247, 2692–4.
27. Newton WA, Jr, Gehan EA, Webber BL, Marsden HB, van Unnik AJ, Hamoudi AB, Tsokos M, Shimada H, Harms D, Schmidt D, Ninfo V, Cavazzana A, Gonzalez-Crussi F, Parham DM, Reiman HM, Asmar L, Beltangady MS, Sachs N, Triche TJ, Maurer HM. Classification of rhabdomyosarcomas and related sarcomas. Pathologic aspects and proposal for a new classification. An Intergroup Rhabdomyosarcoma Study. Cancer 1995, 76, 1073–85.
28. Horn RC, Enterline HT. Rhabdomyosarcoma: a clinicopathological study and classification of 39 cases. Cancer 1958, 11, 181–99.
29. Tsokos M, Webber BL, Parham DM, Wesley RA, Miser A, Miser JS, Etcubanas E, Kinsella T, Grayson J, Glatstein E, Pizzo PA, Triche TJ. Rhabdomyosarcoma: a new classification scheme related to prognosis. Arch Pathol Lab Med 1992, 116, 847–55.
30. Caillaud JM, Gerard-Marchant R, Marsden HB, van Unnik AJ, Rodary C, Rey A, Flamant F. Histopathological classification of childhood rhabdomyosarcoma: a report from the International Society of Paediatric Oncology Pathology Panel. Med Pediatr Oncol 1989, 17, 391–400.
31. Palmer NF, Foulkes MA, Sachs N, Newton WA. Rhabdomyosarcoma: a cytological classification of prognostic significance. Proc Am Soc Clin Oncol 1983, 2, 229 (abstract).
32. Maurer HM, Beltangady M, Gehan EA, Crist W, Hammond D, Hays DM, Heyn R, Lawrence W, Newton WA, Jr, Ortega J, Ragab AH, Raney RB, Ruymann FB, Soule E, Tefft M, Webber B, Wharam M, Vietti TJ. The Intergroup Rhabdomyosarcoma Study-I. A final report. Cancer 1988, 61, 209–20.
33. Atlas TNM. Illustrated guide to the TNM/pTNM classification of malignant tumours. Springer, Berlin, 1997.
34. Cavazzana AO, Schmidt D, Ninfo V, Harms D, Tollot M, Carli M, Treuner J, Betto R, Salviati G. Spindle cell rhabdomyosarcoma. A prognostically favorable variant of rhabdomyosarcoma. Am J Surg Pathol 1992, 16, 229–35.
35. Leuschner I, Newton WA, Jr, Schmidt D, Sachs N, Asmar L, Hamoudi A, Harms D, Maurer HM. Spindle cell variants of embryonal rhabdomyosarcoma of the paratesticular region: a report of the Intergroup Rhabdomyosarcoma Study. Am J Surg Pathol 1993, 17, 221–30.
36. Hays DM. Bladder/prostate rhabdomyosarcoma: results of the multi-institutional trials of the Intergroup Rhabdomyosarcoma Study. Sem Surg Oncol 1993, 9, 520–3.
37. Harms D. Soft tissue sarcomas in the Kiel Paediatric Tumor Registry. In: Current topics in pathology, Vol. 89: soft tissue tumours (ed. D Harms, D Schmidt). Springer, Berlin, 1995, 31–45.
38. Leuschner I, Newton WA, for the IRS Committee. Anaplasia and cross striation are prognostically important morphological features for long-term survival in embryonal rhabdomyosarcoma (RMS). Pediatr Develop Pathol 2000, 3, 398.
39. Schmidt D, Reimann O, Treuner J, Harms D. Cellular differentiation and prognosis in embryonal rhabdomyosarcoma. A report from the Cooperative Soft Tissue Sarcoma Study 1981 (CWS 81). Virchows Arch A 1986, 409, 183–94.

40. Beckwith JB, Palmer NF. Histopathology and prognosis of Wilms' tumor. Results from the first National Wilms' Tumor Study. Cancer 1978, **41**, 1937–48.
41. Kodet R, Newton WA, Jr, Hamoudi A, Asmar L, Jacobs DL, Maurer HM. Childhood rhabdomyosarcoma with anaplastic (pleomorphic) features. A report from the Intergroup Rhabdomyosarcoma Study. Am J Surg Pathol 1993, **17**, 443–53.
42. Harms D. Alveolar rhabdomyosarcoma: a prognostically unfavorable rhabdomyosarcoma type and its necessary distinction from embryonal rhabdomyosarcoma. In: Current topics in pathology, Vol. 89: soft tissue tumours (ed. D Harms, D Schmidt). Springer-Verlag, Berlin, 1995, 273–96.
43. Tsokos M, Miser A, Wesley R, Miser JS, Kinsella TJ, Grayson J, Pizzo PA, Glatstein E, Triche TJ. Solid variant alveolar rhabdomyosarcoma: a primitive rhabdomyosarcoma with poor prognosis and distinct histology. SIOP XVII Meeting, Barcelona, 1984, 71–4.
44. Kodet R. Rhabdomyosarcoma in childhood. An immunohistochemical analysis with myoglobin, desmin and vimentin. Path Res Pract 1989, **185**, 207–13.
45. Koss LG, Czerniak B, Herz F, Wersto RP. Flow cytometric measurement of DNA and other cell components in human tumours: a critical appraisal. Hum Pathol 1989, **20**, 528–48.
46. Osborn M, Debus E, Weber K. Monoclonal antibodies specific for vimentin. Eur J Cell Biol 1984, **34**, 137–43.
47. Altmannsberger M, Weber K, Droste R, Osborn M. Desmin is a specific marker for rhabdomyosarcomas of human and rat origin. Am J Pathol 1985, **118**, 85–95.
48. Carter RL, McCarthy KP, Machin LG, Jameson CF, Philip ER, Pinkerton CR. Expression of desmin and myoglobin in rhabdomyosarcomas and in developing skeletal muscle. Histopathol 1989, **15**, 585–95.
49. Osborn M, Hill C, Altmannsberger M, Weber K. Monoclonal antibodies to titin in conjunction with antibodies to desmin separate rhabdomyosarcomas from other tumor types. Lab Invest 1986, **55**, 101–8.
50. Schmidt RA, Cone R, Haas JE, Gown AM. Diagnosis of rhabdomyosarcoma with HHF35, a monoclonal antibody directed against muscle actins. Am J Pathol 1988, **131**, 19–28.
51. Tsukuda T, McNutt MA, Ross R, Gown AM. HHF35, a muscle actin-specific monoclonal antibody. II. Reactivity in normal, reactive, and neoplastic human tissues. Am J Pathol 1987, **127**, 389–402.
52. Schmidt D. Pathologie der Weichteilsarkome. Radiologe 1992, **32**, 579–83.
53. Schmidt D, Harms D. The applicability of immunohistochemistry in the diagnosis and differential diagnosis of malignant soft tissue tumours. A reevaluation based on the material of the Kiel Paediatric Tumor Registry. Klin Pädiatr 1990, **202**, 224–9.
54. Crocker J, Macartney JC, Smith PJ. Correlation between DNA flow cytometric and nucleolar organizer region data in non-Hodgkin's lymphomas. J Pathol 1988, **154**, 151–6.
55. Eusebi V, Ceccarelli C, Gorza L, Schiaffino S, Bussolati G. Immunohistochemistry of rhabdomyosarcoma. The use of four different markers. Am J Surg Pathol 1986, **10**, 293–9.
56. Dodd S, Malone M, McCulloch W. Rhabdomyosarcoma in children: a histological and immunohistological study of 59 cases. J Pathol 1989, **158**, 13–18.
57. Sheppard MN, Wilkinson M, Bobrow LG. A study to assess the usefulness of troponin T (TT) as a marker in the diagnosis of rhabdomyosarcoma. J Pathol 1987, **151**, 51A.
58. Babai F, Skalli O, Schurch W, Seemayer TA, Gabbiani G. Chemically induced rhabdomyosarcomas in rats. Ultrastructural, immunohistochemical, biochemical features and expression of alpha-actin isoforms. Virchows Arch B 1988, **55**, 263–77.
59. Skalli O, Gabbiani G, Babai F, Seemayer TA, Pizzolato G, Schuerch W. Intermediate filament proteins and actin isoforms as marker for soft tissue tumor differentiation and origin. II. Rhabdomyosarcoma. Am J Pathol 1988, **130**, 515–31.
60. Gattenloehner S, Vincent A, Leuschner I, Tzartos S, Müller-Hermelink HK, Kirchner T, Marx D. The fetal form of the acetylcholine receptor distinguishes rhabdomyosarcoma from other childhood tumours. Am J Pathol 1988, **152**, 437–44.
61. Kahn HJ, Yeger H, Kassim O, Jorgensen AO, MacLennan DH, Baumal R, Smith CR, Phillips J. Immunohistochemical and electron microscopic assessment of childhood rhabdomyosarcoma. Cancer 1983, **51**, 1897–903.
62. Tsokos M, Howard R, Costa J. Immunohistochemical study of alveolar and embryonal rhabdomyosarcoma. Lab Invest 1983, **48**, 148–55.
63. Royds JA, Variend S, Timperley WR, Taylor CB. An investigation of beta enolase as a histologic marker in rhabdomyosarcoma. J Clin Pathol 1984, **37**, 905–10.
64. Mukai M, Hisami I, Torikata C, Kageyama K, Morikawa Y, Shimizu K. Immunperoxidase demonstration of a new muscle protein (Z-protein) in myogenic tumours as a diagnostic aid. Am J Pathol 1984, **114**, 164–70.
65. Davis RL, Weintraub H, Lassar AB. Expression of a single transfected cDNA converts fibroblasts to myoblasts. Cell 1987, **51**, 987–1000.
66. Weintraub H, Davis R, Tapscott S, Thayer M, Krause M, Benezra R, Blackwell TK, Turner D, Rupp R, Hollenberg S, Zhuang Y, Lassar A. The myoD gene family: nodal point during specification of the cell lineage. Science 1991, **251**, 761–6.
67. Momand J, Zambetti GP, Olson DC, George D, Levine AJ. The mdm-2 oncogene product forms a complex with the p53 protein and inhibits p53 mediated transactivation. Cell 1992, **69**, 1237–45.
68. Parham DM, Mukunyadzi P, Dias P, Houghton PJ. MyoD staining in rhabdomyosarcoma (RMS). 3rd International Congress on Soft Tissue Sarcoma in Children and Adolescents, April 30 to May 3, Stuttgart, FRG, 1997, 101.
69. Scrable HJ, Witte D, Shimada H, Seemayer T, Wang-Wuu S, Soukup S, Koufos A, Houghton P, Lampkin B, Cavenee W. Molecular differential pathology of rhabdomyosarcoma. Genes Chromosomes Cancer 1989, **1**, 23–35.
70. Tonin PN, Scrable H, Shimada H, Cavenee WK. Muscle-specific gene expression in rhabdomyosarcomas and stages of human fetal skeletal muscle development. Cancer Res 1991, **51**, 5100–6.
71. Wang NP, Marx J, McNutt MA, Rutledge JC, Gown AM. Expression of myogenic regulatory proteins (myogenin and MyoD1) in small blue round cell tumors of childhood. Am J Pathol 1995, **147**, 1799–810.

72. Dias P, Chen B, Dilday B, Palmer H, Hosoi H, Singer S, Wu C, Li X, Thompson J, Parham D, Qualman S, Houghton P. Strong immunostaining for myogenin in rhabdomyosarcoma is significantly associated with tumours of the alveolar subclass. Am J Pathol 2000, **156**, 399–408.

73. Erlandson RA. The ultrastructural distinction between rhabdomyosarcoma and other undifferentiated sarcomas. Ultrastruct Pathol 1987, **11**, 83–101.

74. Mierau GW, Favara BE. Rhabdomyosarcoma in children: ultrastructural study of 31 cases. Cancer 1980, **46**, 2035–40.

75. Prince FP. Ultrastructural aspects of myogenesis found in neoplasms. Acta Neuropathol 1981, **54**, 315–20.

76. Seidal T, Kindblom LG. The ultrastructure of alveolar and embryonal rhabdomyosarcoma. Acta Path Microbiol Immunol Scand Sect A 1984, **92**, 231–48.

77. Stiller D, Holzhausen HJ. Ultrastrukturelle Organisation diagnostisch relevanter Zellmerkmale in Rhabdomyosarkomen. Zentralbl allg Pathol pathol Anat 1988, **134**, 499–66.

78. Dickman PS, Bodner S, Maurer HM. Electron microscopy in the Third Intergroup Rhabdomyosarcoma Study. Lab Invest 1987, **56**, 2P.

79. Shapiro DN, Parham DM, Douglass EC, Ashmun R, Webber BL, Newton WA, Hancock ML, Maurer HM, Look AT. Relationship of tumor-cell ploidy to histologic subtype and treatment outcome in children and adolescents with unresectable rhabdomyosarcoma. J Clin Oncol 1991, **9**, 159–66.

80. De Zen L, Sommaggio A, d'Amore ES, Masiero L, di Montezemolo LC, Linari A, Madon E, Dominici C, Bosco S, Bisogno G, Carli M, Ninfo V, Basso G. Clinical relevance of DNA ploidy and proliferative activity in childhood rhabdomyosarcoma: a retrospective analysis of patients enrolled onto the Italian Cooperative Rhabdomyosarcoma Study RMS88. J Clin Oncol March 1997, **15**, 1198–1205.

81. Niggli FK, Powell JE, Parkes SE, Ward K, Raafat F, Mann JR, Stevens MCG. DNS ploidy and proliferative activity (S-phase) in childhood soft-tissue sarcomas: their value as prognostic indicators. Br J Cancer 1994, **69**, 1106–10.

82. Pappo AS, Crist WM, Kuttesch J, Rowe S, Ashmun RA, Maurer HM, Newton WA, Asmar L, Luo X, Shapiro DN, for the Intergroup Rhabdomyosarcoma Study Committee. Tumor-cell DNA content predicts outcome in children and adolescents with clinical group III embryonal rhabdomyosarcoma. The Intergroup Rhabdomyosarcoma Study Committee of the Children's Cancer Group and the Paediatric Oncology Group. J Clin Oncol October 1993, **11**, 1901–5.

83. Wijnaendts LC, van der Linden JC, van Diest P, van Unnik AJ, Delemarre JF, Voute PA, Meijer CJ. Prognostic importance of DNA flow cytometric variables in rhabdomyosarcomas. J Clin Pathol 1993, **46**, 948–52.

84. Dias P, Kumar P, Marsden HB, Gattamaneni HR, Kumar S. Prognostic relevance of DNA ploidy in rhabdomyosarcomas and other sarcomas of childhood. Anticancer Res July 1992, **12**, 1173–7.

85. Kilpatrick SE, Teot LA, Geisinger KR, Martin PL, Shumate DK, Zbieranski N, Russel GB, Fletcher CDM. Relationship of DNA ploidy to histology and prognosis in rhabdomyosarcoma. Comparison of flow cytometry and image analysis. Cancer 1994, **74**, 3227–33.

86. Kowal-Vern A, Gonzalez-Crussi F, Turner J, Trujillo YP, Chou P, Herman C, Castelli M, Walloch I. Flow and image cytometric DNA analysis in rhabdomyosarcoma. Cancer Res 1990, **50**, 6023–7.

87. Leuschner I, Schmidt D, Möller R, Harms D. DNA ploidy and nucleolar organizer regions (NOR) in rhabdomyosarcoma (RMS). A report from the Kiel Paediatric Tumor Registry. Med Pediatr Oncol 1991, **19**, 350–1.

88. Anderson J, Gordon A, Pritchard-Jones K, Shipley J. Genes, chromosomes, and rhabdomyosarcoma. Genes Chromosomes Cancer 1999, **26**, 275–85.

89. Koufos A, Hansen MF, Copeland NG, Jenkins NA, Lampkin BC, Cavenee WK. Loss of heterozygosity in three embryonal tumours suggests a common pathogenetic mechanism. Nature 1985, **316**, 330–4.

90. Scrable H, Witte D, Shimada H, Seemayer T, Sheng WW, Soukup S, Koufos A, Houghton P, Lampkin B, Cavenee W. Molecular differential pathology of rhabdomyosarcoma. Genes Chromosomes Cancer 1989, **1**, 23–35.

91. Scrable HJ, Witte DP, Lampkin BC, Cavenee WK. Chromosomal localization of the human rhabdomyosarcoma locus by mitotic recombination mapping. Nature 1987, **329**, 645–7.

92. Magri KA, Ewton DZ, Florini JR. The role of the IGFs in myogenic differentiation. In: Molecular biology and physiology, of insulin and insulin-like growth factors (ed. MK Raizada, D LeRoith). Plenum Press, New York 1991, 57–76.

93. Yun K. A new marker for rhabdomyosarcoma. Insulin-like growth factor II. Lab Invest 1992, **67**, 653–64.

94. Scrable HJ, Johnson DK, Rinchik EM, Cavenee WK. Rhabdomyosarcoma-associated locus and MyoD1 are syntenic but separate loci on the short arm of human chromosome 11. Proc Natl Acad Sci USA 1990, **87**, 2182–6.

95. Huff V, Compton DA, Chao LY, Strong LC, Geiser CF, Saunders GF. Lack of linkage of familial Wilms' tumour to chromosomal band 11p13. Nature 1988, **336**, 377–8.

96. Scrable H, Cavenee W, Ghavimi F, Lovell M, Morgan K, Sapienza C. A model for embryonal rhabdomyosarcoma tumorigenesis that involves genome imprinting. Proc Natl Acad Sci USA 1989, **86**, 7480–4.

97. Sabbioni S, Barbanti-Brodano G, Croce CM, Negrini M. GOK: a gene at 11p15 involved in rhabdomyosarcoma and rhabdoid tumor development. Cancer Res, 1997, **57**, 4493–7.

98. Casola S, Pedone PV, Cavazzana AO, Basso G, Luksch R, d'Amore ES, Carli M, Bruni CB, Riccio A. Expression and parental imprinting of the H19 gene in human rhabdomyosarcoma. Oncogene, 1997, **14**, 1503–10.

99. Schwienbacher C, Sabbioni S, Campi M, Veronese A, Bernardi G, Menegatti A, Hatada I, Mukai T, Ohashi H, Barbanti-Brodano, G, Croce CM, Negrini M. Transcriptional map of 170-kb region at chromosome 11p15.5: identification and mutational analysis of the BWR1A gene reveals the presence of mutations in tumor samples. Proc Natl Acad Sci USA 1998, **95**, 3873–8.

100. Loh WE, Jr, Scrable HJ, Livanos E, Arboleda MJ, Cavenee WK, Oshimura M, Weissman BE. Human chromosome 11 contains two different growth suppressor

100. genes for embryonal rhabdomyosarcoma. Proc Natl Acad Sci USA 1992, **89**, 1755–9.
101. Sotelo-Avila C, Gooch W, III. Neoplasms associated with the Beckwith–Wiedemann syndrome. Perspect Pediatr Pathol 1976, **3**, 255–72.
102. Besnard-Guerin C, Newsham I, Winqvist R, Cavenee WK. A common region of loss of heterozygosity in Wilms' tumor and embryonal rhabdomyosarcoma distal to the D11S988 locus on chromosome 11p15.5. Hum Genet 1996, **97**, 163–70.
103. Bridge JA, Liu J, Weibolt V, Baker KS, Perry D, Kruger R, Qualman S, Barr F, Sorensen P, Triche T, Suijkerbuijk R. Novel genomic imbalances in embryonal rhabdomyosarcoma revealed by comparative genomic hybridization and fluorescence in situ hybridization; an Intergroup Rhabdomyosarcoma Study. Genes Chromosomes Cancer 27:337–344.
104. Hahn H, Wojnowski L, Zimmer AM, Hall J, Miller G, Zimmer A. Rhabdomyosarcomas and radiation hypersensitivity in a mouse model of Gorlin syndrome. Nat Genet 1998, **4**, 619–22.
105. Barr FG, Holick J, Nycum L, Biegel JA, Emanuel BS. Localization of the t(2;13) breakpoint of alveolar rhabdomyosarcoma on a physical map of chromosome 2. Genomics 1992, **13**, 1150–6.
106. Barr FG, Sellinger B, Emanuel BS. Localization of the rhabdomyosarcoma t(2;13) breakpoint on a pysical map of chromosome 13. Genomics 1991, **11**, 941–7.
107. Douglass EC, Valentine M, Etcubanas E, Parham D, Webber BL, Houghton PJ, Houghton JA, Green AA. A specific chromosomal abnormality in rhabdomyosarcoma. Cytogenet Cell Genet 1987, **45**, 148–55.
108. Rowe D, Gerrard M, Gibbons B, Malpas JS. Two further cases of t(2;13) in alveolar rhabdomyosarcoma indicating a review of the published chromosome breakpoints. Br J Cancer 1987, **56**, 379–80.
109. Seidal T, Mark J, Hagmar B, Angervall L. Alveolar rhabdomyosarcoma: a cytogenetic and correlated cytological and histological study. Acta Pathol Microbiol Immunol Scand A 1982, **90**, 345–54.
110. Anderson J, Renshaw J, McManus A, Carter R, Mitchell C, Adams S, Pritchard-Jones K. Amplification of the t(2;13) and t(1;13) translocations of alveolar rhabdomyosarcoma in small formalin-fixed biopsies using a modified reverse transcriptase polymerase chain reaction. Am J Pathol 1997, **150**, 477–82.
111. McManus AP, O'Reilly MA, Jones KP, Gusterson BA, Mitchell CD, Pinkerton CR, Shipley JM. Interphase fluorescence in situ hybridization detection of t(2;13) (q35;q14) in alveolar rhabdomyosarcoma—A diagnostic tool in minimally invasive biopsies. J Pathol April 1996, **178**, 410–14.
112. Reichmuth C, Markus MA, Hillemanns M, Atkinson MJ, Unni KK, Saretzki G, Höfler H. The diagnostic potential of the chromosome translocation t(2;13) in rhabdomyosarcoma: a PCR study of fresh-frozen and paraffin-embedded tumour samples. J Pathol 1996, **180**, 50–7.
113. Shapiro DN, Sublett JE, Li B, Downing JR, Naeve CW. Fusion of PAX3 to a member of the forkhead family of transcription factors in human alveolar rhabdomyosarcoma. Cancer Res 1993, **53**, 5108–12.
114. Parham DM, Shapiro DN, Downing JR, Webber BL, Douglass EC. Solid alveolar rhabdomyosarcomas with the t(2;13). Report of two cases with diagnostic implications. Am J Surg Pathol May 1994, **18**, 474–8.
115. Yule SM, Bown N, Malcolm AJ, Reid MM, Pearson AD. Solid alveolar rhabdomyosarcoma with a t(2;13). Cancer Genet Cytogene 1995, **80**, 107–9.
116. Sublett JE, Jeonr IS, Shapiro DN. The alveolar rhabdomyosarcoma PAX3/FKHR fusion protein is a transcriptional activator. Oncogene 1995, **11**, 545–52.
117. Bennicelli JL, Fredericks WJ, Wilson RP, Rauscherr FJ, III, Barr, FG. Wild type PAX3 protein and the PAX3-FKHR fusion protein of alveolar rhabdomyosarcoma contain potent, structurally distinct transcriptional activation domains. Oncogene 1995, **11**, 119–30.
118. Bennicelli JL, Edwards RH, Barr FG. Mechanism for transcriptional gain of function resulting from chromosomal translocation in alveolar rhabdomyosarcoma. Proc Natl Acad USA 1996, **93**, 5455–9.
119. Weber-Hall S, McManus A, Anderson J, Nojima T, Abe S, Pritchard-Jones K, Shipley J. Novel formation and amplification of the PAX7-FKHR fusion gene in a case of alveolar rhabdomyosarcoma. Genes Chromosomes Cancer 1996, **17**, 7–13.
120. Davis RJ, D'Cruz CM, Lovell MA, Biegel JA, Barr FG. Fusion of PAX7 to FKHR by the variant t(1;13)(p36:q14) translocation in alveolar rhabdomyosarcoma. Cancer Res 1994, **54**, 2869–72.
121. Walther C, Guenet JL, Simon D, Deutsch U, Jostes B, Goulding MD, Plachov D, Balling R, Gruss P. PAX: a murine multigen family of paired box-containing genes. Genomics 1991, **11**, 424–34.
122. Fitzgerald JC, Scherr AM, Barr FG. Structural analysis of PAX7 rearrangements in alveolar rhabdomyosarcoma. Cancer Genet Cytogenet 2000, **117**, 37–40.
123. Davis RJ, Barr FG. Fusion genes resulting from alternative chromosomal translocations are overexpressed by gene-specific mechanisms in alveolar rhabdomyosarcoma. Proc Natl Acad Sci USA 1997, **94**, 8047–51.
124. Kelly KM, Womer RB, Sorensen PH, Xiong QB, Barr FG. Common and variant gene fusions predict distinct clinical phenotypes in rhabdomyosarcoma. J Clin Oncol 1997, **15**, 1831–6.
125. Frascella E, Toffolatti L, Rosolen A. Normal and rearranged PAX3, expression in human rhabdomyosarcoma. Cancer Genet Cytogenet 1998, **102**, 104–9.
126. Epstein JA, Shapiro DN, Cheng J, Lam PY, Maas RL. Pax3 modulates expression of the c-Met receptor during limb muscle development. Proc Natl Acad Sci USA 1996, **93**, 4213–18.
127. Driman D, Thorner PS, Greenberg ML, Chilton-MacNeill S, Squire J. MYCN gene amplification in rhabdomyosarcoma. Cancer 1994, **73**, 2231–7.
128. Kouraklis G, Triche TJ, Wesley R, Tsokos M. Myc oncogene expression and nude mouse tumorigenicity and metastasis formation are higher in alveolar than embryonal rhabdomyosarcoma cell lines. Pediatr Res 1999, **45**, 552–8.
129. Taylor AC, Shu L, Danks MK, Poquette CA, Shetty S, Thayer MJ, Houghton PJ, Harris, LC. P53 mutation and MDM2 amplification frequency in pediatric rhabdomyosarcoma tumors and cell lines. Med Pediatr Oncol 2000, **35**, 96–103.

130. Brinkschmidt C, Poremba C, Schäfer KL, Simon R, Jürgens H, Böcker W, Dockhorn-Dworniczak B. Evidence of genetic alterations in chromosome 11 in embryonal and alveolar rhabdomyosarcoma. Verh Dtsch Ges Pathol 1998, 82, 210–14.
131. Casola S, Pedone PV, Cavazzana AO, Basso G, Luksch R, d'Amore ES, Carli M, Bruni CB, Riccio A. Expression and parental imprinting of the *H19* gene in human rhabdomyosarcoma. Oncogene 1997, 14, 1503–10.
132. Treuner J, Kühl J, Beck J, Ritter J, Spaar HJ, Jürgens H, Keim M, Weinel P, Brandeis W, Reiter A, Bürger D, Niethammer D. New aspects in the treatment of childhood rhabdomyosarcoma: Results of the German Cooperative Soft-Tissue Sarcoma Study (CWS-81). Prog Pediatr Surg 1989, 22, 162–75.
133. Flamant F, Rodary C, Rey A, Praquin MT, Sommelet D, Quintana E, Theobald S, Brunat-Mentigny M, Otten J, Voute PA, Habrand JL, Martelli H, Barrett A, Terrier-Lacombe MJ, Oberlin O. Treatment of non-metastatic rhabdomyosarcomas in childhood and adolescence. Results of the second study of the International Society of Paediatric Oncology: MMT84. Eur J Cancer 1998, 34, 1050–62.
134. Koscielniak E, Jürgens H, Winkler K, Bürger D, Herbst M, Keim M, Bernhard G, Treuner J. Treatment of soft tissue sarcoma in childhood and adolescence. A report of the German Cooperative Soft Tissue Sarcoma Study. Cancer 1992, 70, 2557–67.
135. Harms D, Leuschner I, Krams M, Pilgrim TB, Treuner J. Rhabdomyosarcomas and extraosseous Ewing's sarcomas. Path Res Pract 1998, 194, 215.
136. Kuttesch JF, Parham DM, Luo X, Meyer WH, Bowman L, Shapiro DN, Pappo AS, Crist WM, Beck WT, Houghton PJ. P-glycoprotein expression at diagnosis may not be a primary mechanism of therapeutic failure in childhood rhabdomyosarcoma. J Clin Oncol 1996, 14, 886–900.

11 | Malignant soft tissue tumors of childhood

J. Robert Thomas and David M. Parham

Introduction

Other than rhabdomyosarcoma and peripheral primitive neuroectodermal tumor (PNET), malignant neoplasms arising within extraskeletal soft tissue comprise a small percentage of childhood tumors (1). Their relatively infrequent occurrence can contribute to difficulty in clinical recognition and correct classification. Another factor that hinders our understanding, especially in light of their rarity, is their wide diversity in tumor types, as partially listed in Table 11.1, which also gives data related to relative incidence in a large prospective multiinstitutional study (2, 3). Recent developments in the basic biological understanding of some of these entities will hopefully aid in alleviating some problems in their diagnosis and classification.

The most important predictor of the biologic behavior of these neoplasms is, at the present time, the histologic grade (4). Numerous grading schemes have been proposed for malignant adult and pediatric soft tissue tumors based on various histologic parameters that have included cellularity, cellular pleomorphism, phenotypic differentiation, mitotic activity, necrosis, and other parameters (5–13). The infrequent occurrence in the pediatric age group and the inherent diversity of these neoplasms has made the development of a universal grading scheme difficult. It would appear that, other than the histologic diagnosis, the two best predictors of tumor behavior are mitotic index and the percentage of the tumor that is necrotic. In one prospective study involving only pediatric patients, a grading scheme was devised for soft tissue sarcomas (excluding rhabdomyosarcoma and PNET) (Table 11.2) (4). In this scheme, three grades result from a consideration of histologic diagnosis, age of the patient, and a host of other parameters, which include mitotic index and necrosis. To briefly summarize this scheme, certain histologic tumor phenotypes (such as well-differentiated liposarcoma) are low grade or grade 1, and certain tumor phenotypes (such as pleomorphic and round cell liposarcoma) are high grade or grade 3. Sarcomas not specifically assigned to grade 1 or 3 in this manner are assigned to grade 2 if less than 15% of the tumor is necrotic or if the mitotic count is less than or equal to 5 per 10 high power (400×) fields (hpf), and grade 3 if more than 15% of the tumor is necrotic or if the mitotic count is greater than 5 per 10 hpf. Using this scheme, significant differences in 5-year event-free survival rates were found for patients with grades 1 and 2 versus grade 3 surgically resected tumors (93% versus 52%, respectively, $p = 0.0001$) (3).

In recent years biologic studies have brought the molecular genetic features of soft tissue sarcomas to the forefront of scientific investigation. This research has been most fruitful in revealing chromosomal aberrations that characterize these lesions and the genetic lesions that result, adding an exciting new dimension to sarcoma diagnosis and study. A list of lesions described to date and the so-affected diagnostic entities is seen in Table 11.3. This chapter will offer a brief recounting of this data and how it might be used for diagnosis; biologic studies into the molecular nature of these aberrations and their relationship to tumorigenesis are too robust for detailed discussion.

Synovial sarcoma

Excluding rhabdomyosarcoma and PNET, synovial sarcoma is the most common malignant soft tissue neoplasm in the pediatric population. It comprised almost a third of the malignant soft tissue tumors in the pediatric age group as compiled for a 5-year period by the Pediatric Oncology Group (4). In general, synovial sarcoma is rare under the age of 10 years; however, the tumor has been reported in young children and even in newborns (14–16). It is most common in the 10–20-year-old age group. In 345 cases reviewed at

Table 11.1 Distribution of non-rhabdomyosarcomatous soft tissue tumors by histologic category, Pediatric Oncology Group, 1986–94 (2, 3)

Diagnosis	Resected	Unresectable or metastatic	Total
Synovial sarcoma	29	8	37
MPNST	8	13	21
MFH*	10	5	15
Sarcoma, not otherwise specified	6	6	12
Fibrosarcoma	8	4	12
Leiomyosarcoma	6	3	8
Alveolar soft part sarcoma	2	5	7
Clear cell sarcoma	4	2	6
Epithelioid sarcoma	3	2	5
Hemangiopericytoma	0	4	4
Malignant mesenchymoma	1	2	3
Angiosarcoma/hemangioendothelioma	0	2	2
Liposarcoma	1	0	1
Extraskeletal myxoid chondrosarcoma	1	0	1
Totals	79	56	134

* Includes lesions now known as "angiomatoid fibrous histiocytomas" and previously classified as a form of MFH.

Table 11.2 Pediatric Oncology Group grading schema for soft tissue sarcomas other than rhabdomyosarcoma and PNET (4)

Grade 1
Myxoid and well-differentiated liposarcoma
Deep-seated dermatofibrosarcoma protuberans
Well-differentiated or infantile (age <5 years) fibrosarcoma
Well-differentiated or infantile (age <5 years) hemangiopericytoma
Well-differentiated MPNST

Grade 2
Sarcomas not specifically included in grades 1 or 3 and which have a mitotic index of <5 per 10 hpf, using a 40× objective, and <15% of the tumor shows geographic necrosis. Low cellularity and absence of significant pleomorphism are secondary criteria that can be used in assignment of borderline cases

Grade 3
Pleomorphic or round cell liposarcoma
Extraskeletal mesenchymal chondrosarcoma
Extraskeletal osteosarcoma
Malignant triton tumor
Alveolar soft part sarcoma
Sarcomas not specifically in grade 1 and which have a mitotic index of >4 per 10 hpf or in which >15% of the tumor shows geographic necrosis. High cellularity and significant pleomorphism are secondary criteria that can be used in assignment of borderline cases

the Armed Forces Institute of Pathology, only 12 cases occurred in individuals less than 10 years of age while 94 occurred in individuals between 10 and 20 years of age (17). They typically arise as a palpable mass in the soft tissue of an extremity, lower extremity more commonly than upper, and for unknown reasons they are associated with pain or tenderness in over 50% of the cases. Synovial sarcomas often arise in the vicinity of a large joint and may become adherent to peri-articular aponeuroses and membranes, yet intra-articular cases are extremely rare and comprise less than 5% of the reported tumors. The most common location is around the knee (17).

Pathologic examination typically reveals a partially cystic mass with a surrounding pseudocapsule. There may be areas of necrosis. Synovial sarcomas are composed of two phenotypically distinguishable cell types, an epithelial type and a spindle cell type, and these two

Table 11.3 Cytogenetic and molecular genetic aberrations in pediatric non-rhabdomyosarcomatous soft tissue sarcomas

Sarcoma	Chromosomal abnormality	Gene fusion or deletion
Synovial sarcoma	t(X;18)(p11;q11)	SSX1/SYT; SSX2/SYT
MPNST	No consistent abnormality	NF1 deletions (in NF1 patients)
Infantile fibrosarcoma	t(12;15)(p13;q25), +8, +11, +17, +20	ETV6/NTRK3
DSRCT	t(11;22)(p13;q12)	WT1/EWS
Myxoid liposarcoma	t(12;16)(q13;p11)	CHOP/FUS
Epithelioid sarcoma	del(22q), del(1p)	?
Clear cell sarcoma of tendons and aponeuroses	t(12;22)(q13;q12)	ATF-1/EWS
Extraskeletal myxoid chondrosarcoma	t(9;22)(q22;q12)	CHN/EWS
Extrarenal rhabdoid tumor	del(22q)(11.2)	hSNF5/INI1 deletion?

cell types are present in varying proportions in any given tumor. The epithelial cells are typically cuboidal to columnar and may organize as gland-like structures, or as nests, trabeculae, or cords of cells. The epithelial cells and the pseudoglandular spaces may contain mucin stainable with PAS, mucicarmine, colloidal iron, and alcian blue (17). The spindle cell areas are typically composed of uniform spindle cells which may focally resemble fibrosarcoma but are typically less mitotically active. Biphasic tumors contain both epithelial and spindle cells (Fig. 11.1(a)) and are the most common type of synovial sarcoma (16, 17), but the epithelial component is often subtle in these tumors. Monophasic tumors contain only one cell type, and the monophasic spindle cell type (Fig. 11.1(b)) is more common than the monophasic epithelial type. These tumors may also be poorly differentiated (17). Focal myxomatous change and calcification and chondroid and osseous changes may be present (17). Immunophenotyping typically shows positive staining with antibodies to epithelial membrane antigen (EMA) and low and high molecular-weight keratin (17–23). Keratin can usually be identified in both epithelial and spindle cells, although spindle cell staining may be more subtle. Prior trypsinization of the tissue may increase sensitivity to staining for keratin. Vimentin is typically detected in spindle cells only. Leu-7 (18) and S-100 protein (17, 24) may also be detected in synovial sarcomas, precluding the use of these markers in differentiating these tumors from peripheral nerve sheath tumors.

The major differential diagnoses in the pediatric age group are malignant peripheral nerve sheath tumor (MPNST) and fibrosarcoma. Those cases of synovial sarcoma with obvious biphasic or monophasic epithelial patterns will typically be easily differentiated from these entities, especially when immunostaining for keratin can be demonstrated. MPNSTs may rarely show glandular differentiation (25), but these tumors typically present in a patient with neurofibromatosis type 1 and the glands contain intestinal-type epithelial differentiation with microvilli and goblet cells, features never seen in the glandular elements of synovial sarcoma. As previously noted, S-100 protein may be detected in both synovial sarcoma and MPNST, and is thus not generally useful for distinguishing these two entities. Reticulin staining may highlight epithelioid foci (26).

Differentiating monophasic spindle cell synovial sarcoma from fibrosarcoma can be much more difficult, and relies primarily on a diligent search for an "epithelioid" component, the demonstration of focal calcification (less common in fibrosarcoma) and positive immunostaining for keratin. Another problem arises from the often prominent staghorn vessels present in synovial sarcoma, creating a strong resemblance to hemangiopericytoma. However, the latter lesion may be relatively low grade, particularly in very young children. Thus, it behooves one to strongly consider synovial sarcoma in any pediatric soft tissue lesion resembling hemangiopericytoma and to take the necessary steps to eliminate that possibility.

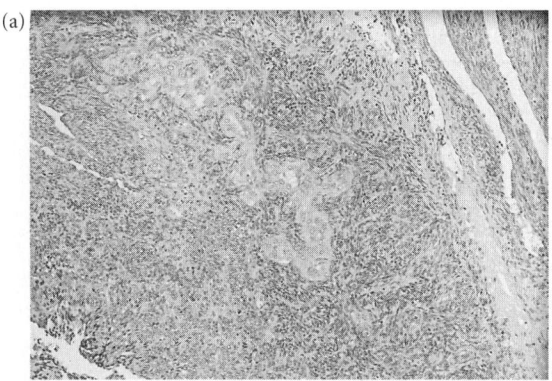 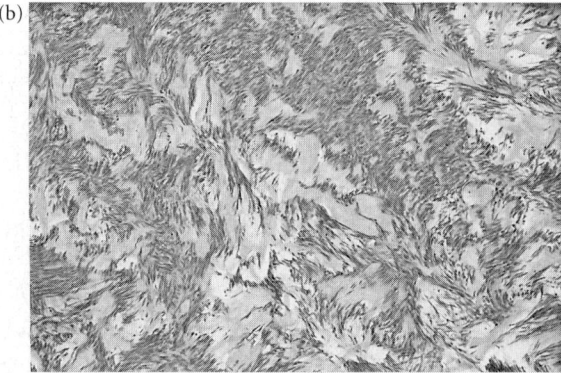

Fig. 11.1 (a) Biphasic synovial sarcoma. Epithelioid tumor cells form pseudoglandular spaces (center) and trabeculae, and are interspersed among spindled tumor cells. (b) Monophasic spindle cell synovial sarcoma. Thick collagen bands, shown here separating monomorphic spindled tumor cells, are sometimes a prominent feature of synovial sarcoma.

Folpe et al. recently described the use of a panel of antibodies which may be useful in distinguishing poorly differentiated synovial sarcoma from other poorly differentiated neoplasms such as PNETs and MPNSTs. They report that most of these tumors can be differentiated using a panel consisting of low and high molecular weight cytokeratins, EMA, type IV collagen, CD99, CD56, and S-100 protein (27).

Clinicopathologic features associated with a favorable outcome include ≤15 years of age, tumor size ≤5 cm, distal location in an extremity, and extensive tumor calcification and ossification (28–30). Mitotic indices of less than 10 mitoses per 10 hpf and negative margins at surgical resection are additional parameters that have been associated with an improved survival rate in synovial sarcoma (30, 31). Factors associated with an unfavorable outcome are essentially those of high-grade tumors and include high mitotic indices and significant tumor necrosis (32–34). Seven-year survival rates of children and adolescents with synovial sarcoma were reported as 63% by Schmidt et al. (16).

Multiple cytogenetic studies of synovial sarcomas have independently confirmed the uniform presence of a characteristic reciprocal translocation, the t(X;18) (p11.2;q11.2) (Fig. 11.2) (35). The exact fusion point delimited by this translocation eluded molecular researchers for several years, until it was determined that there were actually two separate but homologous loci, *SSX1* and *SSX2*, that fuse with the *SYT* on chromosome 18 (36). The protein product of this fusion contains a probable transcriptional activation domain from SYT that replaces a KRAB-homologous region from the SSX genes, resulting in a molecule with altered transcription (36, 37). Detection of the t(X;18) fusion can be accomplished by reverse transcriptase polymerase chain reaction (RT-PCR) or fluorescent *in situ* hybridization (FISH), and the results can be a powerful discriminator in cases with only monophasic features (38). Some data suggest that *SSX1* or *SSX2* involvement correlates with the presence of biphasic versus monophasic histology and good versus bad clinical behavior, respectively (39).

Malignant peripheral nerve sheath tumor

Malignant peripheral nerve sheath tumors are not common in children. According to a survey of soft tissue sarcomas (excluding rhabdomyosarcoma and PNET) treated on a Pediatric Oncology Group study between 1986 and 1991, only 16% were MPNSTs (Table 11.1). Although roughly 50% of these tumors develop in patients with neurofibromatosis type 1 (17, 40, 41), these patients are generally in early adulthood or older when they first present with a MPNST. Patients with neurofibromatosis at the time of diagnosis of MPNST are generally younger than patients without neurofibromatosis (40, 41). Although patients with neurofibromatosis type 1 are at increased risk to develop MPNSTs, the magnitude of the risk has been historically exaggerated and is currently estimated at 2–4% (42, 43).

The classic presentation of MPNST is a fusiform mass that involves a major nerve, often growing along the nerve sheath. These tumors commonly arise in a proximal

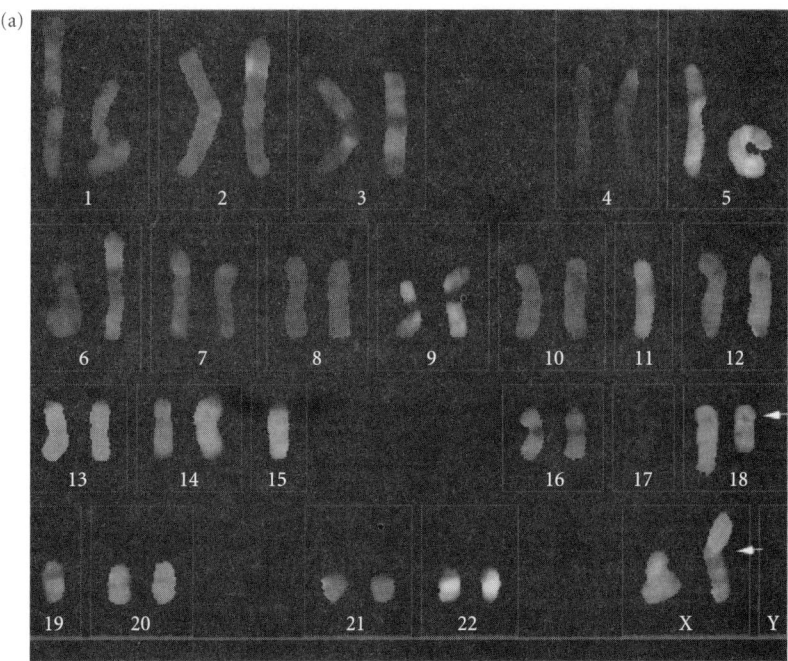

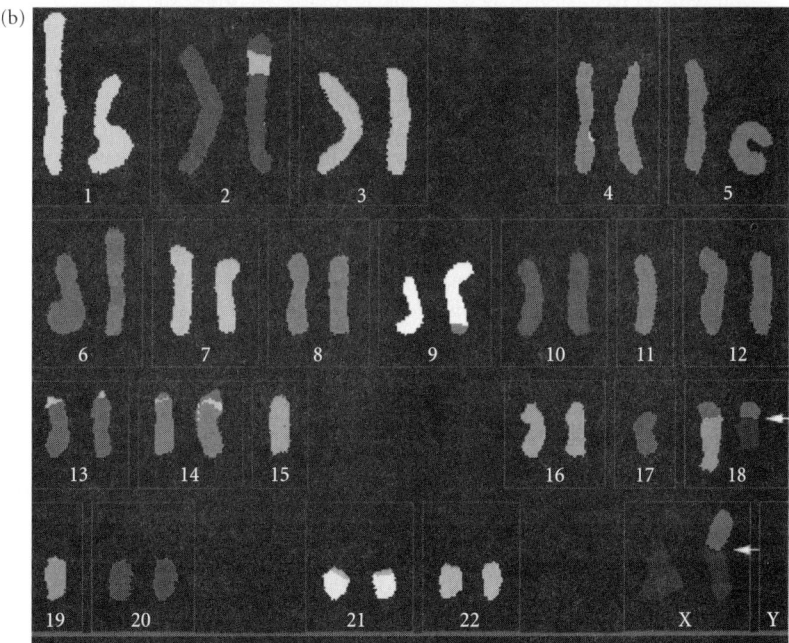

Fig. 11.2 Spectral karyotype of a synovial sarcoma showing the characteristic primary aberration of t(X;18)(p11;q11) (arrows) and secondary aberrations involving chromosomes 3, 9, and 18. (a) Chromosomes in display colors. (b) The same chromosomes in classification colors. See Plate 11.

extremity or the trunk. In neurofibromatosis type 1, these tumors may arise within a neurofibroma, usually one that is within deep soft tissues (17). In some sporadic cases, an association with a nerve is not evident. MPNSTs are a histologically heterogeneous group of tumors, which may reflect their origin from any of the components of the nerve sheath including the schwann cells and fibroblasts. The histologic appearance of these tumors may resemble fibrosarcoma, malignant fibrous histiocytoma (MFH), and synovial sarcoma. Typically, the cells have wavy nuclei, are arranged in fascicles (which may whorl to simulate tactoid corpuscles), and areas of high cell density may alternate with areas of lower cell density due in part to the presence of significant amounts of a myxoid extracellular matrix (Fig. 11.3). Areas of increased cell density are sometimes found in a perivascular distribution, and these areas may show a relative increase in mitoses. Some of these tumors appear as cellular, pleomorphic neurofibromas, and an increased mitotic index offers the best indication of their malignant behavior (17). Likewise, some of these tumors are very poorly differentiated sarcomas and their occurrence in association with neurofibromatosis or in association with a large nerve may be the only clue to the correct diagnosis.

Heterotopic elements may be seen in MPNSTs (40). Bone and cartilage are the most common elements (17). While ectopic skeletal muscle is rare in these neoplasms (17), the presence of rhabdomyoblasts (rhabdomyosarcoma) in an MPNST confers the diagnosis of malignant Triton tumor (17, 44). Muscle-specific actin, desmin, and myoglobin can usually be detected in these cells. Occasionally glandular differentiation is apparent (glandular malignant schwannoma) and confusion with synovial sarcoma may occur (25). A group of tumors that clinically present as MPNSTs and exhibit a predominantly epithelioid appearance have been described and designated epithelioid MPNST (epithelioid malignant schwannoma) (45, 46). These are a histologically heterogeneous group of tumors, composed predominantly of large epithelioid cells with large nucleoli forming nodules and/or cords that may focally merge with a spindle cell component that is indistinguishable from "conventional" MPNST. These tumors usually stain diffusely positive for S-100 protein in contrast to the focal staining seen in conventional MPNST (46). Epithelioid MPNSTs may occur in the dermis and/or subcutaneous tissue, where they are associated with a better prognosis than those occurring in deep soft tissues.

The diagnosis of intermediate to high-grade MPNST is usually not difficult in the setting of neurofibromatosis. Low-grade tumors, however, may be confused with neurofibroma. The presence of mitoses and increased cellularity in the malignant lesions usually allows this distinction to be made, but not always. Coffin and Dehner report that two cases of apparent cellular neurofibroma recurred and one eventually metastasized (47). Nuclear pleomorphism alone is not generally helpful in distinguishing benign and malignant lesions, as it may be present in a neurofibroma with degenerative change.

An appreciation of the characteristic cytologic and nuclear features of the tumor cells and the identification of areas of neural differentiation aid in distinguishing MPNST from fibrosarcoma and synovial sarcoma. Over 50% of MPNSTs are at least focally positive upon immunostaining for S-100 protein (17), which is generally not present in fibrosarcoma. As noted previously, a small percentage of synovial sarcomas may be S-100-positive and thus concomitant keratin staining should be done. MPNSTs (without glandular differentiation) are routinely keratin-negative. The presence of glandular differentiation may cause confusion with synovial sarcoma. The glandular component of MPNST is keratin-positive, but the glands of these tumors show intestinal epithelial differentiation including goblet cells and microvilli (17), features not found in the glandular elements of synovial sarcoma. The distinction between epithelioid MPNST and melanoma may be a difficult one, as both can be diffusely S-100-positive, HMB45-negative, melanin-negative, and biphasic with epithelioid and spindle cell components, and both tumors can also show extracellular type IV collagen deposition (17, 46). Ultrastructural evidence of neural differentiation may be required to establish a diagnosis of MPNST in poorly differentiated cases (48).

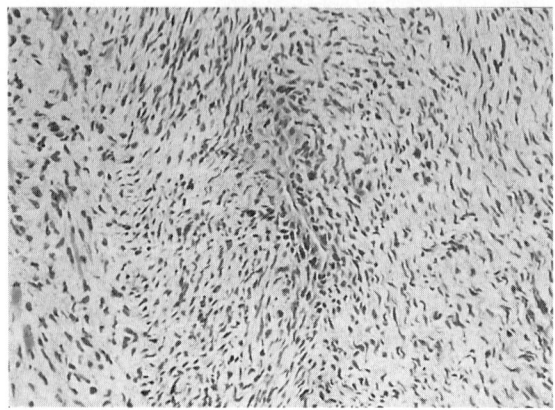

Fig. 11.3 MPNST. Pleomorphic tumor cells are present within a myxomatous stroma. Tumor cells may be seen proliferating around vascular structures (center) in these tumors.

Meis et al. studied various clinicopathologic features in 78 cases of MPNSTs in children 15 years of age. They found that age ≥7 years, tumor size >7.5 cm, tumor necrosis ≥25%, and neurofibromatosis type 1 independently predict a poor prognosis (41). Neurofibromatosis-1-associated MPNSTs are the only ones that are consistently associated with a genetic lesion, a constitutional deletion of the *NF1* gene, located on chromosome 17q11.2. This is a huge gene, approximately 300,000 bp in length, that encodes a protein known as neurofibromin. Neurofibromin is a tumor suppressor protein that modulates the phosphorylation state of the ras protein. Its loss or truncation may allow abnormal growth through altered signal transduction (49). MPNSTs may also be associated with alterations in p53, as demonstrable by immunohistochemical staining (50); this abnormality appears to contribute to increased malignant behavior.

Fibrosarcoma

Fibrosarcomas in the pediatric age group appear to occur as two different entities. Those that arise in children less than 5 years of age have a much better prognosis than those occurring in older children. In one study of 110 cases, the 5-year survival rates for fibrosarcoma in patients under 5 years of age was greater than 90%, whereas the survival rate for older patients approximated that for adults with fibrosarcoma, which in their series was 50% (51). In another study of 48 patients initially presenting at ages ranging from newborn to 4 years, the 5-year survival rate was 84%, although 8 patients developed recurrences (52). For comparison, Scott et al. report 5-year survival rates for fibrosarcoma in adults that range from 58% to 21% depending on the grade of the tumor (53).

Infantile fibrosarcoma

In one series, infantile fibrosarcoma typically presented as a painless, nontender, 1–20 cm mass (52). Most tumors presented during the first year of life and were present at birth in about one-fifth of the cases (congenital fibrosarcoma) (17). The oldest patient was 4 years of age. These tumors appear to occur more commonly on the distal extremities but can occur in the head, neck, and trunk (52, 54).

Infantile fibrosarcomas present a phenotypic spectrum. On one end, tumors may be composed of small immature fibroblasts with little to no extracellular collagen and lacking a well-defined fascicular pattern. On the other end, they may resemble more conventional adult-type tumors, having larger, more mature cells, cytoplasmic borders merging imperceptibly with extracellular collagen, and a well-defined fascicular (herring-bone) pattern. Mitoses are typically present in these tumors. Diffusely scattered lymphocytes are often prominent in infantile fibrosarcomas, a feature not typical of fibrosarcomas arising in the older age groups (17).

Fibrosarcoma may be difficult to differentiate from monophasic spindle-cell synovial sarcoma and MPNST. Synovial sarcomas and MPNSTs are rare under the age of 10 years but do occasionally occur. A diligent search for epithelioid elements (biphasic pattern) may be helpful in excluding synovial sarcoma. Fibrosarcomas are generally negative for S-100 protein and desmin (55), and thus immunostains for these may be helpful in differentiating fibrosarcoma from MPNST and rhabdomyosarcoma, respectively. Fibrosarcomas are also negative for factor VIII-related antigen (55), which can be useful in differentiating tumors with prominent vascularity and/or hemorrhage from angiosarcoma. The differentiation of fibrosarcoma from infantile fibromatosis is more problematic and may be virtually impossible in some cases. In the younger age group (5 years), differentiating these two entities may not be necessary since the treatment of choice for both is wide local excision. Lundgren et al. reported three cases of a tumor with clinicopathologic features of both rhabdomyosarcoma and fibrosarcoma. All three were less than 5 years old (13 months to 3 years). They termed this entity rhabdomyofibrosarcoma. Desmin and muscle-specific actin were detected in the tumor cells that ultrastructurally showed rhabdomyoblastic differentiation (17, 56).

Recent work has indicated the presence of a recurrent, reciprocal translocation in infantile fibrosarcoma, the t(12;15)(p13;q25). This aberration fuses the *ETV6* (also known as the *TEL* gene) on chromosome 12p13 with the *NTRK3* neurotrophin-3 receptor gene (also known as *TRKC*) on chromosome 15q25 (Fig. 11.4) (57). The tumorigenic significance of this unusual combination, which fuses a leukemia gene (*ETV6*) with a nerve growth factor receptor gene (*NTRK3*) to produce a fibroblastic lesion, is unknown at present. Likely, the fusion of the protein tyrosine kinase domain of the NTRK3 protein with the helix-loop-helix domain of the ETV6 protein results in dysregulation of NTRK3 signal transduction. Infantile fibrosarcoma is also cytogenetically characterized by trisomies of 8, 11, 17, and 20, demonstrable by FISH in interphase nuclei (58).

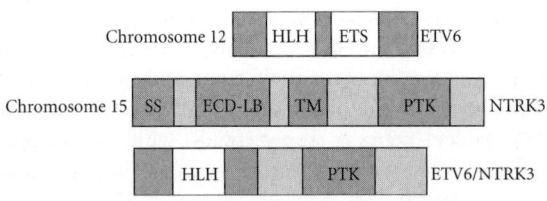

Fig. 11.4 Representation of gene fusion reported seen in infantile fibrosarcoma der(12)t(12;15), resulting from a reciprocal translocation between chromosomes 12 and 15. Abbreviations for genetic loci: HLH = helix-loop-helix; ETS = *ets* family gene; SS = signal sequence; ECD-LB = extracellular domain—ligand binding; TM = transmembrane; PTK = protein tyrosine kinase.

Inflammatory fibrosarcoma, myofibrosarcoma, and inflammatory myofibroblastic tumors

Inflammatory fibrosarcoma has also been termed omental-mesenteric myxoid hamartoma, inflammatory myofibroblastic tumor, inflammatory pseudotumor, and plasma cell granuloma (59–61). It is unclear if cases with the histologic features of this entity represent a single neoplasm or a heterogeneous group of entities. The original characterizations of inflammatory myofibroblastic tumor and inflammatory fibrosarcoma were benign and malignant, respectively, but this distinction appears to be a matter of degrees rather than absolute (62). Most occur in the mesentery or retroperitoneum of children and adolescents (61). Histologically similar tumors also occur in the urinary bladder (63–66). Associated clinical findings include fever, weight loss, anemia, and thrombocytosis (17, 60).

These tumors are typically composed of plump myofibroblasts infiltrated by inflammatory cells, most notably plasma cells, and varying degrees of fibrosis, myxoid change, and calcification may be present (17). The clinical behavior of these tumors is variable. Many of these patients do well following resection of the tumor, but recurrences do occur and metastases to the lung and brain have been reported (61, 67). Myofibroblastic tumors of the bladder have an excellent prognosis (17).

Flow cytometry data on inflammatory myofibroblastic tumors indicate that a substantial proportion are hyperdiploid (68). This phenomenon may explain the apparent transformation of these tumors into malignant lesions (69) and the difficulty in absolute separation of "myofibroblastic tumors" from "inflammatory fibrosarcomas." Clonal cytogenetic changes have also been described (70, 71), again indicating the potential for neoplastic clones to arise from this inflammatory milieu. Epstein–Barr virus infections have been associated with a subset of inflammatory pseudotumors (72).

Myofibrosarcomas are generally high-grade spindle cell lesions that share histologic features of fibrosarcomas, leiomyosarcomas, and MFH. They likely represent a subset of fibrosarcomas but may possess high-grade features and show aggressive clinical behavior. The head and neck of older children appears to be a favored site of origin (73). Differentiating these tumors from rhabdomyosarcoma and leiomyosarcoma can be difficult. Since myofibroblastic tumors may stain with myogenic markers, such as smooth muscle actin and desmin (17), in difficult cases this differentiation is best accomplished by electron microscopy or skeletal muscle-specific stains (e.g. myoglobin, MyoD).

Desmoplastic small round cell tumor

Desmoplastic small round cell tumor (DSRCT) is a malignant neoplasm primarily of adolescents and young adults (74–76), but has also been reported in children (77–79). It is typically an aggressive neoplasm that primarily involves the peritoneum of the abdomen and pelvis (74–76), but has also been reported arising in the male urogenital tract (75, 80, 81), ovary (82), pleura (83, 84), and cranial cavity (85). DSRCT is more common in males than females and presents as a palpable mass associated with clinical signs and symptoms that include fever, nausea and vomiting, abdominal pain and/or distention, constipation, edema of lower extremities, ureteral obstruction, and back, chest, and shoulder pain (17, 74–76).

On gross examination the tumors are typically gray–white, multilobular and firm with areas of necrosis, hemorrhage, and occasionally cystic change (17, 76). DSRCTs are phenotypically varied but the majority are composed of irregular nests of monomorphic, poorly differentiated tumor cells well demarcated from a fibrous stroma. The tumor cells have hyperchromatic nuclei, inconspicuous nucleoli, and little cytoplasm (17, 76). Ordóñez reported that one-third of 39 tumors were phenotypically atypical. Atypical cytologic findings in his series included tumor cells that exhibit spindle cell (two cases), transitional cell (one case), epithelioid (one case), and signet-ring cell (one case) features. Other cases demonstrated the formation of "Homer Wright-like" rosettes by tumor cells (two cases), tubule formation by tumor cells (eight cases), and lack of significant desmoplasia (one case) (76).

Most DSRCTs show immunohistochemical evidence of epithelial, mesenchymal, and neural differentiation (17, 74, 79, 82, 86, 87). In a recent analysis using over 30 different antibodies, DSRCTs were consistently positive for desmin (39 of 39 cases). A majority of tumors were also positive for: EMA (24 of 25 cases), cytokeratin (antibodies to CAM 5.2, AE1 and AE3; 37 of 39 cases), MOC-31 (9 of 10 cases), WT1 protein (8 of 9 cases), vimentin (22 of 27 cases), neuron-specific enolase (18 of 25 cases), Ber-EP4 (5 of 7 cases), CD15 (11 of 16 cases), and CD57 (10 of 15 cases) (87).

The DSRCTs usually can be distinguished from other neoplasms based on their morphologic appearance combined with their rather unique immunophenotypic profile and cytogenetic findings. Differentiation from Ewing's sarcoma involves the demonstration of negative immunostaining with CD99 and lack of cytoplasmic glycogen. Exclusion of rhabdomyosarcoma and neuroblastoma may be aided by demonstrating positive staining with EMA and cytokeratins.

Cytogenetically, DSRCTs are distinguished by the t(11;22)(p13;q12), which fuses the *WT1* gene on chromosome 11p13 with the *EWS* on 22q12 (Fig. 11.5) (88). This unusual combination of a Wilms' tumor gene (*WT1*) with a Ewing's sarcoma gene (*EWS*) may explain the propensity of this tumor to occur on peritoneal surfaces, where WT1 is expressed during embryogenesis (89), and the panoply of phenotypic features seen with immunohistochemistry. Rare cases with the pathologic and clinical features of DSRCT may exhibit the t(11;22) (q24;q12) more typical of Ewing's sarcoma and peripheral neuroectodermal tumors (90). The WT1/EWS fusion can be used as a diagnostic marker utilizing RT-PCR or FISH (91).

Miscellaneous soft tissue malignancies

Besides the more commonly recognized entities listed above, the pediatric patient is host to a variety of unusual and often poorly understood sarcomas. Another

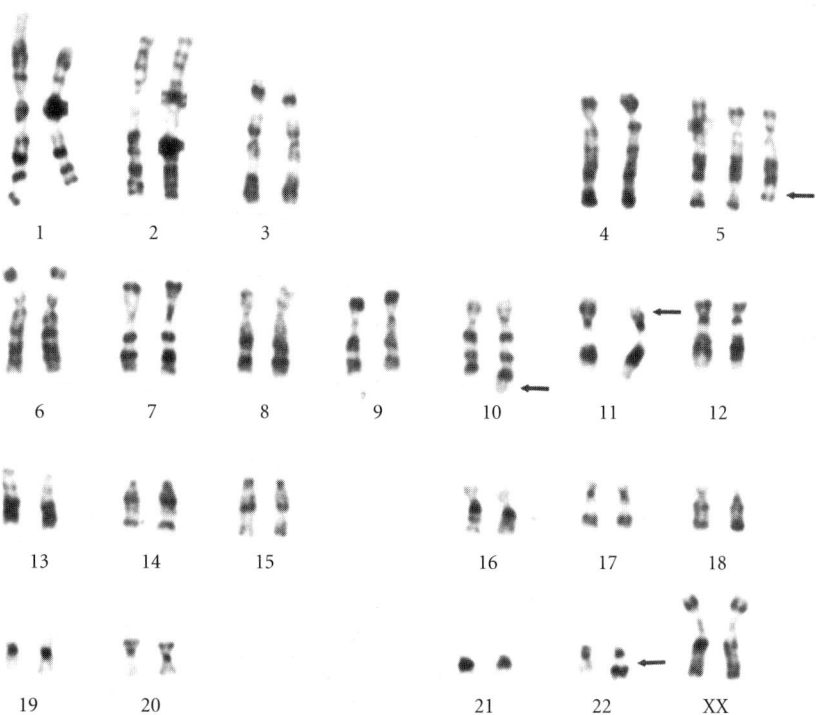

Fig. 11.5 G-band karyotype of a DSRCT showing the characteristic t(11;22)(p13;q12) as the primary chromosome aberration. Secondary chromosome aberrations involving chromosomes 5 and 10 are also present.

observation is that certain soft tissue cancers seen more frequently in adults may rarely arise in children. Examples of the former lesions include putative extrarenal rhabdoid tumors of soft tissue, and examples of the latter include MFH, myxofibrosarcoma, epithelioid sarcoma, alveolar soft part sarcoma, and angiosarcoma. The following section will offer brief morphologic and biologic descriptions of these rare entities. For more detailed discussion, the reader is advised to consult more comprehensive texts such as those by Enzinger and Weiss (17) or Fletcher (92).

Malignant fibrous histiocytoma

Malignant fibrous histiocytoma is a controversial entity at present, with some vociferously denying its existence as a discrete entity (93). At such it is best viewed as an operational definition and not a single lesion, as many examples represent highly dedifferentiated forms of other sarcomas (94). If so accepted, then MFH is the most common sarcoma in adults and one of the rarest ones in children. Only small series have been reported (95). In reviewing literature on pediatric MFH, it is important to not confuse this lesion with angiomatoid fibrous histiocytoma, a relatively more common childhood tumor that initially was published as angiomatoid MFH (96). However, long-term follow-up on a large number of patients has revealed only rare nodal metastases and no tumor-related deaths, so that angiomatoid fibrous histiocytoma is best regarded as a benign lesion at present.

Another point worth considering is that superficial fibrous histiocytomas are common childhood tumors and may contain areas of mitotic activity, necrosis, and pleomorphism. These lesions may recur but do not metastasize (97, 98). Unusual histologic variants, such as the plexiform fibrohistiocytic tumor (99), have been described. As such it is very important to seek consultation on any superficial soft tissue neoplasm for which the diagnosis of pediatric MFH is considered.

Myxofibrosarcoma

Myxoid soft tissue tumors comprise one of the most treacherous entities in sarcoma diagnosis. A gelatinous, myxoid matrix is a common feature of pediatric sarcomas, particularly embryonal rhabdomyosarcomas. Some soft tissue neoplasms are specifically characterized by the abundance of this material, associated with fibroblastic and myofibroblastic cells. The relative benignancy/malignancy of these tumors varies from the benign myxoma of soft tissue to the high-grade myxofibrosarcoma (also referred to as myxoid MFH) (100). Prediction of the outcome of intermediate lesions such as the low-grade fibromyxoid tumor can be quite challenging. Low-grade fibromyxoid tumors predominantly affect young adults and may occur in adolescents (101). Rare pediatric examples of high-grade myxofibrosarcoma have also been described (100). It is important to rule out other sarcomas, such as rhabdomyosarcomas and lipsarcomas. The presence of rhabdomyoblasts would define rhabdomyosarcoma, and lipoblasts definitionally define liposarcoma. However, "pseudolipoblasts" occur in fibromyxoid lesions (102), so that the positive S-100 staining of liposarcoma may be more helpful (103).

Liposarcoma

Liposarcoma is another lesion that is among the most common of adult sarcomas, yet it is exceedingly rare in children. Several small retrospective series of pediatric examples have been published (104, 105). In childhood myxoid liposarcomas are the most commonly occurring variant of this neoplasm (104). As noted above, myxoid liposarcomas must be distinguished from other myxoid tumors such as rhabdomyosarcoma and myxofibrosarcoma. Diagnosis of liposarcoma subtype is critical to predicting outcome, as myxoid liposarcomas are low-grade lesions and round cell liposarcomas are high-grade sarcomas (104, 106). Myxoid liposarcoma is karyotypically characterized by a reciprocal translocation, the t(12;16)(q13;p11) (107); trisomy 8 occurs as a nonrandom secondary change (108). At a molecular level, this genetic anomaly results in the fusion of the *FUS* (or *TLS*) gene on chromosome 16p11 and the *CHOP* gene on chromosome 12q13, making FISH analysis feasible (109).

Grossly, liposarcomas are gelatinous, lobulated masses that infiltrate adjacent soft tissue and can easily disseminate on surgical excision, given their gelatin-like consistency. Microscopically, myxoid liposarcomas have an abundant mucoid ground substance intersected by plexuses of fine capillaries, imparting a chicken yard fence-like appearance. Within this loose stroma are embedded lipoblasts, mesenchymal cells with eccentric ovoid nuclei and coarsely vacuolated cytoplasm. The vacuoles represent nascent lipid droplets that with cell maturation progressively distend the cell and impinge upon the nucleus. Round cell liposarcomas, on the other hand, are highly cellular lesions comprised of dense aggregates of very primitive, round lipoblasts with minimal cytoplasm, again enmeshed in a finely arcuate vasculature. Heterogeneous lesions may contain variable amounts of both myxoid and round cell elements.

Diagnosis of liposarcoma is accomplished by recognition of the histologic features noted above and identification of lipoblasts, with exclusion of other myxoid and round cell neoplasms. S-100 staining may be helpful in this regard (103), and cytogenetic or molecular genetic testing to detect the characteristic t(12;16) translocation or *FUS/CHOP* fusion is definitive (109).

Epithelioid sarcoma

Epithelioid sarcomas are uncommon lesions of children, primarily affecting adolescents. They have a proclivity to occur in distal extremities, particularly the hand. Discovery of lymph nodal metastases may precede clinical recognition of a primary lesion (110). A subset occurs in the head and neck region of young children (111). Epithelioid sarcomas are so named for their resemblance to the squamous epithelial cancers that occur in the respiratory tract and lower female genital tract. An important diagnostic caveat is that their granuloma-like appearance with areas of central necrosis rimmed by epithelioid cells (Fig. 11.6) may invite confusion with benign lesions such as annuloma granulare, rheumatoid nodules, and infections (112). Usually close microscopic inspection will reveal an intercellular stitched appearance created by postfixation stretching of desmosomal junctions, and diagnosis can be confirmed by positive staining with cytokeratins, EMA, CD34, and vimentin (113, 114).

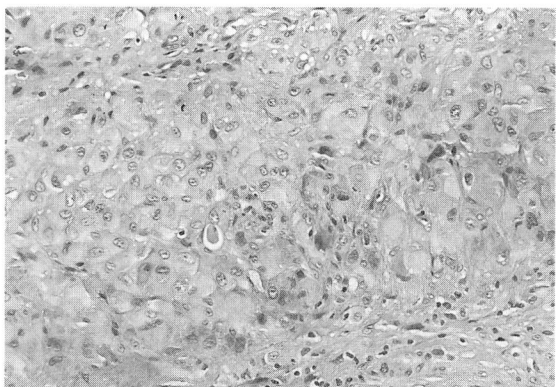

Fig. 11.6 Epithelioid sarcoma. Tumor cells have abundant cytoplasm giving them an epithelioid appearance. Note focal tumor cell necrosis which may be quite pronounced in these tumors.

There is as yet no diagnostic molecular marker, but molecularly epithelioid sarcomas are characterized by alterations on the long arm of chromosome 22 (115–117). Deletion of chromosome 1p, a rather ubiquitous abnormality among neoplasms, has also been described (118).

Alveolar soft part sarcoma

Alveolar soft part sarcoma has been a morphologically distinctive but phenotypically enigmatic lesion since its initial recognition (119). It is another sarcoma affecting all age groups, rarely including children and adolescents. Clinically alveolar soft part sarcoma is characterized by inexorable progression, although survival may be long. There are data to suggest that pediatric examples are more likely to be cured than adult ones (119, 120). All body sites may be involved.

Alveolar soft part sarcomas have a very characteristic histologic appearance, comprising aggregates of cuboidal, eosinophilic cells separated by a fine reticulin framework that subtends these cells into discrete nests or alveoli (Fig. 11.7). In pediatric examples, there may be a more diffuse pattern with less conspicuous nesting (17). The diagnostic *sine qua non* has been the presence of needle-like cytoplasmic crystals identifiable by periodic acid-Schiff stains. By electron microscopy these bodies are rhomboid crystals with a characteristic periodicity. In some cases the crystals are only focally present, and their identification may require some searching. Crystal-deficient cases have been documented (121).

The major controversy in alveolar soft part sarcoma is the cell type these tumors represent, neural versus myogenous. Some lesions stain positively with neural markers (122) and others with muscle markers (123). No feature of myogenous differentiation have been found by electron microscopy, in spite of positivity with desmin and muscle-specific actin stains, although cytoplasmic crystals have been described in ultrastructural studies of intrafusal muscle fibers (124). Rosai and colleagues (123) published a report of immunofluorescent MyoD positivity in these lesions, but later studies found this property to represent non-specific cytoplasmic staining (125). The zellballen-like pattern imparted by the reticulin framework invites a comparison to paragangliomas, possibly explaining the cases with neural positivity. To date there is no final explanation of these enigmatic and divergent phenotypic properties, and cytogenetic studies have not been particularly rewarding (126, 127).

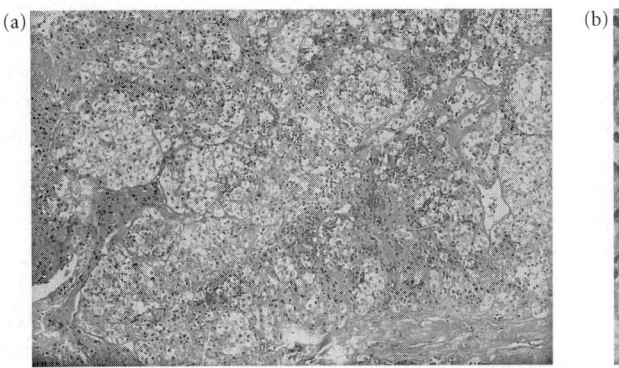 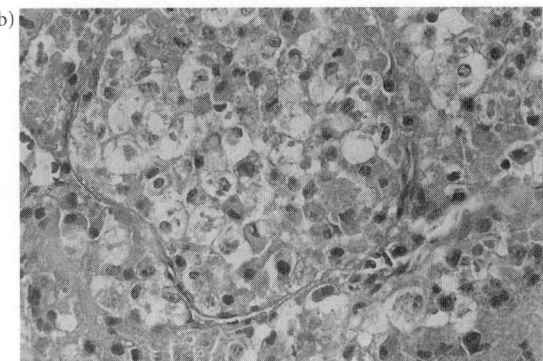

Fig. 11.7 Alveolar soft part sarcoma. (a) Tumor cells form nests separated by fibrovascular tissue (producing an alveolar pattern). (b) Note that the tumor cells are pleomorphic and discohesive.

Clear cell sarcoma of tendons and aponeuroses

Clear cell sarcomas of tendons and aponeuroses (to be distinguished from clear cell sarcoma of kidney, an unrelated entity) are melanocytic neoplasms that have also been called "melanomas of soft parts." However, they are biologically distinct from cutaneous melanomas, as the former tumors are characterized most often by deletions of chromosome 9p (128) and the latter by a reciprocal translocation, the t(12;22)(q13;q12) (129). The 22q12 breakpoint in clear cell sarcomas fuses the EWS gene with the ATF-1 gene on chromosome 12q13, so that these neoplasms share a molecular relatedness with Ewing's sarcomas and peripheral neuroectodermal tumors in possessing a EWS breakpoint (130).

Histologically, clear cell sarcomas have distinctive features not generally seen in cutaneous melanomas. However, this is purely a generalization, as melanomas can exhibit a wide range of morphologic features, and clear cell variants have been described (131). The distinction, then, primarily rests with the strictly soft tissue origin of clear cell sarcoma and the cutaneous derivation of melanomas. Nevertheless, clear cell sarcomas tend to be morphologically homogeneous, comprising relatively large cells with oval nuclei, conspicuous nucleoli, and moderate amounts of clear cytoplasm. In some examples there is a more amphophilic to lightly eosinophilic cytoplasm. Usually there is a vague nesting arrangement. Melanin is usually seen in only rare cells, but special stains such as the Fontana melanin stain may disclose a greater abundance than is visible by routine hematoxylin and eosin. Electron microscopy can be helpful in confirming the melanocytic nature of this tumor by the finding of melanosomes, and as with melanoma immunohistochemical stains are typically positive for S-100 and HMB45 (132).

Extraskeletal myxoid chondrosarcoma

Like clear cell sarcoma, extraskeletal myxoid chondrosarcoma is genetically characterized by a reciprocal translocation, the t(9;22)(q22;q12), that involves the EWS locus on 22q12, in this case fused to the CHN gene on chromosome 9q22 (133). The similarity ends there, as extraskeletal myxoid chondrosarcoma is a morphologically distinctive neoplasm showing none of the histologic features of either clear cell or Ewing's sarcoma. Clinically and biologically, it also is unrelated to myxoid chondrosarcomas of bone, which have different ultrastructural and karyotypic features (134). Extraskeletal myxoid chondrosarcomas are very rare neoplasms that may occur in unusual sites such as the larynx (135). As with pediatric non-rhabdomyosarcomas in general, grade is important in predicting outcome of these tumors (134), which may have a protracted but inexorable course (136). Initially these were listed as de facto low-grade lesions in the Pediatric Oncology Group grading schema (4), but following publication of these recent findings extraskeletal myxoid chondrosarcomas are now part of the two-tiered grade 2 and grade 3 system (Table 11.2).

The chondrocytic nature of extraskeletal myxoid chondrosarcoma was not definitively concluded until relatively recently (137). Prior studies analogized them to chordomas, using the diagnostic term, chordoid sarcoma (137). Microscopically the constituent cells do have an epithelioid appearance; they form small aggregates and trabeculae floating in a sea of abundant mucoid ground substance (hence the name). True hyaline cartilage is rare or non-existent. The cartilagenous nature of the tumor is confirmed by its S-100 positivity (138), and electron microscopy often reveals characteristic intracisternal arrays of microtubules (139). A morphologically similar tumor and even rarer soft tissue tumor is the parachordoma, a true epithelial neoplasm that unlike extraskeletal myxoid chondrosarcoma expresses cytokeratin (140–142). Parachordomas may have clonal cytogenetic aberrations (143, 144).

Angiosarcoma

Angiosarcoma is another soft tissue malignancy that is relatively common in adults, particularly on the sun-exposed skin of the elderly, but exceeding rare in children. Only isolated case reports and a few small series are reported (145). Microscopically pediatric angiosarcomas display the morphologic features typical of adult examples, and they may coexist with more benign lesions such as hemangiomatosis (145). In the authors' experience, the relatively low-grade epithelioid variants of angiosarcoma tend to be more common in pediatric patients than the usual forms. Epithelioid angiosarcomas may be recognized morphologically by their tendency to form intracytoplasmic lumens containing erythrocytes (17). Endothelium-specific markers such as von Willebrand factor (factor VIII-associated protein), Ulex europaeus lectin binding, CD34, and CD31 should be helpful in diagnosis, and a caveat is the occasional positivity of angiosarcomas for cytokeratin (146).

Extrarenal rhabdoid tumor

Extrarenal rhabdoid tumors have been controversial lesions that mostly are the subject of isolated case reports. As such they have spanned the anatomic spectrum of primary sites, and soft tissue lesions are a major group of this rare entity (147–149). In the combined St Jude Children's Research Hospital and National Wilms' Tumor Pathology Center experience (150), soft tissue lesions formed a large percentage of putative rhabdoid tumor cases but generally comprised other sarcoma entities that contained rhabdoid cells. This observation has been made by others (148, 149, 151). Rhabdoid cells, so named from their resemblance to rhabdomyoblasts, are relatively large cells with eccentric nuclei, prominent owl's-eye nucleoli, abundant cytoplasm, and cytoplasmic hyaline inclusions. Ultrastructurally these latter elements comprise whorls of intermediate filaments that stain positively for vimentin with immunohistochemistry. Other markers, usually epithelial proteins, are also positive, and typically these tumors stain for a confusing plethora of phenotypic indicators (150).

Rhabdoid tumors were originally described as renal tumors arising in infants and very young children, and the existence of extrarenal examples has been a matter of debate (152). Nevertheless, young children do occasionally fall prey to apparent rhabdoid tumors that affect organs other than the kidney, so that it is hard to dispute their existence in this patient population. Biologic relatedness is also seen, as both renal and extrarenal rhabdoid tumors are characterized by deletions in chromosome 22q11.2, possibly affecting the *hSNF5/INI1* gene (153). Suffice it to say at this juncture that these are rare tumors usually seen in infants and that diagnosis requires vigorous exclusion of other unrelated entities. The prognosis has been almost universally dismal.

Acknowledgments

The authors thank Dr Jeff Sawyer, Professor of Pathology, University of Arkansas for Medical Sciences, for kindly providing karyotype images for Figs 11.2 and 11.5.

References

1. Pratt CB, Kun LE. Soft tissue sarcomas: new developments in the multidisciplinary approach to treatment. In: Soft tissue sarcomas of children (ed. Pinedo HM, Verweij J, Suit H), Kluwer Academic Publishers, Boston, 1991, 149–65.
2. Pratt CB, Maurer HM, Gieser P, Salzberg A, Rao BN, Parham D, Thomas PR, Marcus RB, Cantor A, Pick T, *et al.* Treatment of unresectable or metastatic pediatric soft tissue sarcomas with surgery, irradiation, and chemotherapy: a Pediatric Oncology Group study. Med Pediatr Oncol 1998, 30(4), 201–9.
3. Pratt CB, Pappo AS, Gieser P, *et al.* The role of adjuvant chemotherapy in the treatment of surgically resected pediatric non-rhabdomyosarcomatous soft tissue sarcomas: a Pediatric Oncology Group study. J Clin Oncol 1999, 17, 1219–26.
4. Parham DM, Webber BL, Jenkins JJ, Cantor AB, Maurer HM. Nonrhabdomyosarcomatous soft tissue sarcomas of childhood: formulation of a simplified system for grading. Mod Pathol 1995, 8, 705–10.
5. Markhede G, Angervall L, Stener B. A multivariate analysis of the prognosis after surgical treatment of malignant soft-tissue tumors. Cancer 1982, 49(8), 1721–33.

6. Myhre-Jensen O, Kaae S, Madsen EH, Sneppen O. Histopathological grading in soft-tissue tumours. Relation to survival in 261 surgically treated patients. Acta Pathol Microbiol Immunol Scand [A] 1983, **91**, 145–50.
7. Costa J, Wesley RA, Glatstein E, Rosenberg SA. The grading of soft tissue sarcomas. Results of a clinicohistopathologic correlation in a series of 163 cases. Cancer 1984, **53**, 530–41.
8. Trojani M, Contesso G, Coindre JM, Rouesse J, Bui NB, de MA, Goussot JF, David M, Bonichon F, Lagarde C. Soft-tissue sarcomas of adults; study of pathological prognostic variables and definition of a histopathological grading system. Int J Cancer 1984, **33**(1), 37–42.
9. Coindre JM, Trojani M, Contesso G, David M, Rouesse J, Bui NB, Bodaert A, De Mascarel I, De Mascarel A, Goussot JF. Reproducibility of a histopathologic grading system for adult soft tissue sarcoma. Cancer 1986, **58**, 306–9.
10. Tsujimoto M, Aozasa K, Ueda T, Morimura Y, Komatsubara Y, Doi T. Multivariate analysis for histologic prognostic factors in soft tissue sarcomas. Cancer 1988, **62**, 994–8.
11. Jensen OM, Hogh J, Ostgaard SE, Nordentoft AM, Sneppen O. Histopathological grading of soft tissue tumours. Prognostic significance in a prospective study of 278 consecutive cases. J Pathol 1991, **163**, 19–24.
12. Hashimoto H, Daimaru Y, Takeshita S, Tsuneyoshi M, Enjoji M. Prognostic significance of histologic parameters of soft tissue sarcomas. Cancer 1992, **70**, 2816–22.
13. Coindre J-M, Bui NB, Bonichon F, De Mascarel I, Trojani M. Histopathologic grading in spindle cell soft tissue sarcomas. Cancer 1988, **61**, 2305–9.
14. Lee SM, Hajdu SI, Exelby PR. Synovial sarcoma in children. Surg Gynecol Obstet 1974, **138**(5), 701–4.
15. Israels SJ, Chan HS, Daneman A, Weitzman SS. Synovial sarcoma in childhood. Am J Roentgenol 1984, **142**(4), 803–6.
16. Schmidt D, Thum P, Harms D, Treuner J. Synovial sarcoma in children and adolescents: a report from the Kiel Pediatric Tumor Registry. Cancer 1991, **67**, 1667–72.
17. Enzinger FM, Weiss SW. Soft tissue tumors, 3 edn. Mosby, St. Louis, 1995.
18. Abenoza P, Manivel JC, Swanson PE, Wick MR. Synovial sarcoma: ultrastructural study and immunohistochemical analysis by a combined peroxidase-antiperoxidase/avidin-biotin-peroxidase complex procedure. Hum Pathol 1986, **17**(11), 1107–15.
19. Corson JM, Weiss LM, Banks-Schlegel SP, Pinkus GS. Keratin proteins and carcinoembryonic antigen in synovial sarcomas: an immunohistochemical study of 24 cases. Hum Pathol 1984, **15**(7), 615–21.
20. Corson JM, Weiss LM, Banks-Schlegel SP, Pinkus GS. Keratin proteins in synovial sarcoma [letter]. Am J Surg Pathol 1983, **7**(1), 107–9.
21. Ordonez NG, Mahfouz SM, Mackay B. Synovial sarcoma: an immunohistochemical and ultrastructural study. Hum Pathol 1990, **21**(7), 733–49.
22. Salisbury JR, Isaacson PG. Synovial sarcoma: an immunohistochemical study. J Pathol 1985, **147**(1), 49–57.
23. Fisher C. Synovial sarcoma: ultrastructural and immunohistochemical features of epithelial differentiation in monophasic and biphasic tumors. Hum Pathol 1986, **17**(10), 996–1008.
24. Fisher C, Schofield JB. S-100 protein positive synovial sarcoma. Histopathology 1991, **19**, 375–7.
25. Woodruff JM. Peripheral nerve tumors showing glandular differentiation (glandular schwannomas). Cancer 1976, **37**, 2399–413.
26. Mackenzie DH. Monophasic synovial sarcoma—a histological entity? Histopathology 1977, **1**(2), 151–7.
27. Folpe AL, Schmidt RA, Chapman D, Gown AM. Poorly differentiated synovial sarcoma: immunohistochemical distinction from primitive neuroectodermal tumors and high-grade malignant peripheral nerve sheath tumors. Am J Surg Pathol 1998, **22**(6), 673–82.
28. Soule EH. Synovial sarcoma. [Review] [16 refs]. Am J Surg Pathol 1986, **10**(Suppl 1), 78–82.
29. Varela-Duran J, Enzinger FM. Calcifying synovial sarcoma. Cancer 1982, **50**, 345–52.
30. Yokoyama K, Shinohara N, Kondo M, Mashima T. Prognostic factors in synovial sarcoma: a clinicopathologic study of 18 cases. Jpn J Clin Oncol 1995, **25**(4), 131–4.
31. Singer S, Baldini EH, Demetri GD, Fletcher JA, Corson JM. Synovial sarcoma: prognostic significance of tumor size, margin of resection, and mitotic activity for survival. J Clin Oncol 1996, **14**(4), 1201–8.
32. Pappo AS, Fontanesi J, Luo X, Rao BN, Parham DM, Hurwitz C, Avery L, Pratt CB. Synovial sarcoma in children and adolescents: the St. Jude Children's Research Hospital experience. J Clin Oncol 1994, **12**(11), 2360–6.
33. Rooser B, Willen H, Hugoson A, Rydholm A. Prognostic factors in synovial sarcoma. Cancer 1989, **63**(11), 2182–5.
34. Mirra JM, Wang S, Bhuta S. Synovial sarcoma with squamous differentiation of its mesenchymal glandular elements. A case report with light-microscopic, ultramicroscopic, and immunologic correlation. Am J Surg Pathol 1984, **8**(10), 791–6.
35. De Leeuw B, Balemans M, Weghuis DO, Seruca R, Janz M, Geraghty MT, Gilgenkrantz S, Ropers HH, Geurts van Kessel A. Molecular cloning of the synovial sarcoma-specific translocation (X;18)(p11.2;q11.2) breakpoint. Hum Mol Genet 1994, **3**, 745–9.
36. Crew AJ, Clark J, Fisher C, Gill S, Grimer R, Chand A, Shipley J, Gusterson BA, Cooper CS. Fusion of SYT to two genes, SSX1 and SSX2, encoding proteins with homology to the Kruppel-associated box in human synovial sarcoma. EMBO J 1995, **14**(10), 2333–40.
37. Fligman I, Lonardo F, Jhanwar SC, Gerald WL, Woodruff J, Ladanyi M. Molecular diagnosis of synovial sarcoma and characterization of a variant SYT-SSX2 fusion transcript. Am J Pathol 1995, **147**(6), 1592–9.
38. Argani P, Zakowski MF, Klimstra DS, Rosai J, Ladanyi M. Detection of the SYT-SSX chimeric RNA of synovial sarcoma in paraffin-embedded tissue and its application in problematic cases. Mod Pathol 1998, **11**(1), 65–71.
39. Kawai A, Woodruff J, Healey JH, Brennan MF, Antonescu CR, Ladanyi M. SYT-SSX gene fusion as a determinant of morphology and prognosis in synovial sarcoma [see comments]. N Engl J Med 1998, **338**(3), 153–60.
40. Hruban RH, Shiu MH, Senie RT, Woodruff JM. Malignant peripheral nerve sheath tumors of the buttock and lower extremity. A study of 43 cases. Cancer 1990, **66**, 1253–65.

41. Meis JM, Enzinger FM, Martz KL, Neal JA. Malignant peripheral nerve sheath tumors (malignant schwannomas) in children. Am J Surg Pathol 1992, **16**, 694–707.
42. Sorensen SA, Mulvihill JJ, Nielsen A, Srensen SA. Long-term follow-up of von Recklinghausen neurofibromatosis. Survival and malignant neoplasms. N Engl J Med 1986, **314**, 1010–15.
43. Woodruff JM. The pathology and treatment of peripheral nerve tumors and tumor-like conditions. CA Cancer J Clin 1993, **43**, 290–308.
44. Woodruff JM, Chernik NL, Smith MC, Millett WB, Foote FW, Jr. Peripheral nerve tumors with rhabdomyosarcomatous differentiation (malignant "Triton" tumors). Cancer 1973, **32**(2), 426–39.
45. Alvira MM, Mandybur TK, Menefee MG. Light microscopic and ultrastructural observations of a metastasizing malignant epithelioid schwannoma. Cancer 1976, **38**(5), 1977–82.
46. Laskin WB, Weiss SW, Bratthauer GL. Epithelioid variant of malignant peripheral nerve sheath tumor (malignant epithelioid schwannoma). Am J Surg Pathol 1991, **15**, 1136–45.
47. Coffin CM, Dehner LP. Cellular peripheral neural tumors (neurofibromas) in children and adolescents: a clinicopathological and immunohistochemical study. Pediatr Pathol 1990, **10**, 351–61.
48. Erlandson RA. Diagnostic transmission electron microscopy of tumors with clinicopathological, immunohistochemical, and cytogenetic correlations. Raven Press, New York, NY, 1994.
49. Feldkamp MM, Lau N, Provias JP, Gutmann DH, Guha A. Acute presentation of a neurogenic sarcoma in a patient with neurofibromatosis type 1—a pathological and molecular explanation. J Neurosurg 1996, **84**(5), 867–73.
50. Halling KC, Scheithauer BW, Halling AC, Nascimento AG, Ziesmer SC, Roche PC, Wollan PC. p53 expression in neurofibroma and malignant peripheral nerve sheath tumor—an immunohistochemical study of sporadic and NF1-associated tumors. Am J Clin Pathol 1996, **106**(3), 282–8.
51. Soule EH, Pritchard DJ. Fibrosarcoma in infants and children: a review of 110 cases. Cancer 1977, **40**, 1711–21.
52. Chung EB, Enzinger FM. Infantile fibrosarcoma. Cancer 1976, **38**, 729–39.
53. Scott SM, Reiman HM, Pritchard DJ, Ilstrup DM. Soft tissue fibrosarcoma: a clinicopathologic study of 132 cases. Cancer 1989, **64**, 925–31.
54. Ummat S, Nasser JG. Fibrosarcoma of the infratemporal fossa in childhood: a challenging problem. J Otolaryngol 1992, **21**(6), 441–6.
55. Wilson MB, Stanley W, Sens D, Garvin AJ. Infantile fibrosarcoma—a misnomer? Pediatr Pathol 1990, **10**, 901–7.
56. Lundgren L, Angervall L, Stenman G, Kindblom L-G. Infantile rhabdomyofibrosarcoma: a high-grade sarcoma distinguishable from infantile fibrosarcoma and rhabdomyosarcoma. Hum Pathol 1993, **24**, 785–95.
57. Knezevich SR, McFadden DE, Tao W, Lim JF, Sorensen PH. A novel ETV6-NTRK3 gene fusion in congenital fibrosarcoma. Nat Genet 1998, **18**(2), 184–7.
58. Schofield DE, Fletcher JA, Grier HE, Yunis EJ. Fibrosarcoma in infants and children: application of new techniques. Am J Surg Pathol 1994, **18**, 14–24.
59. Gonzalez-Crussi F, deMello DE, Sotelo-Avila C. Omental-mesenteric myxoid hamartomas. Infantile lesions simulating malignant tumors. Am J Surg Pathol 1983, **7**, 567–78.
60. Day DL, Sane S, Dehner LP. Inflammatory pseudotumor of the mesentery and small intestine. Pediatr Radiol 1986, **16**(3), 210–5.
61. Meis JM, Enzinger FM. Inflammatory fibrosarcoma of the mesentery and retroperitoneum: a tumor closely simulating inflammatory pseudotumor. Am J Surg Pathol 1991, **15**, 1146–56.
62. Coffin CM, Dehner LP, Meis-Kindblom JM. Inflammatory myofibroblastic tumor, inflammatory fibrosarcoma, and related lesions: an historical review with differential diagnostic considerations. [Review] [94 refs]. Semn Diagn Pathol 1998, **15**(2), 102–10.
63. Coyne JD, Wilson G, Sandhu D, Young RH. Inflammatory pseudotumour of the urinary bladder. [Review] [16 refs]. Histopathology 1991, **18**(3), 261–4.
64. Nochomovitz LE, Orenstein JM. Inflammatory pseudotumor of the urinary bladder—possible relationship to nodular fasciitis. Two case reports, cytologic observations, and ultrastructural observations. Am J Surg Pathol 1985, **9**(5), 366–73.
65. Proppe KH, Scully RE, Rosai J. Postoperative spindle cell nodules of genitourinary tract resembling sarcomas. A report of eight cases. Am J Surg Pathol 1984, **8**(2), 101–8.
66. Albores-Saavedra J, Manivel JC, Essenfeld H, Dehner LP, Drut R, Gould E, Rosai J. Pseudosarcomatous myofibroblastic proliferations in the urinary bladder of children. Cancer 1990, **66**, 1234–41.
67. Tang TT, Segura AD, Oechler HW, Harb JM, Adair SE, Gregg DC, Camitta, BM, Franciosi RA. Inflammatory myofibrohistiocytic proliferation simulating sarcoma in children. Cancer 1990, **65**(7), 1626–34.
68. Biselli R, Ferlini C, Fattorossi A, Boldrini R, Bosman C. Inflammatory myofibroblastic tumor (inflammatory pseudotumor)—DNA flow cytometric analysis of nine pediatric cases. Cancer 1996, **77**(4), 778–84.
69. Donner LR, Trompler RA, White RR. Progression of inflammatory myofibroblastic tumor (inflammatory pseudotumor) or soft tissue into sarcoma after several recurrences. Hum Pathol 1996, **27**(10), 1095–8.
70. Snyder CS, Dell'Aquila M, Haghighi P, Baergen RN, Suh YK, Yi ES. Clonal changes in inflammatory pseudotumor of the lung—a case report. Cancer 1995, **76**(9), 1545–9.
71. Treissman SP, Gillis DA, Lee CL, Giacomantonio M, Resch L. Omental-mesenteric inflammatory pseudotumor. Cytogenetic demonstration of genetic changes and monoclonality in one tumor. Cancer 1994, **73**, 1433–7.
72. Arber DA, Kamel OW, Van de Rijn M, Davis RE, Medeiros LJ, Jaffe ES, Weiss LM. Frequent presence of the Epstein–Barr virus in inflammatory pseudotumor. Hum Pathol 1995, **26**(10), 1093–8.
73. Smith DM, Mahmoud HH, Jenkins JJ, Rao B, Hopkins KP, Parham DM. Myofibrosarcoma of the head and neck in children. Pediatr Pathol Lab Med 1995, **112**, 275–81.
74. Gerald WL, Miller HK, Battifora H, Miettinen M, Silva EG, Rosai J. Intra-abdominal desmoplastic small round-cell tumor: report of 19 cases of a distinctive type of high-grade polyphenotypic malignancy affecting young individuals. Am J Surg Pathol 1991, **15**, 499–513.
75. Ordonez NG, El-Naggar AK, Ro JY, Silva EG, Mackay B. Intra-abdominal desmoplastic small cell tumor: a light microscopic, immunocytochemical, ultrastructural, and flow cytometric study [see comments]. Hum Pathol 1993, **24**(8), 850–65.

76. Ordonez NG. Desmoplastic small round cell tumor: I: a histopathologic study of 39 cases with emphasis on unusual histological patterns. Am J Surg Pathol 1998, 22(11), 1303–13.
77. Basade MM, Vege DS, Nair CN, Kurkure PA, Advani SH. Intra-abdominal desmoplastic small round cell tumor in children: a clinicopathologic study. Pediatr Hematol Oncol 1996, 13(1), 95–9.
78. Variend S, Gerrard M, Norris PD, Goepel JR. Intra-abdominal neuroectodermal tumour of childhood with divergent differentiation. Histopathology 1991, 18, 45–51.
79. Gonzalez-Crussi F, Crawford SE, Sun C-CJ. Intraabdominal desmoplastic small-cell tumors with divergent differentiation: observations on three cases of childhood. Am J Surg Pathol 1990, 14, 633–42.
80. Cummings OW, Ulbright TM, Young RH, Del TA, Fletcher CD, Hull MT. Desmoplastic small round cell tumors of the paratesticular region. A report of six cases. Am J Surg Pathol 1997, 21(2), 219–25.
81. Furman J, Murphy WM, Wajsman Z, Berry AD. Urogenital involvement by desmoplastic small round-cell tumor. [Review] [19 refs]. J Urol 1997, 158(4), 1506–9.
82. Young RH, Eichhorn JH, Dickersin GR, Scully RE. Ovarian involvement by the intra-abdominal desmoplastic small round cell tumor with divergent differentiation: a report of three cases. Hum Pathol 1992, 23, 454–64.
83. Parkash V, Gerald WL, Parma A, Miettinen M, Rosai J. Desmoplastic small round cell tumor of the pleura. Am J Surg Pathol 1995, 19(6), 659–65.
84. Bian Y, Jordan AG, Rupp M, Cohn H, McLaughlin CJ, Miettinen M. Effusion cytology of desmoplastic small round cell tumor of the pleura: a case report. Acta Cytol 1993, 37, 77–82.
85. Tison V, Cerasoli S, Morigi F, Ladanyi M, Gerald WL, Rosai J. Intracranial desmoplastic small-cell tumor. Report of a case. Am J Surg Pathol 1996, 20(1), 112–17.
86. Ordonez NG, Zirkin R, Bloom RE. Malignant small-cell epithelial tumor of the peritoneum coexpressing mesenchymal-type intermediate filaments. Am J Surg Pathol 1989, 13(5), 413–21.
87. Ordonez NG. Desmoplastic small round cell tumor: II: an ultrastructural and immunohistochemical study with emphasis on new immunohistochemical markers. [Review] [98 refs]. Am J Surg Pathol 1998, 22(11), 1314–27.
88. Ladanyi M, Gerald W. Fusion of the EWS and WT1 genes in the desmoplastic small round cell tumor. Cancer Res 1994, 54, 2837–40.
89. Charles AK, Mall S, Watson J, Berry PJ. Expression of the Wilms' tumour gene WT1 in the developing human and in paediatric renal tumours: an immunohistochemical study. Mol Pathol 1997, 50(3), 138–44.
90. Katz RL, Quezado M, Senderowicz AM, Villalba L, Laskin WB, Tsokos M. An intra-abdominal small round cell neoplasm with features of primitive neuroectodermal and desmoplastic round cell tumor and a EWS/FLI-1 fusion transcript. Hum Pathol 1997, 28(4), 502–9.
91. Argatoff LH, O'Connell JX, Mathers JA, Gilks CB, Sorensen PHB. Detection of the EWS/WT1 gene fusion by reverse transcriptase-polymerase chain reaction in the diagnosis of intra-abdominal desmoplastic small round cell tumor. Am J Surg Pathol 1996, 20(4), 406–12.
92. Fletcher CDM. Diagnostic histopathology of tumours. Churchill-Livingstone, Edinburgh, 1995.
93. Fletcher CDM. Pleomorphic malignant fibrous histiocytoma: fact or fiction? A critical reappraisal based on 159 tumors diagnosed as pleomorphic sarcoma. Am J Surg Pathol 1992, 16, 213–28.
94. Brooks JJ. The significance of double phenotypic patterns and markers in human sarcomas: a new model of mesenchymal differentiation. Am J Pathol 1986, 125, 113–23.
95. Zuppan CW, Mierau GW, Wilson HL. Malignant fibrous histiocytoma in childhood: a report of two cases and review of the literature. Pediatr Pathol 1987, 7, 303–18.
96. Costa MJ, Weiss SW. Angiomatoid malignant fibrous histiocytoma: a follow-up study of 108 cases with evaluation of possible histologic predictors of outcome. Am J Surg Pathol 1990, 14, 1126–32.
97. Fletcher CD. Benign fibrous histiocytoma of subcutaneous and deep soft tissue: a clinicopathologic analysis of 21 cases. Am J Surg Pathol 1990, 14, 801–9.
98. Franquemont DW, Cooper PH, Shmookler BM, Wick MR. Benign fibrous histiocytoma of the skin with potential for local recurrence: a tumor to be distinguished from dermatofibroma. Mod Pathol 1990, 3, 158–63.
99. Enzinger FM, Zhang RY. Plexiform fibrohistiocytic tumor presenting in children and young adults. An analysis of 65 cases. Am J Surg Pathol 1988, 12, 818–26.
100. Merck C, Angervall L, Kindblom LG, Oden A. Myxofibrosarcoma. A malignant soft tissue tumor of fibroblastic-histiocytic origin. A clinicopathologic and prognostic study of 110 cases using multivariate analysis. APMIS Supplement 1983, 282, 1–40.
101. Evans HL. Low-grade fibromyxoid sarcoma: a report of 12 cases. Am J Surg Pathol 1993, 17, 595–600.
102. Weiss SW, Enzinger FM. Myxoid variant of malignant fibrous histiocytoma. Cancer 1977, 39(4), 1672–85.
103. Hashimoto H, Daimaru Y, Enjoji M. S-100 protein distribution in liposarcoma: an immunoperoxidase study with special reference to the distinction of liposarcoma from myxoid malignant fibrous histiocytoma. Virchows Arch [A] 1984, 405, 1–10.
104. La Quaglia MP, Spiro SA, Ghavimi F, Hajdu SI, Meyers P, Exelby PR. Liposarcoma in patients younger than or equal to 22 years of age. Cancer 1993, 72, 3114–19.
105. Shmookler BM, Enzinger FM. Liposarcoma occurring in children. An analysis of 17 cases and review of the literature. Cancer 1983, 52, 567–74.
106. Kilpatrick SE, Doyon J, Choong PFM, Sim FH, Nascimento AG. The clinicopathologic spectrum of myxoid and round cell liposarcoma—*A study of 95 cases*. Cancer 1996, 77(8), 1450–8.
107. Sreekantaiah C, Karakousis CP, Leong SPL, Sandberg AA. Cytogenetic findings in liposarcoma correlate with histopathologic subtypes. Cancer 1992, 69, 2484–95.
108. Sreekantaiah C, Karakousis CP, Leong SPL, Sandberg AA. Trisomy 8 as a nonrandom secondary change in myxoid liposarcoma. Cancer Genet Cytogenet 1991, 51, 195–205.
109. Aoki T, Hisaoka M, Kouho H, Hashimoto H, Nakata H. Interphase cytogenetic analysis of myxoid soft tissue tumors by fluorescence *in situ* hybridization and DNA flow cytometry using paraffin-embedded tissue. Cancer 1997, 79(2), 284–93.

110. Sugarbaker PH, Auda S, Webber BL, Triche TJ, Shapiro E, Cook WJ. Early distant metastases from epithelioid sarcoma of the hand. Cancer 1981, 48(3), 852–5.
111. Gross E, Rao BN, Pappo A, Bowman L, Shearer P, Kaste S, Greenwald C, Michalkiewicz E, Pratt C. Epithelioid sarcoma in children. J Pediatr Surg 1996, 31(12), 1663–5.
112. Trotter MJ, Crawford RI, O'Connell JX, Tron VA. Mitotic granuloma annulare—a clinicopathologic study of 20 cases. J Cutan Pathol 1996, 23(6), 537–45.
113. Arber DA, Kandalaft PL, Mehta P, Battifora H. Vimentin-negative epithelioid sarcoma: the value of an immunohistochemical panel that includes CD34. Am J Surg Pathol 1993, 17, 302–7.
114. Ishida T, Oka T, Matsushita H, Machinami R. Epithelioid sarcoma: an electron-microscopic, immunohistochemical and DNA flow cytometric analysis. Virchows Arch A Pathol Anat Histopathol 1992, 421, 401–8.
115. Iwasaki H, Ohjimi Y, Ishiguro M, Isayama T, Kaneko Y, Yoh S, Emoto G, Kikuchi M. Epithelioid sarcoma with an 18q aberration. Cancer Genet Cytogenet 1996, 91(1), 46–52.
116. Sonobe H, Ohtsuki Y, Sugimoto T, Shimizu K. Involvement of 8q, 22q, and monosomy 21 in an epithelioid sarcoma [letter]. Cancer Genet Cytogenet 1997, 96(2), 178–80.
117. Cordoba JC, Parham DM, Meyer WH, Douglass EC. A new cytogenetic finding in an epithelioid sarcoma, t(8;22)(q22;q11). Cancer Genet Cytogenet 1994, 72, 151–4.
118. Stenman G, Kindblom L-G, Willems J, Angervall L. A cell culture, chromosomal and quantitative DNA analysis of a metastatic epithelioid sarcoma: deletion 1p, a possible primary chromosomal abnormality in epithelioid sarcoma. Cancer 1990, 65, 2006–13.
119. Lieberman PH, Brennan MF, Kimmel M, Erlandson RA, Garin-Chesa P, Flehinger BY. Alveolar soft-part sarcoma: a clinico-pathologic study of half a century. Cancer 1989, 63, 1–13.
120. Pappo AS, Parham DM, Cain A, Luo X, Bowman LC, Furman WL, Rao BN, Pratt CB. Alveolar soft part sarcoma in children and adolescents: clinical features and outcome of 11 patients. Med Pediatr Oncol 1996, 26(2), 81–4.
121. Tucker JA. Crystal-deficient alveolar soft part sarcoma. Ultrastruct Pathol 1993, 17, 279–86.
122. Cullinane C, Thorner PS, Greenberg ML, Ng YK, Kumar M, Squire J. Molecular genetic, cytogenetic, and immunohistochemical characterization of alveolar soft-part sarcoma: implications for cell of origin. Cancer 1992, 70, 2444–50.
123. Rosai J, Dias P, Parham DM, Shapiro DN, Houghton P. MyoD1 protein expression in alveolar soft part sarcoma as confirmatory evidence of its skeletal muscle nature. Am J Surg Pathol 1991, 15, 974–81.
124. Carstens PHB. Membrane-bound cytoplasmic crystals, similar to those in alveolar soft part sarcoma, in a human muscle spindle. Ultrastruct Pathol 1990, 14, 423–8.
125. Wang NP, Bacchi CE, Jiang JJ, McNutt MA, Gown AM. Does alveolar soft-part sarcoma exhibit skeletal muscle differentiation—an immunocytochemical and biochemical study of myogenic regulatory protein expression. Mod Pathol 1996, 9(5), 496–506.
126. Kiuru-Kuhlefelt S, El-Rifai W, Sarlomo-Rikala M, Knuutila S, Miettinen M. DNA copy number changes in alveolar soft part sarcoma: a comparative genomic hybridization study. Mod Pathol 1998, 11(3), 227–31.
127. Sreekantaiah C, Li FP, Weidner N, Sandberg AA. Multiple and complex abnormalities in a case of alveolar soft-part sarcoma. Cancer Genet Cytogenet 1991, 55, 167–71.
128. Healy E, Belgaid CE, Takata M, Vahlquist A, Rehman I, Rigby H, Rees JL. Allelotypes of primary cutaneous melanoma and benign melanocytic nevi. Cancer Res 1996, 56(3), 589–93.
129. Mrozek K, Karakousis CP, Perez-Mesa C, Bloomfield CD. Translocation t(12;22)(q13;q12.2–12.3) in a clear cell sarcoma of tendons and aponeuroses. Genes Chromosom Cancer 1993, 6, 249–52.
130. Zucman J, Delattre O, Desmaze C, Epstein A, Stenman G, Speleman F, Fletcher CDM, Aurias A, Thomas G. EWS and ATF-1 gene fusion induced by t(12;22) translocation in malignant melanoma of soft parts. Nat Genet 1993, 4, 341–5.
131. Woodruff JM. Pathology of malignant melanoma—part 1. Clin Bull 1976, 6(1), 15–23.
132. Swanson PE, Wick MR. Clear cell sarcoma: an immunohistochemical analysis of six cases and comparison with other epithelioid neoplasms of soft tissue. Arch Pathol Lab Med 1989, 113, 55–60.
133. Hinrichs SH, Jaramillo MA, Gumerlock PH, Gardner MB, Lewis JP, Freeman AE. Myxoid chondrosarcoma with a translocation involving chromosomes 9 and 22. Cancer Genet Cytogenet 1985, 14, 219–26.
134. Antonescu CR, Argani P, Erlandson RA, Healey JH, Ladanyi, Huvos AG. Skeletal and extraskeletal myxoid chondrosarcoma: a comparative clinicopathologic, ultrastructural, and molecular study. Cancer 1998, 83(8), 1504–21.
135. Wilkinson AH, III, Beckford NS, Babin RW, Parham DM. Extraskeletal myxoid chondrosarcoma of the epiglottis: case report and review of the literature. Otolaryngol Head Neck Surg 1991, 104, 257–60.
136. Saleh G, Evans HL, Ro JY, Ayala AG. Extraskeletal myxoid chondrosarcoma: a clinicopathologic study of ten patients with long-term follow-up. Cancer 1992, 70, 2827–30.
137. Weiss SW. Ultrastructure of the so-called "chordoid sarcoma": evidence supporting cartilaginous differentiation. Cancer 1976, 37, 300–6.
138. Hachitanda Y, Tsuneyoshi M, Daimaru Y, Enjoji M, Nakagawara A, Ikeda K, Sueishi K. Extraskeletal myxoid chondrosarcoma in young children. Cancer 1988, 61, 2521–6.
139. Suzuki T, Kaneko H, Kojima K, Takatoh M, Hasebe K-I. Extraskeletal myxoid chondrosarcoma characterized by microtubular aggregates in the rough endoplasmic reticulum and tubulin immunoreactivity. J Pathol 1988, 156, 51–7.
140. Dabska M. Parachordoma: a new clinicopathologic entity. Cancer 1977, 40, 1586–92.
141. Imlay SP, Argenyi ZB, Stone MS, McCollough ML, Henghold WB. Cutaneous parachordoma. A light microscopic and immunohistochemical report of two cases and

review of the literature. [Review] [38 refs]. J Cutan Pathol 1998, **25**(5), 279–84.
142. Karabela-Bouropoulou V, Skourtas C, Liapi-Avgeri G, Mahaira H. Parachordoma. A case report of a very rare soft tissue tumor. Pathol Res Pract 1996, **192**(9), 972–8.
143. Tihy F, Scott P, Russo P, Champagne M, Tabet JC, Lemieux N. Cytogenetic analysis of a parachordoma. Cancer Genet Cytogenet 1998, **105**(1), 14–19.
144. Limon J, Babinska M, Denis A, Rys J, Niezabitowski A. Parachordoma: a rare sarcoma with clonal chromosomal changes. Cancer Genet Cytogenet 1998, **102**(1), 78–80.
145. Lezama-del VP, Gerald WL, Tsai J, Meyers P, La, Quaglia MP. Malignant vascular tumors in young patients. Cancer 1998, **83**(8), 1634–9.
146. Gray MH, Rosenberg AE, Dickersin GR, Bhan AK. Cytokeratin expression in epithelioid vascular neoplasms. Hum Pathol 1990, **21**, 212–17.
147. Tsuneyoshi M, Daimaru Y, Hashimoto H, Enjoji M. Malignant soft tissue neoplasms with the histologic features of renal rhabdoid tumors: an ultrastructural and immunohistochemical study. Hum Pathol 1985, **16**, 1235–42.
148. Kodet R, Newton WA, Jr., Sachs N, Hamoudi AB, Raney RB, Asmar L, Gehan EA. Rhabdoid tumors of soft tissues: a clinicopathologic study of 26 cases enrolled on the Intergroup Rhabdomyosarcoma Study. Hum Pathol 1991, **22**, 674–84.
149. Kodet R, Newton WA, Jr., Hamoudi AB, Asmar L. Rhabdomyosarcomas with intermediate-filament inclusions and features of rhabdoid tumors: light microscopic and immunohistochemical study. Am J Surg Pathol 1991, **15**, 257–67.
150. Parham DM, Weeks DA, Beckwith JB. The clinicopathologic spectrum of putative extrarenal rhabdoid tumors: an analysis of 42 cases studies with immunohistochemistry and/or electron microscopy. Am J Surg Pathol 1994, **18**, 1010–29.
151. Tsuneyoshi M, Daimaru Y, Hashimoto H, Enjoji M. The existence of rhabdoid cells in specified soft tissue sarcomas: histopathological, ultrastructural and immunohistochemical evidence. Virchows Arch.[A] 1987, **411**, 509–14.
152. Weeks DA, Beckwith JB, Mierau GW. Rhabdoid tumor: an entity or a phenotype. Arch Pathol Lab Med 1989, **113**, 113–14.
153. Versteege I, Sevenet N, Lange J, Rousseau-Merck MF, Ambros P, Handgretinger R, Aurias A, Delattre O. Truncating mutations of hSNF5/INI1 in aggressive paediatric cancer. Nature 1998, **394**(6689), 203–6.

12 | Pediatric renal neoplasms

Pedram Argani and Elizabeth J. Perlman

Introduction

Primary renal tumors account for 6% of cancers in children, surpassed in frequency by leukemias, brain tumors, lymphomas, sarcomas, and neuroblastomas (1). Approximately 500 new pediatric renal neoplasms are diagnosed each year in the United States, over 80% of which are enrolled on a National Wilms Tumor Study (NWTS) clinical protocol (2). The NWTS was started in 1969 with the goal of optimizing therapy for children with renal neoplasms, and has met with great success. Much of this success can be attributed to the accurate subclassification of tumors on the basis of clinical and pathologic features into high- and low-risk types, allowing the intensity of therapy to be modified appropriately. Central pathologic review by Dr J. Bruce Beckwith at the NWTS Pathology Center from 1969 to 1999 has ensured the consistency of pathologic assessments. As a result, children with low-risk tumors (e.g. congenital mesoblastic nephroma) are spared toxic adjuvant therapy, while children with high-risk tumors (e.g. disseminated anaplastic Wilms tumor) receive more intensive therapy. Through four clinical trials, this formula has produced dramatically improved survival rates despite an overall decrease in the intensity of adjuvant therapy employed. In the current trial, molecular biologic parameters are being assessed for their ability to stratify tumors into high- and low-risk types with the goal of potentially optimizing therapy further.

This review will primarily reflect the NWTS approach to classification, staging, and treatment of pediatric renal neoplasms. As such, most of prognostic data cited will be from NWTS trials. The majority of children in European countries are enrolled on the International Society of Pediatric Oncology (SIOP) protocols, an excellent review of which has recently been published (3). A mainstay of the SIOP approach has been the use of pre-operative neoadjuvant chemotherapy, with pathologic features including stage assessed on post-chemotherapy nephrectomy specimens. In contrast, the NWTS approach favors primary nephrectomy, with post-operative chemotherapy based upon pathologic analysis of untreated tumors. As such, the pathologic attributes of tumors are difficult to compare across the two trials. Nonetheless, the SIOP protocols have met with similar success in treating these children.

Classification

Table 12.1 lists the primary malignant renal neoplasms of childhood in decreasing order of frequency. Favorable histology Wilms tumor (WT) and its anaplastic variant comprise the vast majority of cases. Three primary sarcomas, congenital mesoblastic nephroma (CMN), clear cell sarcoma of the kidney (CCSK), and rhabdoid tumor of the kidney (RTK), are sufficiently frequent to have undergone intensive study on NWTS clinical trials. Other rare entities comprise the remaining 5% of cases. These include renal cell carcinomas and other childhood cancers such as lymphoma, primitive neuroectodermal tumor (PNET), synovial sarcoma, and neuroblastoma, which occasionally present as primary renal tumors. This review will cover in detail the four major primary renal tumors of childhood and briefly touch upon three of the less common entities which molecular genetic studies have helped define.

Staging

While the importance of stage has been emphasized for WT, the same set of criteria is used by the NWTS to stage all pediatric renal tumors. These criteria have evolved over the years, and the current NWTS 5 definitions are listed in Table 12.2.

The major recent change has been in the criteria for distinguishing between Stage 1 and Stage 2 for tumors

Table 12.1 Primary renal tumors of childhood (%)

WT, favorable histology	80
WT, anaplastic	4
Congenital mesoblastic nephroma (CMN)	5
Clear cell sarcoma of kidney (CCSK)	4
Rhabdoid tumor of kidney (RTK)	2
Miscellaneous (lymphoma, primitive neuroectodermal tumor (PNET), neuroblastoma, renal cell carcinoma, angiomyolipoma, synovial sarcoma)	5

Table 12.2 NWTS 5 renal tumor staging criteria

Stage 1	Tumor confined to the kidney and completely resected. No penetration of the renal capsule or involvement of renal sinus vessels
Stage 2	Tumor extends beyond kidney but completely resected. Tumor penetrates renal capsule, invades sinus vessels, was biopsied before removal, or spilled locally during removal, but margins are negative
Stage 3	Gross residual tumor, positive surgical margins, tumor spillage involving peritoneal surfaces or lymph node metastases
Stage 4	Hematogenous metastases
Stage 5	Bilateral renal tumors

that involve the medial portion of the kidney (4). This region contains the pelvicalyceal collecting system, perirenal fibroadipose tissue and the major renal vessels, and is referred to as the renal sinus. The previous criterion for Stage 2 status was extension past the hilar plane, an imaginary boundary marked by the medial border of the renal sinus. This plane can be visualized on a gross specimen as a plane connecting the medial borders of the upper and lower poles of the kidney. However, the hilar plane lacks a defining anatomic border, is often distorted by bulky tumors, and can be assessed only on initial gross pathologic examination of the nephrectomy specimen. These factors made the criteria for Stage 2 difficult to apply. Furthermore, the hilar plane has no known biological significance, and could not be evaluated by review pathologists. Therefore, the hilar plane criterion for staging was removed from NWTS 5, and replaced by the criterion of renal sinus vascular invasion. Tumor involvement of any vessel in the renal sinus, regardless of its location in relation to the hilar plane, is a basis for upstaging from Stage 1 to Stage 2. This definition includes vessels located in the radial extensions of the sinus into the renal parenchyma, but excludes other intrarenal vascular invasion. The revised definition has two main advantages. First and foremost, it makes sound biologic sense. The renal sinus veins and lymphatics represent the major portal of venous and lymphatic drainage of the kidney; tumor in these vessels has gained access to the systemic circulation, literally caught in the act of spreading. Identification of tumor in these vessels then indicates that systemic spread may have occurred, and hence a localized Stage 1 designation would be biologically inaccurate. Second, invasion of the sinus vessels can be assessed by secondary reviewers. In histological sections, sinus vessels can be identified by their proximity to the renal medulla and pelvic urothelium or by their proximity to the cortical surfaces of the sinus, which are distinguished from peripheral cortex by their lack of a fibrous renal capsule (5). The new definition appears to have been successful, as survival differences between Stage 1 and 2 WTs have maintained their statistical significance. Preliminary data also indicate that the new criteria can stratify CCSK into stages of high prognostic significance which previous criteria had failed to do (see below).

Wilms tumor (nephroblastoma)

As noted previously, WT is the most common primary malignant renal neoplasm of childhood, comprising approximately 84% of cases. WT affects approximately one of every 8000 infants and children in Europe and North America, with approximately 400 new cases diagnosed each year in the United States (6, 7). The peak incidence is between the years of three and six, though occasional tumors present in adulthood. The usual presentation is that of a unilateral abdominal mass. Five to ten percent of tumors are bilateral; these patients present at a younger mean age (8).

While no significant environmental risk features for WT have been identified, 10% of WT develop in association with one of several well-characterized dysmorphic syndromes (9). These include the WAGR (WT, aniridia, genitourinary malformation, mental retardation) syndrome, which carries a 30% risk of developing WT, and the Denys–Drash syndrome (pseudohermaphroditism, glomerulosclerosis, WT), which carries a risk of greater than 90% of developing WT. Overgrowth syndromes are also implicated, though the risks are less. These include isolated hemihypertrophy (asymmetrical overgrowth) and Beckwith–Wiedemann syndrome (BWS), in which hemihypertrophy is associated with macroglossia, omphalocele, and visceromegaly. In addition, 1% of WT are familial but not syndromic, inherited in an autosomal dominant pattern with incomplete penetrance. These syndromes are discussed further below.

At the beginning of the century, WT was considered one of the most lethal of the solid tumors, curable only in the minority of cases in which it was confined to the kidney and surgically excised (10). The development of effective adjuvant chemotherapy has been one of the major success stories of pediatric oncology, and today WT is considered one of the most curable of the solid tumors, even when disseminated. The overall survival is nearly 90%. As shown below, both microscopic and molecular features can stratify these tumors into subtypes with more sharply defined risks.

Pathology

Wilms tumors are typically lobulated, soft, and friable on cut section, with a variegated appearance that reflects its diversity of cell types, variable necrosis, and cystic change (11). Tumors grow with a pushing border, compressing the adjacent renal parenchyma to form a distinct pseudocapsule. This sharp demarcation from the native kidney distinguishes WT from other renal neoplasms (RTK, CMN) which microscopically infiltrate the native kidney and hence have grossly indistinct borders. WT not infrequently involves the renal vein, and may extend up the inferior vena cava to reach the right atrium. While most WT are unicentric, 11% are multifocal: these tumors are invariably associated with multiple nephrogenic rests. In such cases, the opposite kidney, which presumably harbors similar rests, is at increased risk for subsequent tumor formation (see below).

The classic triphasic histology of WT is composed of three cell types (blastemal, epithelial, and stromal) which are generally arranged so as to recapitulate the entire spectrum of normal renal development (Fig. 12.1). Blastemal cells are undifferentiated small blue cells microscopically, and can be arranged in diffuse or organoid patterns. Epithelial structures such as glomeruli and tubules develop out of condensations of blastema to simulate the nephrogenic zone of the developing kidney. However, larger papillary formations unlike any in the normal developing kidney may be seen, and heterologous squamous or mucinous epithelium may also be present. While stromal differentiation is usually manifest as immature spindled cells, heterologous differentiation commonly yields skeletal muscle, cartilage, osteoid, or fat. Distinction of a WT with prominent heterologous differentiation ("teratoid Wilms tumor") from a true renal teratoma can occasionally be quite challenging. In these cases, the presence of organized organogenesis (which is quite rare) favors a teratoma.

While triphasic histology is the rule, biphasic and monophasic tumors are not uncommon. Monophasic blastemal WT are often highly invasive and raise the differential diagnosis of other small round blue cell tumors, such as PNET, neuroblastoma, and lymphoma, all of which may present in the kidney. Monophasic stromal WT can simulate primary sarcomas such as CCSK and CMN. Other stromal WT show a predominance of skeletal muscle differentiation. This can vary from well-differentiated skeletal muscle (rhabdomyomatous) to poorly differentiated skeletal muscle (rhabdomyoblastic). The distinction of a purely stromal WT

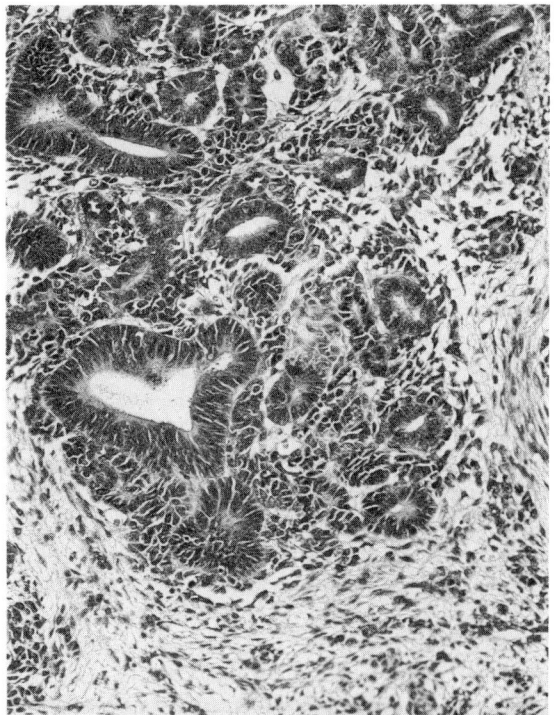

Fig. 12.1 Triphasic favorable histology WT. Spindle cell stroma at the periphery of undifferentiated blastemal cells and epithelially differentiated tubules. 200× magnification.

with exclusive rhabdomyoblastic differentiation from a primary renal rhabdomyosarcoma is often impossible on morphologic grounds. It is generally recommended that such lesions be treated on the basis of their line of differentiation (e.g. as a rhabdomyosarcoma) rather than their putative cell of origin. Finally, a large area of overlap exists among purely tubular and papillary WT and both papillary renal cell carcinomas and metanephric adenomas (12). Cases in which these three patterns merge imperceptibly are not uncommon. Immunohistochemical staining for cytokeratin 7 may be helpful in such cases: diffuse strong staining favors papillary renal cell carcinoma, while WT are only focally positive (J. Bruce Beckwith, unpublished observations).

Some correlations exist between the predominant cell type and the clinical behavior of WT (13). Blastemal rich tumors tend to be extremely invasive and present at high stage, but respond well to chemotherapy. In contrast, predominantly epithelial and rhabdomyomatous WT more frequently present at low stage, reflecting decreased aggressiveness, and hence may be cured by surgery. However, predominantly epithelial WT tend to be resistant to chemotherapy, and when they do present with advanced disease, the prognosis is diminished. While these trends are intriguing, they have not yet been shown to reach statistical significance due to the small number of Stage 4 predominantly epithelial WT available for analysis.

While WTs often contain scattered cysts, tumors which are purely cystic and devoid of any solid nodular growth are also recognized. Such tumors are designated cystic partially differentiated nephroblastoma (CPDN) when their thin septa contain immature nephrogenic elements, and cystic nephroma (CN) when only mature cell types are present. The importance of their distinction from WT is that both CPDN and CN are curable by surgery alone, and are thought to represent the most favorable end of the Wilms spectrum in children. Either lesion can recur if ruptured or incompletely excised, so distinction of CN from CPDN is of little clinical significance. An intriguing familial association between cystic nephroma and the often cystic pleuropulmonary blastoma has recently been documented (14, 15). Also intriguing is the fact that while CN and CPDN show a 2:1 male predominance in children less than 4 years of age, the morphologically identical tumors show a striking 7.5:1 female predominance in those over 30 years of age (16). It is probable that many of the tumors classified as adult CNs represent distinct entities unrelated to WT.

Anaplastic Wilms tumor

The only recognized histologic feature of unfavorable prognosis for WT is the presence of anaplasia, or extreme cytologic atypia (Fig. 12.2). Anaplasia can be present in any of the three cell types in WT, and is defined by the presence of three features: (a) nucleomegaly, defined as nuclei with diameters three times the diameter of a red blood cell in one dimension and two times the diameter in the other direction; (b) hyperchromasia of the enlarged nuclei, signifying polyploidy; (c) atypical (multipolar) mitotic figures. All of the above features must be present. Defined as above, anaplasia is rare in tumors from children less than 2 years of age; its incidence increases until age 5 when it stabilizes at 13% (6). The overall frequency of anaplasia in WT is 5%.

Anaplasia in WT appears to be a marker of resistance to chemotherapy, but not of increased aggressiveness or tendency to disseminate (10). This hypothesis is supported by the fact that localized Stage 1 anaplastic WTs have the same excellent prognosis as Stage 1 favorable histology WT, while Stages 2–4 anaplastic WTs have a markedly diminished prognosis. Only when anaplastic

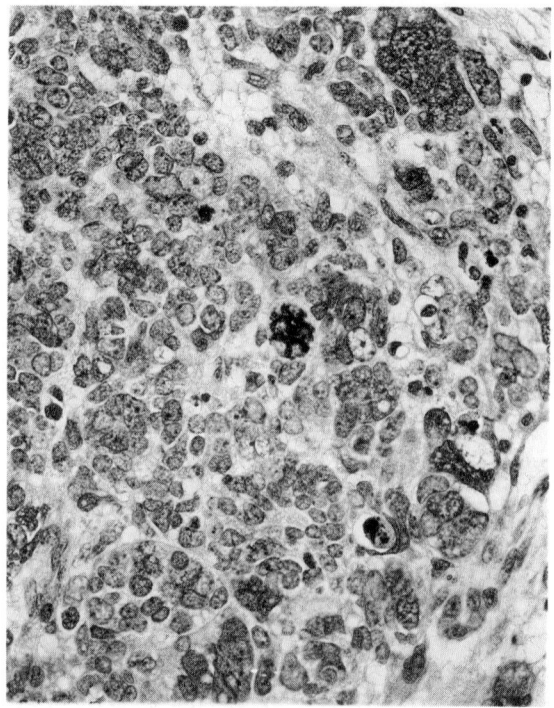

Fig. 12.2 Anaplastic WT. The tumor demonstrates nuclear gigantism, hyperchromasia, and atypical mitoses. 400× magnification.

cells are present in extrarenal sites, and hence response to chemotherapy is needed for their eradication, is the prognosis diminished. Because anaplasia is often not uniformly distributed in a given tumor, a distinction can be made between focal anaplasia and diffuse anaplasia. A nonquantitative but topographical definition currently used makes this distinction prognostically significant (17). By NWTS 5 criteria, focal anaplasia requires that anaplasia be limited to discrete regions within the primary tumor, and that it be surrounded by non-anaplastic tissue. Anaplasia qualifies as diffuse when it is present outside the kidney, when it is identified in a random biopsy, when it is present in a background of severe nuclear atypia (unrest) within the remaining tumor, or when it is present in multiple slides whose precise location cannot be documented. The latter criteria require that pathologists precisely document the site of each tumor section taken, preferably with a gross photograph or diagram (18). When defined as above, the prognostic difference between focal and diffuse anaplasia is highly significant for Stages 2–4. In these patients, the prognosis for WT with focal anaplasia is identical to that for favorable histology WT, while the outcome for WT with diffuse anaplasia is poor.

Nephrogenic rests

Nephrogenic rests, foci of abnormally persistent embryonal tissue, are the recognized precursors to WT (19). Nephrogenic rests are found in almost 1% of unselected pediatric autopsies, but their incidence increases to 35% of kidneys harboring unilateral WT and nearly 100% of kidneys involved by bilateral WT (20). Because the incidence of WT is far less than the incidence of rests, only a small proportion of rests ever transform into WT. Other possible fates include dormancy, sclerosis and subsequent involution, focal or diffuse hyperplasia, and neoplastic transformation into benign adenomatous nodules. The finding of multiple or diffuse nephrogenic rests (nephroblastomatosis) in a kidney bearing WT indicates an increased risk for development of WT in the opposite kidney, which should be considered in planning clinical follow-up (21).

Nephrogenic rests are classified by their position within the renal lobe. Because nephrons are added sequentially to the periphery of the lobe during renal development, the position of a lesion within the lobe reflects the chronology of its development *in utero*. Intralobar nephrogenic rests (ILNR) are randomly distributed but tend to be situated deep within the lobe, likely reflecting an earlier developmental insult to the kidney. These lesions are usually stroma-rich and infiltrate the adjacent renal parenchyma (Fig. 12.3(a)). Perilobar nephrogenic rests (PLNR) are strictly located at the lobar periphery and presumably reflect later developmental disturbances in nephrogenesis. These lesions contain predominantly blastema and tubules and tend to be sharply demarcated from the kidney (Fig. 12.3(b)). Morphologic distinction of the two types of rests is significant because they have different clinical and pathologic associations (22). ILNRs are more strongly linked to the WAGR and Denys–Drash Syndromes and are associated with the development of stroma-rich WT that appear at a younger mean age. PLNRs are associated with BWS and frequently give rise to epithelial and blastemal rich tumors. These observations suggest that the morphologic heterogeneity of WT may reflect differences in its precursor lesions which may in turn reflect distinct underlying genetic abnormalities. Differences between PLNR and ILNR are listed in Table 12.3.

Immunohistochemical stains are rarely needed to confirm the diagnosis of classic WT. When performed, the results are consistent with the pattern of differentiation observed through the light microscope. Hence, areas of tubular differentiation stain for cytokeratin, while areas of muscular differentiation stain as expected for desmin and muscle-specific actin. While appearing undifferentiated microscopically, blastemal cells often exhibit focal cytokeratin immunoreactivity, perhaps indicating early evidence of epithelial differentiation. Along these lines, most blastemal cells show evidence of epithelial differentiation ultrastructurally in the form of desmosomes or cilia (23). A thick flocculent coating of extracellular basement membrane-like material may also surround these cells (24).

Genetics

The Knudson two-hit mutational model for cancer, exemplified by retinoblastoma, was initially proposed to explain the development of WT (25). Using this model, the earlier age of onset of bilateral and familial cases of WT could be accounted for by postulating a germline defect in a single tumor suppressor gene. However, the genetic alterations of WT have proven far more complex than can be accounted for by a single WT gene model. Multiple genes and chromosomal loci have been implicated in the development of WT (25), a fact that is not unexpected given the complexity of nephrogenesis and the fact that at least two distinct precursors (ILNR, PLNR) have been identified. In addition, at least 60% of

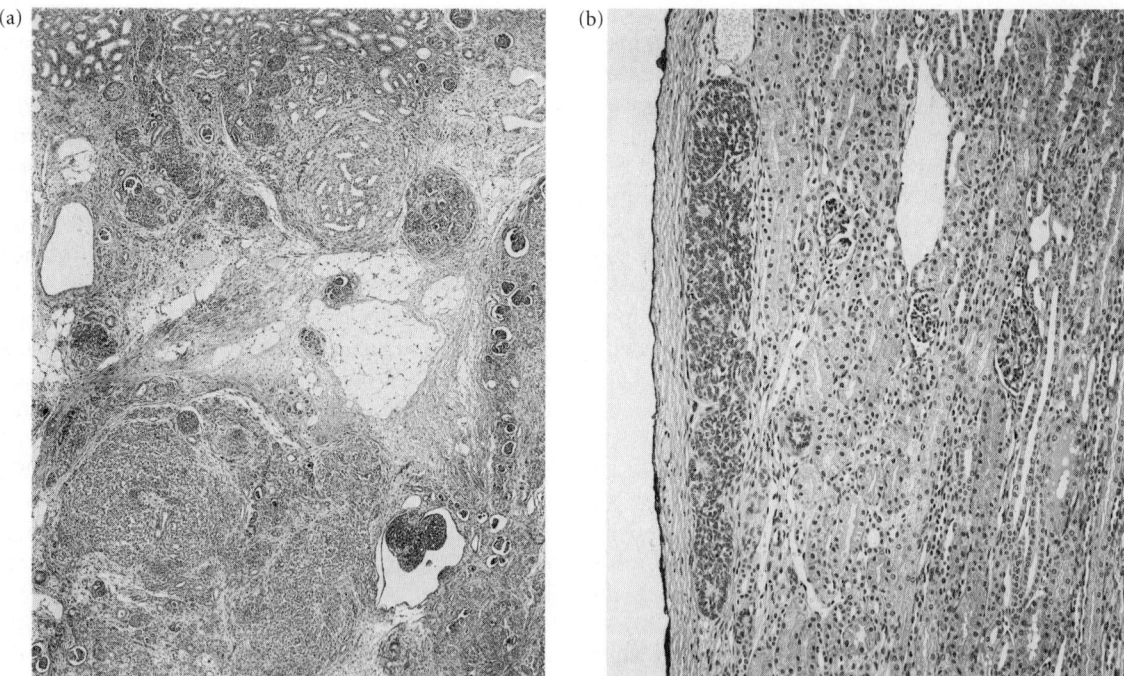

Fig. 12.3 (a) ILNR. The lesion contains mature fat and immature nephrogenic tissue. Note that the lesion irregularly infiltrates among the native renal parenchyma (top of figure). 50× magnification. (b) PLNR. The base of the lesion lies on the renal capsule (left). The lesion contains predominantly blastema and is relatively well demarcated from the native kidney. 160× magnification.

Table 12.3 Nephrogenic rests: perilobar versus intralobar

	Intralobar	Perilobar
Associated syndromes	WAGR, Denys–Drash	BWS
Associated genetic abnormality	WT-1 (11p13)	WT-2 (11p15)
Location within renal lobe	Random, often central	Peripheral
Border with kidney	Infiltrative	Distinct
Dominant component	Stroma	Blastema or tubules
Number	Usually single	Often multiple

tumors arise without morphologic evidence of these precursors, suggesting that some WT may arise via other pathways (26). The following will summarize the data implicating each of the suspected genetic loci.

The first locus implicated in WT development was 11p13, which was found to be the site of constitutional deletions in patients with the WAGR syndrome. Mapping studies by multiple laboratories led to the identification of the responsible gene, named WT-1, in 1990 (27) (28, 29). WT-1 is a transcription factor with a zinc finger protein structure that is thought to play a major role in renal and gonadal development (30). Its normal expression is limited to the developing kidney, gonadal sex cord cells, and mesothelium. Subsequently, patients with Denys–Drash syndrome were found to have constitutional inactivating point mutations in WT-1, while their WTs consistently showed loss of their remaining normal WT-1 allele (31). The incidence of WT is higher and the phenotypic effects are more severe in Denys–Drash syndrome where WT-1 is mutated than in WAGR syndrome where WT-1 is deleted. Therefore, the point mutations in Denys–Drash syndrome are thought to act as dominant negative mutations, creating a dysfunctional protein that interferes with the product of the non-mutated allele (31).

Within the developing kidney, WT-1 expression is restricted to the condensing metanephric blastema, renal vesicles, and glomerular epithelium (32). It is absent in stroma and mature epithelial tubules. It is postulated to arrest the proliferation of blastemal cells and initiate epithelial differentiation at the tip of the ureteric bud. Along these lines, WT-1 is known to function as a repressor of growth promoting genes, such as insulin-like growth factor-2 (IGF-2), that are expressed by blastemal cells (33). A similar pattern of WT-1 expression has been identified in WTs. By both *in situ* hybridization (34) and immunohistochemical staining (32), WT-1 expression has been found in differentiating blastema and immature epithelium, but not stroma.

While WT-1 alterations are strongly linked to development of WT in syndromic cases, its role in sporadic WT appears to be limited. Only one-third of WT show loss of heterozygosity at this locus and only 10% of sporadic WT harbor WT-1 mutations. Of note, microdissection experiments have revealed identical WT-1 mutations in both WT and their associated nephrogenic rests (35), most of which have been ILNRs. Some investigators have demonstrated loss of heterozygosity at WT-1 in both an ILNR and its associated WT (36), suggesting that complete WT-1 inactivation is an early event in Wilms tumorigenesis, perhaps resulting only in the formation of a nephrogenic rest. Subsequent events would be required to produce a WT.

A second WT locus has been localized to chromosome 11p15 (37). Initial evidence was provided by the linkage of the familial BWS cases to this locus (Ping *et al.* 1989) (38). This region shows loss of heterozygosity in approximately 40% of WT; interestingly, the lost allele is nearly always maternal. These results would suggest that the responsible genes in this locus are imprinted, or expressed preferentially from either the maternal or paternal chromosomes. Loss of a growth suppressing gene on the maternal allele or overexpression of a growth promoting gene on the paternal allele could then promote neoplasia. Numerous candidate genes in this region have been identified, though none has been proven to be uniquely responsible for either BWS or WT (39). It is not clear if the same gene will be implicated in both.

One growth promoting gene that maps to 11p15 is IGF-2, which is normally expressed only from the paternal allele (paternally imprinted). IGF-2 is known to be expressed in fetal kidney and over-expressed in WT (40). In 70% of those cases in which loss of heterozygosity does not occur at 11p15, IGF-2 expression has been demonstrated to occur from both parental alleles; hence, the imprinting mechanism is disrupted (Rainier *et al.* 1993) (37, 41). This mechanism may account for the IGF-2 over-expression observed in WTs. By *in situ* hybridization, IGF-2 has been localized preferentially to blastema (40). Its expression diminishes with epithelial differentiation, a pattern which is inverse to that of WT-1 expression.

Two nearby growth suppressing candidate genes in this region, both of which are maternally imprinted, are H19 and $p57^{KIP2}$. H19 codes for a non-translated mRNA which may function to downregulate IGF-2 expression (42). Transfection of H19 into WT cell lines has been shown to suppress tumorogenicity (43). $p57^{KIP2}$ is a cyclin-dependent kinase inhibitor which mediates G1 cell cycle arrest (44). While mutations in $p57^{KIP2}$ are rare in WT (45), reduced expression at the RNA level has been demonstrated in the majority of WT tested (46). However, there are a number of other imprinted genes located at 11p15, and their participation in BWS and WT has yet to be determined. Most recently, LIT1, an imprinted antisense transcript from within the K_vLQT1 gene, was shown to have undergone loss of imprinting and altered expression in most BWS patients (47).

Evidence for the involvement of multiple additional loci in the development of WT comes from familial cases. Linkage studies performed upon these families have thus far excluded involvement of many of the known loci associated with WT, including 11p13 (48), 11p15 (49), and 16q (50) (see below.) In several families, strong linkage has been demonstrated to an as yet uncloned gene mapped to 17q12–17q21 and tentatively designated FWT1 (51). This locus has not been frequently implicated in genetic studies of sporadic WT. While tumors associated with familial cancer predisposition syndromes usually present at a younger age than sporadic cases, these FWT1-linked tumors present at a higher mean age (6 years) than that of sporadic WT. Other cases of familial WT do not show linkage to FWT1, implying that still more as yet undiscovered genes are involved in its pathogenesis (52).

While much effort has focused on the genetic events involved in the pathogenesis of WT, other efforts have targeted the genetic events associated with unfavorable outcome. Anaplasia, a morphologic marker of chemotherapy resistance, has been strongly linked with the presence of p53 mutation. While p53 mutation is rare in favorable histology WT (53, 54), it is found in the majority of anaplastic tumors (55). In one case, a p53 mutation was localized exclusively to the anaplastic portion of a focally anaplastic WT, implying that p53 mutation accompanied anaplastic progression (56).

The fact that p53 mutated tumors are chemotherapy resistant makes biologic sense, given that the normal function of p53 includes mediation of apoptosis in response to the DNA damage effected by chemotherapy. Loss of functional p53 is predicted to disrupt this mechanism of chemotherapy effect (57).

The correlation of anaplasia with p53 over-expression at the immunohistochemical level is strong, though not as strong as with p53 mutational status (58, 59). Occasional non-anaplastic WTs stain strongly for p53. Of interest, these tumors also seem to have a diminished prognosis, suggesting that p53 may be sequestered and inactivated by non-mutational means (60). Alternatively, the morphologic phenotype of anaplasia may not always accompany p53 mutation. Further data are needed to support this hypothesis.

Another possible marker of poor prognosis in WT has been mapped to chromosome 16q. Grundy et al., studying a group of 232 predominantly non-anaplastic tumors on NWTS 3 and 4, found that the 17% of patients with tumor-specific loss of heterozygosity at 16q had a 12-fold higher mortality rate than those without it (61). These differences remained significant when adjusted for histology (anaplasia) and stage. Of note, loss of chromosome 16q had previously been found to be associated with poor prognosis in another tumor, hepatocellular carcinoma (62). Subsequent studies have failed to identify 16q loss of heterozygosity in the rests associated with these tumors (36), suggesting the possibility that 16q loss could represent a relatively late genetic alteration in WT progression. It is hoped that studies like these can identify those children in the favorable histology subgroup who require more intensive chemotherapy to survive, while others can be spared the added toxicity. Identification of the actual genes involved at this locus will provide an additional challenge.

Therapy and prognosis

Primary radical nephrectomy followed by adjuvant chemotherapy and possibly radiation therapy is the mainstay of treatment on the NWTS (8). A random surgical sampling of regional lymph nodes should be performed to exclude metastases. The pathologic features of the untreated tumor, specifically the stage and the presence or absence of anaplasia, dictate the intensity of subsequent therapy. Preoperative chemotherapy is generally used when the primary tumor is unresectable, bilateral, or associated with a tumor thrombus that extends above the hepatic vein. It is also useful when WT develops in a solitary or horseshoe kidney.

Currently on NWTS 5, all Stage 1 and 2 favorable histology tumors and Stage 1 anaplastic tumors are treated identically with 18 weeks of pulse intensive dactinomycin and vincristine. At the beginning of this trial, a subgroup of patients less then 2 years of age with Stage 1 favorable histology tumors weighing less than 550 g were eligible for surgery alone with no adjuvant therapy. This arm of the trial was created because NWTS 4 studies had shown a 2-year relapse-free survival rate of over 95% in such patients. However, a slight increase in relapse rate over that predicted was identified in the first 90 of these patients treated on NWTS 5 without chemotherapy, and this arm of the study was closed in June 1998.

Doxorubicin and radiation therapy are added to the treatment regimen of advanced Stage 3 and 4 favorable histology WT, as well as to Stage 2 through 4 tumors showing focal anaplasia. Radiation is given to the abdominal bed for all of these advanced tumors; additional radiation therapy is given to both lung fields for those with Stage 4 disease. Treatment is markedly intensified for diffuse anaplastic tumors at Stages 2 through 4, with the addition of cyclophosphamide and etoposide to the three drug regimen listed above. Hence, in a diffusely anaplastic WT, the distinction of Stage 1 versus Stage 2 has major therapeutic implications to the patient.

Most relapses of WT occur within 2 years of diagnosis, and hence clinical and radiographic follow-up is concentrated within this window (63). Standard radiographic follow-up includes serial chest X-rays to detect lung metastases and abdominal ultrasonography to rule out local recurrence. The finding of nephrogenic rests in association with a WT may be an indication for increasing the frequency and duration of sonographic surveillance for tumor formation in the opposite kidney.

The prognosis for children with WT is dependent upon both stage and the presence or absence of anaplasia. For children with favorable histology tumors, the effectiveness of modern chemotherapy has considerably decreased the prognostic significance of stage. While Stage 1 favorable histology tumors have a survival rate of over 95%, Stage 4 favorable histology tumors are associated with a diminished but still optimistic survival rate of 81%. No other disseminated non-hematopoetic childhood tumor offers such hope for a cure. The significance of anaplasia, a marker for chemotherapy resistance, is completely dependent upon its stage. The survival rate for localized Stage 1 anaplastic tumors matches that for Stage 1 favorable histology tumors. However, the survival rate for advanced stage diffusely anaplastic tumors is diminished in proportion to stage, despite intensified chemotherapy: 4-year survival rates fall to 70% (Stage 2), 56% (Stage 3), and 17% (Stage 4) (64).

The significance of the location of the anaplastic tumor is verified by the fact that tumors showing focal anaplasia, which by definition must be confined to the kidney, have a similar prognosis as favorable histology WT at any overall stage. Presumably, the anaplastic foci are completely resected in these cases, leaving only responsive favorable histology WT in extrarenal sites. This distinction was emphasized in a comparison of outcomes for patients with focal or diffuse anaplasia in the primary tumor and Stage 4 disease in NWTS 3 and 4. Among eight patients with focal anaplasia, all survived. These patients' metastases were presumably composed of favorable histology tumor. Among 23 patients with diffuse anaplasia, whose metastases presumably contained anaplastic cells, all but one died (17).

Future studies

Future studies will likely result in the more precise mapping of the loci previously implicated in Wilms tumorigenesis, and ultimately lead to the eventual cloning of these genes. The genes involved in tumor progression on 16q, in familial WT on 17q12, and in BWS on 11p15 are prime candidates for such study. Other loci may be uncovered by novel techniques such as comparative genomic hybridization (65) and microarray technologies must also be evaluated. One goal will be to determine what genetic events result in chemotherapy resistance in non-anaplastic tumors. This issue is of considerable clinical significance, since diffuse anaplasia identifies only 30% of children who die of progressive WT. Identification of the loci involved may eventually provide more therapeutic choices for such patients.

Another largely unexplored field of study is the mechanism and frequency of progression of actively proliferating nephrogenic rests to WT. Such knowledge could potentially allow a more precise assessment of the risks to the patient posed by the presence of nephrogenic rests, and rationally guide clinical decisions. This issue is most problematic for children with diffuse hyperplastic nephroblastomatosis, where overzealous surgery could leave a child anephric and dialysis-dependent. Failure to treat such children can allow the remaining functional kidney to become compressed by actively growing rest and lose function. We have generally favored chemotherapy to shrink these rests in such patients, first to prevent renal compression and second to decrease the potential number of targets for induction to WT. A formal study of the efficacy of this approach has not been done.

Congenital mesoblastic nephroma

Initially described by Bolande in 1967 (66), CMN comprise approximately 5% of primary pediatric renal tumors enrolled on the NWTS. However, this may underestimate the incidence of CMN because many are not registered on NWTS protocols, which generally call only for observation after nephrectomy. CMN is a tumor of infancy: over 90% of cases occur during the first year of life, with a rapid decline thereafter. The most common congenital renal neoplasm, CMN is often detected antenatally by maternal ultrasonography. No syndromic associations are known, though kidneys bearing CMNs may show dysplasia (cartilagenous islands), likely resulting from renal obstruction by the tumor during renal development *in utero*.

Congenital mesoblastic nephroma is best considered a low grade sarcoma. While most are cured by complete resection, the tumor's infiltrative borders can make complete excision difficult and sometimes impossible. Incompletely excised CMN may recur locally with alarming rapidity and also rarely metastasizes to distant organs such as the lungs (67) and brain (68).

Pathology

Congenital mesoblastic nephromas are usually centrally located within the kidney, and almost always involve the renal sinus. Three histologic subtypes have been delineated: the classic type initially described by Bolande (24% of cases), the more frequent cellular type (66% of cases), and mixed type (10% of cases) showing both classic and cellular patterns (2).

The classic type of CMN is highly reminiscent of infantile fibromatosis. Tumors are grossly firm and have a whorled appearance. The tumor grows as intersecting fascicles of bland fibroblastic spindle cells with tapered nuclei and pink cytoplasm (Fig. 12.4). The fascicles dissect through the native kidney, entrapping islands of nephrons, and characteristically spread along the underside of the renal capsule when they reach this plane. The tumor entraps the perinephric fat in a fashion identical to fibromatosis. Prominent vascularity is usually found at the tumor's invasive edge, while extramedullary hematopoiesis is often seen within. Mitoses are usually infrequent while necrosis is absent.

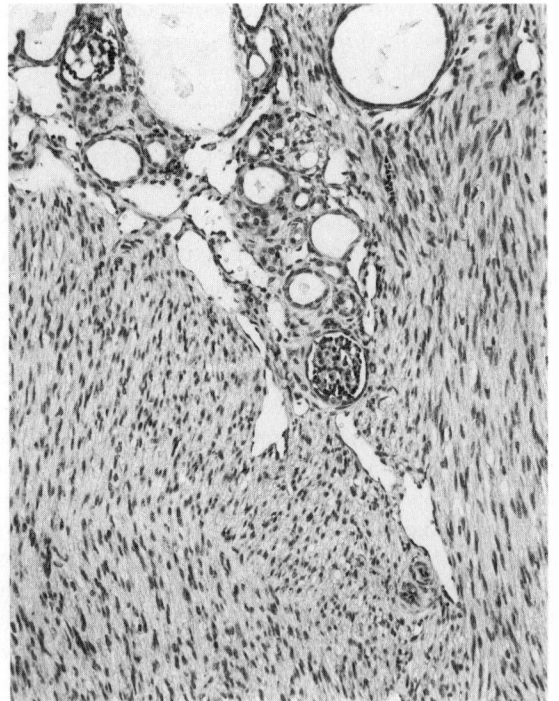

Fig. 12.4 Classic CMN. The tumor grows as fascicles of bland fibroblastic cells which dissect through the native kidney, in this case entrapping an island of glomeruli and associated tubules. 160× magnification.

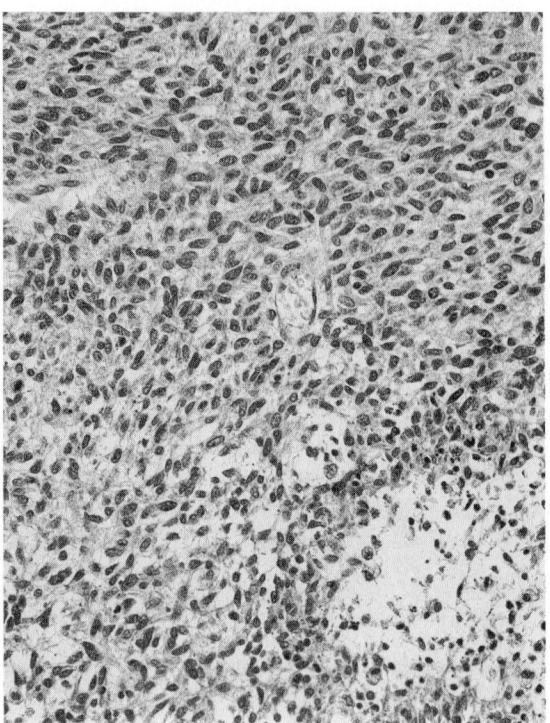

Fig. 12.5 Cellular CMN. The fascicular pattern is less well-formed in this lesion. Mitoses are frequent and palisaded necrosis is evident. 160× magnification.

Table 12.4 Classical versus cellular CMN

	Classical	Cellular
Growth pattern	Fascicular	Fascicular or solid
Border with kidney	Infiltrative	Pushing
Necrosis	No	Frequent
Mitoses	Scattered	Common
Genetic changes	Unknown	t(12;15)(p13;q25), trisomy 11

The cellular type of CMN is remarkably similar to infantile fibrosarcoma. Tumors are often fleshy, feature gross necrosis and hemorrhage, and may be predominantly cystic. The tumor pushes aside the native kidney, only superficially entrapping nephrons. Fascicles are poorly formed and the tumor can adopt a solid, sheet-like growth pattern (Fig. 12.5). Tumor cell nuclei are either hyperchromatic and rounded ("blue cell" appearance) or vesicular and ovoid ("plump cell" appearance). Mitoses and cellularity are high, while necrosis is frequent (Table 12.4). The mixed type of CMN features areas resembling both classical and cellular morphologies. While these transitions may be sharp, most are indistinct and multifocal within a given tumor.

Diagnostic dilemmas can be created by prominent capillary vasculature within some plump cell cellular CMNs, which may mimic the vasculature of CCSK, and focally prominent nucleoli in other cellular CMNs which suggest those of rhabdoid tumor. In addition, treated WTs may acquire a stroma-rich spindle cell appearance similar to that of CMN.

The immunohistochemical profile of CMN reflects its myofibroblastic/fibroblastic nature, which has been demonstrated ultrastructurally (69). Tumor cells are uniformly vimentin positive, usually actin positive, and often desmin positive (70, 71). Cytokeratin and S-100 protein stains are negative.

Genetics

Significant advances have been made in understanding the molecular pathogenesis of the cellular type of CMN. Initial studies demonstrated that while classical CMNs are diploid, cellular CMNs are often aneuploid (70, 72, 73). The most consistent alteration in cellular CMNs has been trisomy for chromosome 11, though similar trisomies for chromosomes 8 and 17 have been identified. Of note, in several individual cases of mixed CMN, a transition from diploidy to aneuploidy was demonstrated in the cellular areas of the tumor, suggesting that aneuploidy may be a marker of histologic progression (70, 72). Interestingly, trisomy 11 had previously been identified in infantile fibrosarcoma, strengthening its morphologic link to cellular CMN.

The linkage of infantile fibrosarcoma and cellular CMN was established when a specific t(12;15)(p13;q25) chromosome translocation, initially discovered in infantile fibrosarcoma (74), was identified in cellular CMN (75–77). This translocation may have been overlooked in past cytogenetic studies of CMN because of the extreme telomeric location and similarities in banding patterns of the exchanged chromosome fragments. The cloning of the resulting gene fusion has allowed more reliable molecular detection assays to be applied. The genes fused by the translocation are the ETV6 gene on 12p13, a member of the ETS transcription factor family previously known to be involved in gene fusions in pediatric B precursor acute lymphoblastic leukemias, and the neurotrophin-3 receptor gene on 15q25 (also known as NTRK3 or TRKC), a membrane-bound protein with tyrosine kinase activity. Using reverse transcriptase polymerase chain reaction (RT-PCR), the ETV6–NTRK3 gene fusion has been detected in 10 of 11 cellular CMNs, 0 of 5 classic CMNs, and, interestingly, 3 of 3 tumors reported as mixed CMNs (76, 77). The absence of the ETV6/NTRK3 fusion in classical CMN correlates with its demonstrated absence in its analog, infantile fibromatosis of soft tissue. In the above-referenced studies, microdissection of the mixed CMNs could not be performed to localize the fusion within different areas of the tumors. In summary, these studies show that the ETV6/NTRK3 gene fusion and the acquisition of polysomies are specific molecular features of the cellular type of CMN.

Treatment and prognosis

As initially stated by Bolande, CMN is best treated by surgical excision alone without the need for adjuvant chemotherapy. NWTS studies have confirmed the excellent prognosis, demonstrating a 98% survival rate that has not been influenced by adjuvant therapy (78). With complete surgical excision, the infants affected by this tumor can be spared the toxicities of chemotherapy that are so dangerous at this age. Less than 5% of CMN recur. While completeness of excision is clearly the most important factor predicting recurrence, adequate margins are often difficult to obtain. This is particularly true of the medial margin, where infiltrating tongues of these sinus-based tumors insidiously penetrate the peri-renal fat. Microscopic foci of tumor are usually present beyond its gross medial confines. In addition, retraction artifact makes the assessment of the medial margin by the pathologist extremely difficult. In these cases of unclear margins, we recommend monthly sonograms for 1 year to monitor for tumor recurrence. The frequency of sonograms is dictated by the ability of the tumor to grow extremely rapidly. The duration of surveillance is dictated by studies showing that most recurrences of CMN will occur within 1 year of nephrectomy, after which time the risk of recurrence becomes negligible (J. Bruce Beckwith, manuscript in preparation). When gross residual tumor is left behind following surgery, adjuvant chemotherapy is indicated (2). CMN in older patients and CMN demonstrating vascular invasion may also be candidates for adjuvant therapy.

While the cellular variant of CMN certainly has a more ominous morphologic appearance than classical CMN, there is little evidence to suggest that histologic subtype alone dictates prognosis in these patients. One retrospective study did find a high incidence of recurrence or metastases (5 out of 18 cases) in cellular CMNs, and proposed are the term "atypical mesoblastic nephroma" (79) to denote an increased potential for aggressive behavior. However, 66% of CMN are of the cellular subtype, and only 5% of CMN recur, so it is apparent that the vast majority of cellular CMN are cured surgically (2).

Future studies

Future studies will center around the oncogenic activity of the ETV6/NTRK3 fusion product in cellular CMN.

This chimeric protein is predicted to contain the N-terminal helix-loop-helix protein dimerization domain of ETV6 and the C-terminal tyrosine kinase domain of NTRK3. While the normal NTRK3 protein requires ligand binding to oligomerize, autophosphorylate, and activate downstream growth pathways, the fusion protein is predicted to be constitutively dimerized and activated (74). In addition, because the fusion product is expressed from the more active ETV6 promoter, it may be over-expressed. The downstream growth promoting targets of the fusion protein will need to be determined. Of particular interest is the potential linkage of the presence of the fusion product to trisomy 11, which has been found in most but not all fusion-positive cases. A variety of imprinted genes, including IGF-2, are localized to chromosome 11p15.5; increase in copy number of the active allele could provide a mechanism of the documented abundant IGF-2 expression in these tumors (80). Of note, a case of mixed CMN with disomy for chromosome 11 but biallelic expression of IGF-2 (loss of imprinting) has been reported, providing another mechanism for IGF-2 over-expression (81).

Another unresolved question is the involvement of the ETV6/NTRK3 fusion transcript in mixed CMN. Given that classic CMN are fusion negative while cellular CMN are fusion positive, one might predict that the fusion transcript would be present only in the cellular portion of a mixed CMN. The fusion transcript could then be a molecular marker of the tumor's progression from classic to cellular morphology. While this hypothesis is appealing, direct proof of it has not yet emerged. Furthermore, no other sarcoma-associated translocation has ever been documented to be acquired in tumor progression.

An additional area requiring further investigation is the recent emergence of reports of "adult mesoblastic nephromas" (82–84). These tumors have been described as circumscribed biphasic lesions with both stromal and epithelial components that occur predominantly near the renal pelvis in adult women. These features are markedly different from the above-discussed pediatric CMNs, which lack a significant gender bias, are infiltrative, and lack a neoplastic epithelial component. In addition, pediatric CMN is non-existent over the age of 3 years of age. It is hard to imagine that a tumor's incidence would drop off so dramatically in childhood, only to return in adulthood. For all of the above reasons, we feel that a histogenic linkage of these adult tumors to pediatric CMN is unlikely. Instead, a relationship may exist with cystic hamartoma of the renal pelvis (85), a biphasic epithelial/stromal tumor that predominantly affects women.

Clear cell sarcoma of the kidney

Initially recognized as a distinct entity by Kidd in 1970 (86), CCSK was described in detail by three independent groups in 1978 (87–89). CCSK comprises 5% of cases registered on the NWTS. Its incidence peaks in the second year of life and slowly declines thereafter. Rare verified adult cases exist. No syndromic associations are known.

Clear cell sarcoma of the kidney has been considered a "unfavorable histology" tumor by the NWTS, following initial trials in which a high mortality rate was observed. Bone has been the most common metastatic site (hence the alternative designation of "bone metastasizing renal tumor of childhood"), in sharp contrast to WTs which rarely spread to bone. Brain and soft tissue metastases are also common in CCSK and unusual for WT. The addition of doxorubicin to NWTS treatment regimens in recent years has dramatically improved the prognosis for children with CCSK (90), leading to a cure rate that now approaches 75% (91).

Pathology

Clear cell sarcomas of the kidney are usually large tumors centered within the renal hilum. Tumors have a mucoid texture, are frequently multicystic, and appear sharply demarcated from the native kidney. However, on microscopic examination, these stromal tumors usually infiltrate and entrap normal renal tissue, sometimes inviting a mistaken perception of a biphasic stromal-epithelial neoplasm such as WT.

The classic morphologic pattern of CCSK is biphasic, composed of nests of plump cord cells located within regularly branching capillary vascular arcades that are lined by spindled septal cells (Fig. 12.6). The cord cells have fine, open chromatin, indistinct cytoplasmic borders, and are surrounded by wisps of extracellular mucopolysaccharide that simulates clear cytoplasm. The regular branching capillary vasculature is highly reminiscent of that of myxoid liposarcoma, while the spindled septal cells resemble fibroblasts.

While most tumors at least focally show the classic pattern, many CCSKs are dominated by one of many variant patterns which lead to confusion with other neoplasms (5, 92). These are the cellular, myxoid, sclerosing, epithelioid, palisading, spindled, storiform, and anaplastic patterns. The diminished extracellular mucopolysaccharide and the subsequent nuclear crowding in the cellular pattern raises the differential diagnosis of other small round blue cell tumors, including blastemal WT and renal PNET. The myxoid pattern

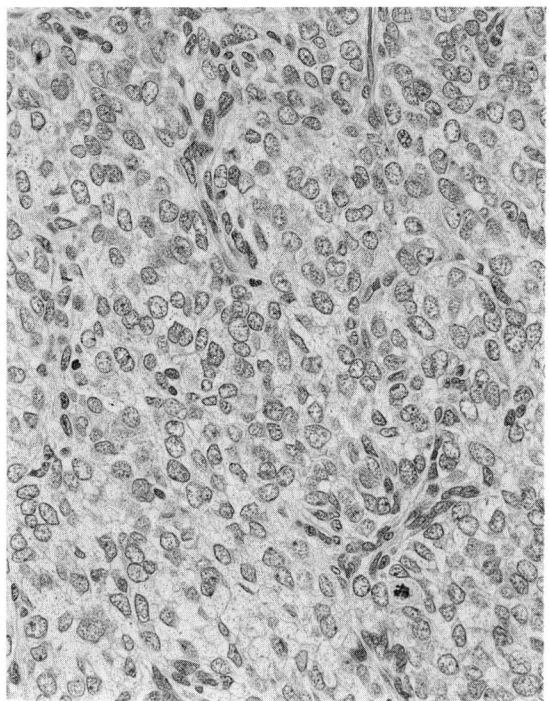

Fig. 12.6 CCSK, classic pattern. Nests (cords) of tumor cells with fine, evenly dispersed chromatin and indistinct cytoplasmic borders are separated by a branching capillary network. 400× magnification.

results from pooling of extracellular mucopolysaccharide material, creating paucicellular pseudocysts that simulate myxoma. Prominent hyaline sclerosis creates an appearance reminiscent of osteosarcoma. Epithelioid patterns feature pseudorosettes which mimic the tubules of WT or trabecular growth that simulates carcinoma. The palisading pattern mimics the verocay bodies seen in schwannoma. Spindled and storiform patterns raise the differential diagnosis of a variety of renal sarcomas. Finally, CCSK can show anaplastic nuclear features identical to those of anaplastic WT.

While CCSK immunoreactivity is limited to vimentin, consistent negativity with other immunostains helps exclude other entities in the differential diagnosis (91). Cytokeratin is uniformly negative, even in epithelioid foci that simulate WT. 013(CD99) is also consistently negative, even in the cellular foci that simulate PNET. Desmin positivity that has been found in CMNs is not seen in CCSK (91).

The ultrastructural appearance of CCSK is that of a primitive mesenchymal cell, with perinuclear cytoplasmic intermediate filaments (probably vimentin) and rudimentary cell junctions (93). Cell processes tend to enfold the prominent extracellular mucopolysaccharide matrix between the cells, imparting the clear cell light microscopic appearance.

Genetics

Remarkably little is known about the molecular genetics of CCSK. Tumor cells have been notoriously difficult to grow in cell culture. To our knowledge, only two publications have reported cytogenetic abnormalities in single tumors which were classified as CCSK (94, 95). However, on critical review, it is not entirely clear to us that these tumors are truly CCSKs. One immunohistochemical study raised the possibility of p53 alterations based upon immunohistochemical detection of p53 in a subset of CCSKs (96). In a large study of CCSKs, we have found limited p53 immunoreactivity in non-anaplastic CCSK, but striking immunoreactivity in two anaplastic CCSKs (91). While requiring direct genetic analysis for confirmation, these results suggest that p53 gene alterations are, as with WT, linked with progression to anaplasia.

Treatment and prognosis

Clear cell sarcoma of the kidneys are optimally treated with nephrectomy and intensive adjuvant therapy. A study of the first three NWTS trials found that the 6-year relapse-free survival rate improved from 25% to 63.5% when doxorubicin was added to a regimen of vincristine, actimomycin D, and radiation therapy. Hence, all tumors are now treated with doxorubicin-containing regimens. Currently, tumors are treated similarly regardless of tumor stage. Patients require prolonged follow-up, as metastases have been reported up to 10 years after diagnosis (97). Bone and brain imaging are used in follow-up to exclude metastases to these sites, while thorough physical examinations can help detect the soft tissue metastases.

Stage has traditionally been de-emphasized as a prognostic factor in CCSK, following NWTS 1 in which 5 of 7 patients classified as Stage 1 by their institution died of tumor. SIOP protocols have met with similar results (98). Based on these results, CCSK has been considered a microscopically disseminated tumor even at seemingly low pathologic stage. We have revisited this concept in a recent review of CCSK on NWTS 1–4 in which tumors were restaged using NWTS 5 criteria. Using these criteria, the pathologic stage of 23% of cases was changed, many going from Stage 1 to 2 on the basis of renal sinus vascular invasion that could be confidently documented in a retrospective slide review. Using the updated staging criteria, the new Stage 1 grouping (25% of patients) had a 98% survival rate (91), compared to 66% for Stages 2 or 3. These data indicate that Stage 1 status is in fact an excellent prognostic factor in CCSK. Using current criteria, the reported Stage 1 patients who died on NWTS 1 were all understaged. Our current view is that CCSK is a slowly growing neoplasm which, when localized, is highly curable. Once it has gained access to the systemic vascular system, the prognosis is diminished and good outcomes require responsiveness to chemotherapy.

Future studies

The outstanding outcome of Stage 1 CCSK patients in NWTS 1–4 may justify a prospective trial of less intensive chemotherapy for this patient subset in future NWTS group studies. The genetic alterations associated with this tumor have remained a mystery, and will likely be the subject of future study. Of note, the majority of CCSKs studied by comparative genomic hybridization showed a normal pattern, suggesting that gene amplification or deletion may not be pathogenic factors (99).

Rhabdoid tumor of the kidney

Rhabdoid tumor of the kidney is a distinctive, highly lethal tumor of infants comprising 2% of NWTS cases (100). Eighty-five percent of cases occur within the first 2 years of life, with a sharp decline thereafter such that the diagnosis is suspect over the age of five. The tumor is usually disseminated at diagnosis, with 80% of patients presenting at Stages 3 or 4 (97). In NWTS studies, 80% of children died of tumor within 1 year of diagnosis. SIOP trials have met with similar results (101).

While no syndromes are associated with RTK, there is an established association with brain tumors, most of which are located in the midline cerebellum (102). Most of these tumors morphologically resemble medulloblastoma or PNET, though gliomas and ependymomas have been reported. In addition, an association of RTK with hypercalcemia mediated via PTH-related peptide has been reported (103).

The diagnosis of renal rhabdoid tumor is complicated by the fact that a variety of renal tumors can show focal rhabdoid features (104). Rhabdoid features are even more prevalent in extrarenal neoplasms making the diagnosis of extra-renal rhabdoid tumor even harder to sustain (105). Nonetheless, the establishment of a common genetic deletion on the long arm chromosome 22 in both renal and extra-renal rhabdoid tumors in infants has linked these two together and solidified the unifying concept of a primary rhabdoid tumor of childhood.

Pathologic features

The RTK is usually a bulky mass which is centered in the renal hilum, universally involving the renal sinus. The grossly indistinct tumor border reflects aggressive microscopic invasion and engulfment of renal parenchyma. Tumor cells rarely pass a blood vessel without invading it. Prominent intrarenal vascular invasion leads to frequent satellite nodules which can be detected grossly. The tumor characteristically grows as sheets of monotonous dyscohesive cells characterized by vesicular nuclei, prominent macronucleoli, and hyaline cytoplasmic inclusions (Fig. 12.7). The latter three cytologic features, while characteristic, are variably developed in different areas of most tumors, with diligent

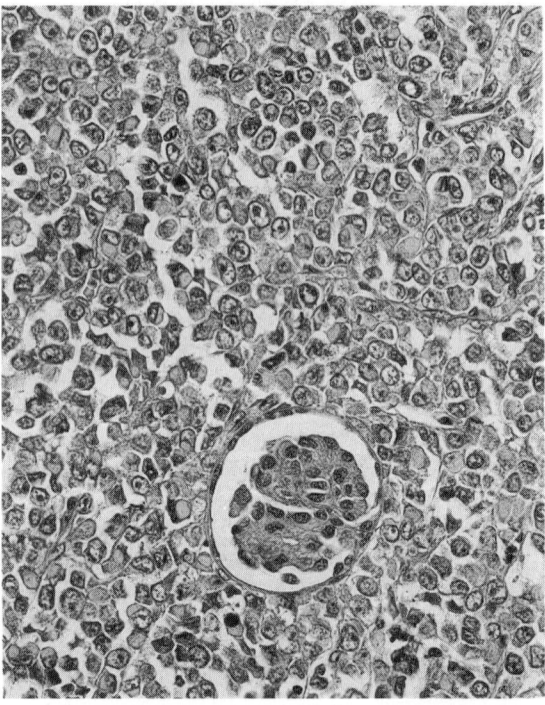

Fig. 12.7 RTK. Sheets of tumor cells surround an entrapped native glomerulus. The cells have vesicular chromatin, prominent nucleoli, and hyaline cytoplasmic inclusions. 400× magnification.

search sometimes required before diagnostic foci are encountered. In addition, a large number of variant patterns have been described, including sclerosing, epithelioid, spindled, vascular, and lymphomatoid, which can simulate other neoplasms (100).

The renal tumors which occasionally show rhabdoid features in some cells and must be distinguished from RTK include cellular CMN, WT, and medullary renal carcinoma. Cellular CMN occasionally shows prominent nucleoli and a diffuse growth pattern, but rarely has hyaline cytoplasmic inclusions. WT may have hyaline cytoplasmic inclusions, but the presence of macronucleoli effectively excludes the diagnosis of WT. Both of these lesions typically show more characteristic foci which make their diagnosis apparent. Importantly, the prognosis for each of these tumors appears to be unaffected by the presence of rhabdoid features, and aggressive therapy triggered by a diagnosis of RTK is contraindicated (104). The recently described medullary renal carcinoma (106) accounts for many of the previously reported RTK in patients over the age of 5 years. Remarkably, this highly lethal tumor is virtually restricted to adolescent patients with sickle cell hemoglobin trait. While perfect phenocopies of rhabdoid cells often predominate, the presence of acute inflammation in the stroma, a reticular "yolk-sac" pattern, and sickled cells in the tissue sections should make the diagnosis evident.

Rhabdoid tumor of the kidney characteristically show a polyphenotypic immunohistochemical staining pattern. While vimentin immunoreactivity is uniform and intense, tumor cells may stain simultaneously with a variety of markers including cytokeratin, EMA, desmin, and neurofilament. Nonspecific trapping of these antibodies by the hyaline inclusions may cause these results. One particularly helpful pattern of staining is the presence of scattered clusters of intensely EMA or cytokeratin positive cells in a background of negative staining; few other pediatric tumors stain in this distinct fashion. Ultrastructurally, the hyaline inclusions correspond to whorled cytoplasmic intermediate filaments, which are variably developed amongst the tumor cells. While rudimentary cell junctions are present, no desmosomes, myogenic contractile proteins, or other features which can help assign specific lineage of differentiation are found (107).

Genetics

Cytogenetic analyses of RTK demonstrated a high frequency of abnormalities on the long arm of chromosome 22. These results were confirmed by molecular analysis in which 80% of 30 RTKs studied showed loss of heterozygosity on chromosome 22q, with a common region of loss between 22q11 and 22q12 (108). These results strongly suggested the presence of a tumor suppressor gene at this locus. Particularly intriguing was the fact that 22q loss had been previously reported in the atypical teratoid/rhabdoid tumor of the brain, another highly lethal tumor of very young children with prominent rhabdoid morphology (109). In addition, 22q11 alterations had been reported in the true primary rhabdoid tumors of soft tissue in infants (110, 111).

A major advance occurred when Versteege et al. mapped the common area of deletion on chromosome 22q11.2 in a series of renal and soft tissue rhabdoid tumors to the hSNF5/INI1 gene (112). In their series of 13 tumors, 6 contained homozygous deletions of this gene while 6 contained truncating mutations in one allele accompanied by loss of the other allele. Confirmation of this finding came from Biegel et al. who studied 18 atypical teratoid/rhabdoid tumors of the brain, 7 RTKs and 4 rhabdoid tumors of soft tissue (113). In this series, all 29 tumors showed hSNF5/INI1 gene alterations; 15 had homozygous deletions of one or more exons while 15 contained mutations. In addition, germ line mutations were demonstrated in four children, supporting the hypothesis that hSNF5/INI 1 is a tumor suppressor gene. This gene product is thought to normally function by altering the conformation of the DNA–histone complex so that transcription factors have access to target genes (112). It is apparent from these studies that disruption of this gene represents the common genetic abnormality linking RTK with other pediatric rhabdoid tumors.

Treatment and prognosis

To date, modern chemotherapy has not altered the dismal prognosis associated with RTK. Combinations of etoposide and cisplatin or ifosfamide are employed, but the results have not been encouraging. As such, intensive experimental protocols are often employed which subject the child to significant toxicity. Few favorable prognostic factors exist, though the minority of adequately staged patients who presented with low stage disease seem to fare better. In NWTS studies, 10 of 20 patients with documented negative lymph nodes survived (100).

Future studies

Future studies will likely examine the possible mechanisms by which loss of function of the hSNF5/INI1 gene is associated with the aggressive malignant behavior of RTK. One might predict loss of function of the specific transcription factors for which hSNF5/INI1 makes the chromatin more accessible. The identity of these transcription factors might shed light on the pathogenesis of RTK and enable a tageted therapy for the tumor. Another unresolved question is the role (if any) of hSNF5/INI1 in other neoplasms, specifically those with rhabdoid features. While the rhabdoid phenotype does not appear to be associated with more aggressive behavior in other primary pediatric renal tumors (104), the rhabdoid phenotype has been associated with marked aggressivity in other pediatric (114) and adult (115) tumors. It has been stated that while a tumor's specific differentiation dictates its epidemiology, the presence of a rhabdoid phenotype dictates its dismal prognosis (115). The intriguing possibility that hSNF5/INI1 is altered in some of these tumors should be addressed.

Another area that demands clarification is the morphologic and molecular relationship between RTK and the midline posterior fossa CNS tumors with which it is associated. While most of these are described as small blue cell tumors such as medulloblastoma or PNET, the atypical teratoid/rhabdoid tumor which shares morphology and the hNF5/INI1 gene deletion with RTK is notorious for having a small cell component that mimics medulloblastoma (116). Is it possible that the brain lesions in patients with RTK in fact represent multifocal rhabdoid tumor? Along these lines, one of the CNS rhabdoid tumors reported by Biegel et al. was diagnosed by three neuropathologists on morphologic grounds as medulloblastoma/PNET, but showed a hSNF5/INI1 gene deletion and resulted in rapid death (113). It is possible that, in cases such as this, the underlying genetic alterations may not be reflected in the morphology of these tumors. In the only reported case in which both the renal rhabdoid tumor and the CNS PNET were compared, the CNS lesion showed loss of heterozygosity in 22q11 while the RTK retained both alleles (117). Such intriguing results merit further study.

Finally, while the delineation of the gene involved on chromosome 22q represents a major advance toward understanding the molecular pathogenesis of RTK, the role of other genes requires study. Of particular interest is the locus on chromosome 11p15.5, the site of the WT-2 gene, which is reported to show loss of heterozygosity in 17% of RTKs (108, 118).

Pediatric renal cell carcinoma

Renal cell carcinoma is rare in children in the absence of a genetic predisposition such as Von–Hippel–Lindau Syndrome (119) or tuberous sclerosis. A subset of these tumors has been found on cytogenetic analysis to have chromosome translocations involving a common breakpoint on chromosome Xp11.2 (120–122). The most common reported translocation has been t(X;1)(p11;q21), though a t(X;17)(p11.2;q25) translocation has also been reported (123). While a detailed clinicopathologic study of this cytogenetically defined subtype of tumor is lacking, the following features seem to be true. First, the tumor tends to affect younger patients than other renal cell carcinomas, though adult cases are on record. Second, the tumor has a distinct male predominance which is intriguing given the involvement of the X chromosome. Third, the tumor has classically been described as having papillary architecture, though cases with predominantly clear cells and solid growth patterns are reported. Given that the genetic alterations associated with papillary (trisomy 7,17) and clear cell (3p deletion) renal cell carcinomas in adults have not been found in the t(X;1)(p11.2;q21) tumors, it seems unwise to place these lesions into either of the above categories. Rather, these tumors appear to represent a genetically distinct tumor type whose morphology may overlap with other genetically disparate adult renal tumors.

The genes fused by the t(X;1)(p11.2;q21) translocation have recently been cloned (124) (125). Xp11.2 harbors the TFE3 gene, a known basic helix-loop-helix transcription factor, which becomes fused to a novel ubiquitously expressed gene of unknown function designated PRCC. While both reciprocal fusion products are expressed, normal TFE3 expression is lost in these tumors. Whether oncogenicity results from either fusion product or from disruption of TFE3 or other genes has yet to be demonstrated.

Primitive neuroectodermal tumor (PNET)

A diagnosis of primary PNET within a visceral organ such as the kidney has traditionally been difficult to prove. The undifferentiated light microscopic appearance of this tumor and the lack of a specific immunohistochemical marker for it has blurred its distinction from blastemal WT. The development of immunohistochemical stains for the MIC2 antigen (CD99) has allowed definitive delineation of primary renal PNETs (126, 127). Several of these cases have been confirmed by detection of the EWS/FLI 1 chimeric RNA transcript that results from the t(11;22)(q24;q12) translocation (128).

The cases of primary renal PNET reported thus far have tended to present with high stage disease. Outcomes have been poor, though this may simply reflect the advanced stage. Most patients have been adolescents or young adults, a significantly older age range than is typical of blastemal WT. In fact, in this age group, PNET is a more likely diagnosis than blastemal WT. These observations may help to explain the long held view among oncologists that adult WTs are more aggressive than those in children. Many of these cases submitted to the NWTS Pathology Center as "adult Wilms tumors" are in fact PNETs (J. Bruce Beckwith, unpublished observations).

Synovial sarcoma

A series of primary renal sarcomas of adolescents and young adults that appeared distinct from WT was identified and reported in abstract form in 1995 as embryonal sarcoma of the kidney (129). These tumors were generally characterized by primitive "embryonal" appearing spindled tumor cells (which led to diagnostic confusion with WT), gross cystification caused by dilation of entrapped renal tubules, and aggressive clinical behavior (130). As initially defined, however, this group seemed heterogeneous. While most cases were composed of bland spindled cells that stained immunohistochemically only with vimentin, a subset showed anaplastic cytology and stained with desmin. Of note, one of the former cases proved to have an t(X;18) translocation which is characteristic of synovial sarcoma on cytogenetic analysis. This observation was particularly intriguing as this and many of the other cases were morphologically compatible with monophasic synovial sarcoma of the kidney. However, fresh frozen tumor, which is traditionally needed to detect the diagnostic SYT–SSX gene fusion that results from the translocation characteristic of synovial sarcoma, was not available from any of these cases.

Using a recently described highly sensitive RT-PCR assay that can detect the SYT–SSX gene fusion in formalin fixed, paraffin-embedded tissue blocks (131), we have found, in the limited number of cases with blocks available, three additional cases of embryonal sarcoma of the kidney with the SYT–SSX gene fusion of synovial sarcoma (132). Eleven additional cases for which confirmatory genetic studies could not be performed, but which were morphologically and immunohistochemically identical to the SYT–SSX positive cases, were also found among the cases previously designated as embryonal sarcoma. These results establish the entity of primary renal synovial sarcoma, and indicate that it composes a large subset of cases previously referred to as embryonal sarcoma of the kidney.

Acknowledgments

We thank Pete Lund and Norman Barker for photographic assistance. We also thank J. Bruce Beckwith, MD, Frederic Askin, MD, and Iradge Argani, MD for reviewing the manuscript and providing helpful comments.

References

1. Robinson LL. General principles of the epidemiology of childhood cancer (ed.). In: Principles and practice of pediatric oncology, 3rd edn (ed. Pizzo PA). Lippincott-Raven Publishers, Philadelphia, 1997, 1–10.
2. Beckwith JB. One. Renal tumors. In: Pathology of solid tumors in children, 1st edn (ed. Stocker JT, Askin FB). Chapman & Hall Medical, New York, 1998, 1–23.
3. Boccon-Gibod LA. Pathological evaluation of renal tumors in children: international society of pediatric oncology approach. Pediatric Devel Pathol 1998, **1**, 243–8.
4. Beckwith JB. National Wilms tumor study: an update for pathologists. Pediatr Dev Pathol 1998, **1**, 79–84.
5. Murphy WM, Beckwith JB, Farrow GM. Tumors of the kidney, bladder, and related urinary structures (third series, fascicle 11. Washington, DC. Armed Forces Institute of Pathology), 1993.
6. Green DM, Coppes MJ, Breslow NE, et al. Wilms tumor. In: Principles and practice of pediatric oncology, 3rd edn (ed. Pizzo PA, Poplack DG). Lippincott-Raven Publishers, Philadelphia, 1997, 733–59.
7. Breslow N, Olshan A, Beckwith JB, Green DM. Epidemiology of Wilms tumor. Med Pediatr Oncol 1993, **21**(3), 172–81.
8. Wiener JS, Coppes MJ, Ritchey ML. Current concepts in the biology and management of Wilms tumor. J Urol 1998, **159**(4), 1316–25.
9. Coppes MJ, Haber DA, Grundy PE. Genetic events in the development of Wilms' tumor. N Engl J Med 1994, **331**(9), 586–90.
10. Beckwith JB. New developments in the pathology of Wilms tumor. Cancer Invest 1997, **15**(2), 153–62.
11. Beckwith JB. Renal neoplasms of childhood. In: Diagnostic surgical pathology, 2nd edn (ed. Sternberg SS). Raven Press, New York, 1994, 1741–66.
12. Davis CJJ, Barton JH, Sesterhenn IA, Mostofi FK. Metanephric adenoma. Clinicopathological study of fifty patients. Am J Surg Pathol 1995, **19**(10), 1101–14.

13. Beckwith JB, Zuppan CE, Browning NG, Moksness J, Breslow NE. Histological analysis of aggressiveness and responsiveness in Wilms' tumor. Med Pediatr Oncol 1996, 27(5), 422–8.
14. Priest JR, Watterson J, Strong L, Huff V, Woods WG, Byrd RL et al. Pleuropulmonary blastoma: a marker for familial disease [see comments]. J Pediatr 1996, 128(2), 220–4.
15. Delahunt B, Thomson KJ, Ferguson AF, Neale TJ, Meffan PJ, Nacey JN. Familial cystic nephroma and pleuropulmonary blastoma [see comments]. Cancer 1993, 71(4), 1338–42.
16. Eble JN, Bonsib SM. Extensively cystic renal neoplasms: cystic nephroma, cystic partially differentiated nephroblastoma, multilocular cystic renal cell carcinoma, and cystic hamartoma of renal pelvis. Semin Diagn Pathol 1998, 15(1), 2–20.
17. Faria P, Beckwith JB, Mishra K, Zuppan C, Weeks DA, Breslow N et al. Focal versus diffuse anaplasia in Wilms tumor—new definitions with prognostic significance: a report from the National Wilms Tumor Study Group. Am J Surg Pathol 1996, 20(8), 909–20.
18. Zuppan CW. Handling and evaluation of pediatric renal tumors. Am J Clin Pathol 1998, 109(4 Suppl 1), S31–S37.
19. Beckwith JB, Kiviat NB, Bonadio JF. Nephrogenic rests, nephroblastomatosis, and the pathogenesis of Wilms' tumor. Pediatr Pathol 1990, 10(1–2), 1–36.
20. Beckwith JB. Precursor lesions of Wilms tumor: clinical and biological implications. Med Pediatr Oncol 1993, 21(3), 158–68.
21. Coppes MJ, Arnold M, Beckwith JB, Ritchey ML, D'Angio GJ, Green DM et al. Factors affecting the risk of contralateral Wilms tumor development: a report from the National Wilms Tumor Study Group. Cancer 1999, 85(7), 1616–25.
22. Beckwith JB. Nephrogenic rests and the pathogenesis of Wilms tumor: developmental and clinical considerations [in process citation]. Am J Med Genet 1998, 79(4), 268–73.
23. Mierau GW, Berry PJ, Malott RL, Weeks DA. Appraisal of the comparative utility of immunohistochemistry and electron microscopy in the diagnosis of childhood round cell tumors. Ultrastruct Pathol 1996, 20(6), 507–17.
24. Mierau GW, Weeks DA, Beckwith JB. Anaplastic Wilms' tumor and other clinically aggressive childhood renal neoplasms: ultrastructural and immunocytochemical features. Ultrastruct Pathol 1989, 13(2–3), 225–48.
25. Knudson AGJ. Introduction to the genetics of primary renal tumors in children. Med Pediatr Oncol 1993, 21(3), 193–8.
26. Gerald WL. The molecular genetics of Wilms tumor: a paradigm of heterogeneity in tumor development. Cancer Invest 1994, 12(3), 350–9.
27. Call KM, Glaser T, Ito CY, Buckler AJ, Pelletier J, Haber DA et al. Isolation and characterization of a zinc finger polypeptide gene at the human chromosome 11 Wilms' tumor locus. Cell 1990, 60(3), 509–20.
28. Gessler M, Poustka A, Cavenee W, Neve RL, Orkin SH, Bruns GA. Homozygous deletion in Wilms tumours of a zinc-finger gene identified by chromosome jumping. Nature 1990, 343(6260), 774–8.
29. Bonetta L, Kuehn SE, Huang A, Law DJ, Kalikin LM, Koi M et al. Wilms tumor locus on 11p13 defined by multiple CpG island-associated transcripts. Science 1990, 250(4983), 994–7.
30. Haber DA, Englert C, Maheswaran S. Functional properties of WT1. Med Pediatr Oncol 1996, 27(5), 453–5.
31. Pelletier J, Bruening W, Kashtan CE, Mauer SM, Manivel JC, Striegel JE et al. Germline mutations in the Wilms' tumor suppressor gene are associated with abnormal urogenital development in Denys–Drash syndrome. Cell 1991, 67(2), 437–47.
32. Grubb GR, Yun K, Williams BR, Eccles MR, Reeve AE. Expression of WT1 protein in fetal kidneys and Wilms tumors. Lab Invest 1994, 71(4), 472–9.
33. Drummond IA, Madden SL, Rohwer-Nutter P, Bell GI, Sukhatme VP, Rauscher FJ. Repression of the insulin-like growth factor II gene by the Wilms tumor suppressor WT1. Science 1992, 257(5070), 674–8.
34. Pritchard-Jones K, Fleming S. Cell types expressing the Wilms' tumour gene (WT1) in Wilms' tumours: implications for tumour histogenesis. Oncogene 1991, 6(12), 2211–9.
35. Park S, Bernard A, Bove KE, Sens DA, Hazen-Martin DJ, Garvin AJ et al. Inactivation of WT1 in nephrogenic rests, genetic precursors to Wilms' tumour. Nat Genet 1993, 5(4), 363–7.
36. Charles AK, Brown KW, Berry PJ. Microdissecting the genetic events in nephrogenic rests and Wilms' tumor development. Am J Pathol 1998, 153(3), 991–1000.
37. Feinberg AP. Multiple genetic abnormalities of 11p15 in Wilms' tumor. Med Pediatr Oncol 1996, 27(5), 484–9.
38. Li M, Squire JA, Weksberg R. Molecular genetics of Wiedemann–Beckwith syndrome [in process citation]. Am J Med Genet 1998, 79(4), 253–9.
39. Hoovers JM, Kalikin LM, Johnson LA, Alders M, Redeker B, Law DJ et al. Multiple genetic loci within 11p15 defined by Beckwith–Wiedemann syndrome rearrangement breakpoints and subchromosomal transferable fragments. Proc Natl Acad Sci, USA 1995, 92(26), 12456–60.
40. Yun K, Molenaar AJ, Fiedler AM, Mark AJ, Eccles MR, Becroft DM et al. Insulin-like growth factor II messenger ribonucleic acid expression in Wilms tumor, nephrogenic rest, and kidney. Lab Invest 1993, 69(5), 603–15.
41. Ogawa O, Eccles MR, Szeto J, McNoe LA, Yun K, Maw MA et al. Relaxation of insulin-like growth factor II gene imprinting implicated in Wilms' tumour. Nature 1993, 362(6422), 749–51.
42. Steenman MJ, Rainier S, Dobry CJ, Grundy P, Horon IL, Feinberg AP. Loss of imprinting of IGF2 is linked to reduced expression and abnormal methylation of H19 in Wilms' tumour [published erratum appears in Nat Genet 1994 Oct, 8(2), 203]. Nat Genet 1994, 7(3), 433–9.
43. Hao Y, Crenshaw T, Moulton T, Newcomb E, Tycko B. Tumour-suppressor activity of H19 RNA. Nature 1993, 365(6448), 764–7.
44. Matsuoka S, Edwards MC, Bai C, Parker S, Zhang P, Baldini A et al. p57KIP2, a structurally distinct member of the p21CIP1 Cdk inhibitor family, is a candidate tumor suppressor gene. Genes Dev 1995, 9(6), 650–62.

45. Orlow I, Iavarone A, Crider-Miller SJ, Bonilla F, Latres E, Lee MH et al. Cyclin-dependent kinase inhibitor p57KIP2 in soft tissue sarcomas and Wilms' tumors. Cancer Res 1996, 56(6), 1219–21.
46. Thompson JS, Reese KJ, DeBaun MR, Perlman EJ, Feinberg AP. Reduced expression of the cyclin-dependent kinase inhibitor gene p57KIP2 in Wilms' tumor. Cancer Res 1996, 56(24), 5723–7.
47. Lee MP, DeBaun MR, Mitsuya K, Galonek HL, Brandenburg S, Oshimura M et al. Loss of imprinting of a paternally expressed transcript, with antisense orientation to KVLQT1, occurs frequently in Beckwith–Wiedemann syndrome and is independent of insulin-like growth factor II imprinting. Proc Natl Acad Sci, USA 1999, 96(9), 5203–8.
48. Huff V, Compton DA, Chao LY, Strong LC, Geiser CF, Saunders GF. Lack of linkage of familial Wilms' tumour to chromosomal band 11p13. Nature 1988, 336(6197), 377–8.
49. Grundy P, Koufos A, Morgan K, Li FP, Meadows AT, Cavenee WK. Familial predisposition to Wilms' tumour does not map to the short arm of chromosome 11. Nature 1988, 336(6197), 374–6.
50. Huff V, Reeve AE, Leppert M, Strong LC, Douglass EC, Geiser CF et al. Nonlinkage of 16q markers to familial predisposition to Wilms' tumor. Cancer Res 1992, 52(21), 6117–20.
51. Rahman N, Abidi F, Ford D, Arbour L, Rapley E, Tonin P, Barton D et al. Confirmation of FWT1 as a Wilms' tumour susceptibility gene and phenotypic characteristics of Wilms' tumour attributable to FWT1. Hum Genet 1998, 103(5), 547–56.
52. Huff V, Amos CI, Douglass EC, Fisher R, Geiser CF, Krill CE et al. Evidence for genetic heterogeneity in familial Wilms' tumor. Cancer Res 1997, 57(10), 1859–62.
53. Malkin D, Sexsmith E, Yeger H, Williams BR, Coppes MJ. Mutations of the p53 tumor suppressor gene occur infrequently in Wilms' tumor. Cancer Res 1994, 54(8), 2077–9.
54. Takeuchi S, Bartram CR, Ludwig R, Royer-Pokora B, Schneider S, Imamura J et al. Mutations of p53 in Wilms' tumors. Mod Pathol 1995, 8(5), 483–7.
55. Bardeesy N, Falkoff D, Petruzzi MJ, Nowak N, Zabel B, Adam M, Aguiar MC et al. Anaplastic Wilms' tumour, a subtype displaying poor prognosis, harbours p53 gene mutations. Nat Genet 1994, 7(1), 91–7.
56. Bardeesy N, Beckwith JB, Pelletier J. Clonal expansion and attenuated apoptosis in Wilms' tumors are associated with p53 gene mutations. Cancer Res 1995, 55(2), 215–19.
57. Kinzler KW, Vogelstein B. Cancer therapy meets p53 [see comments]. N Engl J Med 1994, 331(1), 49–50.
58. Cheah PL, Looi LM, Chan LL. Immunohistochemical expression of p53 proteins in Wilms' tumour: a possible association with the histological prognostic parameter of anaplasia. Histopathology 1996, 28(1), 49–54.
59. Govender D, Harilal P, Hadley GP, Chetty R. p53 protein expression in nephroblastomas: a predictor of poor prognosis. Br J Cancer 1998, 77(2), 314–18.
60. Lahoti C, Thorner P, Malkin D, Yeger H. Immunohistochemical detection of p53 in Wilms' tumors correlates with unfavorable outcome. Am J Pathol 1996, 148(5), 1577–89.
61. Grundy PE, Telzerow PE, Breslow N, Moksness J, Huff V, Paterson MC. Loss of heterozygosity for chromosomes 16q and 1p in Wilms' tumors predicts an adverse outcome. Cancer Res 1994, 54(9), 2331–3.
62. Tsuda H, Zhang WD, Shimosato Y, Yokota J, Terada M, Sugimura T et al. Allele loss on chromosome 16 associated with progression of human hepatocellular carcinoma. Proc Natl Acad Sci, USA 1990, 87(17), 6791–4.
63. D'Angio GJ, Rosenberg H, Sharples K, Kelalis P, Breslow N, Green DM. Position paper: imaging methods for primary renal tumors of childhood: costs versus benefits [published erratum appears in Med Pediatr Oncol 1993, 21(9), 695]. Med Pediatr Oncol 1993, 21(3), 205–12.
64. Green DM, Beckwith JB, Breslow NE, Faria P, Moksness J, Finklestein JZ et al. Treatment of children with stages II to IV anaplastic Wilms' tumor: a report from the National Wilms' Tumor Study Group. J Clin Oncol 1994, 12(10), 2126–31.
65. Getman ME, Houseal TW, Miller GA, Grundy PE, Cowell JK, Landes GM. Comparative genomic hybridization and its application to Wilms' tumorigenesis. Cytogenet Cell Genet 1998, 82(3–4), 284–90.
66. Bolande RP, Brough AJ, Izant RJJ. Congenital mesoblastic nephroma of infancy. A report of eight cases and the relationship to Wilms' tumor. Pediatrics 1967, 40(2), 272–8.
67. Vujanic GM, Delemarre JF, Moeslichan S, Lam J, Harms D, Sandstedt B et al. Mesoblastic nephroma metastatic to the lungs and heart—another face of this peculiar lesion: case report and review of the literature [see comments]. Pediatr Pathol 1993, 13(2), 143–53.
68. Heidelberger KP, Ritchey ML, Dauser RC, McKeever PE, Beckwith JB. Congenital mesoblastic nephroma metastatic to the brain. Cancer 1993, 72(8), 2499–502.
69. O'Malley DP, Mierau GW, Beckwith JB, Weeks DA. Ultrastructure of cellular congenital mesoblastic nephroma. Ultrastruct Pathol 1996, 20(5), 417–27.
70. Pettinato G, Manivel JC, Wick MR, Dehner LP. Classical and cellular (atypical) congenital mesoblastic nephroma: a clinicopathologic, ultrastructural, immunohistochemical, and flow cytometric study. Hum Pathol 1989, 20(7), 682–90.
71. Nadasdy T, Roth J, Johnson DL, Bane BL, Weinberg A, Verani R et al. Congenital mesoblastic nephroma: an immunohistochemical and lectin study. Hum Pathol 1993, 24(4), 413–19.
72. Schofield DE, Yunis EJ, Fletcher JA. Chromosome aberrations in mesoblastic nephroma. Am J Pathol 1993, 143(3), 714–24.
73. Mascarello JT, Cajulis TR, Krous HF, Carpenter PM. Presence or absence of trisomy 11 is correlated with histologic subtype in congenital mesoblastic nephroma. Cancer Genet Cytogenet 1994, 77(1), 50–4.
74. Knezevich SR, McFadden DE, Tao W, Lim JF, Sorensen PH. A novel ETV6-NTRK3 gene fusion in congenital fibrosarcoma. Nat Genet 1998, 18(2), 184–7.
75. Lowery M, Issa B, Pysher T, Brothman A. Cytogenetic findings in a case of congenital mesoblastic nephroma. Cancer Genet Cytogenet 1995, 84(2), 113–15.
76. Knezevich SR, Garnett MJ, Pysher TJ, Beckwith JB, Grundy PE, Sorensen PH. ETV6-NTRK3 gene fusions and trisomy 11 establish a histogenetic link between mesoblastic nephroma and congenital fibrosarcoma. Cancer Res 1998, 58(22), 5046–8.

77. Rubin BP, Chen CJ, Morgan TW, Xiao S, Grier HE, Kozakewich HP. Congenital mesoblastic nephroma t(12;15) is associated with ETV6–NTRK3 gene fusion: cytogenetic and molecular relationship to congenital (infantile) fibrosarcoma. Am J Pathol 1998, 153(5), 1451–8.
78. Howell CG, Othersen HB, Kiviat NE, Norkool P, Beckwith JB, D'Angio GJ. Therapy and outcome in 51 children with mesoblastic nephroma: a report of the National Wilms' Tumor Study. J Pediatr Surg 1982, 17(6), 826–31.
79. Joshi VV, Kasznica J, Walters TR. Atypical mesoblastic nephroma. Pathologic characterization of a potentially aggressive variant of conventional congenital mesoblastic nephroma. Arch Pathol Lab Med 1986, 110(2), 100–6.
80. Sharifah NA, Yun K, McLay J. Insulin-like growth factor II gene expression by congenital mesoblastic nephroma. Diagn Mol Pathol 1995, 4(4), 279–85.
81. Becroft DM, Mauger DC, Skeen JE, Ogawa O, Reeve AE. Good prognosis of cellular mesoblastic nephroma with hyperdiploidy and relaxation of imprinting of the maternal IGF2 gene. Pediatr Pathol Lab Med 1995, 15(5), 679–88.
82. Trillo AA. Adult variant of congenital mesoblastic nephroma. Arch Pathol Lab Med 1990, 114(5), 533–5.
83. Durham JR, Bostwick DG, Farrow GM, Ohorodnik JM. Mesoblastic nephroma of adulthood. Report of three cases. Am J Surg Pathol 1993, 17(10), 1029–38.
84. Truong LD, Williams R, Ngo T, Cawood C, Chevez-Barrios P, Awalt HL et al. Adult mesoblastic nephroma: expansion of the morphologic spectrum and review of literature. Am J Surg Pathol 1998, 22(7), 827–39.
85. Pawade J, Soosay GN, Delprado W, Parkinson MC, Rode J. Cystic hamartoma of the renal pelvis. Am J Surg Pathol 1993, 17(11), 1169–75.
86. Kidd JM. Exclusion of certain renal neoplasms from the category of Wilms tumor. Am J Pathol 1970, 58, 16a-.
87. Morgan E, Kidd JM. Undifferentiated sarcoma of the kidney: a tumor of childhood with histopathologic and clinical characteristics distinct from Wilms' tumor. Cancer 1978, 42(4), 1916–21.
88. Beckwith JB, Palmer NF. Histopathology and prognosis of Wilms tumors: results from the First National Wilms' Tumor Study. Cancer 1978, 41(5), 1937–48.
89. Marsden HB, Lawler W. Bone-metastasizing renal tumour of childhood. Br J Cancer 1978, 38(3), 437–41.
90. Green DM, Breslow NE, Beckwith JB, Moksness J, Finklestein JZ, D'Angio GJ. Treatment of children with clear-cell sarcoma of the kidney: a report from the National Wilms' Tumor Study Group. J Clin Oncol 1994, 12(10), 2132–7.
91. Argani P, Perlman EJ, Breslow N, et al. Clear cell sarcoma of kidney. A review of 351 cases from the National Wilms Tumor Study Pathology Center. Am J Surg 2000, 24(1), 4–18.
92. Beckwith JB, Larson E. Case 7. Clear cell sarcoma of kidney. Pediatr Pathol 1989, 9(2), 211–18.
93. Haas JE, Bonadio JF, Beckwith JB. Clear cell sarcoma of the kidney with emphasis on ultrastructural studies. Cancer 1984, 54(12), 2978–87.
94. Kaneko Y, Homma C, Maseki N, Sakurai M, Hata J. Correlation of chromosome abnormalities with histological and clinical features in Wilms' and other childhood renal tumors. Cancer Res 1991, 51(21), 5937–42.
95. Punnett HH, Halligan GE, Zaeri N, Karmazin N. Translocation 10;17 in clear cell sarcoma of the kidney. A first report. Cancer Genet Cytogenet 1989, 41(1), 123–8.
96. Cheah PL, Looi LM. Implications of p53 protein expression in clear cell sarcoma of the kidney. Pathology 1996, 28(3), 229–31.
97. Charafe E, Penault-Llorca F, Mathoulin-Portier MP, Bladou F, Delpero JR, Prime-Guitton C et al. Clear cell sarcoma of the kidney relapsing after 10 years of asymptomatic evolution. Ann Pathol 1997, 17(6), 400–2.
98. Sandstedt BE, Delemarre JF, Harms D, Tournade MF. Sarcomatous Wilms' tumour with clear cells and hyalinization. A study of 38 tumours in children from the SIOP nephroblastoma file. Histopathology 1987, 11(3), 273–85.
99. Perlman EJ, Schuster AE, Argani P, et al. Genetic analysis of clear cell sarcoma of kidney (CCSK) by comparative genomic hybridization (CGH). [Abstract] Mod Pathol 1999, 12:(1)4P-.
100. Weeks DA, Beckwith JB, Mierau GW, Luckey DW. Rhabdoid tumor of kidney. A report of 111 cases from the National Wilms' Tumor Study Pathology Center. Am J Surg Pathol 1989, 13(6), 439–58.
101. Vujanic GM, Sandstedt B, Harms D, Boccon-Gibod L, Delemarre JF. Rhabdoid tumour of the kidney: a clinicopathological study of 22 patients from the International Society of Paediatric Oncology (SIOP) nephroblastoma file. Histopathology 1996, 28(4), 333–40.
102. Bonnin JM, Rubinstein LJ, Palmer NF, Beckwith JB. The association of embryonal tumors originating in the kidney and in the brain. A report of seven cases. Cancer 1984, 54(10), 2137–46.
103. Papadakis V, Vlachopapadopoulou EA, Levine L. Rhabdoid tumor of the kidney with humoral hypercalcemia and parathyroid hormone-related protein production. Med Pediatr Oncol 1995, 24(2), 133–6.
104. Weeks DA, Beckwith JB, Mierau GW, Zuppan CW. Renal neoplasms mimicking rhabdoid tumor of kidney. A report from the National Wilms' Tumor Study Pathology Center. Am J Surg Pathol 1991, 15(11), 1042–54.
105. Parham DM, Weeks DA, Beckwith JB. The clinicopathologic spectrum of putative extrarenal rhabdoid tumors. An analysis of 42 cases studied with immunohistochemistry or electron microscopy. Am J Surg Pathol 1994, 18(10), 1010–29.
106. Davis CJJ, Mostofi FK, Sesterhenn IA. Renal medullary carcinoma. The seventh sickle cell nephropathy. Am J Surg Pathol 1995, 19(1), 1–11.
107. Haas JE, Palmer NF, Weinberg AG, Beckwith JB. Ultrastructure of malignant rhabdoid tumor of the kidney. A distinctive renal tumor of children. Hum Pathol 1981, 12(7), 646–57.
108. Schofield DE, Beckwith JB, Sklar J. Loss of heterozygosity at chromosome regions 22q11–12 and 11p15.5 in renal rhabdoid tumors. Genes Chromosomes Cancer 1996, 15(1), 10–17.
109. Biegel JA, Rorke LB, Emanuel BS. Monosomy 22 in rhabdoid or atypical teratoid tumors of the brain [letter]. N Engl J Med 1989, 321(13), 906.
110. Perlman EJ, Ali SZ, Robinson R, Lindato R, Griffin CA. Infantile extrarenal rhabdoid tumor. Pediatr Dev Pathol 1998, 1(2), 149–52.

111. White FV, Dehner LP, Belchis DA, Conard K, Davis MM, Stocker JT et al. Congenital disseminated malignant rhabdoid tumor: a distinct clinicopathologic entity demonstrating abnormalities of chromosome 22q11. Am J Surg Pathol 1999, 23(3), 249–56.
112. Versteege I, Sevenet N, Lange J, Rousseau-Merck MF, Ambros P, Handgretinger R et al. Truncating mutations of hSNF5/INI1 in aggressive paediatric cancer. Nature 1998, 394(6689), 203–6.
113. Biegel JA, Zhou JY, Rorke LB, Stenstrom C, Wainwright LM, Fogelgren B. Germ-line and acquired mutations of INI1 in atypical teratoid and rhabdoid tumors. Cancer Res 1999, 59(1), 74–9.
114. Kodet R, Newton WAJ, Sachs N, Hamoudi AB, Raney RB, Asmar L et al. Rhabdoid tumors of soft tissues: a clinicopathologic study of 26 cases enrolled on the Intergroup Rhabdomyosarcoma Study. Hum Pathol 1991, 22(7), 674–84.
115. Wick MR, Ritter JH, Dehner LP. Malignant rhabdoid tumors: a clinicopathologic review and conceptual discussion. Semin Diagn Pathol 1995, 12(3), 233–48.
116. Burger PC, Yu IT, Tihan T, Friedman HS, Strother DR, Kepner JL et al. Atypical teratoid/rhabdoid tumor of the central nervous system: a highly malignant tumor of infancy and childhood frequently mistaken for medulloblastoma: a Pediatric Oncology Group study. Am J Surg Pathol 1998, 22(9), 1083–92.
117. Fort DW, Tonk VS, Tomlinson GE, Timmons CF, Schneider NR. Rhabdoid tumor of the kidney with primitive neuroectodermal tumor of the central nervous system: associated tumors with different histologic, cytogenetic, and molecular findings. Genes Chromosomes Cancer 1994, 11(3), 146–52.
118. Sabbioni S, Barbanti-Brodano G, Croce CM, Negrini M. GOK: a gene at 11p15 involved in rhabdomyosarcoma and rhabdoid tumor development. Cancer Res 1997, 57(20), 4493–7.
119. Leuschner I, Harms D, Schmidt D. Renal cell carcinoma in children: histology, immunohistochemistry, and follow-up of 10 cases. Med Pediatr Oncol 1991, 19(1), 33–41.
120. Dal Cin P, Stas M, Sciot R, De Wever I, Van Damme B, Van den Berghe H. Translocation (X;1) reveals metastasis 31 years after renal cell carcinoma. Cancer Genet Cytogenet 1998, 101(1), 58–61.
121. Meloni AM, Dobbs RM, Pontes JE, Sandberg AA. Translocation (X;1) in papillary renal cell carcinoma. A new cytogenetic subtype. Cancer Genet Cytogenet 1993, 65(1), 1–6.
122. Tonk V, Wilson KS, Timmons CF, Schneider NR, Tomlinson GE. Renal cell carcinoma with translocation (X;1). Further evidence for a cytogenetically defined subtype. Cancer Genet Cytogenet 1995, 81(1), 72–5.
123. Tomlinson GE, Nisen PD, Timmons CF, Schneider NR. Cytogenetics of a renal cell carcinoma in a 17-month-old child. Evidence for Xp11.2 as a recurring breakpoint. Cancer Genet Cytogenet 1991, 57(1), 11–17.
124. Weterman MA, Wilbrink M, Geurts vK. Fusion of the transcription factor TFE3 gene to a novel gene, PRCC, in t(X;1)(p11;q21)-positive papillary renal cell carcinomas. Proc Natl Acad Sci, USA 1996, 93(26), 15294–8.
125. Sidhar SK, Clark J, Gill S, Hamoudi R, Crew AJ, Gwilliam R et al. The t(X;1)(p11.2;q21.2) translocation in papillary renal cell carcinoma fuses a novel gene PRCC to the TFE3 transcription factor gene. Hum Mol Genet 1996, 5(9), 1333–8.
126. Rodriguez-Galindo C, Marina NM, Fletcher BD, Parham DM, Bodner SM, Meyer WH. Is primitive neuroectodermal tumor of the kidney a distinct entity? [see comments]. Cancer 1997, 79(11), 2243–50.
127. Marley EF, Liapis H, Humphrey PA, Nadler RB, Siegel CL, Zhu X et al. Primitive neuroectodermal tumor of the kidney—another enigma: a pathologic, immunohistochemical, and molecular diagnostic study. Am J Surg Pathol 1997, 21(3), 354–9.
128. Quezado M, Benjamin DR, Tsokos M. EWS/FLI-1 fusion transcripts in three peripheral primitive neuroectodermal tumors of the kidney. Hum Pathol 1997, 28(7), 767–71.
129. Arnold MM, Beckwith JB, Faria P, Weeks DA. Embryonal sarcoma of adult and pediatric kidneys [Abstract #409]. Mod Pathol 1995, 8(1), 72A-.
130. Delahunt B, Beckwith JB, Eble JN, Fraundorfer MR, Sutton TD, Trotter GE. Cystic embryonal sarcoma of kidney: a case report. Cancer 1998, 82(12), 2427–33.
131. Argani P, Zakowski MF, Klimstra DS, Rosai J, Ladanyi M. Detection of the SYT–SSX chimeric RNA of synovial sarcoma in paraffin-embedded tissue and its application in problematic cases. Mod Pathol 1998, 11(1), 65–71.
132. Argani P, Faria PA, Epstein JI et al. Primary renal synovial sarcoma. Molecular and morphologic delineation of an entity previously included among embryonal sarcomas of the kidney. Am J Surg Pathol 2000, 24(8), 1087–96.

13 | Bone tumors (excluding Ewing's sarcoma)

Walter C. Bell and Gene P. Siegal

Introduction

It would be impossible in a single chapter to provide in depth and meaningful coverage of the entire spectrum of bone neoplasia. As osteosarcoma accounts for the majority of primary malignant bone tumors of children, we have elected to limit our discussion to this entity.

Epidemiology

Osteosarcoma is the most common primary malignant tumor of bone (excluding hematopoietic malignancies such as myeloma) and is the most common malignant tumor of childhood. Approximately 1000 new cases are diagnosed per year in the United States with a slight male predominance. The peak incidence of osteosarcoma is in the second decade of life with a second smaller peak in individuals over the age of 50 (1). This second peak in older individuals may be largely attributed to secondary forms of osteosarcoma arising, for example, in Paget's disease or post irradiation, or to unusual subtypes such as osteosarcoma of the jaw, which occurs in older individuals (1, 2). The most common sites for the development of osteosarcoma are the metaphyseal regions of the long bones with the distal femur, proximal tibia, and proximal humerus, in that order, representing the three most common sites affected (3–5). Osteosarcoma is less common among African-American individuals as compared to Caucasians, but the incidence among Blacks appears to be increasing with a peak incidence at a slightly younger age that seen in Whites (6).

Diagnosis

Clinical symptoms

The most common presenting symptom of osteosarcoma is pain, often for several months with associated swelling (3). There may be limitation of motion in the adjacent joint. Laboratory studies are not generally helpful in diagnosis, although serum alkaline phosphatase may be elevated (7). Liu and colleagues have suggested that elevated bone-specific alkaline phosphatase may serve as a tumor marker for diagnosis and monitoring of osteosarcoma (8).

Radiologic findings

Radiologic evaluation is invaluable in the proper diagnosis and classification of osteosarcoma. Routine radiographs typically show a lesion with both lytic and blastic features. Commonly, destruction of the cortex is noted with extension through the periostium into the surrounding soft tissue (9, 10, Fig. 13.1). Beneath the

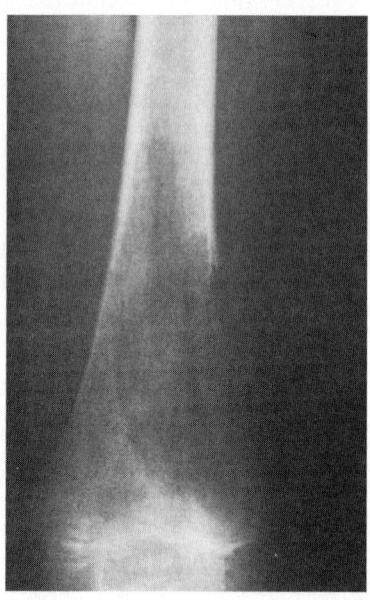

Fig. 13.1 Radiograph of a conventional osteosarcoma involving the distal femur. The intramedullary tumor extends through the cortex to form a soft tissue mass.

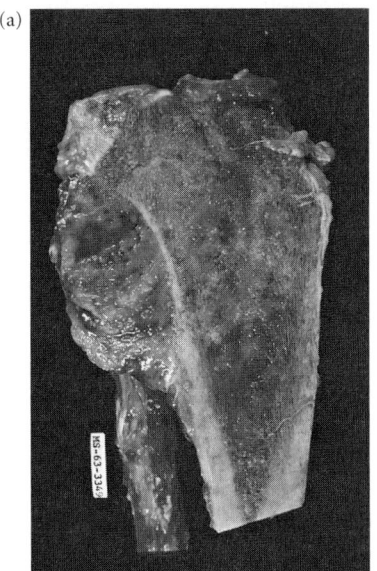 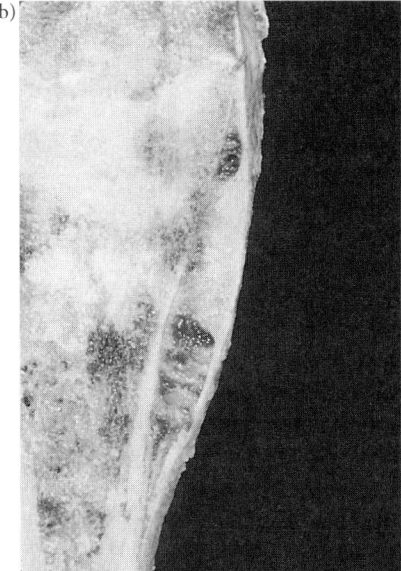

Fig. 13.2 (a) Gross photograph of a conventional osteosarcoma with extension of the intramedullary mass through the cortex to form a soft tissue mass. (b) Conventional osteosarcoma extending through the cortex and lifting the periosteum.

periostium reactive new bone formation may be seen resulting in a "Codman angle", and with extension into soft tissues a radial or "sunburst" pattern may be noted (11). Computed tomography (CT) and magnetic resonance imaging (MRI) evaluation are used primarily to determine extent of disease and involvement of surrounding tissues prior to surgical intervention (12–14).

Gross findings

The gross appearance of osteosarcoma is variable and dependent on subtype (15). Conventional osteosarcoma appears as an expansile lesion arising within the medulla at the metaphysis of a long bone (Fig. 13.2). The tumors extend into the surrounding soft tissue with destruction of the intervening cortex. The cut surface shows varying amounts of bone admixed with chondroid and fibrous appearing soft tissue. Necrosis may be extensive, particularly in resection specimens obtained following preoperative chemotherapy. Conventional osteosarcomas are by and large intramedullary lesions. A family of surface lesions has been defined and characterized and includes among subtypes, parosteal, periosteal, and high-grade surface tumors (Table 13.1).

Table 13.1 Osteosarcoma variants

Types	References
Conventional intramedullary osteosarcoma	
Osteoblastic	15 (see text)
Chondroblastic	15 (see text)
Fibroblastic	15 (see text)
MFH-like	16
Epithelioid	17, 18
Telangiectatic	15, 19–21
Surface osteosarcoma	
Parosteal (including de-differentiated variants)	15, 22, 23
Periosteal	15, 24, 25
High grade surface	15, 26

Histologic findings and classification

The histologic appearance of osteosarcoma is extremely variable with conventional osteosarcoma traditionally divided into osteoblastic, chondroblastic, and fibroblastic subtypes as well as a number of less common subtypes (MFH-like, epitheleoid, telangiectatic) based on the histologic appearance of the mesenchymal component of the tumor (Table 13.1). The unifying histologic feature

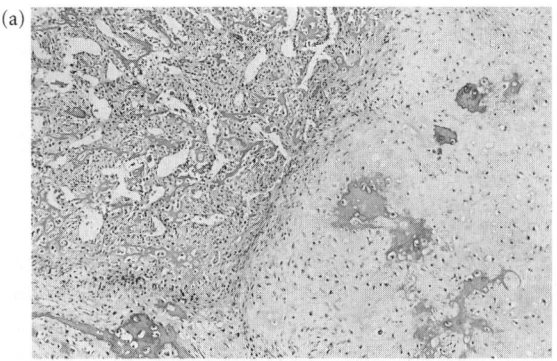 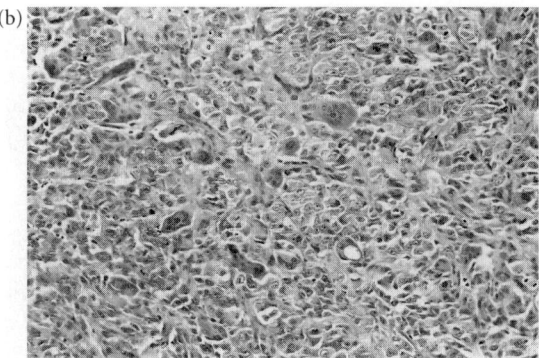

Fig. 13.3 (a) Conventional osteosarcoma with both osteoblastic (left) and chondroblastic (right) features. (b) Osteosarcoma with tumor osteoid and increased tumor giant cells.

among all types and subtypes is the production of tumor osteoid by the malignant cells (Fig. 13.3). Tumors have historically been assigned a histologic grade of I through IV based on the degree of nuclear anaplasia (27). The more recent trend is to classify tumors as either low or high grade. Immunohistochemical staining has historically been of little diagnostic value in osteosarcoma. Fanburg et al. suggest that cytoplasmic staining for osteocalcin may be helpful in distinguishing osteosarcoma from other entities and that staining of extracellular matrix for osteocalcin and osteonectin can aid in differentiating tumor osteoid from collagen (28).

patients with sensitive tumors have a greater than 90% 5-year event free survival. Those with tumors not found to be sensitive (less than 90% tumor necrosis) have a correspondingly poorer prognosis with a 5-year event free survival of approximately 14%.

Metastatic disease at the time of diagnosis is the other major prognostic factor with pulmonary metastasis via a hematogenous route common in this tumor. Among patients without metastatic disease, the overall 5-year disease-free survival is approximately 60% with current therapies. Overall 5-year survival for all patients treated prior to the mid-1980s was approximately 45% (1, 33–35).

Treatment and prognosis

Following biopsy and histologic confirmation of diagnosis, preoperative induction combination chemotherapy is today almost always initiated using a variety of agents including methotrexate, cisplatin, adriamycin, bleomycin, dactinomycin, etoposide, and other agents in various combinations with ifosfimide. Surgery remains the mainstay of treatment, and limb-sparing resections are often achieved followed by multidrug adjuvant chemotherapy (29, 30). Resection of pulmonary metastases has also been shown to be beneficial under certain conditions (31, 32).

Primary tumor resection specimens are examined following induction chemotherapy to determine the extent of tumor necrosis, an indicator of sensitivity of the tumor to chemotherapy and a major prognostic indicator. Tumor necrosis of greater than 90–95% (dependent upon which grading system is selected) indicates sensitivity to the induction chemotherapy, and

Cytogenetic and molecular findings

Introduction

Cytogenetic and molecular studies have, to date, been found to be of limited value in *diagnosing* osteosarcoma. Our understanding of molecular events in osteosarcoma tumorigenesis is in its infancy and is hampered by the rarity of the tumors, difficulty in obtaining tissues suitable for molecular studies following preoperative chemotherapy, and the necessity for decalcification of specimens for tissue processing. However, such investigation is leading to new insights into tumor etiology and may yield important information affecting prognosis and therapy.

DNA analysis and cytogenetics

DNA content analysis of osteosarcomas by flow cytometry has shown a tendency toward aneuploidy, particularly among high-grade tumors (36–39). Bauer *et al.* reported 92 of 96 high-grade osteosarcomas studied were hyperploid while 4 low-grade parosteal osteosarcomas were found to be diploid (39). In general, high-grade bone tumors have proven to be aneuploid, whereas benign and low-grade tumors are diploid (37). The presence of near-diploid stem lines in hyperploid tumors has been associated with an improved prognosis with decreased incidence of pulmonary metastasis and improved relapse-free survival following treatment, suggesting that DNA content analysis may be helpful in predicting response to chemotherapy (40). Not surprisingly, DNA analysis following preoperative chemotherapy has shown a higher frequency of aneuploidy among tumors with poor response (41).

In a recent cytogenetic evaluation of osteosarcoma cases, Bridge *et al.* examined 73 new cases and reviewed 111 cases from the literature (42). They report a variety of complex karyotypic alterations with clonal chromosomal abnormalities identified in 47 of the 73 new cases with tumors ranging from haploid to near hexaploid and two tumors exhibiting multiple clones of differing ploidy. The most frequent chromosomal band rearrangements were at 1p11-13, 1q10-10, 1q21-22, 11p15, 12p13, 17p12-13, 19q13, and 22q11-13. Whole chromosome losses were more frequent than gains with the most frequent numerical abnormalities including +1, −9, −10, −13, and −17.

Partial deletion of the long arm of chromosome 13 was common, and all cases showed a partial loss of the long arm of chromosome 6 suggesting the possibility of a tumor suppressor gene at this site. Parosteal osteosarcomas were shown to be characterized by the presence of ring chromosomes, often as the only abnormality. Other groups (43–45) have previously reported similar complex karyotypes among high-grade tumors and demonstrated this association of parosteal osteosarcoma and ring chromosome formation.

Examination of 11 cases of osteosarcoma by Tarkkanen *et al.* by comparative genomic hybridization showed similar complex changes with extensive genetic aberrations in 10 of the cases (46). High-level amplification regions including 12q12-13, 17p11-12, 3q26 and Xq12 were identified with the most common DNA gains at 8q and Xp. DNA sequence losses were most common at 2q, 6q, 8p, and 10p. One study suggests that patients with copy number increases at 8q or 8cen have a poorer prognosis with shorter overall survival (47). A translocation of chromosomes 11 and 22, the same translocation associated with Ewing's sarcoma, has been reported in small cell osteosarcoma (48). This has led us, and others, to note similarity in immunophenotypes and ultrastructural features between these entities.

Tumor Suppressor Genes

An association between retinoblastoma (RB) and osteosarcoma has long been recognized. Children with hereditary RB are at increased risk of developing osteosarcoma and exhibit up to 1000 times the incidence of osteosarcoma as the general population (49, 50). A number of studies have demonstrated a loss of heterozygosity (LOH) of chromosome 13 in osteosarcomas at the locus of the RB gene (51–54). Belchis *et al.* showed LOH at this locus in 78% (14/18) of cases examined (54). LOH at the RB gene has been suggested as a poor prognostic indicator (55).

The RB gene functions as a tumor suppressor gene and is located on the q14 band of human chromosome 13 (56). The gene product participates in a cell-cycle regulatory pathway that functions to inhibit entry of cells into the S phase possibly by inverse transcriptional regulation of the c-myc and c-fos oncogenes (57, 58). The RB gene product is active in a hypophosphorylated state with virtually all of the protein in an unphosphorylated state in G0/G1 cells (57). Analysis of osteosarcomas by Western-blot techniques shows no RB gene product or a grossly truncated product in approximately 10% of osteosarcoma cases, while DNA sequencing methods show functionally significant alteration of the gene in 60–70% of tumors examined (59–61). As in RB, oncogenesis in osteosarcoma appears to follow Knudson's two-hit hypothesis with loss of function of both RB alleles (51, 62). Penetrance of familial RB is approximately 90–95% while the risk of patients with bilateral RB developing osteosarcoma is only 12% suggesting that additional genetic events are involved in the development of osteosarcoma (61). Other proteins in the cell-cycle regulatory pathway in which the RB protein functions include p16 protein, a cyclin dependent kinase inhibitor, and cyclin dependent kinase 4. Loss of p16 expression has been reported in some osteosarcomas lacking RB mutations, which may allow phosphorylation and, thus, inactivation of the RB protein (58). The p19 protein, a cyclin dependent kinase inhibitor with similar structure and function to p16, has also been shown to be altered in a small percentage of osteosarcomas (63). Similarly, increased expression of CDK4 has been shown in a small percentage of osteosarcomas. This could also theoretically lead to inactivation of the RB protein through increased phosphorylation (64–66, Fig. 13.4).

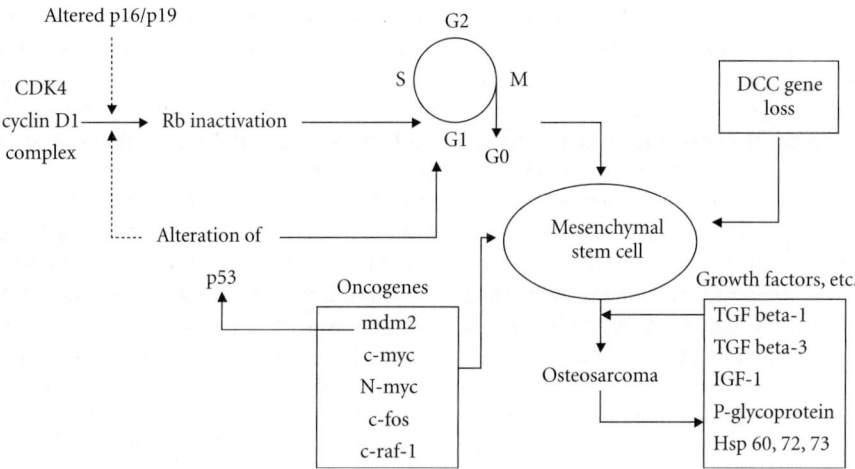

Fig. 13.4 Molecular and biochemical alterations associated with osteosarcoma (see text for specific references).

Scheffer et al. reported complete association between LOH of chromosomes 13 and 17, suggesting that another tumor suppressor gene located on chromosome 17 might be involved in the oncogenesis of osteosarcomas (53). The p53 gene is located on chromosome 17 at position 13.1 and, thus, represents a second tumor suppressor gene implicated in the development of osteosarcomas (67–69). The p53 gene product acts to induce transcription of genes that control cell-cycle arrest and apoptosis (69). Alterations of the p53 gene have been shown in as many as 50% of osteosarcomas with up to 86% of alterations being missence mutations (67, 70). Germline mutations of p53 have been identified in patients with the Li–Fraumeni syndrome who have a high risk of bone sarcomas, and similar new germline mutations are identified in many patients with sporadic osteosarcoma (71, 72). A cyclin-dependent kinase inhibitor, p21, is transcriptionally regulated by p53 and may provide a link between p53 and regulation of phosphorylation of the RB gene product (73–75). A recent study by Goto et al. has shown that osteosarcomas with LOH at the p53 locus are less likely than tumors without this alteration to be sensitive to preoperative chemotherapy, suggesting that identification of p53 gene deletions or alterations may be useful in predicting chemoresistance (76).

Yamaguchi et al. found frequencies of allele loss in osteosarcoma of greater than 60% at 3q (75%), 13q (68%), 17p (72%), and 18q (64%), suggesting that in addition to the RB and p53 genes, two other tumor suppressor genes located at 3q and 18q may be involved in the development of osteosarcoma (77). Kruzelock et al. used polymorphic markers to localize a possible tumor suppressor gene to the region between 3q26.2 and 3q26.3 (78). Horstmann and his colleagues report absent or substantially decreased expression of the deleted in colon cancer (DCC) gene, which has been mapped to 18q21.1, in 14 of 19 high-grade osteosarcomas and 3 of 6 lower grade osteosarcomas (79).

Oncogenes

Altered expression of several oncogenes has been described in osteosarcomas. Amplification of the murine double minute two (MDM2) gene has been reported in as many as 25% of osteosarcomas examined (80). Transcription of the MDM2 gene is regulated by p53 and the MDM2 protein binds p53 forming a stable complex. Increased MDM2 protein production has been suggested as an alternate mechanism for the inactivation of p53 function (81). Ladanyi et al. report that amplification of MDM2 is more frequent in metastatic or recurrent tumors and suggest that amplification may be associated with tumor progression (82).

Expression of erbB-2 has been reported in a subset of osteosarcomas. In cases which express erbB-2 by immunoblot and immunohistochemical analysis, a correlation between expression and early pulmonary metastasis has been demonstrated suggesting erbB-2 expression plays a role in promoting metastatic potential and could potentially serve as a useful prognostic marker (83).

Pompetti et al. examined osteosarcoma samples for expression of c-myc, N-myc, c-fos, H-ras, Ki-ras, and N-ras and identified alterations of c-myc, N-myc, and c-fos (84). These alterations occurred singly and in various combinations both with and without alterations of p53 and Rb. Other studies have also shown amplification of c-myc and c-fos in osteosarcoma with c-fos amplification identified in up to 61% of cases in one study (85–87). Amplification of c-raf-1 has also been reported in one case in which amplification of c-myc was also observed (85).

The sarcoma amplified sequence (SAS) gene is located in the 12q13-15 region along with the MDM2 gene and the gene encoding CDK4. Amplification of this gene has been reported in a number of sarcomas. Noble-Topham et al. reported amplification of the SAS gene in 36% of osteosarcomas and 100% of surface osteosarcomas (7/7) examined suggesting a divergent molecular pathway for tumorigenesis in the surface tumors (88). Others have found increased expression of MDM2 and CDK4 genes and amplification of SAS in central low-grade osteosarcomas (89). That three genes in the 12q13-15 region have been noted to be amplified in some osteosarcomas raises the possibility of a coamplification phenomenon involving this region.

Growth factors and chemoresistance associated genes

Studies have shown a number of growth factors to be elevated in osteosarcoma. Franchi et al. demonstrated high levels of TGF beta-1 in high-grade osteosarcomas and low or absent mRNA in low-grade tumors, suggesting a role for TGF beta-1 in tumor progression (90). A separate study has correlated expression of TGF beta-3 with disease progression (91). Expression of insulin-like growth factor 1 (IGF-1) and its receptor (IGF-R) has been reported in osteosarcomas with no difference in expression between primary and metastatic tumors (92). Additionally, p53 appears to exert negative transcriptional regulation of IGF-1, with increased levels of IGF-1 in selected cell lines with altered p53 (93).

Resistance to high dose methotrexate appears to be related to impaired methotrexate transport by the reduced folate carrier and increased expression of dihydrofolate reductase (94). Chan et al. examined 62 cases of osteosarcoma for expression of P-glycoprotein, which has been shown in other systems to confer resistance to multi-drug chemotherapy (95). They found over-expression in 27 of the cases and those patients with over-expression had a significantly higher recurrence rate than those without increased expression. Baldini et al. similarly demonstrated that increased P-glycoprotein expression at the time of diagnosis is associated with a higher rate of relapse, and that such patients may benefit from additional chemotherapeutic modalities (96). Doxorubicin binding activity appears to be a more sensitive predictor of chemosensitivity than P-glycoprotein status (97).

Trieb et al. examined biopsies of high-grade osteosarcomas from 45 patients by immunohistochemistry on paraffin embedded tissue to evaluate for expression of heat shock proteins (hsp) 60, 72, and 73 which have been shown to play a role in tumor chemoresistance (98). Hsp 72 was over-expressed in 38% of osteosarcomas as compared to 2.9% of benign bone tumors. Those tumors with hsp 72 expression had a better response to induction chemotherapy than osteosarcomas that did not express hsp 72.

Conclusions

The body of knowledge concerning molecular findings in osteosarcoma has grown significantly in the past decade. The association of alterations of p53 and RB are now well established and other tumor suppressor genes and oncogenes apparently involved in carcinogenesis are being identified (Fig. 13.4). As the interrelationships between these alterations are elucidated, our understanding of the biology of osteosarcoma grows, with the promise of leading to more accurate prediction of prognosis. Of particular importance to current practice patterns are those markers that can be determined by immunohistochemical methods on fixed tissues from small initial biopsy specimens. In the future, the expectation is that this greater understanding will lead to an enhanced understanding of tumorigenesis and to new treatment modalities focusing on the molecular basis of disease. Until that day, a full understanding of the histologic subtleties associated with reaching the correct diagnosis, when blended with complete radiologic evaluation and clinical acumen, remains the best course of action to assure the best outcome for patients afflicted with this most serious of malignant diseases (99).

References

1. Dorfman HD, Czerniak B. Bone cancers. Cancer 1995, 75, 203–10.
2. Clark JL, Unni KK, Dahlin DC, Devine KD. Osteosarcoma of the jaw. Cancer 1983, 51, 2311–16.

3. Dahlin DC, Coventry MB. Osteogenic sarcoma. A study of 600 cases. J Bone Joint Surg 1967, **49**, 101–10.
4. Marcove RC, Mike V, Hajek JV, Levin AG, Hutter RV. Osteogenic sarcoma under the age of twenty-one: a review of one hundred and forty-five operative cases. J Bone Joint Surg Am 1970, **52**, 411–23.
5. Taylor WF, Ivins JC, Dahlin DC, Edmonson JH, Pritchard DJ. Trends and variability in survival from osteosarcoma. Mayo Clin Proc 1978, **53**, 695–700.
6. Huvos AG, Butler A, Bretsky SS. Osteogenic sarcoma in the American black. Cancer 1983, **52**, 1959–65.
7. Parham DM, Pratt CB, Parvey LS, Webber BI, Champion J. Childhood multifocal osteosarcoma: clinicopathologic and radiologic correlates. Cancer 1985, **55**, 2653–8.
8. Liu PP, Leung KS, Kumta SM, Lee KM, Fung KP. Bone-specific alkaline phosphatase in plasma as tumour marker for osteosarcoma. Oncology 1996, **53**, 275–80.
9. Lindbom Å, Söderberg G, Spjut HJ. Osteosarcoma: a review of 96 cases. Acta Radiol 1961, **56**, 1–19.
10. Kumar R, David R, Madewell JE, Lindell MM. Radiographic spectrum of osteogenic sarcoma. Am J Roentgenol 1987, **148**, 767–72.
11. Ragsdale BD, Madewell JE, Sweet DE. Radiologic and pathologic analysis of solitary bone lesions. Part II: periosteal reactions. Radiol Clin North Am 1981, **19**, 749–83.
12. De Santos LA, Beernardino ME, Murray JA. Computed tomography in the evaluation of osteosarcoma: experience with 25 cases. Am J Roentgenol 1979, **132**, 535–40.
13. Seeger LL, Eckardt JJ, Bassett LW. Cross-sectional imaging in the evaluation of osteosarcoma: MRI and CT. Semin Roentgenol 1989, **24**, 174–84.
14. Gillespy T, Manfrini M, Rugieri P, Spanier SS, Petterson H, Springfield DS. Staging of intraosseous extent of osteosarcoma: correlation of preoperative CT and MR imaging with pathologic macroslides. Radiology 1988, **167**, 765–7.
15. Dahlin DC, Unni KK. Osteosarcoma of bone and its important recognizable varieties. Am J Surg Pathol 1977, **1**, 61–72.
16. Huvos AG, Heilweil M, Bretsky SS, The pathology of malignant fibrous histiocytoma of bone. A study of 130 patients. Am J Surg Pathol 1985, **9**, 853–71.
17. Hasegawa T, Shibata T, Hirose T, Seki K, Hizawa K. Osteosarcoma with epithelioid features. An immunohistochemical study. Arch Pathol Lab Med 1993, **117**, 295–8.
18. Kramer K, Hicks DG, Palis J, Rosier RN, Oppenheimer J, Fallon MD, Cohen HJ. Epithelioid osteosarcoma of bone. Immunocytochemical evidence suggesting divergent epithelial and mesenchymal differentiation in a primary osseous neoplasm. Cancer 1993, **71**, 2977–82.
19. Farr GH, Huvos AG, Marcove RC, Higinbotham NL, Foote FW, Jr. Telangiectatic osteogenic sarcoma. A review of twenty-eight cases. Cancer 1974, **34**, 1150–8.
20. Huvos AG, Rosen G, Bretsky SS, Butler A. Telangiectatic osteogenic sarcoma: a clinicopathologic study of 124 patients. Cancer 1982, **49**, 1679–89.
21. Mervak TR, Unni KK, Pritchard DJ, McLeod RA. Telangiectatic osteosarcoma. Clin Orthop 1991, **270**, 135–9.
22. Unni KK, Dahlin DC, Beabout JW, Ivins JC. Parosteal osteogenic sarcoma. Cancer 1976, **37**, 2644–75.
23. Okada K, Frassica FJ, Sim FH, Beabout JW, Bond JR, Unni KK. Parosteal osteosarcoma. A clinicopathological study. J Bone Joint Surg Am 1994, **76**, 366–78.
24. Hall RB, Robinson LH, Malawar MM, Dunham WK. Periosteal osteosarcoma. Cancer 1985, **55**, 165–71.
25. Ritts GD, Pritchard DJ, Unni KK, Beabout JW, Eckardt JJ. Periosteal osteosarcoma. Clin Orthop 1987, **219**, 299–307.
26. Wold LE, Unni KK, Beabout JW, Pritchard DJ. High-grade surface osteosarcomas. Am J Surg Pathol 1984, **8**, 181–6.
27. Meister P, Konrad E, Lob G, Janka G, Keyl W, Sturz H. Osteosarcoma: histological evaluation and grading. Arch Orthop Trauma Surg 1979, **94**, 91–8.
28. Fanburg JC, Rosenberg AE, Weaver DL, Leslie KO, Mann KG, Taatjes DJ, et al. Osteocalcin and osteonectin immunoreactivity in the diagnosis of osteosarcoma. Am J Clin Pathol 1997, **108**, 464–73.
29. Glasser DB, Lane JM, Huvos AG, Marcove RC, Rosen G. Survival, prognosis and therapeutic response in osteogenic sarcoma: the Memorial Hospital experience. Cancer 1992, **69**, 698–708.
30. Marcove RC, Sheth DS, Healey J, Huvos A, Rosen G, Meyers P, et al. Limb-sparing surgery for extremity sarcoma. Cancer Invest 1994, **12**, 479–504.
31. Sweetnam R, Ross K. Surgical treatment of pulmonary metastases from primary tumors of bone. J Bone Joint Surg 1967, **49**, 74–9.
32. Belli L, Scholl S, Lwarlowski A. Resection of pulmonary metastases in osteosarcoma. A retrospective analysis of 44 patients. Cancer 1989, **63**, 2546–50.
33. Picci P, Bacci G, Campanacci M, Gasparini M, Pilotti S, Cerasoli S, et al. Histologic evaluation of necrosis in osteosarcoma induced by chemotherapy: regional mapping of viable and nonviable tumor. Cancer 1985, **56**, 1515–21.
34. Rosen G, Capairos B, Huvos AG, Kosloff C, Nirenberg A, Cacavio A, et al. Preoperative chemotherapy for osteogenic sarcoma: selection of postoperative adjuvant chemotherapy based on the response of the primary tumor to preoperative chemotherapy. Cancer 1982, **49**, 1221–30.
35. Raymond AK, Chaula SP, Currasco H, Ayala AG, Fanning CV, Grice B, et al. Osteosarcoma chemotherapy effect: a prognostic factor. Semin Diagn Pathol 1987, **4**, 212–36.
36. Kreicbergs A, Broström L-Å, Cewrien G, Einhorn S. Cellular DNA content in human osteosarcoma. Cancer 1982, **50**, 2476–81.
37. Kreicbergs A, Silverswärd C, Tribukait B. Flow DNA analysis of primary bone tumors. Cancer 1984, **53**, 129–36.
38. Hiddemann W, Roessner A, Wörmann B, Mellin W, Klockenkemper B, Bösing T, et al. Tumor heterogeneity in osteosarcoma. Cancer 1987, **59**, 324–8.
39. Bauer HCF, Kreicbergs A, Silverswärd C, Tribukait B. DNA analysis in the differential diagnosis of osteosarcoma. Cancer 1988, **61**, 2532–40.
40. Look AT, Douglass EC, Meyer WH. Clinical importance of near-diploid tumor stem lines in patients with osteosarcoma of an extremity. N Engl J Med 1988, **318**, 1567–72.
41. Bösing T, Roessner A, Hiddemann W, Mellin W, Grundmann E. Cytostatic effects in osteosarcomas as detected by flow cytometric DNA analysis after preoperative chemotherapy according to the COSS 80/82 protocol. J Cancer Res Clin Oncol 1987, **113**, 369–75.

42. Bridge JA, Nelson M, McComb E, McGuire MH, Rosenthal H, Vergara G, et al. Cytogenetic findings in 73 osteosarcoma specimens and a review of the literature. Cancer Genet Cytogenet 1997, **95**, 74–87.
43. Sinovic JF, Bridge JA, Neff JR. Ring chromosome in parosteal osteosarcoma: clinical and diagnostic significance. Cancer Genet Cytogenet 1992, **62**, 50–2.
44. Mertens F, Mandahl N, Örndal C, Baldetorp B, Bauer HCF, Rydholm A, et al. Cytogenetic findings in 33 osteosarcomas. Int J Cancer 1993, **55**, 44–50.
45. Fletcher JA, Gebhardt MC, Kozadewich HP. Cytogenetic aberrations in osteosarcomas: nonrandom deletions, rings, and double-minute chromosomes. Cancer Genet Cytogenet 1994, **77**, 81–8.
46. Tarkkanen M, Karhu R, Kallioniemi A, Elomaa I, Kivioja AH, Nevalainen J, et al. Gains and losses of DNA sequences in osteosarcomas by comparative genomic hybridization. Cancer Res 1995, **55**, 1334–8.
47. Tarkkanen M, Elomaa I, Blomqvist C, Kivioja A, Kellokumpu-Lehtinen P, et al. DNA sequence copy number increase at 8q: a potential new prognostic marker in high-grade osteosarcomas. Int J Cancer 1999, **84**, 114–21.
48. Noguera R, Navarro S, Triche TJ. Translocation (11;22) in small cell osteosarcoma. Cancer Genet Cytogenet 1990, **45**, 121–4.
49. Kitchin FD, Ellsworth RM. Pleiotropic effects of the gene for retinoblastoma. J Med Genet 1974, **11**(3), 244–6.
50. Abramson DH, Ellsworth RM, Kitchin FD, Tung G. Second nonocular tumors in retinoblastoma survivors. Are they radiation-induced? Ophthalmology 1984, **91**(11), 1351–5.
51. Hansen MF, Koufos A, Gallie BL, Phillips RA, Fodstad O, Brogger A, et al. Osteosarcoma and retinoblastoma: a shared chromosomal mechanism revealing recessive predisposition. Proc Natl Acad Sci, USA 1985, **82**, 6216–20.
52. Dryja TP, Rapaport JM, Epstein J, Goorin AM, Weichselbaum R, Koufos A, et al. Chromosome 13 homozygosity in osteosarcoma without retinoblastoma. Am J Hum Genet 1986, **38**, 59–66.
53. Scheffer H, Kruize YCM, Osinga J, Kuiken G, Oosterhuis JW, Leeuw JA, et al. Complete association of loss of heterozygosity of chromosomes 13 and 17 in osteosarcoma. Cancer Genet Cytogenet 1991, **53**, 45–55.
54. Belchis DA, Meece CA, Benko FA, Rogan PK, Williams RA, Gocke CD. Loss of heterozygosity and microsatellite instability at the retinoblastoma locus in osteosarcomas. Diagn Mol Pathol 1996, **5**, 214–19.
55. Feugeas O, Guriec M, Babin-Boilletot A, Marcellin L, Simon P, Babin S, et al. Loss of heterozygosity of the RB gene is a poor prognostic factor in patients with osteosarcoma. J Clin Oncol 1996, **14**, 467–72.
56. Friend SH, Bernards R, Rogelj S, Weinberg RA, Rapaport JM. A human DNA segment with properties of the gene that predisposes to retinoblastoma and osteosarcoma. Nature 1986, **323**, 643–6.
57. DeCaprio JA, Ludlow JW, Lynch D, Furukawa Y, Griffin J, Piwnica-Worms H, et al. The product of the retinoblastoma susceptibility gene has properties of a cell cycle regulatory element. Cell 1989, **58**, 1085–95.
58. Nielsen GP, Burns KL, Rosenberg AE, Louis DN. CDKN2A gene deletions and loss of p16 expression occur in osteosarcomas that lack RB alterations. Am J Pathol 1998, **153**, 159–63.

59. Benedict WF, Fung YT, Murphree AL. The gene responsible for the development of retinoblastoma and osteosarcoma. Cancer 1988, **62**, 1691–4.
60. Womer RB. The cellular biology of bone tumors. Clin Orthop 1991, **262**, 12–21.
61. Hansen MF. Molecular genetic considerations in osteosarcoma. Clin Orthop 1991, **270**, 237–46.
62. Knudson AG, Jr. Mutation and cancer: statistical study of retinoblastoma. Proc Natl Acad Sci, USA 1971, **68**, 820–3.
63. Miller CW, Yeon C, Aslo A, Mendoza S, Aytac U, Koeffler HP. The p19^{INK4D} cyclin dependent kinase inhibitor gene is altered in osteosarcoma. Oncogene 1997, **15**, 231–5.
64. Maelandsmo GM, Berner JM, Florenes VA, Forus A, Hovig E, Fodstad O, et al. Homozygous deletion frequency and expression levels of the CDKN2 gene in human sarcomas—relationship to amplification and mRNA levels of CDK4 and CCND1. Br J Cancer 1995, **72**, 393–8.
65. Guo W, Lonardo F, Ueda T, Kim T, Huvos A, et al. CDK4 gene amplification in osteosarcomas: reciprocal relationship with INK4A gene alterations and mapping of 12q13 amplicons. Int J Cancer 1999, **80**, 199–204.
66. Benassi M, Molendini L, Gamberi G, Ragazzini P, Sollazzo M, et al. Alteration of pRb/p16/cdk4 regulation in human osteosarcomas. Int J Cancer 1999, **84**, 489–93.
67. Masuda H, Miller C, Koeffler HP, Battifora H, Cline MJ. Rearrangement of the p53 gene in human osteogenic sarcomas. Proc Natl Acad Sci, USA 1987, **84**, 7716–19.
68. Toguchida J, Yamaguchi T, Ritchie B, Beauchamp RL, Dayton SH. Mutation spectrum of the p53 gene in bone and soft tissue sarcomas. Cancer Res 1992, **52**, 6194–9.
69. Hung J, Anderson R. p53: functions, mutations, and sarcomas. Acta Orthop Scand 1997, Supplement **273**, 68–71.
70. Diller L, Kassel J, Nelson CE, Gryka MA, Litwak G, Gebhardt M, et al. p53 functions as a cell cycle control protein in osteosarcomas. Mol Cell Biol 1990, **10**, 5772–81.
71. Li FP, Fraumeni JF, Jr, Mulvihill JJ, Blattner WA, Dreyfus MG, Tucker MA, et al. A cancer family syndrome in twenty-four kindreds. Cancer Res 1988, **48**, 5358–62.
72. Toguchida J, Yamaguchi T, Dayton SH, Beauchamp RL, Herrera GE, Ishizaki K, et al. Prevalence and spectrum of germline mutations of the p53 gene among patients with sarcoma. N Engl J Med 1992, **326**, 1301–8.
73. El-Deiry WS, Tokino T, Velculescu VE, Levy DB, Parsons R, Trent JM, et al. WAF1, a potential mediator of p53 tumor suppression. Cell 1993, **75**, 817–25.
74. Elledge SJ, Harper JW. Cdk inhibitors: on the threshold of checkpoints and development. Curr Opin Cell Biol 1994, **6**, 847–52.
75. Picksley SM, Lane DP. p53 and Rb: their cellular roles. Curr Opin Cell Biol 1994, **6**, 853–8.
76. Goto A, Kanda H, Ishidawa Y, Matsumoto S, Kawaguchi N, Machinami R, et al. Association of loss of heterozygosity at the p53 locus with chemoresistance in osteosarcomas. Jpn J Cancer Res 1998, **89**, 539–47.
77. Yamaguchi T, Toguchida J, Yamamuro T, Kotoura Y, Takada N, Kawaguchi N, et al. Allelotype analysis in osteosarcomas: frequent allele loss on 3q, 13q, 17p, and 18q. Cancer Res 1992, **52**, 2419–23.
78. Kruzelock RP, Murphy EC, Strong LC, Naylor SL, Hansen MF. Localization of a novel tumor suppressor locus on

human chromosome 3q important in osteosarcoma tumorigenesis. Cancer Res 1997, 57, 106–9.
79. Horstmann MA, Pösl M, Scholz RB, Anderegg B, Simon P, Baumgaertl K, *et al*. Frequent reduction or loss of DCC gene expression in human osteosarcoma. Br J Cancer 1997, 75, 1309–17.
80. Miller CW, Aslo A, Won A, Tan M, Lampkin B, Koeffler HP. Alterations of the p53, Rb, and MDM2 genes in osteosarcoma. J Cancer Res Clin Oncol 1996, 122, 559–65.
81. Momand J, Zambetti GP, Olson DC, George D, Levine AJ. The mdm-2 oncogene product forms a complex with the p53 protein and inhibits p53-mediated transactivation. Cell 1992, 69, 1237–45.
82. Ladanyi M, Cha C, Lewis R, Jhanwar SC, Huvos AG, Healey JH. MDM2 gene amplification in metastatic osteosarcoma. Cancer Res 1993, 53, 16–18.
83. Onda M, Matsuda S, Higaki S, Iijima T, Fukushima J, Yokokura A, *et al*. ErbB-2 expression is correlated with poor prognosis for patients with osteosarcoma. Cancer 1996, 77, 71–8.
84. Pompetti F, Rizzo P, Simon RM, Freidlin B, Mew DJ, Pass HI, *et al*. Oncogene alterations in primary, recurrent, and metastatic human bone tumors. J Cell Biochem 1996, 63, 37–50.
85. Ikeda S, Sumii H, Akiyama K, Watanabe S, Ito S, Inoue H, *et al*. Amplification of both c-myc and c-raf-1 oncogenes in a human osteosarcoma. Jpn J Cancer Res 1989, 80, 6–9.
86. Wu JX, Carpenter PM, Gresens C, Keh R, Niman H, Morris JW, *et al*. The proto-oncogene c-fos is overexpressed in the majority of human osteosarcomas. Oncogene 1990, 5, 989–1000.
87. Ladanyi M, Park CK, Lewis R, Jhanwar SC, Healey JH, Huvos AG. Sporadic amplification of the MYC gene in human osteosarcomas. Diagn Mol Pathol 1993, 2, 163–7.
88. Noble-Topham SE, Burrow SR, Eppert K, Dandel RA, Meltzer PS, Bell RS, *et al*. SAS is amplified predominantly in surface osteosarcoma. J Orthop Res 1996, 14, 700–5.
89. Ragazzini P, Gamberi G, Benassi M, Orlando C, Sestini R, *et al*. Analysis of SAS gene and CDK4 and MDM2 proteins in low-grade osteosarcomas. Cancer Det Prev 1999, 23, 129–36.
90. Franchi A, Arganini L, Baroni G, Calzolari A, Capanna R, Campanacci D, *et al*. Expression of transforming growth factor beta isoforms in osteosarcoma variants: association of TGF beta 1 with high-grade osteosarcomas. J Pathol 1998, 185, 284–9.
91. Kloen P, Gebhardt MC, Perez-Atayde A, Rosenberg AE, Springfield DS, Gold LI, *et al*. Expression of transforming growth factor-beta (TGF-beta) isoforms in osteosarcomas: TGF-beta3 is related to disease progression. Cancer 1997, 80, 2230–9.
92. Burrow S, Andrulis IL, Possak M, Bell RS. Expression of insulin-like growth factor receptor, IGF-1, and IGF-2 in primary and metastatic osteosarcomas. J Surg Oncol 1998, 69, 21–7.
93. Ohlsson C, Kley N, Werner H, LeRoith D. p53 regulates insulin-like growth factor-I (IGF-I) receptor expression and IGF-I-induced tyrosine phosphorylation in an osteosarcoma cell line: interaction between p53 and Sp1. Endocrinology 1998, 139, 1101–7.
94. Guo W, Healey J, Meyers P, Laadanyi M, Huvos A, *et al*. Mechanisms of methotrexate resistance in osteosarcomas. Clin Cancer Res 1999, 5, 621–7.
95. Chan HS, Grogan TM, Haddad G, DeBoer G, Ling V. P-glycoprotein expression: critical determinant in the response to chemotherapy. J Natl Cancer Inst 1997, 89, 1706–15.
96. Baldini N, Scotlandi K, Serra M, Picci P, Bacci G, *et al*. P-glycoprotein expressin in osteosarcomas: a basis for risk-adapted adjuvant chemotherapy. J Ortho Res 1999, 17, 629–32.
97. Kusuzaki K, Hirata M, Takeshita H, Murata H, Hashiguchi S, *et al*. Relationship between P-glycoprotein positivity, Doxorubicin binding ability and histologic response to chemotherapy in osteosarcomas. Cancer Lett 1999, 138, 203–8.
98. Trieb K, Lechleitner T, Lang S, Windhager R, Kotz R, Dirnhofer S. Heat shock protein 72 expression in osteosarcomas correlates with good response to neoadjuvant chemotherapy. Hum Pathol 1998, 29, 1050–5.
99. Siegal GP. Primary tumors of bone. In: Stocker T, Askin FB (ed.) Pathology of solid tumors in children. Chapman and Hall, London, 1998, 183–212.

14 Germ cell tumours

Elizabeth S. Gray

Introduction

Germ cell tumours (GCT) are a heterogeneous group of tumours presenting in all age groups including neonates; occurring in a wide range of sites; behaving as entirely benign through to highly malignant; having a variable and intriguing histology; and probably developing from at least two pathogenetic pathways and cell lines. What unites them as an entity is their typical and shared range of histological features and, when present, their shared serological markers. They are also very responsive to the platinum-based group of chemotherapeutic agents. However there is increasing evidence that GCT in infancy and childhood are different in their clinical behaviour, cell of origin, and cytogenetic profile from similar tumours in adolescents and adults.

Epidemiology

Incidence

In the UK National Registry of Childhood Cancer malignant germ cell tumours (MGCTs) account for only 3% of all malignancies in children aged 0–15 years (1). The annual incidence is 2.4/million with gonadal MGCT having an incidence of 1.5/million and non-gonadal MGCT an incidence of 0.9/million. In the United States, the incidence is similar at 2–3/million children/year (2).

The incidence of all GCT is less clear as the more frequent benign forms are not recorded in cancer registers. It is also likely that the majority of immature teratomas (IT), which are of indeterminate behaviour, are not recorded in such registers. From a personally collected series at a primary care hospital in the United States (3) the incidence of all GCT was 4.5/million children. Despite the United Kingdom Children's Cancer Study Group (UKCCSG) asking that all GCT be registered, of 365 cases registered and reviewed only 27% were mature teratomas (MT) and 19% IT with 54% being malignant. These figures are obviously distorted due to under-reporting of benign teratomas.

The sex distribution of MGCT is almost equal apart from sacrococcygeal tumours, which show a striking female preponderance (4). In children MGCT show two incidence peaks, the higher being at 0–4 years and the lower at 10–14 years.

Rising incidence

There is strong evidence of a world-wide increase in the incidence of GCT, best documented in adolescent and adult testicular GCT (5), but also found in paediatric GCT. In a long term study (1957–92) of all malignancies in children under 18 years living in the West Midlands of England the overall incidence of malignant GCT was 2.61/million/year (4). However over the 36 years studied the incidence had increased from 1.61/million to 3.6/million, that is, more than doubled. Another English region has shown a similar increase (6) as has a larger national study in the United Kingdom (7). Although these results could be reflecting more rigorous registration and more accurate pathological diagnosis, ascertainment of cases had always been thorough and all were reviewed by a panel of experienced pathologists using current diagnostic techniques. Only yolk sac tumours (YST) were present in sufficient number to permit statistical analysis and a very significant increase ($p = 0.004$) was found. The number of MGCT of ovary and testis had also increased.

Ethnicity

The frequency of GCT varies in different ethnic populations, for example, Black Americans have a very low incidence of testicular GCT compared to white Americans (8). European immigrant families in Israel (9) showed a relatively high incidence of testicular MGCT in males under 30 years of age, an excess which persisted, but became lower, over two generations, indicating genetic as well as environmental factors in the pathogenesis of this tumour. It seems likely that similar ethnic differences exist in childhood GCT. Asian children in the United Kingdom appeared to be at higher risk of MGCT than non-Asian peers and are 3–4 times more likely to develop MGCT than either Wilms' tumour or neuroblastoma—a very different incidence from Caucasian children in the same region (10). A cofactor could be that the Asian children studied were more likely to live in industrialised urban areas and be exposed to environmental pollutants.

Clinical conditions which increase the risk of GCT

Gonadal GCT is much more common in gonadal dysgenesis, testicular feminisation syndrome, and young adults with undescended testis (11). Trisomy 21 also increases the risk of gonadal MGCT (12). Malformations of the urogenital tract and sacral agenesis are also reported risk factors (13). Klinefelter's syndrome (KS) (47,XXY) is associated with an increased frequency of extragonadal GCT (14), particularly involving the mediastinum and central nervous system (CNS).

Familial factors

A small number of GCT are familial. Some occur as part of the Li–Fraumeni syndrome, but the majority do not. Affected families show a mixture of benign and malignant GCT in both sexes. Siblings were most frequently involved, but cousins and parents were also reported (15).

Associated primary malignancies

In adults a GCT predisposes to a second primary GCT. This is not the case in children. Mediastinal GCT are associated with haemopoietic malignancies, for example, leukaemia (16), myelodysplastic disorders, and mastocytosis, which can arise simultaneously with the GCT and therefore are not due to chemotherapy or irradiation. Moreover cytogenetic markers show that these haemopoietic malignancies arise from the GCT rather than the bone marrow (16). Mast cell proliferation post-mediastinal GCT has shown isochrome 12p, a cytogenetic marker for some GCT (17). Because these blood dyscrasias are particularly common in mediastinal YST, it is suggested they develop from the haemopoietic cells found in hepatoid YST. However blood cell antigens have been found in other GCT tumours apart from YST, for example, embryonal carcinoma (EC)—emphasising that EC cells can transform to embryonal stem (ES) cells. The association is not limited to malignant GCT because an MT of the mediastinum has been associated with autoimmune haemolytic anaemia, cured by excision of the tumour (18).

Environmental

There is considerable epidemiological evidence that environmental factors are important in the pathogenesis of GCT, particularly adult testicular MGCT. The increase in this group of tumours is associated with an increase in male infertility, hypospadias, undescended testis, and diminishing semen quality. Where semen quality is significantly better, as in several US states (19) and Finland (20), rates of both testicular tumours and hypospadias are lower (5). Childhood ovarian and infantile testicular GCT are also increasing (4), so the same environmental factors are probably active in children. The increase in MGCT came almost entirely from children living in the heavily populated, industrialised areas of the region (4). These epidemiological trends point to a new environmental contaminant possibly related to industry and to increased oestrogen-like pollutants (21).

Aetiology and pathogenesis

The aetiology, pathogenesis, and even the cell of origin for most GCT remain enigmatic. The generally accepted theory is that the germ cell is the cell of origin for all of these tumours whatever their site. It is postulated that in both sexes the primordial germ cells (PGC) arise in the yolk sac endoderm and migrate along the paravertebral gonadal ridge in a caudal to cranial fashion. This theory explains the distribution of the GCT along the midline of the body and within the gonads. These PGC undergo molecular genetic changes resulting in the diverse range of tumours, which come under the hubris of GCT. Not everyone accepts this concept. Chaganti and Houldsworth (22) point out that such misplaced PGC have never been reported by embryologists outside the abdominal cavity. Because their detailed cytogenetic studies of the male extragonadal GCT showed no significant difference between the various sites, Chaganti et al. (23) propose a transformation of PGC within the gonad followed by a backward migration of these transformed cells along the gonadal ridge to the various sites of tumour development.

To some extent the adoption of the Chaganti's hypothesis makes it easier to extrapolate from the precursor events in the germ cell of the human male testis to the development of GCT elsewhere, both benign and malignant. This still leaves many unanswered questions particularly in infantile and childhood GCT which, on the basis of histology, epidemiology, and molecular biology have a different aetiology.

Pathogenesis of adolescent and adult testicular GCT

The precursor cellular events in adult and adolescent testicular GCT have been extensively studied. Because adolescents (from 10 years onwards) have the adult type of testicular GCT, the pathogenesis proposed by Rajpert-de Meyts et al. (24) outlined below is likely.

In the fetal testis the precursor cell, the primordial germ cell (PGC), is prevented from going into meiosis by a meiosis-inhibiting factor produced by the Sertoli cells, that is, they suffer a long spell of arrested development, which may be a time of increased susceptibility to adverse environmental factors. This hypothesis is supported by these arrested germ cells over-expressing growth factor receptors for c-kit ligand and sertoli cell factor (SCF) (24). This receptiveness to growth factors may explain tendency to undergo neoplastic transformation to intratubular germ cell neoplasia (ITGCN). Arrested PGC share several immunohistochemical markers, for example, placental alkaline phosphatase (PLAP) with ITGCN (25). They do not however show the cytogenetic abnormality isochrome 12p, found in true ITGCN and in adult MGCT. The arrested PGC gradually differentiate into spermatogonia in the second half of gestation. The PGC remaining at birth disappear in the first year of life except, significantly, in those conditions (gonadal dysgenesis, androgen insensitivity syndrome, and Down's syndrome) with an increased risk of adolescent/adult testicular MGCT. In vitro experiments (26) have shown that murine pluripotenial embryonic cells can be derived from PGC and can then develop into ES cells. This pathway would explain the wide range of tissues found in GCT.

Pathogenesis of infantile testicular GCT

How much of the above is applicable to infantile testicular GCT? There is good evidence—epidemiological, histological, and cytogenetic that the pathogenesis of infantile and childhood tumours is different (27). Despite occasional reports of ITGCN occurring in association with infantile tumours (28), this is very uncommon.

A Danish study (29) found that in 18 testicular GCT in children under 5 years only 2 had possible ITGCN. Some believe that the large germ cells with prominent nuclei and clear cytoplasm, often seen in quantity in seminiferous tubules adjacent to an infantile testicular GCT, are not true ITGCN despite similar morphology. This view is supported by their usual failure to express PLAP or other markers, their diploid DNA, and lack of i(12p). The current opinion (2) is that they represent immature infantile germ cells, their prominence being due to stimulation by paracrine growth factors from the adjacent tumour. Whilst the pathogenesis of infantile GCT is not really understood, it is postulated that infantile YST develops from a PGC at an earlier stage in its transformation when it is still exhibiting mainly stem cell behaviour (1, 5). Adult GCT would arise at a later stage and seminoma would develop from an 'aged' ITGCN cell with almost no stem cell behaviour. Even within the same tubule, there are variations in the immunophenotype of the ITGCN cells with some expressing the phenotype of seminoma cells, others of EC cells, and some cells expressing both patterns (25).

Pathogenesis of extragonadal GCT in males and females

Detailed genetic studies limited to childhood GCT have shown that all paediatric extragonadal and testicular GCT arise by mitotic division of a premeiotic germ cell or a pluripotential somatic cell, that is, extragonadal tumours in the female appear to follow the male pattern of arising in mitotic division and not the ovarian pattern. Moreover it is postulated (22) that in males already transformed PGC carry out a backward migration to the extragonadal sites where they progress to GCT in a fashion similar to that described in the testis. In support of this hypothesis the i(12p) chromosome abnormality has been recorded in occasional mediastinal GCT (30).

Pathogenesis of ovarian GCT

The normal development of germ cells is fundamentally different in the two sexes. In contrast to the male, the female germ cell enters meiosis early in fetal life. Cytogenetic studies (31) have shown multiple genetic origins for adult and paediatric ovarian GCT, namely that 65% are derived from a single germ cell after meiosis I and failure of meiosis II (type ii) or by endoreduplication of a mature ovum (type iii); 35% arise by failure of meiosis I (type i) or at mitotic division of premeiotic germ cells (type iv), which is the male pattern.

Cytogenetics

Teratomas, mature and immature

Almost all the cytogenetic analyses have been carried out in adult GCT, which are similar to GCT in adolescents, but not to GCT in infancy and childhood. Paediatric MT and IT are usually diploid (32). A study of congenital sacrococcygeal teratomas (33) confirmed this and showed that IT had small populations of aneuploid cells in the immature neural and blastematous tissue. Similarily in adult ovarian teratomas, chromosomal abnormalities are much more common in immature than mature tumours.

There is a direct relationship between aneuploidy and the histological grade of IT, aneuploidy being more common in grade 3. Aneuploid grade 3 IT may do less well than euploid grade 3 cases. Although studies on infantile IT from all other sites have been reported as diploid we have seen a congenital retroperitoneal IT (grade 3) in which there was aneuploidy and several cell lines trisomic for chromosome 3. Trisomy for chromosome 3 is the most frequent trisomy reported in IT of the adult ovary, although trisomy for 8, 12, and 14 have also been recorded. If the IT should develop YST, then there is concurrent development of aneuploidy. The isochromosome abnormality i(12p) associated with adult/adolescent testicular MGCT, has not been reported in ovarian IT.

Teratomas of the CNS are different from those in other sites as they have a high incidence of increased copies of the X chromosome and, less frequently, of the Y chromosome. This is interesting as these tumours are more common in KS (47,XXY).

Malignant germ cell tumours

Isochrome 12p—i(12p) is the characteristic cytogenetic abnormality found in adolescent and adult MGCT whether gonadal or extragonadal, whatever the tumour histology. This abnormality, but non-amplified, is also found in ITGCN (34). MGCT may have more than one copy (i.e. amplification) and an increased copy number is associated with a poorer prognosis (35). Isochrome 12p is not found in childhood testicular or ovarian MGCT, nor in YST.

Childhood YST is aneuploid, often near tetraploid. Some series (36) have shown repeated involvement of chromosomes 1, 2, 3, and 6. Comparative genomic hybridisation of four infantile testicular teratomas showed no aberrations in two cases and gains and losses of parts of chromosomes in the remainder. In addition three YST (two pure testicular and one sacrococcygeal) showed a similar range of gains and losses in the same chromosomes, that is, there was a gain of parts of 19q, 20q, and 22, and a loss of parts of 4q and 6q were present in all cases, suggesting a pathogenetic relationship (27).

Staging

Previously rather complex staging criteria, which were site specific and based on adult patients, were used in children with GCT. Children's GCT have proven extremely sensitive to the new chemotherapeutic regimens so there is an opportunity to look afresh at staging. Although Pinkerton (1) states 'the aim of any staging system should be to distinguish patient groups on the basis of outcome and this is clearly not the case with the older systems' that is, an evidence—based approach (Table 14.1), the more traditional anatomical staging classification still forms the basis of most clinical treatments and indeed has recently been further expanded (Table 14.2) in the United States (37).

The weakness of anatomical classifications is the exclusion of potentially useful information derived from serum tumour markers. Alternative classifications have

Table 14.1 Categories of GCT proposed by North American Oncologists (1)

Low risk	IT
	Completely resected gonadal MGCT
	Completely resected sacrococcygeal MGCT
Intermediate risk	Unresectable gonadal
	Extragonadal tumours (apart from sacrococcygeal)
	Metastatic from gonadal primary
	Failed low risk (i.e. those who were treated by surgery alone and have had local recurrence)
High risk	Unresectable extragonadal
	Metastatic from extragonadal primary
	Extensive primary or metastatic disease, both recurring after initial treatment with surgery alone

Table 14.2 Anatomical staging of germ cell tumours (37)

a. Testis:
  I Tumour limited to the testis and completely resected with no tumour spill
    No clinical, radiographic, or histologic evidence of tumour outside the testis
    Tumour markers normal after appropriate half-life decline
    (Normal or unknown markers at diagnosis require a negative ipsilateral
      retroperitoneal node sampling to confirm stage 1; bilaterality does not change stage)
  II Transcrotal orchiectomy with gross spill of tumour, or
    Microscopic disease in scrotum or high in spermatic cord ($= 0.5$ cm from proximal end), or
    Retroperitoneal lymph node involvement ($= 2$ cm), or
    Increased tumour markers after appropriate half-life
  III Retroperitoneal lymph node involvement (>2 cm)
    No visceral or extra-abdominal involvement
  IV Distant metastases including liver

b. Ovary:
  I Tumour is limited to the ovary, peritoneal washings, or ascitic fluid negative for malignant cells
    No clinical, radiographic, or histologic evidence of tumour outside the ovary
    Tumour markers normal after appropriate half-life decline
    Bilaterality does not change stage
  II Microscopic residual or positive lymph nodes (<2 cm)
    Peritoneal washings or ascitic fluid negative for malignant cells
    Tumour markers positive or negative
  III Lymph node involvement or metastatic nodule (>2 cm)
    Gross residual tumour
    Contiguous visceral involvement
    Peritoneal washings or ascitic fluid positive for malignant cells
    Tumour markers positive
  IV Distant metastasis

c. Extragonadal:
  I Complete resection at any site
    Coccygectomy for sacrococcygeal site
    Negative tumour margins
    Tumour markers positive or negative
  II Microscopic residual
    Lymph nodes negative
    Tumour markers positive or negative
  III Gross residual tumour or biopsy only
    Lymph nodes positive or negative
    Tumour markers positive or negative
  IV Distant metastasis, including liver

placed heavy emphasis on the importance of these tumour markers—alpha-fetoprotein (AFP) and human chorionic gonadotropin (HCG) by the Charing Cross Group London (38), and HCG and Lactic dehydrogenase (LDH) by the Group at Memorial Hospital, New York (39).

These numerous classification systems have hindered multinational studies and clinical trials, which are necessary in order to establish optimum treatment for this relatively rare but chemically sensitive group of tumours. In 1997 International Germ Cell Cancer Collaborative Group (40) published an internationally agreed prognostic factor-based classification (Table 14.3). It was based on pooled data worldwide comprising 5862 patients who had developed metastatic GCT arising from any extracranial primary site. Of these cases 562 were under 20 years. All received platinum-based chemotherapy and follow up was for a minimum of 5 years. They found that adverse factors were mediastinal primary, high serum tumour marker levels and presence of non-pulmonary visceral metastases (NPVM). These factors were of course based on a largely adult population and may not be directly applicable to children. The classification

Table 14.3 International malignant germ cell consensus classification (40)

Non-seminoma	Seminoma
Good prognosis	
Testis/retroperitoneal primary *and*	Any primary site *and*
No non-pulmonary visceral metastases *and*	No non-pulmonary visceral metastases *and*
Good markers—all of: AFP < 1000 ng/ml and HCG < 5000 iu/l (1000 ng/ml) and LDH < 1.5 × N	Normal AFP, any HCG, any LDH
Intermediate prognosis	
Testis/retroperitoneal primary *and*	Any primary site *and*
No non-pulmonary visceral metastases *and*	Non-pulmonary visceral metastases *and*
Intermediate markers—any of: AFP = 1000 and = 10,000 ng/ml or HCG = 5000 iu/l and = 50,000 iu/l or LDH = 1.5 × N and = 10 × N	Normal AFP, any HCG, any LDH
Poor prognosis	
Mediastinal primary *or*	
Non-pulmonary visceral metastases *or*	
Poor markers—any of: AFP > 10,000 ng/ml or HCG > 50,000 iu/l (10,000 ng/ml) or LDH > 10 × N	No patients classified as poor prognosis

N = upper limit of normal.

Table 14.4 WHO classification (European in italic script) with grading (41)

1	MT	Grade 0 (Europe—'Benign' Teratoma = Grade 0 'and' includes Grade 1)
2	IT	Grade 1 immature area in one 40 × field/section
		Grade 2 immature area in 2–3 40 × fields/section
		Grade 3 immature area in >4 40 × fields/section
3	Malignant teratoma[1]	i.e. malignant component not of germ cell type (NB rare in children)
4	Mixed malignant germ cell tumour	i.e. malignant component(s) all of germ cell type, e.g. IM + YST + germinoma, etc.
5	EST	YST/infantile EC
6	Germinoma	Seminoma/dysgerminima
7	Choriocarcinoma[2]	NB rare in childhood
8	Adult type EC	NB rare in childhood
9	Gonadoblastoma	
10	Polyembryoma	Very rare in pure form at any age

[1] Malignant PNET can occur in children with teratoma, but is very rare.
[2] Gestational choriocarcinoma (metastatic) can occur in neonates and sexually active adolescents.

has proved robust when tested on more recent data derived from European trials.

Histopathological classification

Most histopathological classifications of GCT are developed from those established for adult testicular GCT and there are at least three very different variants of those! A relatively simple classification (Table 14.4) based on the WHO classification, is appropriate for childhood and applicable to all sites of GCT and is the one currently used by the UKCCSG. The grading system of IT is that used by Norris *et al.* (41). It is essentially the same as that used in North America.

Pathology

Teratoma

Mature teratoma

These tumours are often cystic with firm gritty areas. The cysts may contain fluid but more often contain yellowish greasy material and especially in the ovary tangled hair, which is almost always dark. Malformed teeth, bone, and cartilage may be identified (Fig. 14.1). All three embryonic cell layers should be represented—endoderm, mesoderm, and ectoderm (or neuroectoderm). Rarely only one layer is represented and that is termed a 'monodermal' teratoma. The so-called 'dermoid cyst' is not monodermal as it always has a mesodermal component in addition to the prominent ectoderm and is better classified as a cystic teratoma. The three cell layers show some degree of local organiser activity so that pancreatic tissue will often be next to intestinal type structures, which in turn can show all intestinal muscle layers and include the ganglion cells equivalent to the submucosal and intermyenteric plexuses. Only exceptional tumours show well-developed organ formation or development of segmental structures within an axial skeleton. It is this very rare group of teratomas with an axial structure, which have been offered as examples of 'fetus in fetu' or 'parasitic twin'. In an MT, by definition, all tissue elements must be fully mature, or, in neonates, show the same degree of maturity as in the somatic tissues. If any immature element is present whether mesodermal or neuroectodermal, then it should be classified as IT. If frankly malignant germ cell elements are present within the teratoma, then it must be classified as a malignant mixed GCT with the malignant component described (e.g. teratoma with YST). In adults the malignancy may not be of germ cell origin, for example, squamous carcinoma, and it is then classified as a malignant teratoma. Apart from the rare cases of malignant neuroectodermal tissue or sarcoma in a teratoma, this type of tumour is very unusual in childhood. Truly MT are benign, but extensive sampling is necessary to ensure a focus of YST is not missed. Dehner (42) recommends that one section be taken for every 1 cm of the longest diameter.

Occasionally YST occurs at the site of a previous MT, or as a metastasis following an MT. The assumption is that YST developed in an incompletely excised teratoma, or that a focus of YST was overlooked in the original tumour. Such foci are much more common in high grade IT than in MT.

MT with elevated alpha-fetoprotein (AFP): Elevation of serum AFP at the time of resection indicates foci of YST except in the neonatal period when the physiological level of AFP can be as high as 50,000 ng/ml in neonates (43) falling steadily to normal adult levels by about 6–8 months.

Immature teratoma

These tumours are mainly solid with cystic areas. They often are greyish and soft ('encephaloid') reflecting the large amount of neural tissue present. In this group of tumours all three embryological layers are represented as in MT, but there is immaturity or incomplete differentiation of the tissues. This may affect one or all of the three cell layers, but most usually it is the neuroectodermal element which is immature.

Various studies (44) have shown that the ovary is the most common childhood site (63%), although in children less than 4 years the extragonadal sites followed by testis are more common. Between 4 and 10 years IT are rare except in the ovary. IT is biologically less predictable than MT and in an attempt to predict behaviour a histological grading system for IT of the adult ovary was introduced by Thurlbeck and Scully (45) and modified by Norris et al. (41) (Table 14.4). Follow-up studies in children have shown that ovarian tumours grades 1 and 2 almost always behave in a benign fashion (42) and that those grade 3 tumours, which behave in a malignant fashion usually had foci of YST, which may have been overlooked on the original assessment. The value of applying histological grading to non-ovarian IT has been unclear. One hundred and thirty-five paediatric

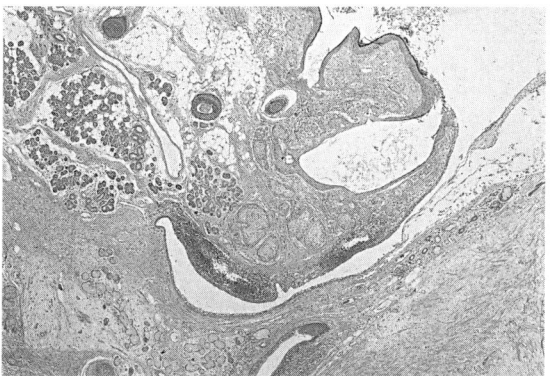

Fig. 14.1 MT. Cyst lined partly by keratinising epithelium with adjacent pilosebaceous units and partly by respiratory type epithelium with sub-epithelial seromucinous glands. All tissues are mature. Haematoxylin and eosin ×66.

GCT in which there was a substantial immature component were graded retrospectively (44). These tumours comprised 60 which were apparently pure IT and 75 with areas of YST. This study showed that histological grading was independent of age. Whatever the site there was a significant correlation between the presence of foci of YST and the grade of the IT, that is, foci were present in 24% of grade 1 rising to 83% of grade 3. Foci of YST were more common in all grades of IT if the child was >3 years. They also found that in ovarian tumours in children >1 year old an elevation of the serum level of AFP at diagnosis of >100 ng/dl correlated very closely with foci of YST. In this series only those IT with foci of YST or elevated serum AFP levels had recurred as frankly malignant YST and therefore these 2 elements should be regarded as prognostic factors for the risk of developing YST. The risk was however very low and they felt that surgery alone was curative in most cases with salvage chemotherapy should there be a malignant recurrence. The grade of IT in itself was non-prognostic but a high grade alerts the pathologist to the increased risk of foci of YST, as does elevation of serum AFP levels. Prior to the Heifetz report the accepted opinion had been that very small areas of yolk sac differentiation within a large teratoma were of doubtful significance, although they could have some malignant potential. Many pathologists would not even mention them, but in contrast Joshi (46) has always regarded foci of YST in an IT as indicating malignancy. Current practice based on the Heifetz (44) study, would be to mention these microfoci in the report to the oncologist (e.g. IT, grade 3, with microfoci of yolk sac differentiation of uncertain significance) in order to indicate the need for particularly careful clinical and serological follow up. It is important that the pathologist remembers that YST can adopt many guises (see section on Yolk sac tumour; Endodermal sinus tumour) including fetal liver with haemopoietic activity. It is prudent to subject suspicious areas to immunohistochemistry for evidence of endodermal differentiation (i.e. AFP, A-1-AT, cytokeratin (CK)) and then to assess whether the positive areas represent differentiated foetal endoderm-derived structures (e.g. intestine) or yolk sac tumourlets. If the area of YST is substantial, then the classification would become mixed MGCT, that is, IT with YST. From the above it is essential that IT are widely sampled, selecting tissue from the most suspicious looking areas—haemorrhagic, mucoid, etc.

Sometimes a high grade IT can have neuroepithelial areas, which appear highly malignant, being densely cellular with a very high mitotic rate, nuclear pleomorphism,

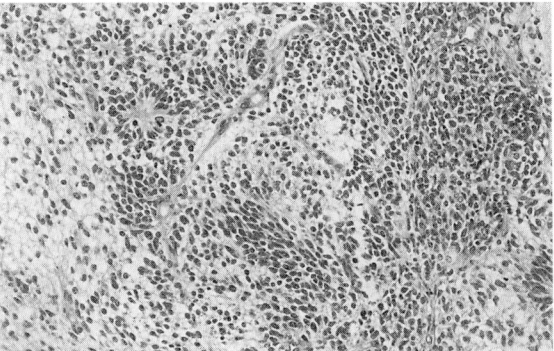

Fig. 14.2 IT. Primitive neural tissue with small dark cells some arranged in rosettes, fibrillary neuropil, and fibrovascular bands. This area resembles a neuroblastoma. Haematoxylin and eosin × 132.

and prominent apoptosis. Despite this appearance, they may not behave in a malignant fashion. This is a very difficult diagnostic problem because of the very occasional case in which this neuroepithelial element metastasises and kills the patient. Unlike germ cell malignancies these malignant neuroepithelial tumours can be chemotherapy-resistant. We have tried using CD99 to select those cases which might behave as primitive neuroectodermal tumour (PNET), but are not convinced of its selectivity in the context of very immature neuroepithelial tissue in an IT. Joshi (46) suggests abnormal mitoses together with nuclear pleomorphism are indicators of malignant as opposed to immature neuroepithelium. Less difficult are areas of immature neuroepithelial tissue which resemble differentiating neuroblastoma rich in neuropil (Fig. 14.2). Such areas are quite common in IT and have little or no metastatic potential. Likewise nephroblastoma-like areas do not carry a bad prognosis, although cases of nephroblastoma following GCT have been reported in young adults, but not so far in childhood (47).

Malignant germ cell tumours

The most common germ cell malignancy in prepubertal children is the YST either in its pure form or in combination with teratoma or with another malignant element. Pure germinomas occur almost exclusively in the ovary or CNS and the testicular form (seminoma) is very rare even in adolescence. Choriocarcinoma is rare and is most commonly found in an ovarian GCT in adolescence along with another malignant germ cell element. Embryonal carcinoma is very rare in pre-adolescence and carcinoma (squamous carcinoma, adenocarcinoma) almost unknown in childhood and adolescence. Rarely sarcomas, such as rhabdomyosarcomas, may be a component in childhood GCT particularly in mediastinal tumours.

Yolk sac tumour; endodermal sinus tumour (EST)

Yolk sac tumours are the most common malignant GCT in infancy and childhood, often existing in a pure form but also being part of an otherwise mature, or more commonly, immature teratoma. Occasionally they are only a tiny component or micro-focus, within an otherwise benign teratomatous tumour. The macroscopic appearance is variable often being mucoid, greyish, and friable with areas of haemorrhage and necrosis.

Histology

The histology is particularly diverse. There are four main histological patterns often seen together in the same tumour. These are pseudopapillary (Fig. 14.3(a)), microcystic or reticular, solid and polyvesicular vitelline. Less common are the hepatoid and endometroid. Schiller Duval bodies (Fig. 14.3(a)), which are the most easily recognised feature in YST are particularly common in areas either of pseudopapillary or of microcystic appearance. Another useful marker is the intra- and extra-cytoplasmic eosinophilic hyaline body (Fig. 14.3(b)), which is strongly Periodic Acid Schiff (PAS) positive and diastase resistant. Strands of similar eosinophilic material may be present in the background stroma and if prominent are

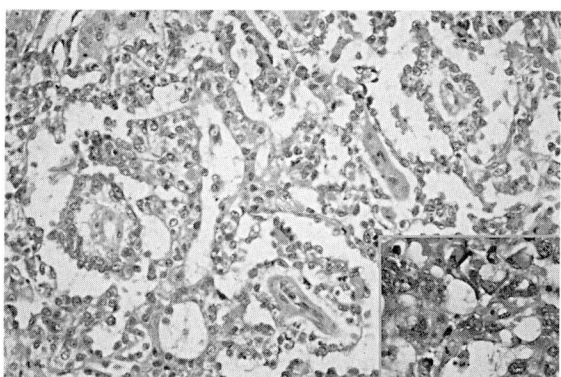

Fig. 14.3 YST. (a) Papillary pattern with single central vessels covered by tumour cells and protruding into a space lined by tumour cells (Schiller Duval bodies). Haematoxylin and eosin × 66. (b) Hyaline bodies both intra- and extra-cellular. Haematoxylin and eosin × 260.

thought to confer a degree of resistance to chemotherapy. Angioblastic or mesenchymal like areas are more difficult to recognise as YST and are particularly found post-chemotherapy and in mediastinal tumours, where they may be the source of post-chemotherapy sarcomas or the associated haemopoietic tumours. Immunohistochemistry: all YST will have areas positive for AFP so that this is a very useful immunohistochemical marker. Unfortunately because it is only present focally, small biopsies may be negative. However the serum AFP will be very elevated in YST. A1AT is also patchily positive in YST and CK CAM 5.2 is strongly positive. The angioblastic form is CK positive, vimentin positive, and often AFP negative. Areas of hepatic differentiation will also stain positively. One of the current controversies is whether these foci are the hepatoid variant of YST (i.e. malignant) or merely represent differentiation towards liver. In the context of an MT, the latter may empirically be considered to be the case, as foci of YST are truly uncommon in that tumour type. Many high grade IT have foci of definite YST and in such tumours hepatic differentiation is best viewed with suspicion. It has been suggested that staining the tissue for Concavalin A would show positivity if it were liver, but be negative if hepatoid YST.

Embryonal carcinoma (EC)

This tumour is very rare in childhood but begins to appear in adolescence usually as a malignant component in a mixed malignant tumour of ovary, testis, or mediastinum. The histology is of sheets of anaplastic epithelial cells which are large, overlapping with indistinct cell margins. Papillary areas may be present.

These cells are usually negative or weakly positive for AFP, usually positive for PLAP, and always positive for CK. Uniquely for an epithelial tumour, their cell membranes are CD30 positive (Fig. 14.4).

Choriocarcinoma (CC)

This is very rare in childhood and is most frequently seen in adolescence as a component within a mixed GCT. In early infancy it has been reported in a pure form and represents a gestational choriocarcinoma metastatic from the mother. In adolescence gestational trohphoblastic malignancy is again a possibility if it is the sole histological pattern. The tumour is very friable, necrotic, and haemorrhagic.

Histological diagnosis depends on identifying two cell layers—cytotrophoblast as well as syncitiotrophoblast,

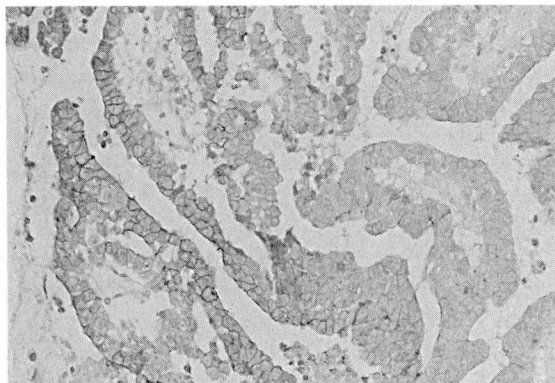

Fig. 14.4 EC (adult type). Looks like anaplastic carcinoma but stains positively for CD30 antigen. Immunoperoxidase ×32.

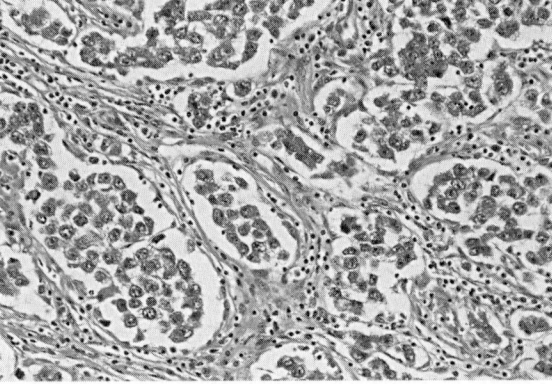

Fig. 14.5 Dysgerminoma. Clear tumour cells are traversed by septa containing lymphocytes. Haematoxylin and eosin ×132.

which are HCG positive. Small clusters of syncitial cells are frequently seen in germinomas but despite being HCG positive these cells do not amount to CC and do not imply the poorer prognosis, which a focus of true CC would indicate. It is these small areas which account for the slight elevations of serum bHCG in some germinomas.

Germinoma

Although a common adult GCT, they are much less common in children in whom they occur in the ovary (dysgerminoma) or in the CNS (germinoma). They may be in the pure form or part of a mixed GCT. The most common site in the adult is the testis (seminoma), but that is virtually unknown in the prepubertal male and rare even in adolescence. We have seen a single case of seminoma in a karyotypically normal 14-year-old male with bilateral undescended testes and preceding ITGCN.

Histologically they are similar to the adult form with large polygonal cells, clear cytoplasm, and distinct nuclear membranes and prominent nucleoli (Fig. 14.5). Often divided into cords and nests by fibrous bands they may have a focal syncitial appearance, which not only mimics that of syncitio-trophoblast but stains positively with bHCG. Lymphocytes may be very conspicuous within the fibrous tissue and also a granulomatous inflammatory reaction. Spermatocytic or anaplastic forms do not occur in paediatric practice.

Immunohistochemistry shows strong membrane staining with PLAP and the syncytial cell clusters may be HCG positive. Unlike gonadal germinomas, those in the CNS are CK and vimentin positive.

Germinomas in childhood are particularly sensitive to modern chemotherapeutic measures.

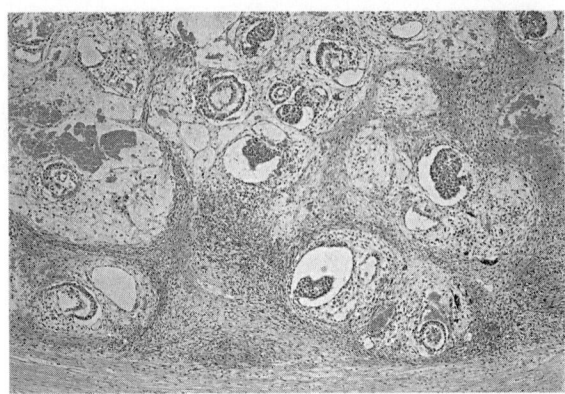

Fig. 14.6 Polyembryoma. Numerous embryoid bodies in varying stages of development. Almost always other areas will show other forms of germ cell malignancy. Haematoxylin and eosin ×26.

Polyembryoma

Embryoid bodies in which the structure of the blastocyst is recapitulated to varying degrees occasionally appear in otherwise typical yolk sac or embryonal carcinoma. Sometimes they dominate the histology such that the tumour is designated a polyembryoma. The case we have seen had several well-differentiated embryoid bodies with an embryonic plate, amniocoele, coelomic cavity, and in the adjacent tissue areas resembling yolk sac and even early trophoblast the latter staining positively with HCG (Fig. 14.6). Polyembryoma has been declared both less and more malignant than YST, but in fact with modern chemotherapy responds in a similar fashion as other MGCT.

Gonadoblastoma

This is included with GCT because at least one cellular component of this tumour arises from the germ cell. The gonadoblastoma is itself benign, but it has a potential (given at about 30%) to develop a malignant GCT, usually a dysgerminoma. Gonadoblastomas are very rare tumours always intragonadal and only arise in the dysgenetic gonads of patients with some Y chromosome material in their karyotype. They are never found in the normal gonads in karyotypically normal subjects, nor are they found in the streak gonads of Turner's syndrome. Because of their potential to develop malignancy they should be removed by bilateral gonadectomy.

Histology of post-chemotherapy tumours

Maturation of previously immature elements (chemotherapeutic retroversion) is common. Necrosis of the tumour is followed by an inflammatory reaction characterised by foamy macrophages and fibrosis. YST is the most chemo-resistant and careful search should be made for foci of viable YST. Immunohistochemistry for CK and AFP are useful. Although mature in histological terms, these tumours still maintain their original cytogenetic abnormality, for example, i(12p) (48).

Serological tumour markers

Alpha feto-protein is a sensitive and specific marker for YST apart from the first 6–8 months of life, when there is a naturally elevated level (up to 50,000 ng/dl at birth falling to normal by 6–8 months). Low elevations of AFP will be found in some cases of IT (<100 ng/dl) and are now thought to represent microscopic foci of YST in these tumours rather than immature choroid plexus tissue, which was the previous explanation. Some workers regard an AFP level as high as 1000 ng/dl as still being acceptably accounted for by small, biologically inactive foci of YST in what is classified as IT. However having decided to treat such cases with modest elevations of AFP as IT (i.e. by surgery) rather than as YST, it is mandatory that the level of AFP is very closely followed for evidence of an increasing serum level. This would be indicative of an active focus of YST. During and following treatment monitoring of the serum level of AFP is useful in assessing the success of the therapy and alerting clinicians to a poor response or to recurrence of the tumour.

Human chorionic gonadotrophin is a useful tumour marker for choriocarcinoma, being elevated in the serum of pure choriocarcinoma (>1000 ng/dl). Levels of <100 ng/dl may be found when syncitial cells form a small component within a mixed MGCT or within a germinoma. Such levels do not alter the diagnosis nor the prognosis. Elevations >100 ng/dl are unusual and suggest the presence of choriocarcinoma (37). In certain mixed GCT both AFP and HCG can be elevated.

Placental Alkaline Phosphatase has been reported as being elevated in the serum of patients with germinoma.

LDH is a non-specific marker for malignancy.

Some of these tumour markers can be used in diagnostic immunohistochemistry (Table 14.5).

Distribution according to site, age, and tumour type

In children involvement of extragonadal sites is much more common (Table 14.6), whereas adults show a reverse pattern. There is a marked difference between the personally collected series, for example, Marsden *et al.* (49) having a high number of gonadal tumours

Table 14.5 Immunohistochemistry and diagnosis

	AFP	CK	PLAP	HCG	CD30
YST	+++	+++	---	---	---
EC	+/-	+++	++/-	---	+++
Germinoma (gonadal)	---	---	+++	+/-	---
Germinoma (CNS)	---	++	+++	---	---
Choriocarcinoma	---	++	---	+++	---

Table 14.6 Sites of paediatric germ cell tumours (modified from Dehner (42))

Site	Berry et al.	Marsden et al.	Bale et al.	6 Studies (Dehner)	
Sacrococcygeum	58	31	51	321	41%
Ovary	10	45	16	221	28%
Testis	7	25	7	56	7%
Mediastinum	5	5	4	46	6%
CNS	5	13	5	43	5%
Retroperineum	1	6	7	34	4%
Neck (thyroid)	3	3	10	23	3%
Head (oral cavity, etc.)	0	1	6	21	3%
Stomach	2	0	0	3	<1%
Female genital tract	0	3	0	3	<1%
Spinal cord, meninges	0	3	0	3	<1%
Bladder, prostate	0	2	0	2	>0%
Liver	0	0	0	2	>0%
Pericardium	0	0	1	1	>0%
Umbilical cord	0	0	0	1	>0%
Total	91	137	107	780	100%

and also of tumours in unusual sites. This may reflect his referral pattern and areas of special interest. Bale et al. (50) and Berry et al. (51) a world apart geographically (Australia and United Kingdom respectively) are very similar in total numbers and in distribution, yet Bale records significantly more tumours in the head and neck (16 cases to 3), possibly resulting from her access to perinatal tumours. Head and neck tumours and large congenital sacrococcygeal tumours usually present in the neonatal period, can result in stillbirth and neonatal death, and are frequently not registered. Very few registers of tumours are completely unbiased or complete.

Gonadal GCT

Ovary

Teratomas

About 60% are MT usually cystic, which can grow to a very large size and present as a mass. They are generally encapsulated. The peak age is between 9 and 11 years. Adequate sampling is essential especially if haemorrhagic or necrotic.

Immature teratomas account for about 10% of tumours especially those in the early teens and they tend to be solid. The histologic grading system devised by Norris et al. (41) can be used, but in itself is not prognostically valuable in children. However there is a direct correlation between grade and the presence of YST. Small foci of YST, if well within the teratoma and in the presence of a very low serum AFP, may have no clinical significance; so if the tumour is stage 1 then surgery with follow-up will suffice. Pathologists should report these foci (focal or multifocal) and estimate their area and relationship to the capsule (37).

Gliomatosis

Any peritoneal nodules should be sampled. These may prove to be deposits of glial tissue—gliomatosis peritonei. Such deposits, when associated with a mature ovarian teratoma should also be mature (grade 0) and in IT the grade of immaturity should be appropriate to the the grade of the primary tumour (44), in which circumstances they do not have a sinister implication and the tumour remains stage 1. If the nodules show any evidence of YST then the primary tumour, although apparently an IT, is actually a mixed malignant tumour and is stage 3 (omental involvement). Similar criteria are applied when the deposits of glial tissue are found in local lymph nodes (*nodal gliomatosis*).

Frequently ovarian teratomas present with acute onset abdominal pain and laparotomy reveals that they have undergone torsion and infarction. Although haemorrhagic and necrotic, they must nonetheless be carefully examined for evidence of a malignant component. If no evidence is found it is still prudent to remind the oncologist that tissue detail was poor because of infarction and therefore small foci of malignancy cannot be completely ruled out. Pre-operative serum tumour marker levels are very useful in such infarcted tumours.

Malignant tumours

These account for 30% of childhood ovarian tumours and are divided equally between pure and mixed forms. Many will have progressed beyond stage 1 by the time of surgery (Table 14.2). YST is the most common malignant element, but in later adolescence dysgerminoma becomes increasingly frequent. The latter is a solid rubbery tumour and unless ruptured, remains encapsulated. The capsule should be widely sampled and any adhesions to adjacent structures should be biopsied and the omentum excised to allow careful pathological examination for microstaging. YST, dysgerminoma, adult type EC, and choriocarcinoma can exist in pure form but are more often part of a mixed tumour.

If the tumour is a dysgerminoma and there is evidence of a preceding gonadoblastoma, then there is gonadal dysgenesis and the other ovary must be assessed and removed because of the risk of bilateral GCT. Occasionally dysgerminoma is bilateral even in the absence of gonadal dysgenesis.

Testis

All testicular GCT should be excised by high inguinal orchidectomy and if a biopsy is performed it should not be transcrotal as that immediately raises the staging of a malignant GCT to stage 2. If the tumour is present within 0.5 mm of the transected spermatic cord margin, then it is stage 2. The tumour should be sampled at 1 block/cm and the relationship of the tumour to the tunica and epididymis be documented. Older children should have 2 blocks of testis adjacent to the tumour sampled to determine the presence of ITGCN. This staging system is current in the United States (37). The staging is presented in Table 14.2.

Pure YST is the most common, usually presents early, and is almost always stage 1. This is the most likely explanation for their excellent prognosis. The peak age is under 4 years. From puberty onwards the pattern of testicular malignancy is that of the young adult, that is, mixed malignant tumours with very occasional pure seminomas. ITGCN is usually found in this age group an indicator of their shared aetiology with adult testicular cancer. We have seen a 14-year-old boy with undecended testis, ITGCN, and invasive seminoma.

MT is biphasic with a first peak in infancy and a second peak in adolescence and young adult life.

Staging of testicular germ cell tumours
Adults and adolescents

The staging system used by the Intergroup Pediatric GCT protocol is shown in Tables 14.2. Retroperitoneal node examination is now not used in the United Kingdom, being superseded by using elevation of tumour markers after orchidectomy as an indicator of residual disease.

Infants

These are biologically different from the above, as they lack i(12p). They are usually YST, MT, or IT. Seminomas do not occur in this age group. Over 80% are stage 1 at diagnosis and do well with orchidectomy and follow-up.

Table 14.7 Distribution according to age and tumour type (1)

Site	Relative incidence (%)	Age	Pathology
Sacrococcyx	35	Neonate	Teratoma: mature 65% Teratoma: immature 5% Malignant (usually yolk sac) 10–30%
Ovary	25	Early teens	Teratoma: mature 65% Teratoma: immature 5% Malignant (usually yolk sac) 30%
Testis	20	Infant and adolescent	Teratoma: mature 20% Malignant 80% (infants—pure yolk sac, adolescents—mixed, occasionally seminoma)
Cranium	5	Child	Teratoma: mature 20–30% Germinoma 20–50%, yolk sac 20–50%
Mediastinum	5	Adolescent	Teratoma: mature 60% Malignant (mixed or pure yolk sac) 40%
Retroperitoneum	5	Infant	Teratoma: mature or immature (occasionally yolk sac)
Head and neck	3	Neonate and infant	Usually mature, occasionally immature, rarely Malignant
Vagina	2	Infant	Usually yolk sac, retroperitoneal

Extragonadal sites

Sacrococcygeal tumours. Overall about 40–60% of tumours occur in this region (52). In neonates they are even more common (80%), especially in females (m:f = 3:1). There is an association with malformations of the sacrum and genitourinary tract. Prenatally they may present with polyhydramnios or be discovered incidently on ultrasound. Intrapartum or neonatal death can result from obstruction of labour or torrential haemorrhage following avulsion. The tumour may be postsacral, presacral, or combined. Those with a postsacral element present earlier and this probably accounts for their better outlook. The frequency of the histological types is shown in Table 14.7. Because they are not encapsulated and may be inaccessible particularly if presacral, they can re-grow (20% in one series). Residual teratoma carries a risk of developing YST (as high as 35%), so complete excision and coccygectomy is required. The pathologist should identify the coccyx and ascertain the adequacy of the excision margins using marker ink. Careful search for YST element is imperative particularly in a high grade IT and a minimum of 10 blocks (42) is recommended. As noted previously natural elevation of serum AFP in early infancy makes this a less useful marker for the presence of YST. YST of the sacrococcyx may be pure or arise within a teratoma. Some are diagnosed de novo, others arise as recurrences following an incompletely excised sacrococcygeal teratoma. Alternatively review of the teratoma may show foci of YST. If presacral they may present late and sometimes only when they produce metastatic disease. We have seen two infants present with pathological bone fractures due to metastases from an unsuspected presacral YST. Both children are alive many years later following repeated salvage chemotherapy.

Mediastinum. The most frequent thoracic site is the anterior mediastinum (7% of all childhood GCT). The frequency is spread equally from birth to adolescence with no gender bias, although males with KS are at increased risk (in the prepubertal male KS can be subtle and the diagnosis overlooked). Most are MT and usually present with respiratory obstruction, infrequently with the effects of hormone secretion from mature endocrine elements, for example, hypoglycaemia, precocious puberty. Mediastinal tumours of childhood are unusual in that they predispose to blood dyscrasias including leukaemia (see above).

Because of their site, excision is hazardous especially if malignant. If there is significant elevation of any of the tumour markers pre-operative chemotherapy is often the safest course. When excision is carried out resection margin assessment is important.

Pericardium and *heart* are rare sites, almost limited to the neonatal period. The tumours are generally IT or MT and because of their position require urgent surgery. *Lung* is another rare site.

Retroperitoneum. GCT are usually found in children under 2 years of age. Unlike sacrococcygeal tumours those in the retroperitoneum are usually IT. They must be particularly carefully searched for YST because complete resection in this site can be difficult. Some retroperitoneal MGCT may be metastatic from an unknown primary. Occasionally they have a very immature blastematous pattern or a primitive embryonal cell type suggesting extrarenal Wilms' or a PNET. We have had a trucut biopsy from a presacral mass thought to be an IT, which showed immature neuroblastoma—like tissue. On excision the tumour was a typical neuroblastoma which demonstrated n-myc amplification.

Stomach. These are rare and generally occur in infants. The histology is of MT and if excised prognosis is good. According to Dehner (42) a malignant childhood GCT of stomach has yet to be described.

Liver and kidney. These are extremely rare sites and teratoma must be distinguished from hepatoblastoma and nephroblastoma. Using strict criteria (42), there should be a range of somatic components without any hepatoblastomatous or nephroblastomatous tissues included. The presence of these elements would suggest that the correct diagnosis be 'teratoid hepatoblastoma' or 'teratoid nephroblastoma.'

Lower genital tract. YST occur rarely in the infantile uterus and vagina.

Head and neck

Nasopharynx, mouth, orbit, and *cervico-thyroid* are well reported and are frequently congenital. A particular example being the 'epignathus', which arises in basicranial region to protrude through the midline of the palate and fills the mouth. It is usually an IT and if excised the outlook is good, but if very large it can obstruct breathing and cause death. The so-called 'hairy polyp' of the newborn palate often is reported as a teratoma, but is actually a choristoma with no malignant potential (42).

Central nervous system

Germ cell tumours in this site account for 5% of all childhood cases. They almost always occur in the midline structures of the CNS particularly in the pineal or suprasellar regions. They tend to present at puberty and show distinct site related gender differences: pineal gland tumours are more common in boys and the suprasellar region rather more common in girls. The histological classification used in other sites can be applied. Malignant GCT are more common, with the most frequent being pure germinoma, followed by teratoma, mature and immature and YST, pure or part of a mixed GCT.

Germinomas usually present in the pure form in pubertal males especially in the pineal gland. They are more common in the Far East and in males with chromosomal abnormality. Some may show such a prominent lymphocytic or granulomatous reaction that diagnosis is difficult. YST occur predominantly in young children and favour the pineal gland.

Teratomas, both mature and immature, occur in the CNS and are much more common in children than in adults. An overall male predominance is present. They can occur in neonates and we have seen a baby with prenatal hydrocephalus so gross as to obstruct labour and result in stillbirth. The cause turned out to be a large unsuspected suprasellar MT. It is important to identify high grade IT as in the CNS they appear to be more aggressive and prone to recurrence. Therapy for germinomas and non-germinomas in the CNS is similar.

Treatment

Prior to any treatment, *all* paediatric tumours, including those not thought to be GCT, should have the serum levels of the common tumour markers established. The standard serum tumour markers for GCT are AFP, HCG, and LDH (non-specific). Serum PLAP is very rarely relevant in paediatric practice. The usefulness is twofold: it is helpful to the pathologist with a difficult case and it is essential to the oncologist when interpreting the pathologist's diagnosis and when deciding on the appropriate treatment.

Pre-treatment biopsy; fine needle aspirate

If the serum markers are not raised and the tumour is stage 1, then a needle biopsy might be justified to establish the diagnosis. Prior to the biopsy other factors must be considered: the biopsy may not produce representative tissue and if the tumour is malignant, then upstaging could result. Fine needle aspirate is another possibility. Surgery is the treatment of choice in stage 1 and even in stage 2. In stage 3 some oncologists especially in North America would accept that surgical de-bulking has value. After surgical removal the appropriate serum markers should be checked allowing for their half-life, so that the excision is proven to be complete. Even after apparently complete excision of a benign teratoma serum markers should be monitored for several years. Because in 'good prognosis' patients the survival rate is over 90%, the aim of the new treatment trials is to reduce toxicity while maintaining efficacy. In contrast, in 'poor prognosis' patients survival can be as low as 50%, so the goal is to increase efficacy.

Tjan- Heijnen *et al.* (53) have produced an excellent overview of current worldwide treatment protocols for adult GCT. They advocate basing future treatment protocols on the internationally agreed classification of GCT (Table 14.3). This may eventually be adopted for use in children.

In a recent UK review by Mann *et al.* (54) 184 children with extracranial MGCT of whom 47 were treated by surgery alone and 137 received chemotherapy the overall 5-year survival was 93.2% and for those requiring chemotherapy it was 90.9%. These excellent results demonstrate the exquisite sensitivity of GCT to modern chemotherapy, which in this series comprised carboplatin, etopiside, and bleomycin. The protocol followed was to treat MT and IT by surgery alone, but to follow up with serum levels of AFP and/or ultrasound examination. If YST developed chemotherapy was given. Even if pre-treatment histology suggested an MT or IT, if the serum AFP was raised, then chemotherapy was started on the assumption that a focus of YST existed, which had not been detected by the pathologist.

Stage 1 malignant tumours were treated by complete surgical removal with a watch and wait policy and monitoring clinically and with scanning and serum AFP levels. Recurrences were treated by chemotherapy. All but one patient with stage 1 had a tissue diagnosis before treatment. In this solitary case the AFP level was so high and the child's condition so poor that chemotherapy was immediately instituted and the residual chemotherapeutically retroverted teratomatous tissue resected. A similar approach is advised in surgically inaccessible mediastinal or retroperitoneal YST. All stage 2 and stage 3 tumours had chemotherapy. The high cure rates are encouraging but continuing efforts are being made to reduce side-effects. Many of the complications of earlier treatments were due to radiotherapy, which is no longer used in the United Kingdom except for intracranial tumours.

The response to platinum based therapy has been dramatic, but recently there have been reports (55) of the emergence of late relapses (LR) from 2 to 32 years after the primary GCT. The majority of LR were also GCT, but were relatively refractory to chemotherapy. Twenty percent were malignant non-GCT.

Although there is much yet to understand about the pathogenesis of GCT, their response to modern chemotherapy is so gratifyingly successful that they are now regarded as being amongst the most favourable of childhood malignancies. Nonetheless long-term follow-up remains necessary even after an apparent cure.

References

1. Pinkerton CR. Malignant germ cell tumours in childhood. European Journal of Cancer 1997, 33, 895–902.
2. Hawkins EP, Perlman EJ. Germ cell tumors. In: Pediatric neoplasia: morphology and biology (ed. DM Parham). Lippincott-Raven, Philadeldpia, 1996, 297–330.
3. Hawkins EP. Pathology of germ cell tumors in children. Crit Rev Oncol-Hematol 1990, 10, 165–79.
4. Muir KR, Parkes SE, Lawson S, Thomas AK, Cameron AH, Mann JR. Changing incidence and geographical distribution of malignant paediatric germ cell tumours in the West Midlands Health Authority region, 1957–1992. Br J Cancer 1995, 72, 219–23.
5. Skakkebaek NE, Rajpert-De Meyts E, Jorgensen N, Carlsen E, Petersen PM, Giwercman A, Andersen AG, Jensen JK, Andersson AM, Muller J. Germ cell cancer and disorders of spermatogenesis: an environmental connection? APMIS 1998, 106, 3–12.
6. Birch JM, Marsden HB, Swindell R. Prenatal factors in the origin of germ cell tumours of childhood. Carcinogenesis 1982, 3, 75–80.
7. Mann JR, Stiller CA. Changing patterns of incidence and survival in children with germ cell tumours (GCTs). Adv Biosci 1994, 91, 59–64.
8. Moul JW, Schanne FJ, Thompson IM, Frazier HA, Peretsman SA, Wettlaufer JN, Rozanski TA, Stack RS, Kreder KJ, Hoffman KJ. Testicular cancer in blacks. A multicenter experience. Cancer 1994, 73, 388–93.
9. Parkin DM, Iscovich J. Risk of cancer in migrants and their descendants in Israel: 11. Carcinomas and germ cell tumours. Int J Cancer 1997, 70, 654–60.
10. Powell JE, Parkes SE, Cameron AH, Mann JR. Is the risk of cancer increased in Asians in the UK? Archives of Diseases of Childhood 1994, 71, 398–403.
11. Moller H, Prener A, Skakkebaek NE. Testicular cancer, cryptorchidism, inguinal hernia, testicular atrophy and genital malformations: case-control studies in Denmark. Cancer Causes and Control 1996, 7, 264–74.
12. Braun DL, Green MD, Rausen AR, David R, Wolman SR, Greco MA, Muggia FM. Down's syndrome and testicular cancer: a possible association. Am J Pediatr Hematol Oncol 1985, 27, 208–10.
13. Bale PM. Sacrococcygeal abnormalities and tumors in children. Perspect Pediatr Pathol 1984, 8, 9–56.
14. Hasle H, Mellengaard A, Nielsen J, Hansen J. Cancer incidence in men with Klinefelter's syndrome. Br J Cancer 1995, 71, 416–20.
15. Huddart RA, Thompson CM, Houlston R, Nicholls EJ, Horwich A. Familial predisposition to both male and female germ cell tumours? (letter) J Med Genet 1996, 33, 86.
16. Ladanyi M, Samaniego F, Reuter VE, Motzer RJ, Jhamvar SC, Bosl GJ. Cytogenetic and immunohistochemical evidence for the germ cell origin of a subset of acute leukemias associated with mediastinal germ cell tumors. J Nat Cancer Inst 1990, 82, 221–7.
17. Chariot P, Monnet I, Gaulard P, Abd-Alsamad I, Ruffie P, De Cremoux H. Systemic mastocytosis following mediastinal germ cell tumor: an association confirmed. Hum Pathol 1993, 24, 111–12.
18. Levasseur P, Reynard J, Paquet J, Darteville P. Acute autoimmune hemolytic anemia and mediastinal mature teratoma in a 6-year-old child: excision and cure of the anemia. Ann Chir 1988, 42, 170–2.
19. Fisch H, Golubhoff ET, Olson JH, Feldshuh J, Broder SJ, Barad DH. Semen analysis in 1283 men from the United States over a 25 year period: no decline in quality. Fertil Steril 1996, 65, 1009–14.
20. Vierula M, Niemi M, Keiski A, Saaranen M, Saariskoski S, Suominen J. High and unchanged sperm counts of Finnish men. Int J Androl 1996, 19, 11–17.
21. Toppari J, Larsen JC, Christiansen P, Giwercman A, Grandjean P, Guillette LJ, Jegou B. Male reproductive health and environmental xenoestrogens. Env Health Perspect 1996, 104, 741–803.
22. Chaganti RSK, Houldsworth J. The cytogenetic theory of the pathogenesis of human adult male germ cell tumours. A review article. APMIS 1998, 106, 80–4.
23. Chaganti RSK, Rodriguez E, Mathew S. Origin of adult male mediastinal germ cell tumours. The Lancet 1994, 45, 1130–2.
24. Rajpert-De Meyts E, Jorgensen N, Brondum-Nielsen K, Muller J, Skakkebaek NE. Developmental arrest of germ cells in the pathogenesis of germ cell neoplasia. APMIS 1998, 106, 198–206.
25. Rajpert-De Meyts E, Kvist M, Skakkebaek, NE. Heterogeneity of expression of immunohistochemical tumour markers in testicular carcinoma-in-situ: pathogenetic evidence. Virchows Arch 1996, 428, 133–9.
26. Matsui Y, Zsebo K, Hogan BML. Derivation of pluripotential stem cells from murine primordial germ cells in culture. Cell 1992, 70, 841–7.
27. Looijenga LHJ, Oosterhuis JW. Pathogenesis of testicular germ cell tumours. Rev Reprod 1999, 4, 90–100.
28. Ramani P, Yeung CK, Habeebu SSM. Testicular intertubular neoplasia in adolescents and children with intersex. Am J Surg Pathol 1993, 17, 1124–33.
29. Jorgensen N, Muller J, Giwercman A, Visfeldt J, Moller H, Skakkebaek NE. DNA content in germ cells adjacent to germ cell tumours in childhood: probably a different origin for infantile and adolescent germ cell tumours. J Pathol 1995, 176, 269–78.
30. dal Cin P, Drochmans A, Moerman P, Van den Berghe H. Isochrome 12p in mediastinal germ cell tumor. Cancer Genet Cytogenet 1989, 42, 243–51.

31. Surti U, Hoffner L, Chakravarti A, Ferrell RE. Genetics and biology of human ovarian teratomas. 1. Cytogenetic analysis and mechanism of origin. Am J Hum Genet 1990, **47**, 635–43.
32. Hoffner L, Deka R, Chakravarti, A, Surti U. Cytogenetics and the origin of pediatric germ cell tumors. Cancer Genet Cytogenet 1994, **74**, 54–8.
33. Herrmann ME, Thompson K, Wojcik EM, Martinez R, Husain AN. Congenital sacrococcygeal teratoma: effect of gestational age on size, morphologic pattern, ploidy, p53 ret expression. Pediatr Dev Pathol 2000, **3**, 240–8.
34. Voss AM, Oosterhuis JW, de Jong B, Buist J, Koops HS. Cytogenetics of carcinoma-in-situ of the testis. Cancer Genet Cytogenet 1990, **46**, 75–81.
35. Bosl GJ, Dmitrovsky E, Reuter VE, Samaniego F, Rodriguez E, Geller NL, Chaganti RS. Isochromosome of chromosome12: clinically useful marker for male germ cell tumors. J Nat Cancer Inst 1989, **81**, 1874–8.
36. Perlman EJ, Cushing B, Hawkins E, Griffin CA. Cytogenetic anlysis of childhood endodermal sinus tumors: a Pediatric Oncology Group study. Pediatr Pathol 1994, **14**, 695–708.
37. Perlman EJ, Hawkins EP. Pediatric germ cell tumors: protocol update for pathologists. Pediatr Dev Pathol 1998, **1**, 328–35.
38. Newlands ES, Bagshawe KD, Begent RHJ, *et al.* Current optimum management of anaplastic germ cell tumours of the testis and other sites. Br J Urol 1986, **58**, 307–14.
39. Bosl GJ, Geller NL, Cirrincoine C, Vogelzang NJ, Kennedy BJ, Witmore WF, Vugrin D, Scher H, Nisselbaum J, Golbey RB. Multivariate analysis of prognostic variables in patients with metastatic testicular cancer. Cancer Res 1983, **43**, 3403–7.
40. International Germ Cell Cancer Collaborative Group (IGCCCG). The international Germ Cell Classification: a prognostic factor-based staging system for metastatic germ cell cancer. J Clin Oncol 1997, **15**, 594–603.
41. Norris HJ, Zirkin HJ, Benson WL. Immature (malignant) teratoma of the ovary: a clinical and pathological study of 58 cases. Cancer 1976, **37**, 2359–72.
42. Dehner LP. Gonadal and extragonadal germ cell neoplasms: teratomas in childhood. In: Pathology of neoplasms in children and adolescents (ed. M Finegold, JL Pennington). W B Saunders, Philadelphia, 1986, 282–312.
43. Tsuchida Y, Endo Y, Saito S. Evaluation of alpha-fetoprotein in early infancy. J Pediatr Surg 1978, **13**, 155–6.
44. Heifetz SA, Cushing B, Giller R, Shuster JJ, Stolar CJH, Vinocur CD, Hawkins EP. Immature teratomas in children: pathologic considerations. A report from the combined Pediatric Oncology Group/ Children's Cancer Group. Am J Surg Pathol 1998, **22**, 1115–24.
45. Thurlbeck WM, Scully RE. Solid teratoma of the ovary: a clinico-pathologic analysis of nine cases. Cancer 1960, **13**, 804–11.
46. Joshi VV. Classification and grading of teratomas in children. In: Common problems in pediatric pathology. Igaku-Shoin, New York, 1994, 333–57.
47. Michael H, Hull MT, Foster RS, Sweeney CJ, Ulbright TM. Nephroblastoma-like tumors in patients with testicular germ cell tumors. Am J Surg Pathol 1998, **22**, 1107–14.
48. Van Echten J, van der Vloedt WS, van de Pol M, Dam A, te Meerman GJ, Schraffordt Koops H, Sliejfer DT, de Jong B. Comparison of the chromosomal pattern of primary testicular nonseminomas and residual mature teratomas after chemotherapy. Cancer Genet Cytogenet 1997, **99**, 59–67.
49. Marsden HB, Birch JM, Swindell R. Germ cell tumours of childhood: a review of 137 cases. J Clin Pathol 1981, **34**, 879–83.
50. Bale PM, Painter DM, Cohen D. Teratomas in childhood. Pathology 1975, **7**, 209–18.
51. Berry CL, Keeling JW, Hilton C. Teratomata in infancy and childhood: a review of 91 cases. J Pathol 1969, **98**, 241–52.
52. Gonzalez-Crussi F, Winkler RF, Mirkin DL. Sacrococcygeal teratomas in infants and children. Relationship of histology and prognosis. Arch Pathol Lab Med 1978, **102**, 420–5.
53. Tran-Heijnen VCG, Oosterhof GDN, De Wit R, De Mulder PHM. Treatment in germ cell tumours: state of the art. Eur J Surg Oncol 1997, **23**, 110–22.
54. Mann JR, Raafat F, Robinson K., Imeson J, Gornall P, Phillips M, Sokal M, Gray E, McKeever P, Oakhill A. UKCCSG germ cell tumour (GCT) studies: improving outcome for children with malignant extracranial non-gonadal tumours—carboplatin, etopiside, and bleomycin are effective and less toxic than previous regimens. Med Pediatr Oncol 1998, **30**, 217–27.
55. Michael H, Lucia J, Foster RS, Ulbright TM. The pathology of late recurrence of testicular germ cell tumors. Am J Surg Pathol 2000, **24**, 257–73.

15 | Liver tumors

Milton J. Finegold

Incidence and epidemiology

The 1988 International Agency for Research on Cancer survey of childhood cancer in 50 countries during the 1970s revealed an incidence of liver cancer that ranged from 0.4 per million children aged 0–14 years in France and Jamaica to about 4.0 in Hong Kong, Shanghai, Taiwan, and Fiji (1). This 10-fold difference reflects the high carrier rate for Hepatitis B virus (HBV) in the latter countries, leading to hepatocarcinoma. The rate for hepatocarcinoma ranged from 0.1 per million in Manchester, England, New York City Whites and Puerto Rico to 2.1 in Hong Kong and Japan. For hepatoblastoma, which has no association with HBV infection (however, see Fig. 15.1), the range of incidence was 0.3–0.4 in Osaka and Manchester (from 1954 to 1970) to 1.0 in the United States to 2.6 among males in Slovenia.

During the period 1971–83, the West Midlands Regional Children's Tumor Registry in Manchester observed an increased incidence of hepatoblastoma from 0.4 to 1.0 per million (1). This change might be explained by Ikeda's observation in Japan that hepatoblastomas account for 58% of all malignancies occurring in surviving premature infants who weighed less than 1000 g at birth (2). Further analysis of the Japanese Children's Cancer Registry data revealed that 15 of 303 (5%) hepatoblastomas between 1985 and 1995 occurred in post-premature infants weighing less than 1500 g (3). This rate was greater than 10× that for all live borns. The relative risk for hepatoblastoma for children who weighed less than 1000 g at birth was 15.64 versus 2.53 for those 1000–1499 g versus 1.21 for 2000–2499 g (4). Of 77 children with hepatoblastoma in the German registry (5), 3 (4%) were prematures who required parenteral nutrition, a treatment that has been life-saving for many small prematures but has been reported to lead to cirrhosis in many survivors and in two cases to hepatocarcinoma (6, 7). It has not previously been associated with hepatoblastoma.

Of 15 children with hepatoblastoma at the Children's Hospital of Michigan from 1988 to 1998, 6 (40%) occurred in premature infants born at 26–36 weeks of gestation (8). Another 26-week premature developed hepatocarcinoma 9 years later. The US National Cancer Institute Surveillance, Epidemiology and End-Result (SEER) program includes approximately 14% of the population and it revealed an average annual percent increase in the incidence of hepatoblastoma from 1973 to 1992 of 5.2 (9). Interestingly this was particularly true for females, contrary to the usual ratio of hepatoblastomas in males being 2.4 to 1 (10) (Table 15.1). The Children's Cancer Group, prompted by Ikeda's report, found that 13.9% of 72 patients with hepatoblastoma in their series for whom birth weights were recorded were premature (11). Ten of the eighteen patients weighed less than 1000 g at birth. Thus, there was a 16- to 23-fold excess of extreme prematures in the hepatoblastoma population.

The SEER data has also revealed a significant increase in the incidence of hepatocellular carcinoma in the period 1991–95 (2.4 per 100,000 persons) versus 1976–80 (1.4) (12). This increase was greatest in the 40–60-year-old population and represented a 70% increase in White males and 50% increase in Black males. Twenty-three percent of cases occurred in other ethnic groups, including many immigrants. There was no breakdown of cases in childhood in this report.

Etiology

The causes of hepatocellular neoplasms are, with a few exceptions, still mysterious despite many well-documented associations (reviewed in Weinberg and Finegold 1983) (13). The clearest pathogenetic factor is HBV, which has induced hepatocarcinoma in the sons of chronic carrier mothers in Asia in as little as

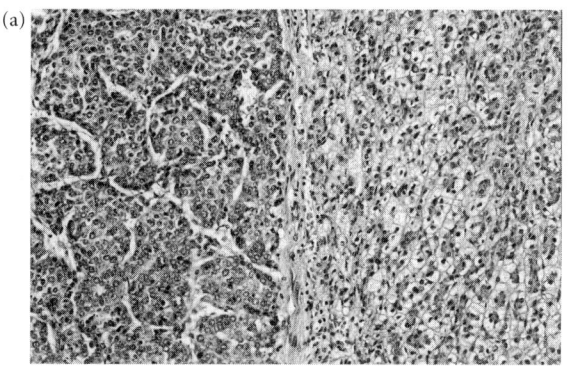 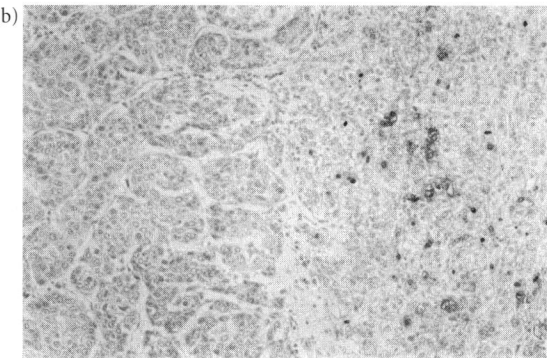

Fig. 15.1 (a) Hepatocarcinoma and hepatoblastoma side-by-side in a 15-year-old boy from Asia with perinatally acquired Hepatitis B infection. (b) Hepatitis B core antigen (black deposits in nuclei) is abundant in fetal hepatoblastoma cells, absent from the carcinoma. Surface antigen was demonstrable only in non-neoplastic hepatocytes, which rarely contained Hbcore Ag as well.

Table 15.1 Hepatoblastomas. Pediatric Oncology Group—1986–95 (10 years)

Age	
0–6 months	28
6–12 months	49
1–2 years	52
>5 year	8
Gender	
Males	111
Females	67
Treatment	
Primary resection	69
Resection after chemo	45
Biopsy only	55
Other features	
FAP	3 males 1 female
BWS	2 females
Umbilical hernia	1 female
Fetal hydantoin syndrome	1
Prematurity, hypothyroidism	1
Precocious puberty/virilization	2
Hypercholesterolemia	2

4 years (14). With vaccination at birth, the incidence of hepatocarcinoma in childhood in Taiwan has decreased 50% from 1981–86 to 1990–94 (15). Vaccination obviously will have enormous benefit in eradicating the chronic carrier state and preventing carcinoma in adults. Hepatitis C virus is now responsible for the majority of hepatocarcinomas in Japan and other countries with excellent public health programs. Unlike Hepatitis B, it has not been responsible for childhood hepatocarcinoma, because it appears to act via chronic inflammation with repeated episodes of injury and regeneration providing for accumulation of somatic mutations. When hepatitis B infection is acquired after the perinatal period, it also takes 20 or more years to be carcinogenic but in the very young, whose livers are growing rapidly, it is capable of integrating into host DNA and producing neoplasia very quickly (14). Integration sites for HBV-DNA vary considerably but some of them involve human loci that may be relevant to the process of carcinogenesis, such as Cyclin A (16, 17). Mutations in the viral genome itself may be important in carcinogenesis in adults (18); this has not been evaluated in children. Among the data of great interest emerging from studies of mice carrying Hepatitis B surface antigen genes is the observation that the p-glycoprotein MDR3/MDR1, a gene responsible for drug resistance, is activated (19). The role of aflatoxin in causing mutations of p53 will be discussed in the section on molecular genetics.

The particularly vulnerability of male children to get hepatocellular neoplasms remains an enigma (20). It is true not only for perinatally acquired HBV infection but also for hepatocarcinomas arising in children with autosomal recessive disease, such as glycogen storage disease type 1 (21) and for hepatoblastomas in families with familial polyposis (22). A partial explanation from studies of experimental carcinogenesis is that only male mice expressing the TGF α gene develop hepatocarcinoma (23). TGF α is a strong stimulus to hepatocyte replication and normally is expressed much more in younger individuals (24). TGF α is produced by more than 65% of hepatocarcinomas, providing for autocrine stimulation (25). It is also expressed strongly in fetal hepatoblastoma cells that have low proliferative activity (26), supporting a paracrine role for this molecule. Disruption of the pRB/E2F pathway and inhibition of apoptosis were observed in TGFα and c-myc transgenic mice (27).

The role of sex steroids in hepatocellular neoplasms is well known, primarily because of the frequent development of the previously rare adenoma in women taking early oral contraceptives containing large quantities of estrogen. One study found fibrolamellar carcinoma in two young women exposed to estrogens (28) but this has not been observed subsequently. However, endogenous abnormalities in sex hormone metabolism may also contribute, as observed in two boys age 15 and $17\frac{1}{2}$ with failure to enter puberty and gynecomastia who developed fibrolamellar carcinomas having high levels of aromatase in the tumor (29, 30). Exogenous androgens are also implicated, especially in patients with Fanconi's anemia, most of whom have had benign adenomas but hepatocellular carcinomas have also been observed (31–33).

Several chronic cholestatic syndromes have been precursors to hepatocarcinoma, including long-term use of parenteral nutrition (vide supra), and extra-hepatic biliary atresia. Of 109 orthotopic liver transplants in children reported from France, 3 had hepatocarcinoma, one of whom had extrahepatic biliary atresia and another Byler syndrome (34). Adenomatous hyperplasia, which may be a pre-neoplastic lesion, was observed in 11 more biliary atresia livers out of 80 cases (14%). The genetic basis for neonatal "giant cell" hepatitis (35, 36) and other chronic cholestatic syndromes associated with carcinoma (37) is becoming better defined by progress in molecular genetics (see section below and Table 15.2).

Table 15.2 Constitutional genetic disease leading to liver tumors*

Disease	Tumor type	Chromosome location	Gene	Reference
Familial adenomatous polyposis	Hepatoblastoma, adenoma hepatocarcinoma, biliary adenoma	5q21.22	APC	(22, 45–49)
BWS	Hepatoblastoma Hemangioendothelioma	11p15.5	p57KIP2 others	(50–52)
Li–Fraumeni syndrome	Hepatoblastoma Undifferentiated sarcoma	17p13	P53, others	(53, 54)
Trisomy 18	Hepatoblastoma	18		(55, 56)
Glycogen storage disease type I	Hepatocellular adenoma, carcinoma, hepatoblastoma	17	Glucose-6-phosphatase	(39, 40)
Hereditary tyrosinemia	Hepatocarcinoma	15q23-25	Fumarylacetoacetate hydrolase	(57)
Alagille syndrome	Hepatocarcinoma	20p12	Jagged-1	(58, 59)
Other familial cholestatic syndromes	Hepatocarcinoma	? 18q21-22 ? 2q24		(60–62)
Neurofibromatosis	Hepatocarcinoma Malignant Schwannoma Angiosarcoma	17q11.2	NF-1	(63–66)
Ataxia-telangiectasia	Hepatocellular carcinoma	11q22-23	ATM	(67, 68)
Fanconi anemia	Hepatocarcinoma, fibrolamellar CA adenoma	1q42,3p, 20q13.2-13.3, others	FAA, FAC, others (20%)	(31, 32, 69, 70)
Tuberous sclerosis	Angiomyolipoma	9q34 16p13	TSC 1 TSC 2	(71, 72)

* α-1-antitrypsin deficiency and hereditary hemochromatosis are not listed because hepatocarcinomas do not occur until adulthood. One 15-year-old with Wilson's disease had HCC discovered when transplanted (73). One 11-month-old with glycogen storage disease type 4 (brancher enzyme deficiency) had a hepatocellular adenoma discovered after transplantation (41). Five families with autosomal dominant transmission of infantile hemangiomas have shown linkage to 5q 31-33. Three candidate genes involved in blood vessel growth are mapped to this region; fibroblast growth factor receptor, platelet-derived growth factor receptor beta, and fms-related tyrosine-kinase-4 (74). No sporadic tumors have been reported yet with mutations in this region.

However, the carcinomas in these cases have not been included in the many molecular and cytogenetic studies of hepatocarcinoma described below.

Hepatocarcinoma has also occurred with high frequency in children with hereditary tyrosinemia type 1 (fumarylacetoacetate hydrolase deficiency) but treatment with a chemical that can block an enzyme upstream in the catabolic pathway (4-hydroxydioxygenase) prevents the accumulation of toxic metabolites and both the acute liver failure and carcinogenesis in almost every treated patient (38). The other metabolic disease responsible for hepatocellular neoplasia is glycogen storage disease type 1, which has been responsible for adenomas most often but on rare occasions for focal nodular hyperplasia and occasionally for hepatocarcinoma in adolescents and young adult males (21, 39). Two siblings with GSD 1A, aged 12 and 19, developed hepatoblastoma (40). Both patients had multiple tumors, at least one of which was an adenoma. Interestingly, neither patient had increased serum alpha-fetoprotein (α-FP). Recently a hepato carcinoma was found in a case of brancher enzyme deficiency (Type IV GSD) (41).

Several constitutional genetic abnormalities are associated with hepatocellular neoplasia, including the Beckwith–Wiedemann syndrome (BWS), familial adenomatous polyposis and Trisomy 18 (Table 15.2) (10). In addition, occasional patients have had umbilical hernia, undescended testes, renal dysplasia, agenesis of the gallbladder, or other minor malformations (42). Environmental or drug exposure has been evaluated by the Children's Cancer Group (43). Seventy-five sets of parents of children with hepatoblastoma were compared with those of age-matched controls and there was a significant excess of maternal exposure before and during pregnancy to metals used in welding and soldering, lubricating oils, and protective greases. Paternal exposure to metals was also greater. A congenital hepatoblastoma was found in a stillborn fetus at 23 weeks whose mother was an artist exposed to volatile hydrocarbons (44).

Classification

There is a great diversity among liver tumors, reflecting the several cell types comprising the organ and the differences in genetic and environmental factors leading to excessive and unregulated growth. Malignancies of hepatocytes, which make up 60% of the cells in the fully grown liver and a smaller fraction in the fetus because of the many hematopoietic cells, are the major form of disease. In a survey of 1256 liver tumors compiled from eight series that included all cell types, 43% were hepatoblastomas and 23% hepatocarcinomas (13). *Hepatoblastomas* are themselves highly diverse, ranging from well-differentiated glycogen-rich cells that are almost indistinguishable from those of the normal liver in mid to late gestation to small undifferentiated cells that are never recognized in the developing liver because they are either very rare or short-lived but contain intermediate filaments reflecting both mesenchymal and epithelial gene expression (75). This raises the possibility that they are the malignant form of the putative liver "stem cell" (76, 77). Twenty percent of hepatoblastomas contain mature mesenchymal derivatives, most often osteoid but also cartilage and striated muscle in rare instances. These "mixed" hepatoblastomas (78) support the concept that an undifferentiated stem cell with multipotentiality can become malignant.

Among the *hepatocarcinomas* there is a variant that occurs more often in younger people including children, the *fibrolamellar carcinoma* (79). Unlike typical hepatocarcinomas, there is very rarely evidence of chronic inflammation and cirrhosis, no synthesis of α-FP and production of transcobalamin and neurotensin (80). The latter product suggests a neuroendocrine origin for this tumor, which is supported by some ultrastructural and immunohistochemical studies (81). Primary *carcinoids* of the liver also occur infrequently but they attest to the presence in the liver of neuroendocrine cells (82–84). Such cells are seen in mixed hepatoblastomas, where some of them express chromogranin, serotonin, and somatostatin (85).

The liver of young infants may also develop *germ cell tumors*, either pure yolk sac tumors or teratomas, or rarely as discrete tumors combined with hepatoblastoma (86, 87). This further attests to the presence in the liver of multipotential stem cells and there are many otherwise typical mixed hepatoblastomas that contain ganglion cells, dendritic melanocytes, and cells containing glial fibrillary acidic protein, leading to their designation as "*teratoid*" (Fig. 15.2) (88, 89).

Cholangiocarcinomas are very rare in childhood but a few cases have occurred in patients with biliary tract disease, such as Caroli's and sclerosing cholangitis (60).

The *undifferentiated or embryonal sarcoma*, which accounted for 6% of cases in our compilation, is usually not fully undifferentiated but contains diverse derivatives reflecting a mesenchymal origin, such as fibrosarcomatous, liposarcomatous, pericytomatous, and areas indistinguishable from malignant fibrous histiocytomas (53, 90). However, immunohistochemical evidence of

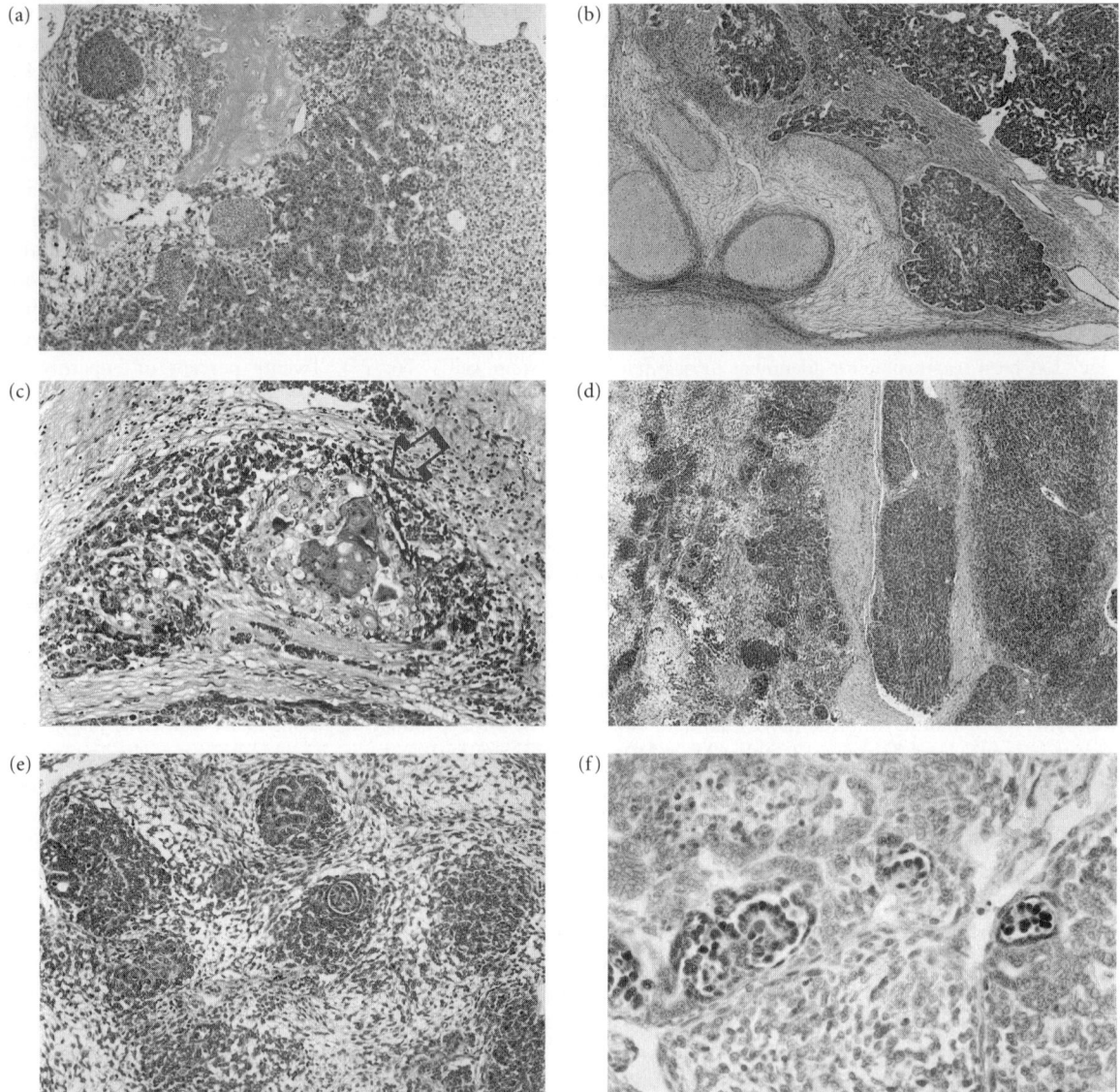

Fig. 15.2 Teratoid hepatoblastoma. (a) Mixed hepatoblastomas are defined as having mesenchymal derivatives in addition to epithelial elements. There is osteoid at the top center, surrounded by diverse epithelial cells. (b) Islands of mature cartilage lie in a background of loose fibrous tissue with adjacent nodules of epithelial cells. (c) A nest of squamous epithelium with central keratinization has melanocytes with long dark processes (arrow). (d) Within the hepatoblastoma a region indistinguishable from Wilms tumor is present on the left side of the low power photomicrograph. (e) The Wilms tumor region contains blastema, tubules, and glomeruli. (f) The epithelial cells of the glomeruli contain the WT-1 protein, as revealed by intense nuclear staining. Blastemal and tubular epithelial cells, as well as the hepatoblastoma were unstained. (This case was referred for POG review by Dr S. Harawi and M. Goldfisher of the Hackensack Hospital, New Jersey. They generously permitted its inclusion in this chapter.)

epithelial cells in some of these tumors (53, 60, 91–95) suggests that it also may arise from the putative "stem cell." The later age of presentation of the sarcomas (Table 15.3) and different cytogenetics in the few examples of each tumor that have been analyzed (Table 15.4) do not support an origin from the small cell undifferentiated component of hepatoblastoma, however. Instead, several examples of sarcoma developing after or together with

Table 15.3 Neoplasia of the liver in children—usual age of presentation

Age	Benign	Malignant
Infancy (0–1 year)	Hemangioendothelioma (HE) Mesenchymal hamartoma (MH) Teratoma	Hepatoblastoma, especially small cell undifferentiated Rhabdoid tumor Yolk sac tumor Langerhans histiocytosis Megaloblastic leukemia Disseminated neuroblastoma
Early childhood (1–3 year)	HE MH Inflammatory pseudotumor (Myofibroblastic)	Hepatoblastoma Rhabdomyosarcoma
Later childhood (3–10 year)	Angiomyolipoma	Angiosarcoma Hepatocarcinoma (HCC) Embryonal (undifferentiated) sarcoma
Adolescence (10–16 year)	Adenoma Biliary cystadenoma	Fibrolamellar HCC Hodgkin's disease/lymphoma leiomyosarcoma

Table 15.4 Cytogenetic abnormalities in pediatric liver tumors other than hepatoblastoma and hepatocarcinoma

Tumor	Patient	Karyotype	Reference
Hemangioendothelioma	6 month—M	del 6q(q21;q27)	(201)
Mesenchymal hamartoma	3 year—M	t(15;19) (q15;q13.4)	(202)
	2 year—F	t(11;19) (q13;q13.4)	(203)
	6 month—M	t(11;19) (q13;q13.4)	(204)
Undifferentiated (embryonal) sarcoma*	6 year—M	Dicentric telomeric association (4;22) (p16;q13) Tricentric fusion 22p;10p del (1) (q32;p35); −2; −20; many others	(205)
	5 year—F	Aneuploidy 61–76; many rearrangements (5 cells); 46XX (11 cells)	(206)
(Arising in mesenchymal hamartoma)	15 year—F	51–55XX +1, +19q13; der(5), t(5;7); −20, many others	(96)
Inflammatory pseudotumor (myofibroblastoma, plasma cell granuloma) (nonhepatic)	2–11 years 5—F 4—M	4/9 Hyperdiploid; low S-phase	(139)

* One of 16 cases reported by Lack et al. 1991 (53) occurred in a child in a Li–Fraumeni family. The tumor was not analyzed for p53 abnormalities.

a benign *mesenchymal hamartoma* have been reported (92, 96–98). The latter tumor, which usually presents in infancy but has been reported in many case reports in adults, consists of proliferating fibroblasts, a myxoid stroma and cysts of bile ducts and it comprised 6% of cases in our compilation. The histology of the mesenchymal hamartomas in cases that were associated with sarcomas concurrently or later, or those that recurred, was not distinguishable from those that resolved or were cured. The cytogenetic findings in mesenchymal hamartomas (Table 15.4) also do not support a relationship to the small undifferentiated cells of hepatoblastoma. Another rare highly malignant neoplasm having features of both mesenchymal and epithelial cells is the *Rhabdoid tumor*, which occurs in young infants (99, 100). Rhabdoid cells have been observed in otherwise typical hepatoblastomas (60). *Rhabdomyosarcomas* associated with the intra and extrahepatic biliary tree occur rarely and in middle years of childhood (10, 101).

Another form of benign mesenchymal hamartoma in the liver of children is the *angiomyolipoma*, which occurs in 24% of mainly female patients with tuberous sclerosis (102). *Angiosarcomas* of the liver in childhood are very infrequent but noteworthy because of their occurrence in five instances in children who had the relatively common (13% of our survey) *hemangioendothelioma* in infancy (60, 103). Nothing unusual was detected histologically in the primary tumor in the cases that later had angiosarcomas.

Benign tumoral proliferation of hepatocytes in children takes two forms, the *adenoma* and *focal nodular hyperplasia*, each of which contributed 2% to our compilation. These differ histologically and in origin, with adenomas being a bland proliferation of hepatocytes and in those patients exposed to estrogens particularly, large telangiectatic vessels, whereas fibronodular hyperplasia consists of proliferation of hepatocytes around a central fibrous scar and is a probable reaction to focal ischemic injury. *Bile duct adenomas* are very infrequent in childhood but cystadenomas may have their origin in mesenchymal hamartomas (13). The benign tumors are well-reviewed in Patterson (104).

Natural history and spread

The usual age of presentation of hepatic neoplasms is shown in Table 15.3. Fifty-six percent of hepatoblastomas are detected in the first year and 20% in the first six months (Table 15.1). Small cell undifferentiated hepatoblastomas and rhabdoid tumors are especially prevalent in young infants and are almost always fatal.

The typical presentation of a hepatic tumor is a palpable mass, regardless of age or cell of origin. Jaundice is infrequent except for Rhabdomyosarcomas and inflammatory pseudotumors (myofibromas). In infants, failure to thrive may precede discovery and pain, vomiting and diarrhea may also be primary manifestations. Occasionally hypercholesterolemia is found in hepatoblastoma patients, especially in infants with fetal histology, and those with higher levels all died (105, 106). Precocious puberty secondary to chorionic gonadotropin or testosterone secretion has been observed in 6% boys with hepatoblastoma (104, 107, 108). Hypercalcemia may be found with hepatocarcinomas. Osteoporosis is observed with both malignancies. Thrombocytosis has been present in 25–65% of patients with hepatoblastoma (104). Congestive heart failure occurs in 15% of patients with hemangioendotheliomas and mesenchymal hamartomas when large vascular channels are present (109). The spread of hepatic neoplasms to the peritoneal cavity occurs when tumors breach the capsule. Metastases to hilar nodes and the lungs are the usual sites of dissemination.

Staging

The US Children's Oncology Group Staging system is shown in Table 15.5. The COG study is also using the SIOPEL pretreatment grouping system for surgical staging (Fig. 15.3) (110, 111).

Histopathological diagnostic features; immunocytochemistry

The histopathology of pediatric liver tumors has been well described and illustrated by Abenoza *et al.* (112), Haas *et al.* (113), Ishak and Glunz (78), Lack *et al.* (53),

Table 15.5 Staging of hepatoblastoma

Stage I "Favorable histology" tumors are those which are completely resected and have a typical histology of a purely fetal histologic pattern with a low mitotic index (<2 per hpf). *(Stratum I)*

Stage I (other histology) are completely resected tumors with a histologic picture other than purely fetal with low mitotic index. *(Stratum 2)*

Stage II tumors are grossly resected tumors with evidence of microscopic residual. Such tumors are rare, and patients with this stage have not fared differently from those with Stage I tumors in previous protocols. Resected tumors with preoperative (intra-operative) rupture are classified as Stage II. *(Stratum 2)*

Stage III (unresectable) tumors are those which are considered by the attending pediatric surgeon to be not resectable without undue risk to the patient. This includes partially resected tumors with measurable tumor left behind. It does not include grossly resected tumors with microscopic disease at the margins, or resected tumors with pre-operative/intra-operative rupture. Lymph node involvement is considered to constitute Stage III disease, and may require evaluation with a second laparotomy after the initial four courses of chemotherapy. *(Stratum 3)*

Stage IV tumors are those which present with measurable metastatic disease to lungs or other organs. *(Stratum 3)*

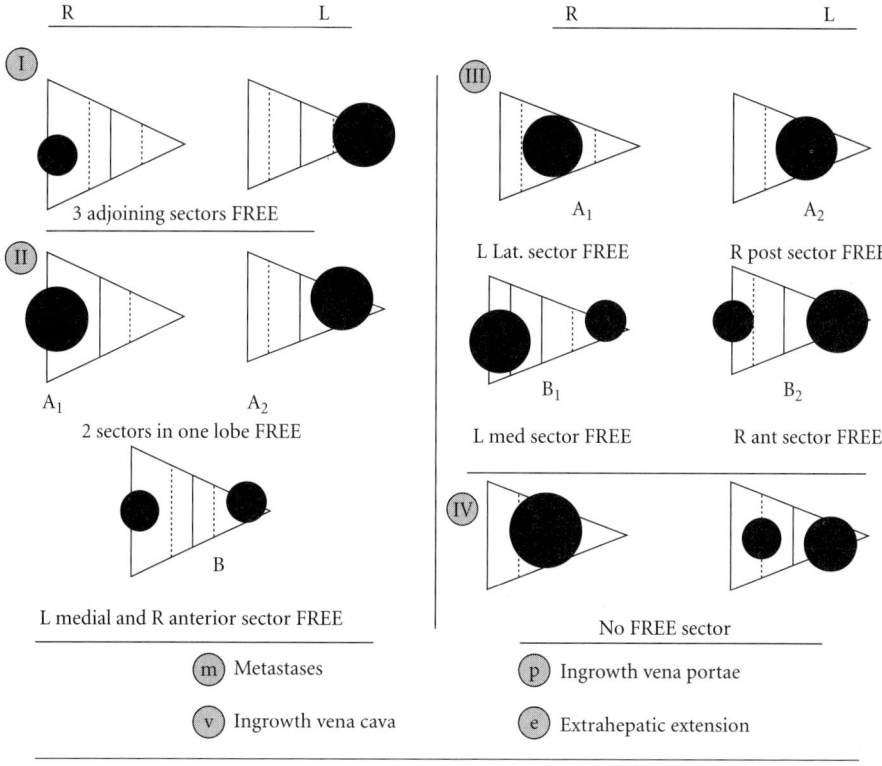

Fig. 15.3 SIOPEL schema for pretreatment evaluation of hepatoblastoma location (111).

Manivel et al. (89), Parham et al. (93, 100) Patterson (104), Ruck et al. (75, 85), Scheimberg et al. (99), Selby et al. (109), and Weinberg and Finegold (60). Therefore, this discussion and the accompanying illustrations are focussed on histologic features that have not been fully appreciated and unusual and instructive cases.

Hepatocarcinomas in children may occur rarely as early as 6 months and several hepatoblastomas have been reported as adults, so it is inappropriate to rely on age to distinguish between them (60). Both histological patterns may occur together, as in Fig. 15.1 from a patient with perinatally acquired Hepatitis B infection. HBV DNA integration was found in a 4-month-old boy's hepatoblastoma (114) but this has not been repeated or confirmed since. However, 7 of 17 hepatoblastomas in adults were associated with chronic hepatitis or cirrhosis (115). The macrotrabecular component of a hepatoblastoma can be indistinguishable from a small cell hepatocarcinoma (Fig. 15.4(d)) and no immunohistochemical stains can differentiate them (116). However, immunostaining for MIB1 has proven useful in predicting the doubling time for small hepatocarcinomas (117). Histochemistry for biliary epithelial Cytokeratin staining was useful in recognizing underlying biliary dysgenesis in a 15-year-old with a typical hepatocarcinoma (Fig. 15.5). When 290 hepatocarcinomas were analyzed for biliary cytokeratins (CK 19, AE1–AE3), 29.3% were positive (118). None of those patients survived more than 27 weeks, versus 22.6% survival of the cytokeratin negative tumors. The positive tumors were more active in DNA synthesis and less well differentiated. Well-differentiated carcinoma displayed positive staining for TGF α in 29/53 small nodules whereas epidermal growth factor receptor was positive in poorly differentiated lesions (119).

The *fibrolamellar carcinoma*, which occurs in late childhood and adolescents as well as young adults, is noteworthy for cytokeratin 8 and 18 positivity, which is consistent with a hepatocytic origin. Some tumors have immunochemical and electron microscopic evidence of neural differentiation (81), which correlates with neurotensin secretion, but even in these cases most of the tumor cells stain and look like hepatocytes. The stroma of fibrolamellar carcinomas is also similar to aggressive forms of ordinary hepatocarcinoma, with large amounts of tenascin and scarce basement membrane

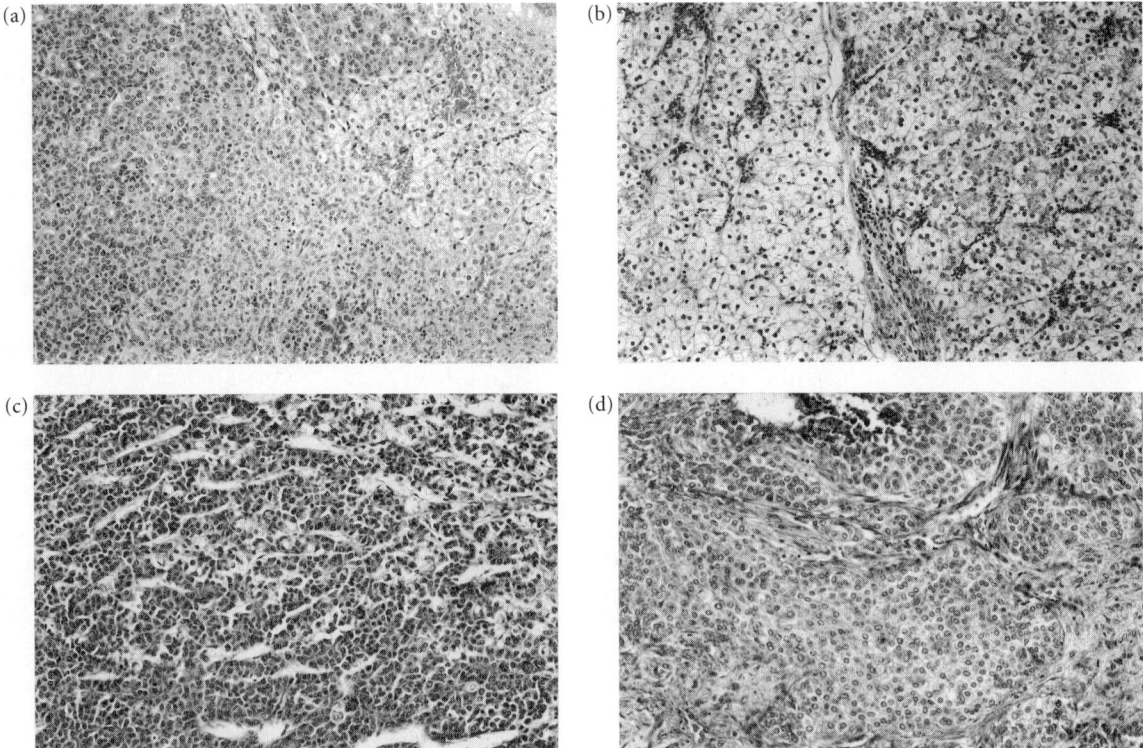

Fig. 15.4 (a) Hepatoblastoma in a 5-month-old girl with BWS and hemihypertrophy. A mixture of epithelial cells having variable degrees of differentiation is observed, with well-differentiated fetal cells on the right, embryonal-type cells on the left, and small undifferentiated or blastemal cells in the center. (b) Well-differentiated fetal epithelium may have clear cytoplasm secondary to abundant glycogen or lipid. It is organized in cords (2 cells thick) as in the developing liver. This tumor arose in a 2-year-old with familial adenomatous polyposis. When mitoses are few, as in this case, prognosis is favorable without chemotherapy in Stage I tumors. (c) Embryonal epithelium from a hepatoblastoma with t1;4 translocation in addition to Trisomy 2, 8, and 20. The small cells form cords and primitive tubules resembling those of the liver at 6–7 weeks gestation. Mitoses are abundant. (d) Macrotrabecular growth pattern in the same hepatoblastoma as (c). Nests of relatively uniform small tumor cells with no sinusoids or cords. This pattern resembles the small cell variant of hepatocarcinoma closely and was initially thought to confer a poor prognosis but that hypothesis has not been sustained.

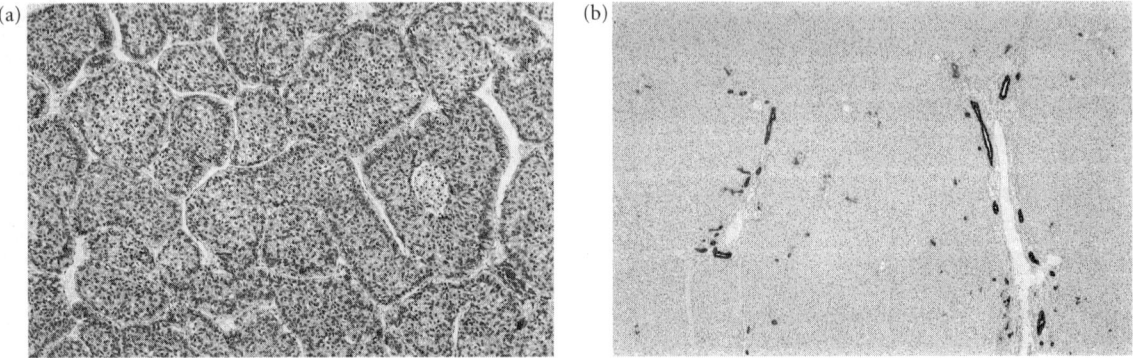

Fig. 15.5 (a) Hepatocarcinoma of the classical trabecular moderately differentiated type in a 15-year-old boy with underlying biliary dysgenesis. (b) Cytokeratin 7 immunohistochemistry reveals many small bile ducts distributed throughout the lobule. There was no cholestasis or history of liver dysfunction prior to the appearance of a mass lesion.

proteins. The tumor cells also express cell adhesion molecules characteristic of hepatocytes and no N-cadherin or N-CAM (120). CD44, an integral membrane protein, is not detectable by immunohistochemistry in normal hepatocytes but was strongly positive in two fibrolamellar carcinomas (and less intense in 12 of 32 usual hepatocarcinomas) (121). Image analysis of tissue sections revealed tetraploidy in 6/12 and aneuploidy in 6/12 fibrolamellar carcinomas (122). Nine of eleven fibrolamellar carcinomas had diffuse and intense positivity for TGF β by immunohistochemistry compared to three of fourteen usual hepatocarcinomas (123). The authors speculate about the possible contribution of TGF β to the lamellar fibrosis characteristic of this tumor.

Hepatoblastoma histology was first thoroughly described by Ishak and Glunz in 1967 (78) and then correlated with prognosis by Kasai and Watanabe in 1970 (124). It can be very diverse (Fig. 15.4) and epithelial cells reflecting different degrees of maturation can be intimately intermingled (Fig. 15.4(a)) or in separate nodules. This feature makes it hazardous to draw conclusions about the character of a hepatoblastoma from a small biopsy, to base chemotherapy on such samples when primary resection is possible, and to draw negative conclusions about the value of histology in prognosis when thorough evaluation has not occurred. For example, in the very extensive report on histology and prognosis from the US Children's Cancer groups in 1989 (125), three of 28 Stage I pure fetal histology patients died of progressive disease. Subsequent review of all the histologic slides from the referring institutions revealed the presence of islands of small undifferentiated cells (Fig. 15.6) in the original tumor and these are the cells that resist the usual chemotherapeutic regimens and almost always metastasize and kill the child (126). The failure of most authors and study groups to subdivide hepatoblastomas composed of fetal epithelium into those with minimal mitotic activity (Fig. 15.4(b)) versus those with significant proliferation that we have called "crowded fetal" (Fig. 15.7) may help to account for the impression that the prognosis of pure fetal histology is not significantly better than the more common other types of differentiation (127). This interpretation is likely to be erroneous, as discussed under Prognosis factors below.

Flow cytology or image analysis of hepatoblastomas for DNA content and S-phase fractionation confirms the histologic data that pure fetal hepatoblastomas with low mitotic rates have a favorable prognosis. In Hata's series (128) diploid tumors had 100% 5-year survival versus 20% for aneuploid lesions. The corresponding data from Germany was 72% 6-year survival for diploid tumors with low S-phase versus 47% for aneuploid tumors (129). Six of the seven pure fetal tumors in this series were diploid and the fetal regions of tumors with diverse epithelium were also diploid, whereas embryonal epithelium was aneuploid. Ten of fifteen diploid hepatoblastomas survived in Zerbini's series (130), compared to three of eight aneuploid tumors. The one small cell undifferentiated tumor was aneuploid, but in Krober's series (131), the small cell tumor was diploid. In his series, all fetal regions in nine hepatoblastomas were diploid and embryonal regions aneuploid.

(a) 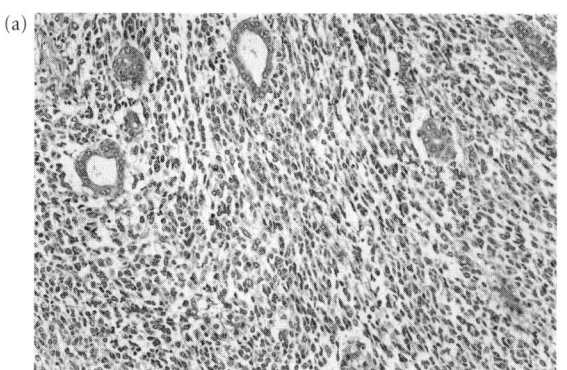 (b)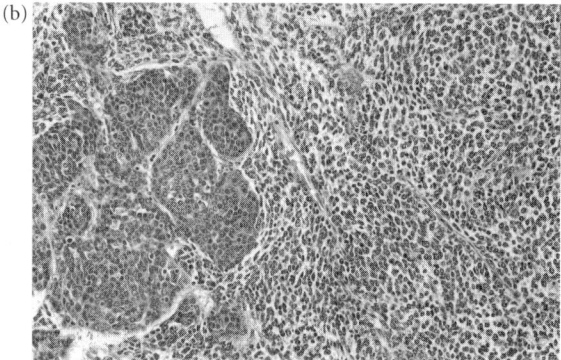

Fig. 15.6 (a) Small cell undifferentiated hepatoblastoma. This neoplasm grows like a sarcoma, infiltrating extensively and sparing bile ducts. The cells are small and undifferentiated, contain intermediate filaments of epithelial type (cytokeratins) and mesenchymal type (Vimentin) and display variable mitotic activity, yet they metastasize early and fail to respond to chemotherapeutic regimens effective for other forms of hepatoblastoma. (b) Small undifferentiated cells may be part of an otherwise typical hepatoblastoma. Failure to see them in a small pre-chemotherapeutic biopsy may lead to an unexpected recurrence and fatal outcome.

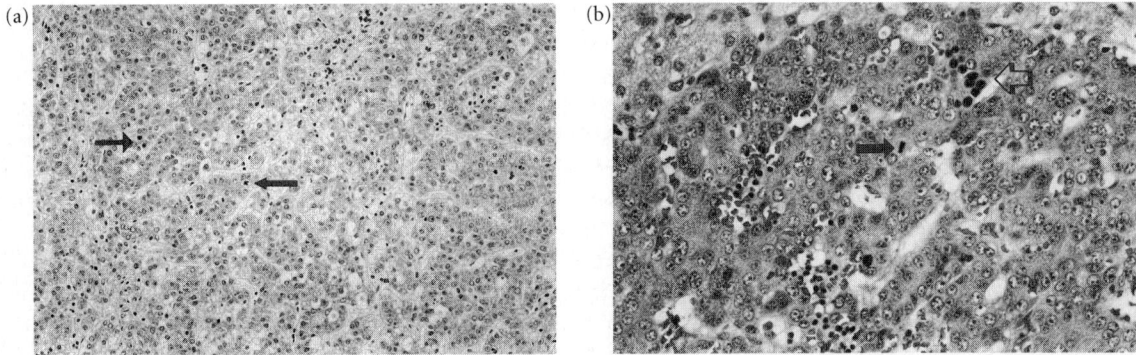

Fig. 15.7 (a) "Crowded fetal" or mitotically active fetal hepatoblastoma. The hepatocytes contain less glycogen than the fetal hepatocytes in Fig. 15.4(b) but are the same size with relatively small regular nuclei and the same cord architecture. Only the presence of greater than two mitoses per 400× microscopic field (arrows) separates the two, but the distinction may be meaningful prognostically. This tumor metastasized to the lungs. (b) Another "crowded fetal" hepatoblastoma at higher magnification. In this case cords are more than two cells thick and the nuclei are slightly larger. In addition to mitoses (arrows), there are collections of hematopoietic cells (open arrow), which may be seen with all types of epithelium in hepatoblastoma.

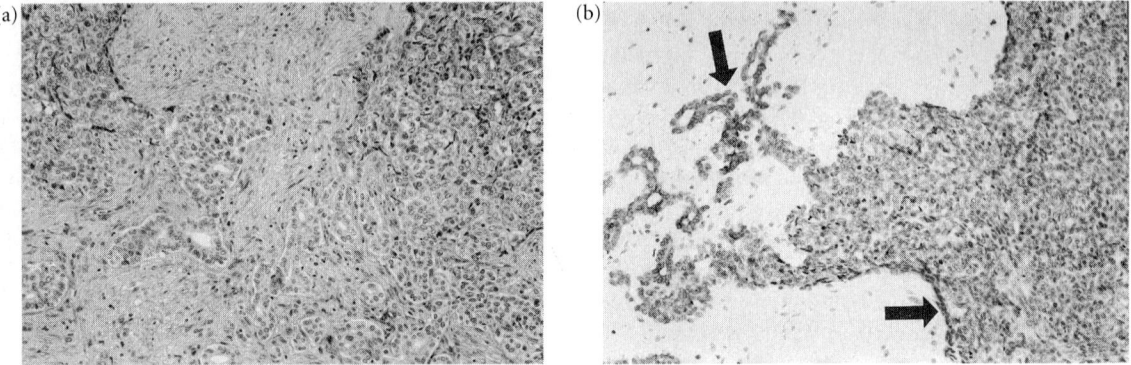

Fig. 15.8 "Cholangioblastic" histology in a hepatoblastoma. (a) H&E stained section reveals nests of relatively mature ductal structures at the margins of typical fetal epithelial hepatoblastoma nodules. (b) Cytokeratin staining with antibodies to biliary epithelium (CK 7 and 19) darkens the cytoplasm of the ductular cells (arrows) but leaves the hepatocytes unstained and pale. (See Zimmermann A. Hepatoblastoma with cholangioblastic features. Med Pediatr Oncol 2002, 39, 487–91).

The MIB-1 labeling index is a measure of DNA synthesis and mitotic activity. When it was less than 10%, survival was much better than when it exceeded 10% and the index rose with more aggressive Stage III and IV tumors (132). PCNA is another protein reflecting DNA synthesis that is detectable immunohistochemically and Rugge (133) found a close correlation between low levels of PCNA staining, diploidy, low S-phase by flow cytometry, and fetal histology. As in hepatocarcinoma, high expression of TGF α (and low PCNA and Cyclin A) was found in fetal cells and the opposite was true for all three proteins in embryonal hepatoblastoma (26).

In some hepatoblastomas, ductular differentiation that is mature, unlike that in embryonal regions, may be seen (Fig. 15.8) (75). We have designed this pattern as *cholangioblastic* (88). The prognostic significance of this pattern of differentiation has not been evaluated but in hepatocarcinomas the presence of biliary epithelial cytokeratins confers a worse prognosis (118). Approximately 20% of hepatoblastomas are *mixed*, with mesenchymal derivatives as well as neoplastic epithelial cells being present in varying proportions and degrees of intermingling (Fig. 15.2(a), (b). Although the presence of osteoid is regarded as evidence of mesenchymal cell lineage, the cells within the lacunae contain epithelial membrane antigen and their ultrastructure is typical of epithelial cells (112). Chromogranin A was also demonstrated in the cells surrounded by osteoid as well as in fetal and embryonal regions in two mixed hepatoblastomas (85). Some of the cells were also positive for serotonin and somatostatin, indicating *neuro-endocrine* differentiation. Five percent of the hepatoblastomas in the 10-year POG series (Table 15.6) were not only mixed but contained mature neural derivatives and melanocytes as well, leading to the term "*teratoid*" (89). A recent example is depicted in Fig. 15.2, in which there was, in addition, an unequivocal Wilm's tumor in the midst of the hepatic mass (Fig. 15.2(d)–(f)). Simultaneous Wilm's tumor of the kidney and hepatoblastoma in the liver has been reported (134) and both embryonal tumors occur in BWS but there are no prior examples of the sort described here. To date, there seems to be no association of any histologic type with any of the many cytogenetic and molecular genetic defects observed in hepatoblastomas except for the *small cell undifferentiated tumor*, but very few have been studied (Tables 15.7 and 15.8). The latter cells as well as the spindled mesenchymal cells express the polysialated form of NCAM strongly, unlike other cells in hepatoblastoma (135). They share with embryonal epithelium the expression of CD44 and common acute lymphoblastic leukemia antigen (Calla). Only fetal epithelium contained E-cadherin.

Metastases to the liver of infants of neuroblastoma, lymphoma, and pancreaticoblastoma can be mistaken for the small cell undifferentiated variant of hepatoblastoma as might a *primary embryonal rhabdomyosarcoma*. In the West Midlands Regional Tumor Registry covering a period of 30 years, 14% of the original diagnoses of childhood liver tumors were erroneous (10) and so were 10.6% of the 123 cases submitted for review in the US Pediatric Oncology Group trial from 1986 to 1989 (Table 15.9). Several errors involved *hemangioendotheliomas*, which can be relatively solid and cellular (109). In some cases of hemangioendothelioma, elevated serum α-FP and misinterpretation of imaging studies (136) may have misled the pathologist. One of the hemangioendothelioma patients in Germany died from complications of chemotherapy. The reverse also occurred, with four hepatoblastoma cases being called hemangioendothelioma after review. In total, 6/26 liver tumors in infants under 3 months of age were misdiagnosed initially. Hopefully, newer imaging techniques (137) may improve differential diagnosis. Another neoplasm that can lead to confusion where only a small biopsy is taken from a diffusely enlarged liver of an infant is *megakaryoblastic leukemia*, which may present without significant numbers of circulating blasts. A useful clue is hepatic and bone marrow fibrosis secondary to platelet-derived growth factor (88).

Non-neoplastic proliferations have to be distinguished from hepatic adenomas and well-differentiated carcinomas. *Nodular regeneration* of the liver occurs in children and may simulate a neoplasm radiologically. The phenomenon has occurred in association with anticonvulsant drug therapy, congenital malformation syndromes and immunodeficiencies, so thorough history and physical examination may provide clues when interpreting a difficult biopsy (138). The *inflammatory pseudotumor*, or plasma cell granuloma frequently occurs in or near the liver and presents as a mass lesion but will be readily recognized in a biopsy. Its name has been changed to *inflammatory myofibroblastoma* because of flow cytologic data showing hyperdiploidy in 4/9 cases and the recent demonstration of ALK1 and p80 expressions in association with 2p23 abnormalities (138a). Although S-phase fraction was low, three of those four recurred or metastasized (139). None of them arose from the liver.

Table 15.6 Stage and histopathology: 189 hepatoblastomas—1986–95

Stage	Well-differentiated fetal*	"Crowded" fetal [>2 mitoses/Hpf]	Embryonal	Macro trabecular	Teratoid	Small cell undifferentiated	Mixed	Total
I	5	4	14	9	1	3	8	44 (23%)
II	—	2	7	3	2	1	4	19 (10%)
III	6	10	24	11	3	3	20	77 (41%)
IV	2	12	11	12	3	1	8	49 (26%)
Total	13 (7%)	28 (15%)	56 (30%)	35 (18%)	9 (5%)	8 (5%)	40 (21%)	189

The hypothesis that well-differentiated fetal hepatoblastoma with low mitotic rate does not require adjuvant chemotherapy when completely excised was confirmed in POG/CCG protocol (POG 9645) (296).

Table 15.7 Cytogenetic abnormalities in hepatoblastomas

Abnormality	No. of cases	Histopathology	Reference
Trisomy 20 only	3	2 mixed mesenchymal and epithelial (fetal, or fetal and embryonal)	(165)
		1 embryonal epithelium mainly	(166)
Trisomy 2 only	2	1 mixed/fetal, embryonal	(167)
		1 mainly fetal, foci of embryonal	(166)
+20 and +2			
1. +20, dup 2 (q21-35)			(168)
2. +20, dup 2 (q23-25)			(169)
3. +20, dup 2q 21-37, der (4) (t2;4)(q21;q35)		Mixed	(170)
4. (dup) (2) (q21;q33)	9	Fetal	(171)
5. der (2) (t2;2) (p25,q21); der (22) t(1;22) (q22;p13)		Mixed	(172)
6. dup (2) (q23;q35)		Mixed/fetal	(173)
7. +1 (p32)		Embryonal	(174)
+20, +2, +8	7	Mixed/fetal and embryonal	(168)
(dupl 2) (q21;q35), i (8) (q10)		Mixed/fetal	(169)
der (2) (+1;2) (q21;q36)		Embryonal	(174)
+20, +2, +8,t1;4	5	Fetal/embryonal	(175)
der (4) (t1;4) (q12;q34)	(3)	Mixed/fetal	
(q25;q32)	(1)	Mixed, macrotrabecular epithelium	
t (1,4) q21;q32)	(1)	Embryonal	(174)
+20, +8 (50xy, +16, +22 also)	1	Embryonal	(174)
+20, 2q+, dup(4)(q12;q26)	1		(176)
+20, partial Trisomy 2 der (9) ins (9;2) (p22;q21;qter)	1 (FISH vs G-banding) 2-constitutional	1-fetal and embryonal	(177)
+20 and −2 del (2) (p21), der 2(+1;2) (q23;p21)	1	Fetal	(170)
+20 dup (2) (q23 pter), +8 T(1;11); constitutional Trisomy 18	1	Fetal, embryonal and foci of small cell undifferentiated	(55)
Trisomy 18 (1 constitutional mosaic)	2	1-fetal and embryonal	(178)
		1-fetal	(56)
45xx, −12, −15, der 12 (t12,15) (q24;q13)	1	Fetal	(174)
i (8) (q10) (premature with hemihypertrophy)	1	Mixed/fetal	(167)
del (15) (q11;q13)	1 (Prader–Willi)		(179)
t(10;22) (q26;q11)	1	Small cell undifferentiated	(180)
del (1) (q12)	1		(172)
del (17) (p12)	1	Mixed/fetal, embryonal	(166)
Normal karyotype	3	2 embryonal, 1 fetal	(174)
+1q (1q 32 in one)	6/9	This is the first report of CGH applied to hepatoblastomas. The abstract does not indicate how many cases had multiple abnormalities or the histopathology	(181)
+2 (2q 14–22 in one)	6/9		
+20	3/9		
+17	3/9		
−11	2/9		

Table 15.8 Hepatocarcinoma—chromosomal abnormalities

Region	% of tumors affected	Abnormality	Method	Reference
1p 35-36	30	LOH (20%↑) (10 microsatellite polymorphisms)	Microsatellite markers	(184)
1p	30	LOH (well-differentiated <2 cm)	Microsatellite markers	(185)
	30	↓ copies <2 cm)	CGH	(187)
1q	72	↑ copies	Comparative genomic hybridization (CGH)	(186)
	58	↑ copies		(187)
	68	LOH	Microsatellite markers	(188)
4q	70	↓ copies	CGH	(187)
4q	43	↓ copies	CGH	(186)
4q	77	LOH	Microsatellite polymorphism	(189)
4q (12-13)	33	LOH	Microsatellite polymorphism	(148)
4q (12-23)	67	LOH	RFLP	(190)
4q (26-27)		Deletion	Microsatellite markers	(191)
5q (35-qter)	70	LOH	RFLP	(192)
6p	33	↑ copies	CGH	(187)
6q	37	↓ copies	CGH	(187)
8p	41	↑ copies	Polymorphic markers	(193)
8p	63.6	LOH	Polymorphic markers	(188)
8p	65	↓ copies	CGH	(187)
8p	37	↓ copies	CGH	(186)
8p 21.3-p22	45	LOH (more often in aggressive tumors)	RFLP	(194)
8p 23	42	LOH	Microsatellite markers	(195)
8q	60	↑ copies	CGH	(187)
8q	48	↑ copies	CGH	(186)
8q	77.3	LOH	Polymorphic markers	(188)
8q 24-ptr	41	↑ copies	Polymorphic markers	(193)
11p	42	LOH	RFLP	(196)
13q	50	LOH	RFLP	(196)
	35	LOH	CGH	(17)
	37	↓ copies	CGH	(187)
16p	22	LOH	RFLP	(197)
16q	54	↓ copies	CGH	(187)
16q	30	↓ copies	CGH	(186)
16q (22.1-23.2)	52	LOH (advanced tumor stage)	RFLP	(198)
16q 22-23	70	LOH	Microsatellite polymorphism	(189)
17p	51	↓ copies	CGH	(187)
17p	49	LOH	CGH	
17q	33	↑ copies	CGH	(187)
17q	30	↑ copies	CGH	(186)
20p	37	↑ copies	CGH	(186)

Biochemical tests and tumor markers

Serum α-FP is the most useful indicator of hepatocellular neoplasia. It is markedly elevated in 80–90% of hepatoblastomas and 60–70% of carcinomas. Lesser degrees of elevation in infants can be due to variations in the rate of decline after birth or increased secretion from regenerating hepatocytes adjacent to hemangioendotheliomas (140, 141) or mesenchymal hamartomas (142). Therefore, it is unacceptable practice to institute chemotherapy for mass lesions of the liver based solely on imaging studies and serum α-FP. α-FP also can be elevated in *yolk sac tumors*, which may occur as primary tumors in the liver. On the contrary, α-FP will not be increased when hepatoblastomas are primarily composed of the small cell undifferentiated type or in most fibrolamellar carcinomas. Expression of this oncofetal protein appears to result from hypomethylation of the 5′ terminal region (143). Enhancement of the specificity of serum α-FP determinations by determining the degree of fucosylation has been advocated in Japan for cirrhotic adults with suspected hepatocarcinoma (144, 145) and may prove useful in children as well. As the

Table 15.9 Other P.O.G accessions in 10 years

Hepatocarcinoma: 20 (4 fibrolamellar)
  9 males, 11 female
  2 HBV with cirrhosis
  1 underlying biliary dysgenesis
  7 mixed HCC/HBoma
Other tumors
  Hemangioendothelioma   2
  Metastatic neuroblastoma   1
  Undifferentiated sarcoma   1
  Metastatic pancreaticoblastoma   1
  Adenoma   1
  Undifferentiated malignancy—? metastatic   3

Table 15.10 Blood tests for detection of liver tumors

Tumor product	Tumor	Reference
α-FP	Hepatoblastoma	(150)
	Hepatocarcinoma (HCC)	(143)
	Hemangioendothelioma	(141)
	Mesenchymal hamartoma	(151)
	Yolk sac tumor	(87)
Fucosylated α-FP	Hepatoblastoma	(143)
	HCC	(144)
Hepatocyte growth factor	Hepatoblastoma after therapy	(152)
Ferritin	HCC	(25)
Heavy chain (1,2,3,6p21-6 cm, 11,14,20, Xq23-25-qter)		(153)
Light chain (19q 13.3-qter)		
Descarboxy prothrombin	HCC	(154)
	Hepatoblastoma	(155)
Chorionic gonadotropin	Hepatoblastoma	(156)
	Teratoma	
	Choriocarcinoma	(157)
Neurotensin	Fibrolamellar carcinoma	(158)
Vitamin B12 binding capacity	Fibrolamellar carcinoma	(78)
ICAM-1	HCC	(159)
		(160)
Platelet-derived endothelial growth factor	HCC	(161)
Matrix matalloproteinase-9	HCC	(162)
TGF α	HCC	(163)
VEGF	HCC (metastases)	(164)

Table 15.11 Hepatocarcinoma—molecular genetics

Gene/locus	Tumors	Abnormality	Reference
APC (5q 21)	29	6 LOH (25/29 had LOH for 1 tumor supressor, 17/29 had LOH for 2–4; all advanced stage)	(211)
β-catenin (3p22-21.3)	31	8 activating mutations	(212)
	75	14 activating mutations	(213)
BRCA2 (13q12–13)	60	3 mutations (2 missense germline)	(214)
CD44	32	12+ membrane staining (strongest in 2 fibrolamellar CA)	(121)
CDKN2A (MTS1/p16) (9p21)	17	4 microsatellite alterations at 9q21–24	(215)
	13	7 LOH at D9S 1604	(216)
	14	4 LOH at D9S171	(217)
	30	1 homozygous deletion	(218)
	26	4 hemizygous germ-line point mutation with loss of wild type allele in tumor of 2/4	
CDKN2B (p15/MT52)	30	7 exon 1 or 2, homozygous deletion	(217)
C-met (7q31)	18	8 over-expression	(219)
C-met	62	Over-expression gives worse prognosis (33.3% 5-year survival in high expressors 10/30; 80.2 5-year survival with low expressors 26/32) No mutation	(220)
C-met (exon 15–19)	16 adults 10 children	3 missense mutations	(221)
C-myc (8q24)	77	28-amplification; younger patients have worse outcome	(222)
Cox 2	56	Inceased expression in well-differentiated tumors	(223)
Cyclin A (4q27)	31	12 over-expression; correlated with shorter survival	(224)
Cyclin D1 (11q)	45	5 amplification-advanced stage tumors (4/5 also had Int-2 amplified; No LOH for 13q (Rb locus) in these 5	(225)
E-cadherin (16q22.1)	24	14-reduced expression due to hypermethylation of promoter	(226)
FAS (CD95)/FAS-L (CD95L)	22	14-decreased FAS expression, over-expression of FAS-L in 3/7	(227)
HIC-1 (17p13.3)	21	19 hypermethylation at D17S5. Also found in 44% of noncancerous tissues of these patients with cirrhosis or chronic hepatitis	(228) (229)
	15	9 LOH at D17S5	
	21	9 ↓ mRNA (RT-PCR) in all cases with P53 mutation	
IGF 2 + H19 (11p15.5)	3	Loss of imprinting; no decrease in H19 expression	(230)
IGF2R/MGP (6q25-qter)	3	2 LOH (5/34 deletion of dinucleotide repeat marker)	(231)
MDM2 (12q13–14)	23	6 over-expression (1 had P53 mutation; 11 of 17 other patients had P53 mutation)	(232)
Macrophage metalloelastase 9	40	25 increased expression in hepatocytes, associated with angiostatin expression and better prognosis	(233)
Mitogen-activated protein kinase (MAPK/ERK)	26	15 activation (also c-fos + cyclin D1 expression)	(234)
p16^{INK4}	32	11 absence of p16 protein, no decrease in mRNA	(235)
p21 (6p21.2)	21	8 decreased mRNA (in 5 p53 was mutated, 6 HCV+)	(236)
P53 (17p13.1)	Hundreds	67% in Aflatoxin regions are mutated, codon 249. 15% or less in other regions; LOH in 60% of patients from Shanghai with HBV	(237) (238) (239)

Table 15.11 (continued)

Gene/locus	Tumors	Abnormality	Reference
Rb	15	11 LOH (nontumorous tissue had LOH in 20/31 cirrhotic nodules)	(240)
	29	10 LOH	(211)
Telomerase (3q 26.3)	29	11+ (3/7 well-differentiated; 12/13 mod diff)	(241)
	10	10+ (also + in 2 adenomatous hyperplastic nodules)	(242)
	26	22+ (16 had abnormal telomere length; 11 shorter, 5 longer)	(243)
	24	23+ (activity in nontumor tissue predicted early recurrence)	(244)
TGF α	53	29+ well-differentiated	(245)
TGF β	6	6 marked increase in mRNA and protein	(246)

incidence of HBV-related hepatocarcinoma has fallen in Japan, the proportion of patients with serum α-FP >100 ng/ml has declined from 57.2% in 1980 to 32.3% in 1993 (146). Hepatitis C infected patients with carcinoma have a much lower frequency of high α-FP. α-FP is elevated in patients with hereditary tyrosinemia type I and ataxia-telangiectasia prior to the development of hepatocarcinoma. Screening of the population of Shanghai by serum α-FP detected subclinical hepatocellular carcinoma in 263 persons over 33 years (147). Unlike patients with symptoms, 81.4% had resectable tumors (versus 46.8%) and 60.5% of those resected survived 5 years (versus 36.8%).

Table 15.10 shows a list of many proposed blood assays for the detection of hepatic malignancies. Other than chorionic gonadotropin, none are used widely thus far because of relatively low specificity and predictive value. The known chromosomal loci for these secretory products have not been demonstrably altered in any of the cytogenetic or molecular genetic studies of hepatocellular neoplasia (Tables 15.11 and 15.12), except for loss of heterozygosity (LOH) at the α-FP locus, (4q12, q13) in 33% of African Blacks and Japanese with hepatocarcinoma (148). Fine needle aspiration for histologic examination is more useful for questionable lesions (149).

Cytogenetics

Constitutional genetic abnormalities associated with *Hepatoblastoma* are listed in Table 15.2. Only Trisomy 18, some cases of BWS, and in some cases deletions of 20p in Alagille's syndrome are recognizable by karyotyping, the remainder requiring molecular genetic methods for detection. In the tumors themselves, karyotyping has revealed a recurrent pattern of defects, as shown in Table 15.7. Twenty-nine of forty reported cases have Trisomy 20 and twenty-six have complete or partial Trisomy 2. Thirteen of the cases had Trisomy 8 but never as the sole abnormality, unlike 20 and 2. +20 is a feature of benign soft tissue tumors (182) and congenital fibrosarcomas and Wilms tumors and +8 is seen with progression of Ewing's and rhabdomyosarcoma (174) as well as benign fibrous tumors (182). 2q abnormalities are also observed in rhabdomyosarcoma (171). Abnormalities in chromosome 1 also occurred with modest frequency with eight cases of translocations (4 having +1;4, 2 with 1q12 translocation or deletion). Translocation involving 4q32 is interesting because it occurs in 10% of hepatocarcinomas and is an integration site for HBV (175). LOH for loci on 1q and 1p has been shown (Table 15.11) in 7/32 hepatoblastomas each and LOH in both arms was found in three cases (183). This is the only region where cytogenetic and molecular data coincide. Using comparative genomic hybridization (CGH) +1q was found in 6/9 hepatoblastomas and +2 in six (181). Only 3/9 cases had +20 with this method. Three had +17, which may reflect p53, HIC 1 or neurofibromin loci but has not been observed by karyotyping. The only small cell undifferentiated hepatoblastoma karyotyped thus far had t(10;22) (180), which was never seen in other hepatoblastomas, suggesting that these cells are not a precursor to fetal and embryonal cells in the tumors. There is no other correlation of karyotypes with histology.

Chromosome 1, 4, 8, 16, and 17 abnormalities have been observed in *Hepatocarcinomas*, relying mainly on CGH and microsatellite polymorphisms (Table 15.8). Fifty-eight percent to seventy-two percent of HCC had increased copies of 1q (186, 187). The high incidence of 8q excess may account for increased c-myc expression as it is located at 8q24 (187). The data for 8p differs depending on the method of analysis. Using polymorphic markers, Fujiwara et al. (193) found increased

Table 15.12 Gene expression in hepatoblastoma

Gene/chromosomal region	No. of tumors	Overexpression or loss of imprinting	Normal	Decreased expression	Loss of heterozygosity	Reference
P53						
17p13 (exons 4–8)	7		7			(256)
	15	10 (immunohistochemistry-IH)	5			(257)
	10	1-macrotrabecular	9			(258)
(exons 5–9)	10	1-(IH)	[8 codon 157 mutations]			(259)
(exons 5–9)	38		38			(249)
	21	9 (IH)	12			(130)
11p	11p	2			2	(260)
11p telomeric region	1				1	(261)
Insulin (11p 15–15.1)						
Calcitonin (11p13–15)						
11p15 (2 non-overlapping regions)	6				4 different loci (1/1 maternal)	(262)
IGF 2 (11p 15.5)	3					(263)
11P15.5	21	1	3		9 (all maternal)	(264)
						(265)
IGF 2 (11P 15.5)	11	Embryonal epithelium mRNA *in situ*			LOH	(266)
IGF 2Bp						
IGF 2	3	3 (1 LOI) (↓ methylation)			3 (↑ methylation)	(267)
H 19						(268)
IGF 2	5	1				(119)
Insulin (11p15)	3	1			1 clone of tumor LOH 1 clone of tumor-No LOH	(269)
APC						
5q21	11	11	10	1 (FAP germline)		(270)
	13 (10% of coding region examined)		(8 mutations, 7 missense point)		4/7	(45)
	1				Maternal allele lost; LOH for 11p15 also	(271)

Table 15.12 (continued)

Gene/chromosomal region	No. of tumors	Overexpression or loss of imprinting	Normal	Decreased expression	Loss of heterozygosity	Reference
Cyclin-related						
CDKN2A	14		14			(272)
9p21 (CDKN2A)						
1p32 (CDKN2C)						
Cyclin D; 11q13	7	4 (CD2,CD3)		4 (CD1)		(273)
Cyclin D1	17	13 (11 both)	4			
CDK4	17	15 (11 both)	2			
p16/CDKN2A	17		17			
RB q13,14	17		17			
Cyclin A, 4q27	9	Embryonal				(26)
TGF α 2p13	9	Fetal		Fetal		(26)
β-catenin 3p22-p21-3	52	25	27			(274)
Chromosome 1q	32				7—both 3	(181)
Chromosome 1p	32				7—both 3	
MDM2, 12q13–14	38		38			(249)
BRCA2, 13q12–13	3	3				(275)
C-met, 7q31	28		No mutations			(276)
						(115)

copies in 41% of cases, whereas decreased copies were shown by CGH (186, 187). Fluorescence in situ hybridization (FISH) showed that polysomy for chromosome 1 was the most common abnormality in HCC and Trisomy 8 was next (199). The most frequent abnormalities found by CGH were of 4q, with decreased copies in 43–70% (186, 187) and LOH in 77% of cases (189). 6q, where many HCC have LOH or decreased copies, is not a site of abnormality in hepatoblastomas. Interestingly, +20, +8, and i(8,q10), as well as rearrangement of 1, were found in cytogenetic analysis of a metastatic fibrolamellar carcinoma, among several other abnormalities (200). i(8,q10) was reported in one hepatoblastoma from a premature infant with hemihypertrophy (167). An abnormality of chromosome 1 in a near triploid fibrolamellar carcinoma was reported (29).

Chromosomal aberrations in hepatic neoplasms of mesenchymal origin are shown in Table 15.4. It is particularly interesting that in contrast to hepatoblastoma in which triploidy for chromosomes 20 and 2 are the most common findings, those chromosomes are frequently lost in the undifferentiated or embryonal sarcoma (96, 206). It is also noteworthy that mesenchymal hamartomas, which some authors attribute to a vascular accident in utero (142), have a characteristic translocation involving t(19q 13.4). This suggests a neoplastic process rather than a post-injury reparative phenomenon. This is supported by Justrabo et al.'s (151) finding of aneuploidy in a mesenchymal hamartoma. This is noteworthy because some recent publications advocate conservative management, such as marsupialization of cysts without resection (207). Failure of marsupialization does not necessarily lead to sarcoma but to recurrence (208, 209). Although several cases of mesenchymal hamartoma have been reported to evolve into a sarcoma, the translocation has yet to be observed in sarcomas.

Molecular genetics

The rapidly expanding application of molecular genetic analyses of *Hepatocarcinoma* has provided much data and considerable stimulation but thus far the significance of the information explosion in explaining carcinogenesis has been limited. Table 15.11 shows the genes that have received the most attention and it is clear that for most genes the proportion of carcinomas in which abnormalities of expression have been demonstrated is generally under 50% and that many of the defects occur only in advanced stage of disease, when many secondary mutations have accumulated (210).

The most important and consistent finding has been codon 249 mutations in p53, which was found in 67% of patients exposed to aflatoxin in Mexico, Mozambique, South China, and Africa (237, 247). The frequency of p53 mutations elsewhere in the world is lower and involves other loci in the gene. LOH for p53 was found in 57% of hepatocarcinomas and 63% of adjacent cirrhotic nodules, indicating premalignant loss of the tumor suppressor in some cases (239). The importance of p53 is to regulate cell division via p21 WAF by sensing abnormalities in the DNA and preventing defective cells from dividing. p53 also activates expression of HIC-1, a recently discovered candidate for tumor suppression in nearby chromosomal region (17p 13.3) (228). HIC-1 in mRNA is markedly reduced in precancerous liver nodules of chronic hepatitis and cirrhosis and even more so in hepatocarcinoma, especially in poorly differentiated tumors (229). This is due to hypermethylation at the D17S5 locus on 17p. There was LOH at the locus in 54% of carcinomas. Reduced expression of E-cadherin in hepatocarcinomas also was attributable to methylation of the promoter on 16q 22.1 (226). The Mdm2 proto-oncogene was overexpressed in 6/23 hepatocarcinomas (232). Mdm2 is known to down-regulate p53 activity by competing with it but it appears to have a p53 independent role in carcinogenesis because transgenic mice deficient in p53 also develop many sarcomas (248). No amplification of Mdm2 was found in 19 hepatoblastomas (249). When p53 mutations in other loci were detected in a group of hepatocarcinomas that were treated by surgical excision, mean patient survival was reduced from 60 to 15 months, compared to patients with wild-type p53 in their tumors (250). The presence of antibody to p53 in the serum of patients with hepatocarcinoma (32% of 86 patients) was predictive of shorter survival (251).

Independent clonal origin of multiple hepatocarcinomas in the same liver has been demonstrated by different patterns of LOH in the separate tumors (252). When LOH for a particular locus is observed in *non-cirrhotic* livers, it may have more significance. That is the case for 5q LOH in five of seven patients from England (193). Nine cirrhotic patients with hepatocarcinoma failed to show this abnormality but both groups had LOH at 17p13 (the p53 and HIC 1 loci). The 5q locus was at q35-qter, distant from the APC and MCC genes at 5q 21–22 (253).

Telomerase activity which is not detectable in normal liver, was increased in 17% of nontumoral tissue from patients with hepatocarcinoma and was present in 38% of the tumors (241). It was more prevalent in moderately differentiated than well-differentiated tumors. Eighty-six percent of large regenerative nodules in patients without carcinoma had telomerase activities equal to carcinomas (254). Telomerase activity in the nontumoral tissues was associated with early recurrence (244). In 63% of hepatocarcinomas, telomere length differed from normal tissues, with 44% being shorter and 19% longer (243). LOH for DNA mismatch repair gene loci has recently been reported (255).

Unlike hepatocarcinomas, in which p53, Mdm2, p21, and c-met are frequently mutated, the major loci involved in *Hepatoblastoma* involve the 11p15 region where the Beckwith–Wiedemann gene, Insulin-like growth factor 2 (IGF2), insulin, calcitonin, and H19 are located. The cyclin A and D and CDK4 genes, and β-catenin are also frequently altered in expression (Table 15.12). None of the loci that are over-expressed, under-expressed or show LOH are on the chromosomes that are most often altered in hepatoblastomas (Table 15.7). The first application of CHIP technology to screen for mRNA expression in hepatoblastomas confirmed the high expression of IGF2 that is well known using more traditional methods (275). However, it also revealed a surprise, which was BRCA2 expression in three cases. BRCA2 is constitutionally mutated in familial breast and ovarian cancers and was mutated in 3 of 60 hepatocarcinomas (214). It is an inhibitor of p53 function. Antibody to BRCA2 stained 6/6 hepatoblastomas but not fetal liver (275). Interestingly, no APC expression was found with CHIP probes in the three tumors.

Children with the BWS have a relative risk of having a hepatoblastoma of 2280 (276), particularly in patients with hemihypertrophy. Eight percent of tumors in BWS are hepatoblastomas (262). The development of an embryonal malignancy in BWS patients is not as ominous as in other children. Vaughan et al. (277) found 100% disease-free survival in 13 affected children. Two of the tumors were advanced stage hepatoblastomas that responded completely to chemotherapy. One patient with hepatoblastoma had an interstitial deletion of 11p but 19 of 28 other BWS patients had no constitutional karyotypic abnormality (50). Of the nine cases with aberrations, six had triplication for 11p15. The p57KIP2 gene is located at 11p15.5 and is a negative regulator of cell proliferation. This is an imprinted gene with expression of only the maternal allele in normal cells. Mutation in the maternal allele has been observed in only 4 of 49 BWS patients (51, 278). Mice whose p57KIP2 gene has been knocked out develop abdominal wall defects, cleft palate, skeletal alterations, adrenal cytomegaly, and renal medullary dysplasia, partially replicating BWS in humans (279). However, they live only a few days and no tumors have been seen. Transgenic mice that over-express IGF2 have many features of BWS, including overgrowth, visceromegaly, omphalocele, cardiac, and adrenal defects (280). Using 14 polymorphic markers on chromosome 11, Byrne et al. (262) were able to demonstrate LOH in 2 non-overlapping loci of 11p15 in 4 of 6 hepatoblastomas, one of which was in a BWS child. Albrecht et al. (264) also found LOH for 11p15.5 in 6 of 18 hepatoblastomas, one of which was from a BWS patient. This suggested loss of a tumor suppressor while preserving the growth-stimulation activity of IGF2. Interestingly, Tomlinson (271) found LOH for 11p15 markers in a hepatoblastoma from a child with FAP who had lost the maternal APC gene in the tumor while retaining a mutant allele from the father. This work refines the first observation of LOH of 11p in diverse tumors of BWS patients by Koufos et al. (260). There have been many studies of gene expression in the 11p15 region (Table 15.12). Insulin and IGF2 are stimulants of embryonal cell growth, so their up-regulation or loss of imprinting in a few hepatoblastomas is suggestive of an early genetic contribution to fetal oncogenesis. Drut et al. (281) have observed hepatic hemangioendotheliomas in an infant with BWS. It is a unique report thus far.

Hepatoblastoma occurs in children of families with heritable polyposis (FAP) at a frequency 1000–2000× that of the population at large. Nevertheless, no karyotypic alterations in tumors have been detected at 5q21 and most reports of molecular analysis of the APC gene in hepatoblastomas fail to show mutations (270). However, Oda et al. (45) found mutations in APC in 8/13 sporadic hepatoblastomas, with no abnormality in the nontumoral liver.

The kinds of germline mutations of APC in patients with hepatoblastoma are not different from families without liver tumors and all the survivors of hepatoblastoma have later developed colonic polyposis (22). However, the APC gene has 16 different transcripts with some tissue specific expression, so we may expect to learn more about the hepatoblastoma-related mutation in the future (282). The APC protein regulates β-catenin, a cadherin-binding protein involved in intercellular adhesion (283). When APC is mutated, β-catenin accumulates in cells and activating mutations in β-catenin have been observed in 48% of hepatoblastomas (274) and in 20–26% of hepatocarcinomas (212, 213), so this is a clue to oncogenesis in hepatocytes.

Other hepatobiliary tumors are being reported in FAP cases, including hepatocarcinoma in a $9\frac{1}{2}$-year-old boy and fibrolamellar carcinoma in a 15-year-old girl (46), adenoma in a 2-year-old with biallelic inactivation of the APC gene in the tumor (47), bile duct adenoma (48), and gallbladder adenomatous proliferation and dysplasia (49).

Data on the expression of cyclins in hepatoblastoma are emerging. Using quantitative RT-PCR for mRNA and Western blotting for proteins, Iolascon et al. (272) found significant down-regulation of cyclin D1 in four of seven tumors whereas cyclin D2 and D3 were overexpressed versus non-neoplastic tissue. With immunohistochemistry, cyclin D was overexpressed in comparison to adjacent nontumoral liver in 13/17 cases, and cdk4 was increased in 15 of 17. In 11 patients both were over-expressed (273).

The overexpression of p53 in hepatoblastomas and other liver malignancies, when detected immunohistochemically, does not signify mutations in the gene (257). In fact, other authors found infrequent or no p53 overexpression in hepatoblastomas (130, 249, 256, 284).

p53 mutations were found in 9% of angiosarcomas not associated with vinyl chloride exposure (285). Kras-2 mutations were seen in 5/19 sporadic angiosarcomas and in 2/5 patients who had thorotrast exposure (286).

Prognostic factors

Resectability is the key prognostic feature for all liver tumors. Unfortunately 67% hepatoblastomas were not amenable to primary surgery (41% Stage III and 26% Stage IV) in the last 10 years of Pediatric Oncology Group accessions (Table 15.6). The figure was 70% in the prior US Intergroup study (113). For hepatocarcinoma in the latter study, primary resection was possible in only 21%, and the Stage III and IV tumors are much less susceptible to chemotherapy than hepatoblastomas. On the other hand, in the most recent Intergroup study all seven children with hepatocarcinoma who had Stage I disease survived disease-free (287). Happily, chemotherapeutic regimens based mainly on *cis*-platinum have made it possible to perform resections of as many as 92% of hepatoblastomas whose initial presentation involved so much of the liver or vital structures at the hilum that surgical excision could not be performed (5, 110, 288). Although some Stage IV hepatoblastomas have been cured by chemotherapy, the prognosis of metastatic disease remains very poor.

The second most important prognostic feature in the initial evaluation of all liver tumors is mitotic activity, whether measured in routine histologic sections (13, 113), by diploidy in flow cytometry (128, 129, 131, 133), or by immunohistochemical stains for DNA synthesis (133). This is equally relevant for sarcomas, which tend to be aneuploid (91, 96) and inflammatory myofibroblastoma (139).

For *Hepatoblastomas*, it has become evident that Kasai and Watanabe's (124) early observation that fetal histology has a favorable prognosis and small cell undifferentiated tumors (which they called "anaplastic") are rarely cured has been verified in many studies. Weinberg and Finegold (13) found that 6 of 6 patients with pure fetal histology and low mitotic activity were cured by surgery alone. After 16 years and hundreds of hepatoblastomas undergoing review in Intergroup studies in the United States and Germany, there have been up to 92% survivors with no evidence of disease (47 of 51) of Stage I and II fetal histology tumors and not all of these cases were fully evaluated for mitotic activity (86). One hundred percent of pure fetal tumors (17 patients) in the German HB89 study are alive with no evidence of disease (5). Therefore, the current US Intergroup study treats Stage I fetal hepatoblastomas with low mitotic rates by surgery alone. None of the patients with the small cell undifferentiated tumor (5% of the POG series—Table 15.6) have survived despite three being Stage I at presentation. Two reported survivors are unusual for late presentation at 2 and 5 years (289), as most cases occur in the first 6 months after birth. The prognosis of boys presenting with precocious puberty (108) or infants with hypercholesterolemia secondary to hepatoblastoma (106) appears much worse than ordinary hepatoblastomas.

For *hepatocarcinomas*, several molecular genetic observations about prognosis have been reported and some have already been discussed (circulating antibody to p53 mutations and telomerase activity in adjacent nontumoral liver, and biliary epithelial markers predict shorter survival). In addition, over-expression of c-met, cyclin A, and c-myc predict reduced survival (220, 222, 224). Over-expression of matrix metalloproteinase 9 appeared to correlate with local invasiveness (290), whereas the expression of human macrophage metalloelastase, which stimulates angiostatin production, enhanced survival (233). Vascular endothelial growth factor (VEGF) expression as measured by RT-PCR for mRNA was found in 39 of 51 hepatocarcinomas and the highest levels were found in poorly encapsulated tumors with vascular invasion (291), which confers a worse prognosis. Jin-no et al. (164) confirmed this by measuring VEGF in the circulation of patients with chronic liver disease and hepatocarcinoma. The highest levels were in patients with metastases. This was also true for serum levels of ICAM-1 (160). The impression that *Fibrolamellar carcinomas* have a significantly better prognosis (78, 79) because of a higher frequency of resectability and the absence of cirrhosis has not been supported in the most recent US Intergroup study (79a).

Treatment strategies

Prior to the discovery of NTBC (2-(2-nitro-4-trifluoromethyl benzoyl)-1-3-cyclohexane dione), an inhibitor of the 4-hydroxy dioxygenase in the catabolic pathway of tyrosine metabolism, children with mutant fumaryl acetoacetate hydrolase developed hepatocarcinoma at a very high rate (up to 37%), as early as 12 months of age. Therefore, many patients had orthotopic liver transplants and survival rates ranged from 80% (292) to 92% (293). Children with low glomerular filtration rates required renal transplantation as well. Since 1992, over 200 patients have been treated with NTBC beginning prior to age 2 and 2 have developed hepatocarcinoma (38). One was a 1-year-old who had the tumor at presentation with liver dysfunction. The second was diagnosed at 5 months and the carcinoma was recognized at 15 months. What will happen to the others remains uncertain, as our studies of long-term NTBC treatment of FAH-deficient mice revealed delayed onset of carcinoma in greater than 50% (294). This is the only example of a direct chemical approach to the prevention of hepatocarcinoma, based on the elimination or reduction of toxic and mutagenic metabolites generated within hepatocytes themselves.

Vaccination for HBV, as discussed earlier, will have profound benefits in preventing hepatocarcinoma, once it can be delivered to populations at great risk, and the major efforts to treat and ultimately vaccinate for hepatitis C will hopefully prove fruitful soon. Meanwhile, screening programs using serum α-FP and ultrasound have proven very valuable in detecting hepatocarcinomas early and allowing resections (81.4% versus 46.8% in symptomatic patients) (147). Such screening should be performed in all children with the genetic conditions listed in Table 15.2 and possibly in survivors of extreme prematurity. But for the present, we must deal with treatment of established tumors by surgical excision of both the primary tumor and metastases (125).

As stated earlier (Prognostic factors, vide supra), the excellent results obtained for Stage I pure fetal tumors by surgery alone in the past or with a short course of doxorubin in the recently completed POG trial has led to the current US Intergroup protocol of surgery alone for those cases with low mitotic activity. This approach is not universally accepted, with some centers advocating biopsy and chemotherapy prior to surgery, regardless of histologic findings (295) and others considering chemotherapy based solely on elevated serum α-FP and imaging studies (111). We strongly disagree with this because (a) small biopsies may fail to disclose all components of a hepatoblastoma and the presence of small undifferentiated cells has led to recurrence and fatality in at least four patients thought to have pure fetal tumors (113, 126), (b) misinterpretation of histology has occurred with sufficient frequency to be alarming (10, 136) (Table 15.9) so review by experienced pathologists can be helpful in selecting treatment, (c) the reliability of imaging, especially in infants is questionable (136), and (d) toxicity of doxorubin and cisplatin is not insignificant (296), so their avoidance, when possible, is desirable (296a).

The great improvement in adjunctive chemotherapy for hepatoblastoma following the introduction of *cis*-platinum in the mid-1980s has led to increasing resectability and cure of Stage III but little benefit for Stage IV tumors. The Children's Cancer Group used *cis*-platinum and continuous IV doxorubicin to convert initially unresectable hepatoblastoma to excision in 20 of 33 children, with 19 of the 20 being cured (297). Concurrently the Pediatric Oncology Group achieved similar results with cisplatin, vincristine, and fluorouracil (24 of 31 Stage III patients (67%) having a complete remission after chemotherapy and surgery) (298). When the two regimens were compared in a subsequent joint study, the results were once again similar but the frequency of complications was less with the POG protocol (296). Similar results emerged from the German HB 89 protocol which added Ifosphamide to cisplatin and doxorubicin (299), the Nagoya University experience (300), and the SIOPEL study involving 91 institutions in 30 European countries (111). Even three of the tiniest premature babies with Stage III disease in Ikeda's report (3) were cured by chemotherapy with cisplatin, doxorubicin, VP-16, and cyclophosphamide. Once again, well-differentiated fetal histology was superior to embryonal differentiation in long-term survival, regardless of stage (5/8 versus 1/7). The effect of chemotherapy on the histology of the resected tumors was to increase the quantity of osteoid and mature mesenchymal tissue (301, 302). In the latter report, the presence of vascular invasion, proportion of surviving embryonal epithelium, extent of tumor necrosis, amount of viable mesenchymal tissue and mitotic activity in the epithelial component were of prognostic significance. In the new Intergroup protocol for Hepatoblastoma, Amofostine will be evaluated for its capacity to protect against renal complications (303).

Efforts to obtain complete surgical removal of hepatoblastomas without transplantation can be heroic and successful as in Uotani et al.'s (304) use of inferior vena cava (IVC) atrial venovenous bypass to perform a trisegmentectomy and removal of a completely occluded IVC below the hepatic veins. Their 11-month-old with a massive tumor has no evidence of disease at 39 months.

Postoperative combination chemotherapy with intravenous epirubicin and hepatic arterial infusions of cisplatin in 30 patients who had apparently complete resection of hepatocarcinoma produced a worse outcome than in patients treated by surgery alone (305). These cirrhotic patients may have had second malignancies rather than recurrences. Efforts to ablate intrahepatic tumors in adults with transhepatic freezing or heat, lipiodol delivery of chemotherapy, and ethanol infusions have all yielded temporary reduction in tumor burden but no cures. Busuttil and Farmer (306) reviewed the results of surgical resection for carcinoma in 1954 patients from 15 centers. Only 3–30% of patients could be resected and 1164 of 1864 (62%) had cirrhosis. The 5-year actuarial survival averaged 33 months.

Chemotherapy has proven more useful for sarcomas in recent reports than earlier studies (89, 101). In reviewing the literature in 1990, Leuschner et al. (95) found that 37.5% (15 of 40) patients with undifferentiated sarcomas had no evidence of disease at an average of 37.5 months. Recurrences occurred between 6 and 29 months and deaths at average duration of 11.9 months. The improvement was related to the use of doxorubicin and cisplatin (307). Walker et al. (97) were able to save three of four children with embryonal sarcoma, two with surgical resection alone. Four additional cures were achieved by Urban et al. (308) using chemotherapy containing cisplatin, doxorubicin, ifosphamide, and vincristine, plus in one patient 40 Gy of external photon radiation to achieve resectability. Oncologists at Texas Children's Hospital used the same combination of drugs to cure a 4-year-old girl of angiosarcoma of the liver (309). Multidrug chemotherapy was successful in a case of primary yolk sac tumor of the liver (310).

Treatment of hemangioendotheliomas remains difficult and unpredictable. Six of eleven tumors in Holcomb et al.'s series (311) responded to corticosteroids alone with complete regression of the tumor and a 14-year-old also survived with steroids and 2000 R of external irradiation. Two younger children treated with the same combination died of congestive heart failure because of unresponsiveness of the tumor. Some tumors have responded to cyclophosphamide and some to interferon-γ and some have been treated by hepatic artery ligation or embolization (109). Special compression sutures to produce rapid alleviation of shunts and congestive failure were recently reported (312). No reports have emerged as yet on trials of angiostatic agents for these tumors. When all other treatments fail, orthotopic liver transplantation (OLT) has been used (313). However, in two girls from Birmingham, England, there was a vertebral metastases 29 and 36 months after the transplant and ultimately death due to a type 2 hemangioendothelioma indistinguishable from the original tumor (313, 314)

Orthotopic liver transplantation has been used for all types of hepatic tumors, with relatively good results, at least initially. In 1991, Koneru et al. (289) reported that 6 of 12 hepatoblastomas transplanted at 8 US centers survived 24 to 70 months with no evidence of disease. Microscopic evidence of vascular invasion and embryonal or small cell undifferentiated tumors had a worse prognosis. The recurrence rate for all OLT for all malignancies in the liver was 40% in Penn's 1991 review of 637 patients (315). Eighty-seven percent of those recurrences were fatal. The fatality rate was least for hepatoblastomas (33%) and hepatocarcinomas discovered incidentally (13%) and highest for angiosarcoma (64%). When Starzl's group in Pittsburgh reviewed their experience with children (316), five of six hepatoblastomas and four of nine hepatocarcinomas were alive with no evidence of disease at 1.3 ± 0.5 years and 2.3 ± 1.2 years. In Toronto (317), seven of eight patients were disease-free at 1–5 years post OLT. Four of five hepatoblastomas survived. The sole fatality was related to metastatic disease in the lung and a failure of the primary tumor to respond to chemotherapy prior to the transplant. A second patient with lung metastases survived when they were resected after the OLT. The patients were able to stop chemotherapy after OLT and their frequency of graft rejection has been lower than other OLT recipients.

Current and future research

From the information previously discussed, some urgent needs have to be addressed, including (a) a more appropriate therapeutic regimen for undifferentiated small cell hepatoblastoma [should retinoids be tried to induce maturation?], (b) more effective medical therapy for hepatocarcinomas and sarcomas, (c) new methods for predicting which hemangioendotheliomas will fail to respond to steroids and which of those that have responded will recur or convert to angiosarcoma, (d) methods for detecting the potential for recurrence or sarcomatous transformation of mesenchymal hamartomas.

Data from research for experimental animals and *in vitro* studies have provided some insights that may help to address those issues. Germain and colleagues (318), for example, found that modifications of the media in which embryonal rat liver cells were grown could induce either hepatocellular or bile duct differentiation. Ponder (319) has recently reviewed the plasticity of post-natal hepatocytes in relation to carcinogenesis and the use of gene markers to trace both development and neoplastic transformation. She found that both hepatocarcinomas and cholangiocarcinomas will occur after transfection of an oncogene (K-ras) into hepatocytes. The OV-6 monoclonal antibody first produced by Dunsford and Sell (320) has proven to be a useful marker for the possible precursor cell in human fetal liver and in children with chronic cholestatic liver disease due to extrahepatic atresia and α-1-antitrypsin deficiency (321). Whether or not this is the cell that develops into small cell undifferentiated hepatoblastoma or the more differentiated cells is not yet known.

The role of TGF α in hepatocarcinogenesis is interesting. Over-expression in male transgenic mice leads to hepatocarcinoma, as discussed under "Etiology." Castration of the mice reduced the incidence of tumors in males sevenfold but ovariectomy increased tumor formation 6× (23). Possibly, gene transfer with an antisense construct to TGF α, as was done with IGF antisense cDNA in rats with hepatomas (322), will have a significant effect on tumor growth. Hepatocyte growth factor expression in the liver of transgenic mice prevented malignancy induced by c-myc, so it may be a useful adjunct as well (323, 324).

The potential of gene therapy for liver tumors has been nicely reviewed by Ruiz *et al.* (325). Restoring p53 to a mutant-containing rat carcinoma cell line has been achieved by intrahepatic artery delivery of an adenovirus vector suppressed tumor growth (326). Retroviral transfer of tumor necrosis factor α by direct injection of mouse hepatocarcinomas led to significantly longer survival (327), as did interleukin-2 in an adenoviral vector (328). Other recent applications include antisense RNA to inhibit HBV replication (329), use of the α-FP promoter to direct cytosine deaminase to murine hepatoma, whereupon 5-fluorocytosine injections can kill the transduced cells (330), and monoclonal antibodies to cell surface glycoproteins to deliver genes into cells (331).

The use of oral acyclic retinoids to reduce the occurrence of secondary hepatocarcinomas seems highly effective. Muto *et al.* (332) have followed their patients for a median period of 62 months and the difference in estimated 6-year survival was 74% for the treated group versus 46% in a placebo group. This encouraging data is why we have suggested retinoid use for small cell undifferentiated hepatoblastomas. Thus, there are many diverse initiatives, employing many new modalities and the latest scientific discoveries to treat hepatic tumors and we have reason to be optimistic about the future.

Acknowledgments

The author is grateful to Virginia Bates for preparing the manuscript, including the complex tables, and to Lottie Cade for assistance with literature searches. Colleagues in the Pediatric Oncology Group, particularly Edwin C. (Pete) Douglass, provided both the clinical data and tissue samples that informed and stimulated the author. Joel Haas, Pathologist to the Children's Cancer Group and long-time collaborator and friend, provided valuable commentary and editing.

References

1. Parkin DM, Stiller CA, Draper GJ, Bieber CA, Terracini B, Young JL. International incidence of childhood cancer. IARC, Lyon, 1988, 358 pp.
2. Ikeda H, Matsuyama S, Tanimura M. Association between hepatoblastoma and very low birth weight: a trend or a chance. J Pediatr 1997, 130, 557–60.
3. Ikeda H, Hachitanda Y, Tanimura M, Maruyama K, Koizumi T, Tsuchida Y. Development of unfavorable hepatoblastoma in children of very low birth weight. Cancer 1998, 82, 1789–96.
4. Tanimura M, Matsui I, Abe J, Ikeda H, Kobayashi N, Ohira M, *et al.* Increased risk of hepatoblastoma among immature children with a lower birth weight. Cancer Res 1998, 58, 3032–5.
5. vonSchweinitz D, Byrd DJ, Hecker H, Weinel P, Bode U, Burger D, *et al.* Efficiency and toxicity of Ifosfamide, Cisplatin and Doxorubicin in the treatment of childhood hepatoblastoma. Eur J Cancer 1997, 33, 1243–9.

6. Patterson K, Kapur S, Chandra RS. Hepatocellular carcinoma in a noncirrhotic infant after prolonged parenteral nutrition. J Pediatr 1985, **106**, 797–800.
7. Vileisis RA, Sorensen K, Gonzalez-Crussi F, Hunt CE. Liver malignancy after parenteral nutrition. J Pediatr 1982, **100**, 88–90.
8. Ribons LA, Slovis TL. Hepatoblastoma and birth weight. J Pediatr 1998, **132**, 750.
9. Ross JA, Gurney JG. Hepatoblastoma incidence in the United States from 1973 to 1992. Med Pediatr Oncol 1998, **30**, 141–2.
10. Mann JR, Kasthuri N, Raafat F, Pincott JR, Parkes SE, Muir KR, et al. Malignant hepatic tumors in children, incidence, clinical features and aetiology. Paediatr Perinat Epidemiol 1990, **4**, 276–89.
11. Feusner J, Buckley J, Robison L, Ross J, vanTornout J. Prematurity and hepatoblastoma: more than just an association? J Pediatr 1998, **133**, 585–6.
12. El-Serag HB, Mason AC. Rising incidence of hepatocellular carcinoma in the United States. N Engl J Med 1999, **340**, 745–50.
13. Weinberg AG, Finegold MJ. Primary hepatic tumors of childhood. Hum Pathol 1983, **14**, 512–37.
14. Tanaka T, Miyamoto H, Hino O, Kitagawa T, Iizuka T, Sakamoto H, et al. Primary hepatocellular carcinoma with hepatitis B virus-DNA integration in a 4-year old boy. Hum Pathol 1986, **17**, 202–4.
15. Chang MH, Chen CJ, Lai MS, Hsu HM, Wu TC, Kong MS, et al. Universal hepatitis B vaccination in Taiwan and the incidence of hepatocellular carcinoma in children. Taiwan Childhood Hepatoma Study Group, N Engl J Med 1997, **336**, 1855–9.
16. Wang J, Chenivesse X, Henglein B, Brechot C. Hepatitis B virus integration in a cyclin A gene in a hepatocellular carcinoma. Nature 1990, **343**, 555–7.
17. Nishida N, Fukula Y, Ishizaki K, Nakao K. Alteration of cell cycle-related genes in hepatocarcinogenesis. Histol Histopathol 1997, **12**, 1019–25.
18. Baptista M, Kramvis A, Kew M. High prevalence of 1762^T 1764^A mutations in the basic core promoter of Hepatitis B virus isolated from black Africans with hepatocellular carcinoma compared with asymptomatic carriers. Hepatology 1999, **29**, 946–53.
19. Kuo MT, Zhao J, Teeter LD, Ikeguchi M, Chisari FV. Activation of multidrug resistance (P-glycoprotein) *mdr 3/mdr1a* gene during the development of hepatocellular carcinoma in hepatic B virus transgenic mice. Cell Growth Differ 1992, **3**, 531–40.
20. Finegold MJ. Liver tumors. In: Pediatric gastrointestinal disease, Vol. 2 (ed. Walker WA, Durie PR, Hamilton JR, Walker-Smith JA, Watkins JB). Mosby, St Louis, 1996, pp. 1102–16.
21. Coire EI, Qizilbash AH, Castelli MF. Hepatic adenomata in type 1a glycogen storage disease. Arch Pathol Lab Med 1987, **111**, 166–9.
22. Giardiello FM, Peterson GM, Brensinger JF, Luce MC, Cayouette MC, Bacon J, et al. Hepatoblastoma and APC gene mutation in familial adenomatous polyposis. Gut 1996, **39**, 867–9.
23. Takagi H, Sharp R, Hammermeister C, Goodrow T, Bradley MO, Fausto N, et al. Molecular and genetic analysis of liver oncogenesis in transforming growth factor alpha transgenic mice. Cancer Res 1992, **19**, 5171–7.
24. Sandgren EP, Luetteke NC, Qui TH, Palmiter RD, Brinster RL, Lee DC. Transforming growth factor alpha dramatically enhances oncogene-induced carcinogenesis in transgenic mouse pancreas and liver. Mol Cell Biol 1993, **1**, 320–30.
25. Sirica AE. The role of cell types in hepatocarcinogenesis. CRC Press, Boca Raton, 1992.
26. Kiss A, Szepesi A, Lotz G, Nagy P, Schaff Z. Expression of transforming growth factor-alpha in hepatoblastoma. Cancer 1998, **83**, 690–7.
27. Santoni-Rugui E, Jensen MR, Thorgeirsson SS. Disruption of the pRb/E2F pathway and inhibition of apoptosis are major oncogenic events in liver constitutively expressing c-myc and transforming growth factor alpha. Cancer Res 1998, **58**, 123–34.
28. Malt RA, Galdabini JJ, Jeppson BW. Abnormal sex-steroid milieu in young adults with hepatocellular carcinoma. World J Surg 1983, **7**, 247–52.
29. Hany MA, Betts DR, Schmugge M, Schonle E, Niggli FK, Zachmann M, et al. A childhood fibrolamellar hepatocellular carcinoma with increased aromatose activity and a near triploid karyotype. Med Pediatr Oncol 1997, **28**, 136–8.
30. Agarwal VR, Takayama K, VanWyk JJ, Sasano H, Simpson ER, Bulum SE. Molecular basis of severe gynecomastia associated with aromatase expression in a fibrolamellar carcinoma. J Clin Endocrin Metab 1998, **83**, 1797–850.
31. LeBrun DP, Silver MM, Freedman MH, Phillips MJ. Fibrolamellar carcinoma of the liver in a patient with Fanconi anemia. Hum Pathol 1991, **22**, 396–8.
32. Abbondanzo SL, Herbert JM, Klappenbach RS, Gootenberg JE. Hepatocellular carcinoma in an 11-year-old girl with Fanconi's anemia. Am J Pediatr Hematol Oncol 1986, **8**, 334–7.
33. Chandra RS, Kapur SP, Kelleher J. Benign hepatocellular tumors in the young. Arch Pathol Lab Med 1984, **108**, 168–71.
34. Fabre M, Gauthier F, Martin V, Hadchoudel M, Yandza T, Chardot D. Hepatocarcinoma and preneoplastic lesions in chronic advanced liver disease in children. SIOP XXVI Meeting, 1998, 233 (Abstract).
35. Moore L, Bourne AJ, Moore DJ, Preston H, Byard RW. Hepatocellular carcinoma following neonatal hepatitis. Pediatr Pathol Lab Med 1997, **17**, 601–10.
36. McGoldrick JP, Boston VE, Glasgow JFT. Hepatocellular carcinoma associated with congenital macronodular cirrhosis in a neonate. J Pediatr Surg 1986, **21**, 177–9.
37. Ugarte N, Gonzalez-Crussi F. Hepatoma in siblings with progressive familial cholestatic cirrhosis of childhood. Am J Clin Path 1981, **76**, 172–7.
38. Holme E, Lindstedt S. Non-transplant treatment of tyrosinemia. Clin Liver Dis 2000, **4**, 805–14.
39. Limmer J, Fleig WE, Leupold D, Bittner R, Ditschuneit H, Beger H. Hepatocellular carcinoma in type 1 glycogen storage disease. Hepatology 1988, **8**, 531–7.
40. Ito E, Sato Y, Kawauchi K, Munakata H, Kamata Y, Yodono H, et al. Type 1A glycogen storage disease with hepatoblastoma in siblings. Cancer 1987, **59**, 1776–80.
41. de Moor RA, Schweizer JJ, van Hoek B, Wasser M, Vink R, Maaswinkel-Mooy PD. Hepatocellular carcinoma in glycogen storage disease type IV. Arch Dis Child 2000, **82**, 479–80.
42. Hartley AL, Birch JM, Kelsey AM, Morris Jones PH, Harris M, Blair V. Epidemiological and familial aspects of hepatoblastoma. Med Pediatr Oncol 1990, **18**, 103–9.

43. Buckley JD, Sather H, Ruccione K, Rogers PCJ, Haas JE, Henderson BE, et al. A case-control study of risk factors for hepatoblastoma. Cancer 1989, **64**, 1169–76.
44. Robinson HB, Bolande RP. Fetal hepatoblastoma with placental metastases. Pediatr Pathol 1985, **4**, 163–7.
45. Oda H, Imai Y, Nakatsuru Y, Hata J, Ishikawa T. Somatic mutations of the APC gene in sporadic hepatoblastomas. Cancer Res 1996, **56**, 3320–3.
46. Gruner BA, DeNapoli TS, Andrews W, Tomlinson G, Bowman L, Weitman SD. Hepatocellular carcinoma in children associated with Gardner syndrome or familial adenomatous polyposis. J Pediatr Hematol Oncol 1998, **20**, 274–8.
47. Bala S, Wunsch PH, Ballhausen WG. Childhood hepatocellular adenoma in familial adenomatous polyposis: mutations in adenomatous polyposis coli gene and p53. Gastroenterology 1997, **112**, 919–22.
48. Futami H, Furuta T, Hanai H, Nakamura S, Baba S, Kaneko E. Adenoma of the common human bile duct in Gardner's syndrome may cause relapsing acute pancreatitis. J Gastroenterol 1997, **32**, 558–61.
49. Walsh N, Qizilbash A, Banerjee R, Waugh GA. Biliary neoplasia in Gardner's syndrome. Arch Pathol Lab Med 1987, **111**, 76–7.
50. Haas OA, Zoubek A, Grumayer ER, Gadner H. Constitutional interstitial deletion of 11p11 and pericentric inversion of chromosome 9 in a patient with Wiedemann–Beckwith syndrome and hepatoblastoma. Cancer Genet Cytogenet 1986, **23**, 95–104.
51. Hatada I, Ohashi H, Fukushima Y, Kaneko Y, Inoue M, Komoto Y, et al. An imprinted gene p57KIP2 is mutated in Beckwith–Wiedemann syndrome. Nat Genet 1996, **14**, 171–3.
52. Orozco-Florian R, McBride JA, Favara BE, Steele A, Brown SJ, Steele P. Congenital hepatoblastoma and Beckwith–Wiedemann syndrome. Pedi Path 1991, **11**, 131–42.
53. Lack EE, Schloo BL, Azumi N, Travis WD, Grier HE, Kozakewich HPW. Undifferentiated (embryonal) sarcoma of the liver. Am J Surg Pathol 1991, **15**, 1–16.
54. Srivastava S, Zou Z, Pirollo K, Blattner W, Chang EH. Germ-line transmission of a mutated p53 gene in a cancer-prone family with Li–Fraumeni syndrome. Nature 1990, **348**, 747–9.
55. Bove KE, Soukup S, Ballard ET, Ryckman F. Hepatoblastoma in a child with trisomy 18: cytogenetics, liver anomalies and literature review. Pediatr Pathol Lab Med 1996, **16**, 253–62.
56. Teraguchi M, Nogi S, Ikemoto Y, Ogino H, Kohdera U, Sakaida N, et al. Multiple hepatoblastomas associated with trisomy 18 in a 3-year-old girl. Pediatr Hematol Oncol 1997, **14**, 463–7.
57. Phaneuf D, Labelle Y, Berube D, Arden K, Cavenee W, Gagne R, Tanguay RM. Cloning and expression of the cDNA encoding human fumarylacetoacetate hydrolase, the enzyme deficient in hereditary tyrosinemia: assignment of the gene to chromosome 15. Am J Hum Genet 1991, **48**, 525–35.
58. Oda T, Elkahloun AG, Pike BL, Okajima K, Krantz ID, Genin A, et al. Mutations in the human Jagged 1 gene are responsible for Alagille syndrome. Nat Genet 1997, **16**, 235–42.
59. Kaufman SS, Wood P, Shaw Jr, Markin RS, Gridelli B, Vanderhoof JA. Hepatocarcinoma in a child with the Alagille syndrome. Am J Dis Child 1987, **141**, 698–700.
60. Weinberg AG, Finegold MJ. Primary hepatic tumors in childhood. In: Pathology of neoplasia in children and adolescents (ed. Finegold M). W.B. Saunders, Philadelphia, 1986, 347–8.
61. Alonso EM, Snover DC, Montag A, Freese DK, Whitington PF. Histologic pathology of the liver in progressive familial intrahepatic cholestasis. J Pediatr Gastroenterol Nutr 1994, **18**, 128–33.
62. Bull LN, Carlton VEH, Stricker NL, Baharloo S, DeYoung JA, Freimer NB, et al. Genetic and morphological findings in progressive familial intrahepatic cholestasis (Byler Disease [PFIC-1] and Byler syndrome): evidence for heterogeneity. Hepatology 1997, **26**, 155–64.
63. Young SJ. Primary malignant neurilemmoma (Schwannoma) of the liver in a case of neurofibromatosis. J Pathol 1975, **117**, 151–3.
64. Lederman SM, Martin EC, Laffey KT, Lefkowitch JH. Hepatic neurofibromatosis, malignant schwannoma, and angiosarcoma in von Recklinghausen's disease. Gastroenterology 1987, **92**, 234–9.
65. Wallace MR, Marchuk DA, Andersen LB, Letcher R, Odeh HM, Saulino AM, et al. Type 1 neurofibromatosis gene: identification of a large transcript disrupted in three NFI patients. Science 1990, **249**, 181–6.
66. Cawthon RM, Weiss R, Xu G, Viskochil D, Culver M, Stevens J, et al. A major segment of the neurofibromatosis type 1 gene: cDNA sequence, genomic structure, and point mutations. Cell 1990, **62**, 193–201.
67. Weinstein S, Scottolini AG, Loo SYT, Caldwell PC, Bhagavan NV. Ataxia-telangiectasia with hepatocellular carcinoma in a 15 year old girl and studies of her kindred. Arch Pathol Lab Med 1985, **109**, 1000–4.
68. Savitsky K, Bar-Shira A, Gilad S, Rotman G, Ziv Y, Vanagaite L, et al. A single ataxia telangiectasia gene with a product similar to PI-3 kinase. Science 1995, **268**, 1749–53.
69. Whitney M, Thayer M, Reifsteck C, Olson S, Smith L, Jakobs PM, et al. Microcell mediated chromosome transfer maps the Fanconi anaemia group D gene to chromosome 3p. Nat Genet 1995, **11**, 341–3.
70. Pulsipher M, Kupfer GM, Naf D, Suliman A, Lee JS, Jakobs P, et al. Subtyping analysis of Fanconi anemia by immunoblotting and retroviral gene transfer. Mol Med 1998, **4**, 468–79.
71. Green AJ, Smith M, Yates JRW. Loss of heterozygosity on chromosome 16 p 13.3 in hamartomas from tuberous sclerosis patients. Nat Genet 1994, **6**, 193–6.
72. Green AJ, Johnson PH, Yates JRW. The tuberous sclerosis gene on chromosome 9q34 acts as a growth supressor. Hum Mol Genet 1994, **3**, 1833–4.
73. Jaffe R. Liver transplant pathology in pediatric metabolic disorders. Pediatr Dev Pathol 1998, **1**, 102–17.
74. Walter JW, Blei F, Anderson JL, Orlow SJ, Speer MC, Marchuk DA. Genetic mapping of a novel familial form of infantile hemangioma. Am J Med Genet 1999, **82**, 77–83.
75. Ruck P, Xiao JC, Kaiserling E. Small epithelial cells and the histogenesis of hepatoblastoma. Electron microscopic, immunoelectron microscopic and immunohistochemical findings. Am J Pathol 1996, **148**, 321–9.

76. Michalopoulos GK, DeFrances MC. Liver regeneration. Science 1997, **276**, 60–6.
77. Sell S. Cellular origin of cancer: dedifferentiation or stem cell maturation arrest? Environ Health Perspect 1993, **101**(Suppl 5), 15–26.
78. Ishak KG, Glunz PR. Hepatoblastoma and hepatocarcinoma in infancy and childhood. Cancer 1967, **20**, 396–422.
79. Fahri DC, Shikes RH, Murari PJ, Silverberg SG. Hepatocellular carcinoma in young people. Cancer 1983, **52**, 1516–25.
79(a). Katzenstein HM, Krailo MD, Malogolowkin MH et al. Fibrolamellar carcinoma in children and adolescents. Cancer 2003, **97**, 2006–12.
80. Paradinas FJ, Melia WM, Wilkinson ML, Portmann B, Johnson PJ, Murray-Lyon IM, et al. High serum vitamin B12 binding capacity as a marker of the fibrolamellar variant of hepatocellular carcinoma. Br Med J 1982, **285**, 840–2.
81. Garcia de Davila MT, Gonzalez-Crussi F, Mangkornkanok M. Fibrolamellar carcinoma of the liver in a child: ultrastructural and immunohistologic aspects. Pediatr Pathol 1987, **7**, 319–31.
82. Andreola S, Lombardi L, Audisio RA, Mazzaferro V, Koukouras D, Doci R, et al. A clinicopathologic study of primary hepatic carcinoid tumors. Cancer 1990, **65**, 1211–18.
83. Barsky SH, Linnoila I, Triche TJ, Costa J. Hepatocellular carcinoma with carcinoid features. Hum Pathol 1984, **15**, 892–4.
84. Sioutos N, Virta S, Kessimian N. Primary hepatic carcinoid tumor. Am J Clin Pathol 1991, **95**, 172–5.
85. Ruck P, Harms D, Kaiserling E. Neuroendocrine differentiation in hepatoblastoma. An immunohistochemical investigation. Am J Surg Pathol 1990, **14**, 847–55.
86. Conrad RJ, Gribbin D, Walker NI, Ong TH. Combined cystic teratoma and hepatoblastoma of the liver. Probable divergent differentiation of an uncommitted hepatic precursor cell. Cancer 1993, **72**, 2910–13.
87. Cross SS, Variend S. Combined hepatoblastoma and yolk sac tumor of the liver. Cancer 1992, **69**, 1323–6.
88. Finegold MJ. Tumors of the liver. Semin Liver Dis 1994, **14**, 270–81.
89. Manivel C, Wick MR, Abenoza P, Dehner LP. Teratoid hepatoblastoma. Cancer 1986, **57**, 2168–74.
90. Aoyama C, Hachitanda Y, Soto JK, Said JW, Shimada H. Undifferentiated (embryonal) sarcoma of the liver. Am J Surg Path 1991, **15**, 615–24.
91. Chou P, Mangkornkanok M, Gonzalez-Crussi F. Undifferentiated (embryonal) sarcoma of the liver, ultrastructure, immunochemistry and DNA ploidy analysis of two cases. Pedi Path 1990, **10**, 549–62.
92. deChadarevian JP, Pawel BR, Faerber EN, Weintraum WH. Undifferentiated (Embryonal) sarcoma arising in conjunction with mesenchymal hamartoma of the liver. Mod Pathol 1994, **7**, 490–3.
93. Parham DM, Kelly DR, Donnelly WH, Douglass EC. Immunohistochemical and ultrastructural spectrum of hepatic sarcomas of childhood: evidence for a common histogenesis. Mod Pathol 1991, **4**, 648–53.
94. Miettinen M, Kahlos T. Undifferentiated (embryonal) sarcoma of the liver. Cancer 1989, **64**, 2096–103.
95. Leuschner I, Schmidt D, Harms D. Undifferentiated sarcoma of the liver in childhood. Hum Pathol 1990, **21**, 68–76.
96. Lauwers GY, Grant LD, Donnelly WH, Meloni AM, Foss RM, Sandberg AA, et al. Hepatic undifferentiated (embryonal) sarcoma arising in a mesenchymal hamartoma. Am J Surg Pathol 1997, **21**, 1248–54.
97. Walker NI, Horn MJ, Strong RW, Lynch SV, Cohen J, Ong TH, et al. Undifferentiated (embryonal) sarcoma of the liver. Cancer 1992, **69**, 52–9.
98. Corbally MT, Spitz L. Malignant potential of mesenchymal hamartoma: an unrecognized risk. Pediatr Surg Int 1992, **7**, 321–2.
99. Scheimberg I, Cullinane C, Kelsey A, Malone M. Primary hepatic malignant tumor with rhabdoid features. A histological, immunocytochemical, and electron microscopic study of four cases and a review of the literature. Am J Surg Pathol 1996, **20**, 1394–400.
100. Parham DM, Peiper SC, Robicheaux G, Ribeiro RC, Douglass EC. Malignant rhabdoid tumor of the liver. Arch Pathol Lab Med 1988, **112**, 61–4.
101. Horowitz ME, Etcubanas E, Webber BL, Kun LE, Rao BN, Vogel RJ, et al. Hepatic undifferentiated sarcoma and rhabdomyosarcoma in children. Results of therapy. Cancer 1987, **59**, 396–402.
102. Jozwiak S, Pedich M, Rajszys P, Michalowicz R. Incidence of hepatic hamartomas in tuberous sclerosis. Arch Dis Child 1992, **67**, 1363–5.
103. Awan S, Davenport M, Portmann B, Howard ER. Angiosarcoma of the liver in children. J Pediatr Surg 1996, **31**, 1729–32.
104. Patterson K. Liver tumors and tumor like masses. In: Pediatric neoplasia, morphology and biology (ed. Parham DM). Lippincott-Raven, Philadelphia, 331–61.
105. Hanawa Y, Ise T, Hasegawa H, Sano R. Serum cholesterol in children with hepatoma. Jpn J Clin Oncol 1971, **12**, 129–36.
106. Muraji T, Woolley MM, Sinatra F, Siegel SM, Isaacs H. The prognostic implication of hypercholesterolemia in infants and children with hepatoblastoma. J Pediatr Surg 1985, **20**, 228–30.
107. Watanabe I, Yamaguchi M, Kasai M. Histologic characteristics of gonadotropin-producing hepatoblastoma: a survey of seven cases from Japan. J Pediatr Surg 1987, **22**, 406–11.
108. Galifer RB, Sultan C, Margueritte G, Barnean G. Testosterone producing hepatoblastoma in a three year old boy with precocious puberty. J Pediatr Surg 1985, **20**, 713–14.
109. Selby DM, Stocker JT, Waclawiw MA, Hitchock CL, Ishak KG. Infantile hemangioendothelioma of the liver. Hepatology 1994, **20**, 39–45.
110. Reynolds M. Pediatric liver tumors. Semin Surg Oncol 1999, **16**, 159–72.
111. Vos A. Primary liver tumors in children. Eur J Surg Oncol 1995, **21**, 101–5.
112. Abenoza P, Manivel JC, Wick MR, Hagen K, Dehner LP. Hepatoblastoma: an immunohistochemical and ultrastructural study. Hum Pathol 1989, **18**, 1025–35.
113. Haas JE, Muczynski KA, Krailo M, Ablin A, Land V, Vietti TJ, et al. Histopathology and prognosis in childhood

113. hepatoblastoma and hepatocarcinoma. Cancer 1989, 64, 1082–95.
114. Hino O, Kitagawa T, Hirama T, Yokoyama S. Hepatitis B virus DNA integration in hepatoblastoma. Lancet 1984, 1, 462–3.
115. Kuniyasu H, Yasui W, Shimamoto F, Fujii K, Nakahara M, Asahara T. Hepatoblastoma in an adult associated with c-met proto-oncogene imbalance. Pathol Int 1996, 46, 1005–10.
116. Fasano M, Theise ND, Nalesnik M, Goswami S, Garcia de Davila MT, Finegold MJ, et al. Immunohistochemical evaluation of hepatoblastomas with use of the hepatocyte-specific marker, hepatocyte paraffin 1, and the polyclonal anti-carcinoembryonic antigen. Mod Pathol 1998, 11, 934–8.
117. Saito Y, Matsuzaka Y, Doi M, Sugitani T, Chiba T, Abei M, et al. Multiple regression analysis for assessing the growth of small hepatocellular carcinoma: the M1B-1 labelling index is the most effective parameter. J Gastroenterol 1998, 33, 229–35.
118. Wu PC, Fang JW, Lau VK, Lai CL, Lo CK, Lau JY. Classification of hepatocellular carcinoma according to hepatocellular and biliary differentiation markers. Clinical and biological implications. Am J Pathol 1996, 149, 1167–75.
119. Rainer S, Dabry CJ, Feinberg AP. Loss of imprinting in hepatoblastoma. Cancer Res 1995, 55, 1836–8.
120. Scoazec JY, Flejou JF, DiErrico A, Fiorentino M, Zamparelli A, Bringuier AF, et al. Fibrolamellar carcinoma of the liver: composition of the extracellular matrix and expression of cell–matrix and cell–cell adhesion molecules. Hepatology 1996, 24, 1128–36.
121. Washington K, Telen MJ, Gottfried MR. Expression of cell adhesion molecule CD44 in primary tumors of the liver: an immunohistochemical study. Liver 1997, 17, 17–23.
122. Orsatti G, Greenberg PD, Rolfes DB, Ishak KG, Paronetto F. DNA ploidy of fibrolamellar carcinoma by image analysis. Hum Pathol 1994, 25, 936–9.
123. Orsatti G, Hytiroglou P, Thung SN, Ishak KG, Paronetto F. Lamellar fibrosis in the fibrolamellar variant of hepatocellular carcinoma: a role for transforming growth factor beta. Liver 1997, 17, 152–6.
124. Kasai M, Watanabe I. Histologic classification of liver-cell carcinoma in infancy and childhood and its clinical evaluation. A study of 70 cases collected in Japan. Cancer 1970, 25, 551–63.
125. Feusner J, Krailo M, Haas JE, Campbell JR, Lloyd DA, Albin AR. Treatment of pulmonary metastases of initial stage I hepatoblastoma in childhood. Cancer 1993, 71, 759–864.
126. Haas JE, Feusner JH, Finegold MJ, Small cell undifferentiated histology may be unfavorable. Cancer 2007, 92, 3130–4.
127. Dehner LP, Manivel JC. Hepatoblastoma: an analysis of the relationship between morphologic subtypes and prognosis. Am J Pediatr Hematol Oncol 1988, 10, 301–7.
128. Hata Y, Ishizu H, Ohmori K, Hamada H, Sasaki F, Uchino J, et al. Flow cytometric analysis of the nuclear DNA content of hepatoblastoma. Cancer 1991, 68, 2566–70.
129. Schmidt D, Wischmeyer P, Leuschner I, Sprenger E, Langenau E, vonSchweinitz D, Harms D. DNA analysis in hepatoblastoma by flow and image cytometry. Cancer 1993, 72, 2914–19.
130. Zerbini MCN, Sredni ST, Grier H, Cristofani LM, Latorre MRDO, Hollister KA, et al. Primary malignant epithelial tumors of the liver in children: a study of DNA content and oncogene expression. Pediatr Dev Pathol 1998, 1, 270–80.
131. Krober S, Ruck P, Xiao JC, Kaiserling E. Flow cytometric evaluation of nuclear DNA content in hepatoblastoma: further evidence for the inhomogeneity of the different subtypes. Path Int 1995, 45, 501–5.
132. Ara T, Fukuzawa M, Oue T, Komoto Y, Kusafuka T, Imura K, Okada A. Immunohistochemical assessment of the MIB-1 labeling index in human hepatoblastoma and its prognostic relevance. J Pediatr Surg 1997, 32, 1690–4.
133. Rugge M, Sonego F, Pollice L, Perilongo G, Guido M, Basso G, Ninfo V, et al. Hepatoblastoma: DNA nuclear content, proliferative indices, and pathology. Liver 1998, 18, 128–33.
134. Fraumeni J, JF, Miller RW, Hill JA. Primary carcinoma of the liver in childhood: an epidemiologic study. J Natl Cancer Inst 1968, 40, 1087–99.
135. vonSchweinitz D, Leuschner I, Gluer S, Pietsch T. Expression of cell adhesion molecules and common acute lymphoblastic leukemia antigen in hepatoblastoma. Virchows Arch 1996, 429, 239–41.
136. vonSchweinitz D, Gliier S, Mildenberger H. Liver tumors in neonates and very young infants: diagnostic pitfalls and therapeutic problems. Eur J Pediatr Surg 1995, 5, 72–6.
137. Mortele KJ, Mergo PJ, Urrutia M, Ros PR. Dynamic gadolinium-enhanced MR findings in infantile hepatic hemangioendothelioma. J Comput Assist Tomogr 1998, 22, 714–17.
138. Moran CA, Mullick FG, Ishak KG. Nodular regenerative hyperplasia of the liver in children. Am J Surg Pathol 1991, 15, 449–54.
138(a). Cessna MH, Zhou H, Sanger WG et al. Expression of ALK1 and p80 in inflammatory myofibroblastic tumor and its mesenchymal mimics: a study of 135 cases. Mod Pathol 2002, 15, 931–8.
139. Biselli R, Ferlini C, Fattorossi A, Boldrini R, Bosman C. Inflammatory myofibroblastic tumor (inflammatory pseudotumor). Cancer 1996, 77, 778–84.
140. Han SJ, Tsai CC, Tsai HM, Chen YJ. Infantile hemangioendothelioma with highly elevated alpha-fetoprotein level. Hepatogastroenterology 1998, 45, 459–61.
141. Seo IS, Min KW, Mirkin LD. Hepatic hemangioendothelioma of infancy associated with elevated alphafetoprotein and catecholamine by-products. Pediatr Pathol 1988, 8, 625–31.
142. Lennington WJ, Gray Jr, Page DL. Mesenchymal hamartoma of liver. Am J Dis Child 1993, 147, 193–6.
143. Peng SY, Lei PL, Chu JS, Lee PH, Tsung PT, Chen DS, et al. Expression and hypomethylation of alpha-fetoprotein gene in unicentric and multicentric human hepatocellular carcinomas. Hepatology 1993, 17, 35–41.
144. Tsuchida Y, Honna T, Fukui M, Sakaguchi H, Ishiguro T. The ratio of fucosylation of alpha-fetoprotein in hepatoblastoma. Cancer 1989, 63, 2174–6.
145. Aoyagi Y. Molecular discrimination between alpha-fetoprotein from patients with hepatocellular carcinoma and non-neoplastic liver diseases by their carbohydrate structures (Review). Int J Oncol 1994, 4, 369–83.

146. Furui J, Furukawa M, Kanematsu T. The low positive rate of serum alpha-fetoprotein levels in hepatitis C virus antibody-positive patients with hepatocellular carcinoma. Hepatogastroenterology 1995, 42, 445–9.
147. Tang ZY, Yu YQ, Zhou XD, Yang BH, Ma ZC, Lin ZY. Subclinical hepatocellular carcinoma: an analysis of 391 patients. J Surg Oncol 1993, Suppl 3, 55–8.
148. Leon M, Kew M. Loss of heterozygosity in chromosome 4q12-q13 in hepatocellular carcinoma in Southern African Blacks. Anticancer Res 1996, 16, 349–51.
149. Dekmezian R, Sneige N, Popok S, Ordonez NG. Fine-needle aspiration cytology of pediatric patients with primary hepatic tumors. Diagn Cytopathol 1988, 4, 162–8.
150. Ishak KG. Primary hepatic tumors in childhood. In: Progress in liver disease, Vol. 5 (ed. Popper H, Schaffner F). Grune & Stratton, New York, 1980, 636.
151. Justrabo E, Martin L, Yazji N, Couillault JP, Gounot E, Olsson NO, et al. Hepatic mesenchymal hamartoma in children. Immunohistochemical, ultrastructural and flow cytometric case study. Gastroenterol Clin Biol 1998, 22, 964–8.
152. vonSchweinitz D, Fuchs J, Gluer S, Pietsch T. The occurrence of liver growth factor in hepatoblastoma. Eur J Pediatr Surg 1998, 8, 133–6.
153. McGill JR, Naylor SL, Sakaguchi AY, Moore CM, Boyd D, Barrett KJ, et al. Human ferritin H&L sequences lie on ten different chromosomes. Hum Genet 1987, 76, 66–72.
154. Mita Y, Aoyagi Y, Yanagi M, Suda T, Suzuki Y, Asakura H. The usefulness of determining des-gamma-carboxy prothrombin by sensitive enzyme immunoassay in the early diagnosis of patients with hepatocellular carcinoma. Cancer 1998, 82, 1643–8.
155. Motohara K, Endo F, Matsudo I, Iwamasa T. Acarboxy prothrombin (PIVKA-II) as a marker of hepatoblastoma in infants. J Pediatr Gastroenterol Nutr 1987, 6, 42–5.
156. Nakagawara A, Ikeda K, Tsuneyoshi M, Daimaru Y, Enjoji M, Watanabe I, et al. Hepatoblastoma producing both alpha-fetoprotein and human chorionic gonadotropin. Cancer 1985, 56, 1636–42.
157. Kim SN, Chi JG, Kim YW, Dong ES, Shin HY, Ahn HS, et al. Neonatal choriocarcinoma of liver. Pediatr Pathol 1993, 13, 723–30.
158. Collier NA, Bloom SR, Hodgson HJF, Weinbren K, Lee YC, Blumgart LH. Neurotensin secretion by fibrolamellar carcinoma of the liver. Lancet 1984, 1, 538–40.
159. Taketomi A, Takenaka K, Matsumata T, Shimada M, Higashi H, Shirabe K, et al. Circulating intercellular adhesion molecule-1 in patients with hepatocellular carcinoma before and after hepatic resection. Hepatogastroenterology 1997, 44, 477–83.
160. Hamazaki K, Gochi A, Shimmura H, Kaihara A, Muruo Y, Doi T, et al. Serum levels of circulating intercellular adhesion molecule 1 in hepatocellular carcinoma. Hepatogastroenterology 1996, 43, 229–34.
161. Jin-no K, Tanimuzu M, Hyodo I, Nishikawa Y, Hosokawa Y, Endo H, et al. Circulating platelet-derived endothelial cell growth factor increases in hepatocellular carcinoma patients. Cancer 1998, 82, 1260–70.
162. Hayasaka A, Suzuki N, Fujimoto N, Iwama S, Fukuyama E, Kanda Y, et al. Elevated plasma levels of matrix metalloproteinase-9 (92-kd type IV collagenase/gelatinase B) in hepatocellular carcinoma. Hepatology 1996, 24, 1058–62.
163. Tomiya T, Gujiwara K. Serum transforming growth factor alpha level as a marker of hepatocellular carcinoma complicating cirrhosis. Cancer 1996, 77, 1056–60.
164. Jin-no K, Tanimizu M, Hyodo I, Nishikawa Y, Hosokawa Y, Doi T, et al. Circulating vascular endothelial growth factor (VEGF) is a possible tumor marker for metastasis in human hepatocellular carcinoma. J Gastroenterol 1998, 33, 376–82.
165. Mascarello JT, Jones MC, Kadota RP, Krous HF. Hepatoblastoma characterized by trisomy 20 and double minutes. Cancer Genet Cytogenet 1990, 47, 243–7.
166. Tonk VS, Wilson KS, Timmons CF, Schneider NR. Trisomy 2, trisomy 20, and del(17p) as sole chromosomal abnormalities in three cases of hepatoblastoma. Genes Chromosomes Cancer 1994, 11, 199–202.
167. Bardi G, Johansson B, Pandis N, Bekassy AN, Kullendorff CM, Hagerstrand I, Heim S. i(8q) as the primary structural chromosome abnormality in a hepatoblastoma. Cancer Genet Cytogenet 1991, 51, 281–3.
168. Pavelka K. Consistent chromosome aberrations in hepatoblastoma: a common pathway of genetic alterations in embryonal malignancies. Appl Cytogenet 1990, 16, 74.
169. Fletcher JA, Kozakewich HP, Pavelka K, Grier HE, Shamberger RC, Korf B, Morton CC. Consistent cytogenetic aberrations in hepatoblastoma: a common pathway of genetic alterations in embryonal liver and skeletal muscle malignancies? Genes Chromosomes Cancer 1991, 3, 37–43.
170. Soukup S, Lampkin B. Trisomy 2 and 20 in two hepatoblastomas. Genes Chromosomes Cancer 1991, 3, 231–4.
171. Rodriguez E, Reuter VE, Mies C, Bosl GJ, Chaganti RSK. Abnormalities of 2q: a common genetic link between rhabdomyosarcoma and hepatoblastoma? Genes Chromosomes Cancer 1991, 3, 122–7.
172. Dressler LG, Duncan MH, Varsa EE, McConnell TS. DNA content measurement can be obtained using archival material for DNA flow cytometry. A comparison with cytogenetic analysis in 56 pediatric solid tumors. Cancer 1993, 72, 1033–41.
173. Swarts S, Wisecarver J, Bridge JA. Significance of extra copies of chromosome 20 and the long arm of chromosome 2 in hepatoblastoma. Cancer Genet Cytogenet 1991, 91, 65–7.
174. Sainati L, Leazl A, Stella M, Montaldi A, Perilongo G, Rugge M, et al. Cytogenetic analysis of hepatoblastoma: hypothesis of cytogenetic evolution in such tumors and results of a multicentric study. Cancer Genet Cytogenet 1998, 104, 39–44.
175. Schneider NR, Cooley LD, Finegold MJ, Douglass EC, Tomlinson GE. The first recurring chromosome translocation in hepatoblastoma: der(4)t(1;4)(q12;q34). Genes Chromosomes Cancer 1997, 19, 291–4.
176. Anneren G, Nordlinder H, Hedborg F. Chromosome aberrations in an alpha-fetoprotein producing hepatoblastoma. Genes Chromosomes Cancer 1992, 4, 99–100.
177. Balogh E, Swanton S, Kiss C, Jakab ZS, Seeker-Walker LM, Olah E. Fluorescence in situ hybridization reveals trisomy 2q by insertion into 9p in hepatoblastoma. Cancer Genet Cytogenet 1998, 102, 148–50.
178. Tanaka K, Uemoto S, Asonuma K, Katayama T, Utsunomiya H, Akiyama Y, et al. Hepatoblastoma in a 2-year old girl with trisomy 18. Eur J Pediatr Surg 1992, 2, 298–300.

179. Hashizume K, Nakajo T, Kawarasaki H, Iwanaka T, Kanamori Y, Tanaka K, et al. Prader-Willi syndrome with del (15) (q11, q13) associated with hepatoblastoma. Acta Paediatr Jpn 1991, **33**, 718–22.
180. Hansen K, Bagtas J, Mark HF, Homans A, Singer DB. Undifferentiated small cell hepatoblastoma with a unique chromosomal translocation: a case report. Pediatr Pathol 1992, **12**, 457–62.
181. Spellerberg A, Perlman E. Genetic analysis of hepatoblastomas by comparative genomic hybridization. Lab Invest 1998, **78**, 7P.
182. Bridge JA, Swarts SJ, Buresh C, Nelson M, Degenhardt JM, Spanier S, et al. Trisomies 8 and 20 characterize a subgroup of benign fibrous lesions arising in both soft tissue and bone. Am J Pathol 1999, **154**, 729–33.
183. Kraus JA, Albrecht S, Wiestler OD, vonSchweinitz D, Pietsch T. Loss of heterozygosity on chromosome 1 in human hepatoblastoma. Int J Cancer 1996, **67**, 467–71.
184. Yeh SH, Chen PJ, Chen HL, Lai MY, Wang CC, Chen DS. Frequent genetic alterations at the distal region of chromosome 1p in human hepatocellular carcinomas. Cancer Res 1994, **54**, 4188–92.
185. Kuroki T, Fujiwara Y, Tsuchiya E, Nakamori S, Imaoka S, Kanematsu T, et al. Accumulation of genetic changes during development and progression of hepatocellular carcinoma: loss of heterozygosity of chromosome arm 1p occurs at an early stage of hepatocarcinogenesis. Genes Chromosomes Cancer 1995, **13**, 163–7.
186. Wong N, Lai P, Lee SW, Fan S, Pang E, Liew C, et al. Assessment of genetic changes in hepatocellular carcinoma by comparative genomic hybridization analysis. Am J Pathol 1999, **154**, 37–43.
187. Marchio A, Meddeb M, Pineau P, Danglot G, Tiollais P, Bernheim A, et al. Recurrent chromosomal abnormalities in hepatocellular carcinoma detected by comparative genomic hybridization. Genes Chromosomes Cancer 1997, **18**, 59–65.
188. Piao Z, Park C, Park JH, Kim H. Allelotype analysis of hepatocellular carcinoma. Int J Cancer 1998, **75**, 29–33.
189. Yeh SH, Chen PJ, Lai MY, Chen DS. Allelic loss on chromosomes 4q and 16q in hepatocellular carcinoma: association with elevated alpha-fetoprotein production. Gastroenterology 1996, **110**, 184–92.
190. Buetow KH, Murray JC, Israel JL, London WT, Smith M, Kew M, et al. Loss of heterozygosity suggests tumor suppressor gene responsible for primary hepatocellular carcinoma. Proc Natl Acad Sci 1989, **86**, 8852–6.
191. Chou YH, Chung KC, Jeng LB, Chen TC, Liaw YF. Frequent allelic loss on chromosomes 4q and 16q associated with human hepatocellular carcinoma in Taiwan. Cancer Lett 1998, **123**, 1–6.
192. Ding SF, Habib NA, Dooley J, Wood C, Bowles L, Delhanty JD. Loss of constitutional heterozygosity on chromosome 5q in hepatocellular carcinoma without cirrhosis. Br J Cancer 1991, **64**, 1083–7.
193. Fujiwara Y, Monden M, Mori T, Nakamura Y, Emi M. Frequent multiplication of the long arm of chromosome 8 in hepatocellular carcinoma. Cancer Res 1993, **53**, 857–60.
194. Emi M, Fujiwara Y, Ohata H, Tsuda H, Hirohashi S, Koike M, et al. Allelic loss at chromosome band 8 p21.3-p22 is associated with progression of hepatocellular carcinoma. Genes Chromosomes Cancer 1993, **7**, 152–7.
195. Nagai H, Pineau P, Tiollais P, Buendia MA, DeJean A. Comprehensive allele typing of human hepatocellular carcinoma. Oncogene 1997, **14**, 2927–33.
196. Wang HP, Rogler CE. Deletions in human chromosome arms 11p and 13q in primary hepatocellular carcinomas. Cytogenet Cell Genet 1988, **48**, 72–8.
197. Sakai K, Nagahara H, Abe K, Obata H. Loss of heterozygosity on chromosome 16 in hepatocellular carcinoma. J Gastroenterol Hepatol 1992, **7**, 288–92.
198. Tsuda H, Zhang W, Shimosato Y, Yokota J, Terada M, Sugimura T, et al. Allele loss on chromosome 16 associated with progression of human hepatocellular carcinoma. Proc Natl Acad Sci 1990, **87**, 6791–4.
199. Nasarek J, Werner M, Nolte M, Klempnauer J, Georgii A. Trisomy 1 and 8 occur frequently in hepatocellular carcinoma but not in liver cell adenoma and focal nodular hyperplasia. A fluorescence in situ hybridization study. Virchows Arch 1995, **427**, 373–8.
200. Lowichik A, Schneider NR, Tonk V, Ansari MQ, Timmons CF. Report of a complex karyotype in recurrent metastatic fibrolamellar hepatocellular carcinoma and a review of hepatocellular carcinoma cytogenetics. Cancer Genet Cytogenet 1996, **88**, 170–4.
201. Ito H, Yamasaki T, Okamoto O, Tahara E. Infantile hemangioendothelioma of the liver in patient with interstitial deletion of chromosome 6q: report of an autopsy case. Am J Med Genet 1989, **34**, 325–9.
202. Speleman F, De Telder V, De Potter KR, Dal Cin P, Van Daele S, Benoit Y, et al. Cytogenetic analysis of a mesenchymal hamartoma of the liver. Cancer Genet Cytogenet 1989, **40**, 29–32.
203. Bove KE, Blough RI, Soukup S. Third report of t(19q)(13.4) in mesenchymal hamartoma of liver with comments on link to embryonal sarcoma. Pediatr Dev Pathol 1998, **1**, 438–42.
204. Mascarello JT, Krous HF. Second report of a translocation involving 19q13.4 in a mesenchymal hamartoma of the liver. Cancer Genet Cytogenet 1992, **58(2)**, 141–2.
205. Sawyer JR, Roloson GJ, Bell JM, Thomas JR, Teo C, Chadduck WM. Telomeric associations in the progression of chromosome aberrations in pediatric solid tumors. Cancer Genet Cytogenet 1990, **90**, 1–13.
206. Iliszko M, Czauderna P, Babinska M, Stoba C, Roszkiewica A, Limon J. Cytogenetic findings in an embryonal sarcoma of the liver. Cancer Genet Cytogenet 1998, **102**, 142–4.
207. Barnhart DC, Hirschi RB, Garver KA, Geiger JD, Harmon CM, Coran AG. Conservative management of mesenchymal hamartoma of the liver. J Pediatr Surg 1997, **32**, 1495–8.
208. Murray JD, Ricketts RR. Mesenchymal hamartoma of the liver. Ann Surg 1998, **64**, 1097–103.
209. Meinders AJ, Simons MP, Heij HA, Aronson DC. Mesenchymal hamartoma of the liver: failed management by marsupialization. J Pediatr Gastroenterol Nutr 1998, **26**, 353–5.
210. Unsal H, Yakicier C, Marcais C, Kew M, Volkmann M, Zentgraf H, et al. Genetic heterogeneity of hepatocellular carcinoma. Proc Natl Acad Sci 1994, **91**, 822–6.
211. Piao Z, Kim H, Jeon BK, Lee WJ, Park C. Relationship between loss of heterozygosity of tumor suppressor genes

211. and histologic differentiation in hepatocellular carcinoma. Cancer 1997, 80, 865–72.
212. deLaCoste A, Romagnolo B, Billuart P, Renard CA, Buendia MA, Soubrane O, et al. Somatic mutations of the beta-catenin gene are frequent in mouse and human hepatocellular carcinomas. Proc Natl Acad Sci 1998, 95, 8847–51.
213. Miyoshi Y, Iwao K, Nagasawa Y, Aihara T, Sasaki Y, Imaoka S, et al. Activation of the beta-catenin gene in primary hepatocellular carcinomas by somatic alterations involving exon 3. Cancer Res 1998, 58, 2524–7.
214. Katagiri T, Nakamura Y, Miki Y. Mutations in the BRCA2 gene in hepatocellular carcinomas. Cancer Res 1996, 56, 4575–7.
215. Bonilla F, Orlow I, Cordon-Cardo C. Mutational study of p16CDKN2/MTS1/INK4A and p57KIP2 genes in hepatocellular carcinoma. Int J Oncol 1998, 12, 583–8.
216. Biden Y, Young J, Buttenshaw R, Searle J, Cooksley G, Xu DB, et al. Frequency of mutation and deletion of the tumor suppressor gene CDKN2A (MTS1/p16) in hepatocellular carcinoma from an Australian population. Hepatology 1997, 25, 593–7.
217. Lin YW, Chen CH, Huang GT, Lee PH, Wang JT, Chen DS, et al. Infrequent mutations and no methylation of CDKN2A (P16/MTS1) and CDKN2B (p15/MTS2) in hepatocellular carcinoma in Taiwan. Eur J Cancer 1998, 34, 1789–95.
218. Chaubert P, Gayer R, Zimmermann A, Fontolliet C, Stamm B, Bossman F, et al. Germ-line mutations of the p16INK4 (MTS1) gene occur in a subset of patients with hepatocellular carcinoma. Hepatology 1997, 25, 1376–81.
219. Boix L, Rosa JL, Ventura F, Castells A, Bruix J, Rodes J, et al. c-met overexpression in human hepatocellular carcinoma. Hepatology 1994, 19, 88–91.
220. Ueki T, Fujimoto J, Suzuki T, Yamamoto H, Okamoto E. Expression of hepatocyte growth factor and its receptor c-met proto-oncogene in hepatocellular carcinoma. Hepatology 1997, 25, 862–6.
221. Park WS, Dong SM, Kim SY, Na EY, Shin MS, Pi JH, et al. Somatic mutations in the kinase domain of the Met/hepatocyte growth factor receptor gene in childhood hepatocellular carcinomas. Cancer Res 1999, 59, 307–10.
222. Peng SY, Lai PL, Hsu HC. Amplification of the c-myc gene in human hepatocellular carcinoma: biologic significance. J Formos Med Assoc 1993, 92, 866–70.
223. Koga H, Sakisaka S, Ohishi M, Kawaguchi T, Taniguchi E, Sasatomi K, et al. Expression of cyclooxygenase-2 in human hepatocellular carcinoma: relevance to tumor dedifferentiation. Hepatology 1999, 29, 688–96.
224. Chao Y, Shih YL, Chiu JH, Chau GY, Lui WY, Yang WK, et al. Overexpression of cyclin A but not Skp2 correlates with the tumor relapse of human hepatocellular carcinoma. Cancer Res 1998, 58, 985–90.
225. Nishida N, Fukuda Y, Komeda T, Kita R, Sando T, Furukawa M, et al. Amplification and overexpression of the cyclin D1 gene in aggressive human hepatocellular carcinoma. Cancer Res 1994, 54, 3107–10.
226. Kanai Y, Ushijima S, Hui AM, Ochiai A, Tsuda H, Sakamoto M, et al. The E-cadherin gene is silenced by CpG methylation in human hepatocellular carcinomas. Int J Cancer 1997, 71, 355–9.

227. Strand S, Hofmann WJ, Hug H, Muller M, Otto G, Strand D, et al. Lymphocyte apoptosis induced by CD 95 (APO-1/FAS) ligand-expressing tumor cells—a mechanism of immune evasion. Nature Med 1996, 2, 1361–6.
228. Wales MM, Biel MA, Deiry WE, Nelkin BD, Issa JP, Cavenee WK, et al. P53 activates expression of HIC-1, a new candidate tumor supressor gene on 17p 13.3. Nature Med 1995, 1, 570–7.
229. Kanai Y, Hui A, Sun L, Ushijima S, Sakamoto M, Tsuda H, et al. DNA hypermethylation at the D17S5 locus and reduced HIC-1 mRNA expression are associated with hepatocarcinogenesis. Hepatology 1999, 29, 703–9.
230. Kim KS, Lee YI. Biallelic expression of the H19 and IGF2 genes in hepatocellular carcinoma. Cancer Lett 1997, 119, 143–8.
231. Piao Z, Choi Y, Park C, Lee WJ, Park JH, Kim H. Deletion of the M6P/IGF2r gene in primary hepatocellular carcinoma. Cancer Lett 1997, 120, 39–43.
232. Qiu SJ, Ye SL, Wu ZQ, Tang ZY, Liu YK. The expression of the mdm2 gene may be related to the aberration of the p53 gene in human hepatocellular carcinoma. J Cancer Res Clin Oncol 1998, 124, 253–8.
233. Rivas MJ, Arii S, Furutani M, Harada T, Mizumoto M, Nishiyama H, et al. Expression of human macrophage metalloelastase gene in hepatocellular carcinoma: correlation with angiostatin generation and its clinical significance. Hepatology 1998, 28, 986–93.
234. Ito Y, Sasaki Y, Horimoto M, Wada S, Tanaka Y, Kasahara A, et al. Activation of mitogen-activated protein kinases/extracellular signal-regulated kinases in human hepatocellular carcinoma. Hepatology 1998, 27, 951–8.
235. Hui AM, Sakamoto M, Kanai Y, Ino Y, Gotoh M, Yokota J, et al. Inactivation of $p16^{INK4}$ in hepatocellular carcinoma. Hepatology 1996, 24, 575–9.
236. Hui A, Kanai Y, Sakamoto M, Tsuda H, Hirohashi S. Reduced $p21^{WAF1/CLP1}$ expression and p53 mutation in hepatocellular carcinomas. Hepatology 1997, 25, 575–9.
237. Soini Y, Chia SC, Bennett WP, Groopman JD, Wang JS, DeBenedetti VM, et al. An aflatoxin-associated mutational hot spot at codon 240 in the p53 tumor suppressor gene occurs in hepatocellular carcinomas from Mexico. Carcinogenesis 1996, 17, 1007–12.
238. Slagle BL, Zhou YZ, Butel JS. Hepatitis B virus integration event in human chromosome 17p near the p53 gene identifies the region of the chromosome commonly deleted in virus-positive hepatocellular carcinomas. Cancer Res 1991, 51, 49–54.
239. Kishimoto Y, Shiota G, Kamisaki Y, Wada K, Nakamoto K, Yamawaki M, et al. Loss of the tumor supressor p53 gene at the liver cirrhosis stage in Japanese patients with hepatocellular carcinoma. Oncology 1997, 54, 304–10.
240. Ashida K, Kishimoto Y, Nakamoto K, Wada K, Shiota G, Hirooka Y, et al. Loss of heterozygosity of the retinoblastoma gene in liver cirrhosis accompanying hepatocellular carcinoma. J Cancer Res Clin Oncol 1997, 123, 489–95.
241. Nouso K, Urabe Y, Higashi T, Nakatsukasa H, Hino N, Ashida K, et al. Telomerase as a tool for the differential diagnosis of human hepatocellular carcinoma. Cancer 1996, 78, 232–6.
242. Miura N, Horikawa I, Nishimoto A, Ohmura H, Ito H, Hirohashi S, et al. Progressive telomere shortening and

242. telomerase reactivation during hepatocellular carcinogenesis. Cancer Genet Cytogenet 1997, **93**, 56–62.
243. Kojima H, Yokosuka O, Imazeki F, Saisho H, Omata M. Telomerase activity and telomere length in hepatocellular carcinoma and chronic liver disease. Gastroenterology 1997, **112**, 493–500.
244. Ohta K, Kanamaru T, Morita Y, Hayashi Y, Ito H, Yamamoto M. Telomerase activity in hepatocellular carcinoma as a predictor of postoperative recurrence. J Gastroenterol 1997, **32**, 791–6.
245. Kira S, Nakanishi T, Suemori S, Kitamoto M, Watanabe Y, Kajiyama G. Expression of transforming growth factor alpha and epidermal growth factor receptor in human hepatocellular carcinoma. Liver 1997, **17**, 177–82.
246. Ito N, Kawata S, Tamura S, Takaishi K, Shirai Y, Kiso S, et al. Elevated levels of transforming growth factor beta messenger RNA and its polypeptide in human hepatocellular carcinoma. Cancer Res 1991, **51**, 4080–3.
247. Yumoto Y, Hanafusa T, Hada H, Morita T, Ooguchi S, Shinji N, et al. Loss of heterozygosity and analysis of mutation of p53 in hepatocellular carcinoma. J Gastroenterol Hepatol 1995, **10**, 179–85.
248. Jones SN, Hancock AR, Vogel H, Donehower LA, Bradley A. Overexpression of Mdm2 in mice reveals a p53-independent role for Mdm2 in tumorgenesis. Proc Natl Acad Sci 1998, **95**, 15608–12.
249. Ohnishi H, Kawamura M, Hanada R, Kaneko Y, Tsunoda Y, Hongo T, et al. Infrequent mutations of the TP53 gene and no amplification of the MDM2 gene in hepatoblastomas. Genes Chromosomes Cancer 1996, **15**, 187–90.
250. Honda K, Sbisa E, Tullo A, Papeo PA, Saccone C, Poole S, et al. p53 mutation is a poor prognostic indicator for survival in patients with hepatocellular carcinoma undergoing surgical tumor ablation. Br J Cancer 1998, **77**, 776–82.
251. Shiota G, Kishimoto Y, Suyama A, Okubo M, Katayama S, Harada K, et al. Prognostic significance of serum anti-p53 antibody in patients with hepatocellular carcinoma. J Hepatol 1997, **27**, 661–8.
252. Tsuda H, Oda T, Sakamoto M, Hirohashi S. Different pattern of chromosomal allele loss in multiple hepatocellular carcinomas as evidence of their multifocal origin. Cancer Res 1992, **52**, 1504–9.
253. Ding SF, Delhanty JD, Dooley JS, Bowles L, Wood CB, Habib A. The putative tumor supressor gene on chromosome 5q for hepatocellular carcinoma is distinct from the MCC and APC genes. Cancer Detect Prev 1993, **17**, 405–9.
254. Hytiroglou P, Kotoula V, Thung SN, Tsokos M, Fiel MI, Papadimitriou CS. Telomerase activity in precancerous hepatic nodules. Cancer 1998, **82**, 1831–8.
255. Macdonald GA, Greenson JK, Saito K, Cherian SP, Appelman HD, Boland CR. Microsatellite instability and loss of heterozygosity at DNA mismatch repair gene loci occurs during hepatic carcinogenesis. Hepatology 1998, **28**, 90–7.
256. Debuire B, Paterlini P, Pontisso P, Basso G, May E. Analysis of the p53 gene in European hepatocellular carcinomas and hepatoblastoma. Oncogene 1993, **8**, 2303–6.
257. Kennedy SM, Macgeogh C, Jaffe R, Spurr NK. Overexpression of the oncoprotein p53 in primary hepatic tumors of childhood does not correlate with gene mutations. Hum Pathol 1994, **25**, 438–42.
258. Chen L, Agarwal S, Zhou W, Zhang R, Chen J. Synergistic activation of p53 by inhibition of Mdm2 expression and DNA damage. Proc Natl Acad Sci 1998, **95**, 195–200.
259. Oda T, Nakatsuru Y, Imai Y, Sugimura H, Ishikawa T. A mutational hot spot in the p53 gene is associated with hepatoblastomas. Int J Cancer 1995, **60**, 786–90.
260. Koufos A, Hansen MF, Copeland NG, Jenkins NA, Lampkin BC, Cavenee WK. Loss of heterozygosity in three embryonal tumors suggests a common pathogenic mechanism. Nature 1985, **316**, 330–4.
261. Little MH, Thompson DB, Hayward NK, Smith PJ. Loss of alleles on the short arm of chromosome 11 in a hepatoblastoma from a child with the Beckwith–Wiedemann syndrome. Hum Genet 1988, **79**, 186–9.
262. Byrne JA, Simms LA, Little MH, Algar EM, Smith PJ. Three non-overlapping regions of chromosome arm 11p allele loss identified in infantile tumors of adrenal and liver. Genes Chromosomes Cancer 1993, **8**, 104–11.
263. Davies SM. Maintenance of genomic imprinting at the IGF2 locus in hepatoblastoma. Cancer Res 1993, **53**, 4781–3.
264. Albrecht S, vonSchweinitz D, Waha A, Kraus JA, vonDeimling A, Pietsch T. Loss of maternal alleles on chromosome arm 11p in heptoblastoma. Cancer Res 1994, **54**, 5041–4.
265. Montagna M, Menin C, Chieco-Bianchi L, D'Andrea E. Occasional loss of constitutive heterozygosity at 11p15.5 and imprinting relaxation of the IGFII maternal allele in hepatoblastoma. J Cancer Res Clin Oncol 1994, **120**, 732–6.
266. Akmal SN, Yun K, MacLay J, Higami Y, Ikeda T. Insulin-like growth factor 2 and insulin-like growth factor binding protein 2 expression in hepatoblastoma. Hum Pathol 1995, **26**, 846–51.
267. Li X, Kogner P, Sandstedt B, Haas OA, Ekstrom TJ. Promoter-specific methylation and expression alterations of igf2 and h19 are involved in human hepatoblastoma. Int J Cancer 1998, **75**, 176–80.
268. Li X, Adam G, Cui H, Sandstedt B, Ohlsson R, Ekstrom TJ. Expression, promoter usage and parental imprinting status of insulin-like growth factor II (IGF2) in human hepatoblastoma: uncoupling of IGF2 and H19 imprinting. Oncogene 1995, **11**, 221–9.
269. Simms LA, Reeve AE, Smith PJ. Genetic mosaicism at the insulin locus in liver associated with childhood hepatoblastoma. Genes Chromosomes Cancer 1995, **13**, 72–3.
270. Kurahashi H, Takami K, Oue T, Kusafuka T, Okada A, Tawa A, et al. Biallelic inactivation of the APC gene in hepatoblastoma. Cancer Res 1995, **55**, 5007–11.
271. Tomlinson GE. Hepatoblastoma in a child with familial polyposis has loss of the normal maternal allele, 1999 (Abstract).
272. Iolascon A, Giordani L, Moretti A, Basso G, Borriello A, Della Ragione F. Analysis of CDKN2A, CDKN2B, CDKN2C, and cyclin Ds gene status in hepatoblastoma. Hepatology 1998, **27**, 989–95.
273. Kim H, Ham EK, Kim YI, Chi JG, Lee HS, Park SH, et al. Overexpression of cyclin D1 and cdk4 in tumorigenesis

of sporadic hepatoblastomas. Cancer Lett 1998, **131**, 177–83.
274. Koch A, Denkhaus D, Albrecht S, Leuschner I, vonSchweinitz D, Pietsch T. Childhood hepatoblastomas frequently carry a mutated degradation targeting box of the β-catenin gene. Cancer Res 1999, **59**, 269–73.
275. Schofield D, Jackson G, Wetzel J, Triche T. Patterns of gene expression in hepatoblastoma and hepatocellular carcinoma. Lab Invest 1999, **79**, 5P(Abstract).
276. DeBaun MR, Tucker MA. Risk of cancer during the first four years of life in children from the Beckwith–Wiedemann syndrome registry. J Pediatr 1998, **132**, 398–400.
277. Vaughan WG, Sanders DW, Grosfeld JL, Plumley DA, Rescoria FJ, Scherer III, LR, et al. Favorable outcome in children with Beckwith–Wiedemann syndrome and intraabdominal malignancy tumors. J Pediatr Surg 1995, **30**, 1042–5.
278. Lee MP, DeBaun M, Randhawa G, Reichard BA, Elledge SJ, Feinberg AP. Low frequency of p57KIP2 mutation in Beckwith–Wiedemann syndrome. Am J Hum Genet 1997, **61**, 304–9.
279. Zhang P, Liegeois NJ, Wong C, Finegold M, Hou H, Thompson JC, et al. Altered cell differentiation and proliferation in mice lacking p57KIP2 indicates a role in Beckwith–Wiedemann syndrome. Nature 1997, **387**, 151–8.
280. Eggenschwiler J, Ludwig T, Fisher P, Leighton PA, Tighlman SM, Efstratindis A. Mouse mutant embryos over expressing IGF-II exhibit phenotypic features of the Beckwith–Wiedemann and Simpson–Golabi–Behmel syndromes. Genes Dev 1997, **11**, 3128–42.
281. Drut R, Drut RM, Toulouse JC. Hepatic hemangioendotheliomas, placental choriangiomas, and dysmorphic kidneys in Beckwith–Wiedemann syndrome. Pediatr Pathol 1992, **12**, 197–203.
282. Santoro IM, Groden J. Alternative splicing of the APC gene and its association with terminal differentiation. Cancer Res 1997, **57**, 488–94.
283. Munemitsu S, Albert I, Souza B, Rubinfeld B, Polakis P. Regulation of intracellular β-catenin levels by the adenomatous polyposis coli (APC) tumor-suppressor protein. Proc Natl Acad Sci 1995, **92**, 3046–50.
284. Chen TC, Hsieh LL, Kuo TT. Absence of p53 gene mutation and infrequent overexpression of p53 protein in hepatoblastoma. J Pathol 1995, **176**, 243–7.
285. Soini Y, Welsh JA, Ishak KG, Bennett WP. p53 mutations in primary hepatic angiosarcomas not associated with vinyl chloride exposure. Carcinogenesis 1995, **16**, 2879–81.
286. Przgodzki RM, Finkelstein SD, Keohavong P, Zhu D, Bakker A, Swalsky PA, et al. Sporadic and thorotrast-induced angiosarcomas of the liver manifest frequent and multiple point mutations in K-ras-2. Lab Invest 1997, **76**, 153–9.
287. Douglass E, Ortega J, Feusner M, Reynolds M, King D, Finegold MJ, et al. Hepatocellular carcinoma (HCA) in children and adolescents: results from the Pediatric Intergroup Hepatoma study (CCG 8881/POG 8945). Proc Am Soc Clin Oncol 1994, **13**, 420 (Abstract).

288. Reynolds M, Douglass EC, Finegold M, Cantor A, Glicksman A. Chemotherapy can convert unresectable hepatoblastoma. J Pediatr Surg 1992, **27**, 1080–4.
289. Koneru B, Flye MW, Busuttil RW, Shaw BW, Lorber MI, Emond JC, et al. Liver transplantation for hepatoblastoma. Ann Surg 1991, **213**, 118–21.
290. Arii S, Mise M, Harada T, Furutani M, Ishigami S, Niwano M, et al. Overexpression of matrix metalloproteinase 9 gene in hepatocarcinoma with invasive potential. Hepatology 1996, **24**, 316–22.
291. Li XM, Tang ZY, Zhou G, Lui YK, Ye SL. Significance of vascular endothelial growth factor mRNA expression in invasion and metastasis of hepatocellular carcinoma. J Exp Clin Cancer Res 1998, **17**, 13–17.
292. Mieles LA, Esquivel CO, Van Thiel DH, Koneru B, Mokowka L, Tzakis AG, et al. Liver transplantation for tyrosinemia. A review of 10 cases from the University of Pittsburgh. Dig Dis Sci 1990, **35**, 153–7.
293. Paradis K. Tyrosinemia: the Quebec experience. Clin Invest Med 1996, **19**, 311–16.
294. Grompe M, Overturf K, al-Dhalimy M, Finegold M. Therapeutic trials in the murine model of hereditary tyrosinaemia type I: a progress report. J Inherit Metab Dis 1998, **21**, 518–31.
295. Ehrlich PE, Greenberg ML, Filler RM. Improved long-term survival with preoperative chemotherapy for hepatoblastoma. J Pediatr Surg 1997, **32**, 999–1002.
296. Ortega JA, Douglass EC, Feusner J, et al. Randomized comparison of cisplatin/vincristine/fluorouracil and cisplatin/continuous infusion doxorubicin for treatment of pediatric hepatoblastoma. A report from the Children's Cancer Group and the Pediatric Oncology Group. J Clin Oncol 2000, **18**, 2665–75.
296(a). Finegold MY. Chemotherapy for suspected hepatoblastoma without efforts at surgical resection is a bad practice. Med Pediatr Oncol 2002, **39**, 484–6.
297. Ortega JA, Krailo MD, Haas JE, King DR, Ablin AR, Quinn JJ, et al. Effective treatment of unresectable or metastatic hepatoblastoma with cisplatin and continuous infusion doxorubicin chemotherapy: a report from the Children's Cancer Study Group. J Clin Oncol 1991, **9**, 2167–76.
298. Douglass EC, Reynolds M, Finegold M, Cantor A, Glicksman A. Cisplatin, vincristine, and fluorouracil therapy for hepatoblastoma: a Pediatric Oncology Group study. J Clin Oncol 1993, **11**, 96–9.
299. vonSchweinitz D, Hecker H, Harms D, Bode U, Weinel P, Burger D, et al. Complete resection before development of drug resistance is essential for survival from advanced hepatoblastoma—a report from the German Cooperative Liver Tumor Study. J Pediatr Surg 1995, **30**, 845–52.
300. Seo T, Ando H, Watanabe Y, Harada T, Ito F, Kaneko K, et al. Treatment of hepatoblastoma: less extensive hepatectomy after effective preoperative chemotherapy with cisplatin and adriamycin. Surgery 1998, **123**, 407–14.
301. Saxena R, Leake JL, Shafford EA, Davenport M, Mowat AP, Pritchard J, et al. Chemotherapy effects on hepatoblastoma. A histological study. Am J Surg Pathol 1993, **17**, 1266–71.
302. Heifitz SA, French M, Correa M, Grosfeld JL. Hepatoblastoma: the Indiana experience with

pre-operative chemotherapy for inoperable tumors; clinicopathological considerations. Pediatr Pathol Lab Med 1997, **17**, 857–74.
303. Capizzi RL. Protection of normal tissues from the cytotoxic effects of chemotherapy by Amifostine (ethyol): clinical experiences. Semin Oncol 1994, **21** (Suppl 11) 8–15.
304. Uotani H, Yamashita Y, Masuko Y, Shimoda M, Murakami A, Sakamoto T, et al. A case of resection under the IVC-atrial venovenous bypass of a hepatoblastoma after intra-arterial chemotherapy. J Pediatric Surg 1998, **33**, 639–41.
305. Lai EC, Lo CM, Fan ST, Liu CL, Wong J. Postoperative adjuvant chemotherapy after curative resection of hepatocellular carcinoma is a randomized control trial. Arch Surg 1998, **133**, 183–8.
306. Busuttil RW, Farmer DG. The surgical treatment of primary hepatobiliary malignancy. Liver Transpl Surg 1996, **2**, 114–30.
307. Kim DY, Kim KH, Jung SE et al. Undifferentiated sarcoma of the liver: combination treatment by surgery and chemotherapy. J Pediatr Surg 2002, **37**, 1419–23.
308. Urban CE, Mache CJ, Schwinger W, Pakisch B, Ranner G, Riccabona M, et al. Undifferentiated (Embryonal) sarcoma of the liver in childhood. Cancer 1993, **72**, 2511–16.
309. Gunawardena SW, Trautwein LM, Finegold MJ, Ogden AK. Hepatic angiosarcoma in a child: successful therapy with surgery and adjuvant chemotherapy. Med Pediatr Oncol 1997, **28**, 139–43.
310. Whelan JS, Stebbings W, Owen RA, Calne R, Clark PI. Successful treatment of a primary endodermal sinus tumor of the liver. Cancer 1992, **70**, 2260–2.
311. Holcomb GW, III, O'Neill JA, Jr, Mahboubi S, Bishop HC. Experience with hepatic hemangioendothelioma in infancy and childhood. J Pediat Surg 1988, **23**, 661–6.
312. Rokitansky AM, Jakl RJ, Gopfrich H, Voitl P, Anzbock W, Wassipaul M, et al. Special compression sutures: a new surgical technique to achieve a quick decrease in shunt volume caused by diffuse hemangiomatosis of the liver. Pediatr Surg Int 1998, **14**, 119–21.
313. Calder CJ, Raafat F, Buckels JAC, Kelly DA. Orthotopic liver translantation for type 2 hepatic infantile haemangioendothelioma. Histopathology 1996, **28**, 271–3.
314. Achilleos OA, Buist LJ, Kelly DA, Raafat F, McMaster P, Mayer AD, et al. Unresectable hepatic tumors in childhood and the role of liver transplantation. J Pediatr Surg 1996, **31**, 1563–7.
315. Penn I. Hepatic transplantation for primary metastatic cancers of the liver. Surgery 1991, **110**, 726–35.
316. Tagge EP, Tagge DU, Reyes J, Tzakis A, Iwatsuki S, Starzl TE, et al. Resection, including transplantation, for hepatoblastoma and hepatocellular carcinoma: impact on survival. J Pediat Surg 1992, **27**, 292–7.
317. Bilik R, Superina R. Transplantation for unresectable liver tumors in children. Transplant Proc 1997, **29**, 2823–35.
318. Germain L, Blouin MJ, Marceau N. Biliary epithelial and hepatocytic cell lineage relationships in embryonic rat liver as determined by the differential expression of cytokeratins, α-fetoprotein, albumin and cell surface-exposed components. Cancer Res 1988, **48**, 4909–18.
319. Ponder KP. Analysis of liver development, regeneration and carcinogenesis by genetic marking studies. FASEB J 1996, **10**, 673–84.
320. Dunsford HA, Sell S. Production of monoclonal antibodies to preneoplastic liver cell populations induced by chemical carcinogens in rat and to transplantable Morris hepatomas. Cancer Res 1989, **49**, 4887–93.
321. Crosby HA, Hubscher SG, Joplin RE, Kelly DA, Strain AJ. Immunolocalization of OV-6, a putative progenitor cell marker in human fetal and diseased pediatric liver. Hepatology 1998, **28**, 980–5.
322. Ellouk-Achard S, Djenabi S, De Oliveira GA, Desauty G, Duc HT, Zohair M, et al. Induction of apoptosis in rat hepatocarcinoma cells by expression of IGF-I antisense c-DNA. J Hepatol 1998, **29**, 807–18.
323. Tsunoda Y, Shibusawa M, Tsunoda A, Gomi A, Yatsuzuka M, Okamatsu T. Antitumor effect of hepatocyte growth factor on hepatoblastoma. Anticancer Res 1998, **18**, 4339–42.
324. Thorgeirsson SS, Santoni-Rugui E. Interaction of c-myc with transforming growth factor alpha and hepatocyte growth factor in hepatocarcinogenesis. Mutat Res 1997, **376**, 221–34.
325. Ruiz J, Qian C, Prieto J. Gene therapy of liver tumors: principles and applications. Digestion 1998, **59**, 92–6.
326. Anderson SC, Johnson DE, Harris MP, Engler H, Hancock W, Huang WM, et al. p53 gene therapy in a rat model of hepatocellular carcinoma: intra-arterial delivery of a recombinant adenovirus. Clin Cancer Res 1998, **4**, 1649–59.
327. Cao G, Kuriyami S, Du P, Sakamoto T, Kong X, Masui K, et al. Complete regression of established murine hepatocellular carcinoma by in vivo tumor necrosis factor α gene transfer. Gastroenterology 1997, **112**, 501–10.
328. Huang H, Chen SH, Kosai K, Finegold MJ, Woo SL. Gene therapy for hepatocellular carcinoma: long-term remission of primary metastatic tumors in mice by interleukin-2 gene therapy in vivo. Gene Ther 1996, **3**, 980–7.
329. zu Putlitz J, Weiland S, Blum HE, Wands JR. Antisense RNA complementary to hepatitis B virus specifically inhibits viral replication. Gastroenterology 1998, **115**, 702–13.
330. Kanai F, Lan KH, Shiratori Y, Tanaka T, Ohashi M, Okudaira T, et al. In vivo gene therapy for alpha-fetoprotein-producing hepatocellular carcinoma by adenovirus-mediated transfer of cytosine deaminase gene. Cancer Res 1997, **57**, 461–5.
331. Mohr L, Schauer JI, Boutin RH, Moradpour D, Wands JR. Targeted gene transfer to hepatocellular carcinoma cells in vitro using a novel monoclonal antibody-based gene delivery system. Hepatology 1999, **29**, 82–9.
332. Muto Y, Moriwaki H, Ninomiya M, Adachi S, Saito A, Takasaki KT, et al. Prevention of second primary tumors by an acyclic retinoid, polyprenoic acid, in patients with hepatocellular carcinoma. New Engl J Med 1996, **340**, 1046–7.

16 Carcinoma

Catherine J. Cullinane and John J. O'Leary

Introduction

In childhood carcinomas are rare, with an annual incidence for most sites nearly always under 1/1 million (1). In a US study the annual age adjusted rate for all carcinomas in adults was about 434 per 100,000 but only 1.4 per 100,000 in children (2). In their review of paediatric cancer during a 10-year period in the United Kingdom, McWhirter and colleagues found that carcinoma represented about 2% of all childhood malignancies (3). Another UK study estimated the age standardized rate as 2.4 per million per year. However, over the 30-year study period the incidence increased from 1.5 to 3.3 per million (4). The incidence and type of carcinoma in children differs from that in adults, where skin, lung, colon, and breast are the most common. In children the types of carcinoma most frequently seen include thyroid, colon, nasopharyngeal, adrenocortical, melanoma, salivary, liver, and renal, although the incidence varies throughout the world (1–3). Causation of paediatric carcinomas is likely to be multifactorial, with genetic and environmental factors playing a role in certain cases as discussed below. Although many of the carcinomas are encountered frequently in adults, childhood cases can be challenging for clinicians and pathologists due to their rarity, often different epidemiology, pattern of behaviour and morphology. In this chapter we discuss several of the carcinomas likely to be encountered in paediatric practice. Renal and liver carcinomas are discussed in Chapters 12 and 15, respectively.

Thyroid carcinoma

Although the thyroid is one of the commonest sites of carcinoma in children, the annual incidence in most population-based registries is low, <1/1million, but noted to be relatively higher in the United States (1, 2). Less than 2% of childhood malignant tumours are of thyroid origin and these account for less then 12% of paediatric carcinomas (2, 4). Thyroid carcinoma is more common in females than males (2–3:1) and the incidence increases with age in both sexes (5). In childhood the majority arise in female adolescents. Non-malignant disease of the thyroid gland is more common in children than cancer with nodular hyperplasia and benign adenomas outnumbering malignant tumours (6). However, carcinoma appears to arise more frequently in these conditions, especially solitary nodules, in children than in adults (7).

As in adults papillary carcinoma is the most common type of thyroid malignancy in children. In a series of 154 paediatric thyroid carcinomas in England and Wales 68% were papillary, 11% follicular, and 17% medullary (8). These findings are broadly similar to those in other series (7, 9–11). Pure follicular carcinoma is rare and most follicular tumours are solid/follicular variant of papillary carcinoma. An apparent recent increase of medullary carcinoma (MTC) in young patients is attributed to screening of families with multiple endocrine neoplasia (MEN 2) familial cancer syndromes (8). Presentation is either as a mass in the thyroid or cervical adenopathy. Patients are generally euthyroid.

Papillary thyroid carcinoma (PTC) varies in size and extent of thyroid involvement may be multifocal and is rarely encapsulated (12). It shows a mixture of papillae with fibrovascular cores covered by a layer of cuboidal or columnar cells, and follicles, the latter predominant in the follicular variant (Fig. 16.1(a) and (b)). Characteristically papillary carcinoma cells are round or oval with nuclear grooves and frequent intranuclear cytoplasmic inclusions. In paraffin sections the nuclei typically have a clear, empty appearance. This is not apparent on frozen sections or cytological preparations. There may be abundant fibrous stroma, a chronic inflammatory cell infiltrate, and psammoma bodies, which are precipitated calcium. Immunohistochemically the cells are positive for thyroglobulin and low molecular weight cytokeratins.

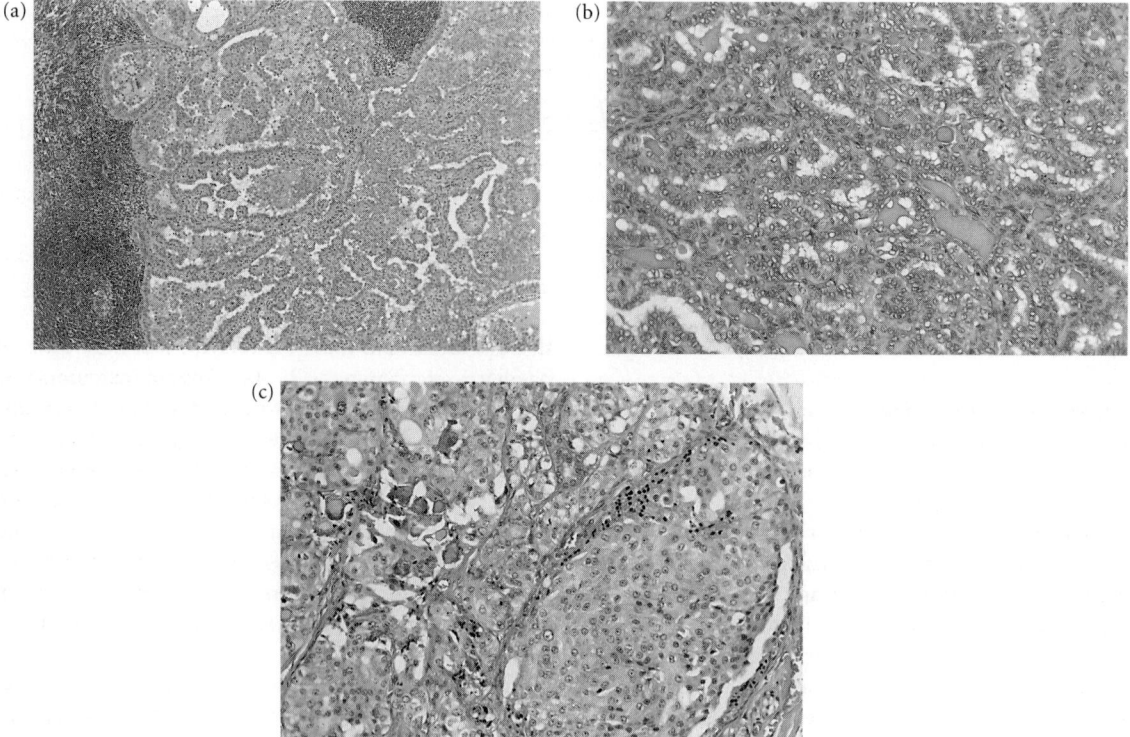

Fig. 16.1 (a) Metastasis of papillary carcinoma of thyroid in a cervical lymph node (haematoxylin and eosin, H&E). (b) The characteristic cells of PTC line papillae or follicles and have round or oval nuclei that are optically clear and frequently grooved (H&E). (c) In this MTC of thyroid from a child with MEN 2B there are lobules of large cells with abundant cytoplasm and round nuclei containing a prominent nucleolus. Focal calcification is also present (H&E).

In children most PTC are moderately or well differentiated. Fine needle aspiration cytology shows fragments of papillae with overlapping cells, dusty chromatin, nuclear grooves, and intranuclear inclusions.

It is a more aggressive disease in childhood than in adults, with a greater prevalence of extrathyroid extension and metastatic spread. Lymph node metastases are present in 60–80% of children at presentation and 10–25% have distant metastases, usually in the lungs, occasionally in bones and liver (11, 13–15). In their report comparing papillary carcinoma in children and adults Zimmerman and colleagues noted that in children mean tumour size was greater (3 cm compared to 2 cm), extrathyroid spread commoner (24% compared to 15%), and lymph node metastases at presentation more frequent (89% compared to 3%) as were distant metastases (6% compared to 2%) (16).

Follicular thyroid carcinoma (FTC) is composed of follicles lined by cells that lack characteristic features of papillary carcinoma cells (12). Minimally invasive FTC are encapsulated nodules resembling adenomas but with a greater tendency for microfollicular, solid, and trabecular growth patterns. The diagnosis of malignancy rests on demonstration of full capsular invasion and vascular permeation. The widely invasive follicular carcinomas are more mitotically active and pleomorphic, with greater infiltration of surrounding thyroid gland. Hurthle-cell carcinoma is a variant of FTC with abundant cytoplasmic mitochondria imparting a granular appearance to the cytoplasm. The immunohistochemical profile of FTC is similar to that of adenomas, normal thyroid follicles and PTC being positive for thyroglobulin and low molecular weight cytokeratins. Aspiration cytology preparations are hypercellular, with syncytial cellular aggregates, microfollicles, and crowded hyperchromatic nuclei with nucleoli. Lymph node involvement is less common than with PTC and metastases to the lungs and bone stem from haematological spread.

The major risk factor for papillary carcinoma in children is previous radiation exposure (17). Prior to the

1960s this reflected radiation treatment of benign head and neck conditions resulting in thyroid neoplasms in about 2% of patients. One-third of these were malignant and most presented in adulthood (18, 19). Abandonment of this practice resulted in a marked decrease in the incidence of childhood thyroid cancer. Radiation therapy for malignancy in children is also associated with secondary thyroid cancer (20, 21). The Chernobyl nuclear accident in 1986 resulted in a dramatic increase (up to 100-fold) in thyroid cancers in children in the Ukraine, Belarus, and Western Russia (22). The minimal latency period for papillary carcinoma was 4 years in exposed children (23). Histologically these papillary carcinomas were classic type or solid/follicular and sclerosing variants with a high prevalence of the solid/follicular type.

The majority of papillary carcinomas are diploid, aneuploidy is reported in 10% of paediatric carcinomas compared to less than 3% in adult disease (16). Aneuploidy has been associated with a higher frequency of recurrence (24). *RET-PTC* gene rearrangements (*PTC-1, PTC-2, PTC-3*) are characteristic of papillary carcinoma. The *RET* proto-oncogene on chromosome 10 encodes the tyrosine kinase receptor of the glial cell line derived neurotrophic factor (GDNF) family of growth factors (22). Fusion of *RET* with *H4* gene, the gene for R1a subunit of protein kinase A or *RFG* (*ELE1*) gene generates *RET-PTC-1*, *RET-PTC-2*, or *RET-PTC-3* chimeric genes, respectively. *RET* gene rearrangements are common in sporadic childhood tumours (45%) and are predominantly *RET-PTC-1*, similar to pattern in adults but more frequent (25). In post-Chernobyl childhood cases however the prevalent rearrangement is *RET-PTC-3* (22, 26). Mutations of *RET-PTC-3* are found in 58% of radiation associated tumours, compared to 18% in sporadic childhood tumours (26). Mutations of *RET-PTC-1* are more common in sporadic tumours (47%) than secondary tumours (16%). The prevalence of the different *RET* gene rearrangements also varies with the histological variants of papillary carcinoma (26). *RET-PTC-3* compared to *RET-PTC-1* predominate in the solid/follicular variant (73% versus 7%) compared to (19% versus 38%) in typical papillary carcinoma. It is postulated that the *RET-PTC-3* may be radiation-induced and could be associated with more aggressive disease (25). No definite correlation between *RET-PTC* gene rearrangements and clinical outcome has been established. Mutations in *RAS* genes are uncommon in childhood sporadic tumours, although they have a similar frequency to that in adult differentiated tumours. They do not appear to be present in paediatric radiation-associated thyroid cancer (27). Multiple chromosomal aberrations are encountered in post-radiation tumours (28).

Familial non-medullary thyroid cancer is occasionally associated with familial adenomatous polyposis (FAP), Peutz Jeghers syndrome (PJS), ataxia telangiectasia, Cowden's disease, and multiple endocrine neoplasia type 1 (MEN 1) (17).

The appropriate treatment of non-medullary thyroid carcinoma has been debated but the current favoured regime includes radical thyroidectomy and excision of all suspect nodes followed by thyro-ablative radioiodine therapy and TSH suppressive L-thyroxine treatment (13, 15, 29). Serum thyroglobin is used to monitor and detect relapse. The prognosis is very good in children in spite of the tumour's more aggressive behaviour. Papillary carcinoma and minimally invasive FTC have a much better outcome than widely invasive FTC (13). Age is a significant prognostic factor. Sixty percent of adults with distant metastases died within 15 years compared to 15% of children with distant disease (16). Other reviews of paediatric thyroid cancer cite survival of 100% at 10 years and over 90% at 20 years (14, 15). Relapse (neck, nodal, or lung) is relatively common, occurring in approximately 30% of patients in the first 10 years following diagnosis. It is associated with male gender, distant disease at diagnosis, incomplete surgical excision and less differentiated tumours (15, 16). Relapse is treated by radioiodine therapy with surgery in some cases. However late relapses or death up to 33 years after initial diagnosis may occur (14). Therefore long-term follow-up is mandatory.

Medullary carcinoma arises from the neural crest derived, calcitonin secreting C-cells of the thyroid gland (12). It is rare in adults and children and may be sporadic or familial. Sporadic tumours are usually unilateral, whereas familial are bilateral, multicentric, and preceded by C-cell hyperplasia. In children MTC is usually associated with Multiple Endocrine Neoplasia type 2 (MEN 2) syndrome and familial medullary thyroid carcinoma (FMTC) (30). MEN 2 and FMTC are due to germline mutations in the *RET* proto-oncogene. MEN 2A is characterized by MTC, phaeochromocytoma, and parathyroid adenoma, and MEN 2B by MTC, phaeochromocytoma, gastrointestinal ganglioneuromatosis, and a marfanoid habitus. In MEN 2 and FMTC characteristic mutations are present in 3 codons of the *RET* proto-oncogene in family members at risk of thyroid disease. In MEN 2A the majority of mutations are in codon 634 of the *RET* proto-oncogene resulting in substitution of arginine for cysteine. Mutations associated with FMTC are evenly distributed between codons 618, 620, and 634. Mutation in codon 918 is found in MEN 2B, which is also associated more frequently with *de novo* mutations than in MEN 2A and FMTC. In sporadic MTC a somatic mutation in codon 918 is common (31, 32).

Tumours that arise in MEN 2 and FMTC are preceded by C-cell hyperplasia with increased C-cells in thyroid follicles, which progress to nodular C-cell hyperplasia and subsequently invade the stroma as MTC (12). MTC is non-encapsulated and typically shows a lobular, trabecular, or sheet-like arrangement of polygonal or spindle cells with round nuclei, speckled chromatin, and amphophilic or eosinophilic cytoplasm (Fig. 16.1(c)). However it frequently mimics other types of thyroid carcinoma. Stromal amyloid and fibrosis are less common in FMTC compared to sporadic tumours (33). The cells are positive for low molecular weight keratins, vimentin, neuron specific enolase, chromogranin, synaptophysin, carcinoembryonic antigen (CEA), and calcitonin. Electron microscopy reveals membrane-bound granules. It metastasises to lymph nodes and also to lungs, bone, and liver (34).

MTC in patients with MEN 2B presents earlier than in those with MEN 2A and FMTC but is more aggressive with greater incidence of metastatic disease and poorer prognosis (34, 35). Significant progress has been made in the past two decades in early diagnosis and treatment of MEN 2 associated MTC and FMTC. Screening methods include serum calcitonin measurement and nowadays genetic testing for *RET* mutations, the latter permitting earlier predictive testing in children even before onset of C-cell hyperplasia (31, 32, 36). The recommended treatment is total thyroidectomy and central neck node dissection before the age 6 years in MEN 2A and after the age of 1 year in MEN 2B (37). Early recognition of gene carriers and preventative thyroidectomy provides the opportunity to cure or prevent development of this disease.

Nasopharyngeal carcinoma

This rare tumour shows a distinct geographical and ethnic pattern of occurrence. A bimodal distribution is seen in the United States with the first incident peak occurring in adolescence (38). It is one of the most common carcinomas in childhood (2, 4). In the white population of Europe, North America, and Oceania it represents well under 1% of paediatric cancer, whereas in parts of Africa it accounts for up to 30% of malignancy in 10–14-year-old Black children (1). In the United States the incidence among Black children is nine times higher than in White children. It is commoner in boys than girls with the vast majority of childhood cases presenting in the second decade (39, 40–43). Local extension and metastases to cervical nodes are usual at presentation. Painless cervical lymphadenopathy is the most common presenting symptom. Headache and nasal and ear symptoms are also frequent (39, 41, 45).

Nasopharyngeal carcinoma (NPC) is classified by the World Health Organization (WHO) into squamous cell carcinoma, non-keratinizing carcinoma subtype A differentiated, and non-keratinizing subtype B undifferentiated (formerly WHO types I, II, and III, respectively) (44). Lymphoepithelioma refers to an undifferentiated tumour with prominent lymphocytic infiltrate. The majority of NPCs in patients less than 20 years old are non-keratinizing and undifferentiated (43, 45–48). This contrasts with the situation in adults where most are keratinizing squamous cell carcinomas (48). The histological type of tumour varies according to patient origin with keratinizing tumours being more common in US White, Hispanic, and Chinese ethnic groups, whereas the undifferentiated type is more common in those of Hong Kong and Japanese origin (48).

Non-keratizing, undifferentiated NPC is composed of cells with oval or round vesicular nuclei and prominent nucleoli. They are arranged in nests and sheets, and have a syncytial appearance due to lack of distinct cell margins (Fig. 16.2). They are positive for cytokeratins and epithelial membrane antigen. In lymph node metastases sinusoidal infiltration is common and initially may suggest a histiocytic proliferation.

The risk factors for NPC are Epstein–Barr virus (EBV) infection, genetic susceptibility (as histocompatability antigen (HLA) linkage appears to be important and may explain racial variation in incidence), and environmental agents (49). The association of EBV with NPC is well established (50). It is always present in undifferentiated NPC and in most non-keratizing NPC in China (50). The viral infection of the epithelial cells in NPC is latent and associated with a particular pattern of EBV gene expression. At least 11 EBV genes coding nuclear proteins are expressed in latent infection and of these EBNA-1 (Epstein–Barr nuclear antigen), LMP 1 and LMP 2 (latent membrane protein), and two non-coding RNAs (the EBER RNAs) are expressed in NPC (50). EBV DNA has been demonstrated in the cytoplasm of tumour cells in 9 of 11 paediatric NPCs by *in situ* hybridization (42). EBER is usually detected

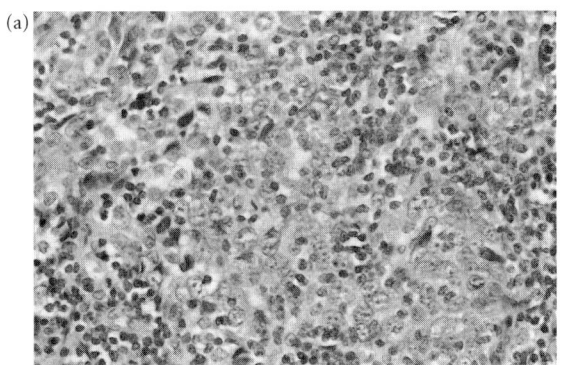 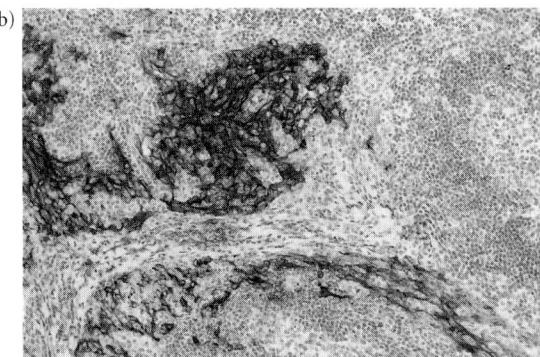

Fig. 16.2 (a) NPC with nests of large cells with indistinct cell borders, abundant cytoplasm, and oval nuclei with prominent nucleoli (H&E). (b) Positive immunohistochemical reaction for cytokeratin antibody highlights the sinusoidal infiltration by NPC in a cervical lymph node (anti-cytokeratin immunohistochemistry).

by *in situ* hybridization and LMP by immunohistochemistry. How EBV infection promotes oncogenesis is not fully explained. Dietary agents have been linked with an increased incidence of NPC in adults in China and United States (51, 52).

Genetic events also appear to be important in genesis and progression of NPC, at least in adults. Abnormalities of chromosome 11 occur in NPC and in a study of Taiwanese cases loss of heterozygosity (LOH) was found in 60% at loci D11S912 (23%) and D11S934 (20%), both of which are located within 11q23-24. Microsatellite instability (MSI(+)) is exhibited in 46% of tumours, with 17% occurring in the transforming growth factor beta-receptor type II (*TGF-beta RII*) gene within exon 3, which is also on chromosome 11. LOH appears to be associated with early stage NPC and correlates with tumour size while MSI(+) is associated with progressive disease (53). In a recent study of Chinese patients with NPC a high frequency LOH (60% or more) was observed on 12 chromosome arms (1p, 2p, 2q, 3p, 3q, 5q, 9p, 9q, 11q, 13q, 14q, and 17q), with the highest LOH frequency (91%) on 3p. Less frequent LOH was noted on a variety of other chromosome arms. High serum antibody titers of IgA against virus capsid antigens (VCA) and early antigen (EA) of EBV were associated with high frequency LOH on 16q and 19q13. It is suggested that aggressiveness and progression of NPC may be associated with high frequency LOH on 9p21, 16q, and 19q, with possible interaction between allelic loss and EBV infection in the genesis of NPC. High frequency LOH on 4q21 and 14q correlates with undifferentiated NPC (54).

The overall 5-year survival rate in a study which included adults and children was 44% with a much better outcome in undifferentiated non-keratizing tumours, around 65% compared to 35% for those with keratizing tumours (48). In paediatric series the overall 5-year survival rate varies from 50% to 65% (42, 43, 55). In adults a number of possible prognostic factors such as p53 and tumour cell proliferation markers have been investigated with variable results (56, 57). Their role in paediatric NPC is not established. Advanced stage at diagnosis is more common in children (42, 45, 46, 58). Metastatic spread is the major factor in prognosis as disseminated disease has a poor prognosis (38, 42, 58). Bone is the most common site for distant metastases (45). Race also has a bearing on prognosis as Black American children have a better outcome (42). The tumour is highly radiosensitive and radiotherapy is the main stay of treatment particularly in Stage 1 and 2 tumours. The addition of chemotherapy is associated with an improved outcome especially in advanced Stages 3, 4 (55, 58).

Intestinal carcinoma

Colorectal cancer is the second most common malignancy in adults but is rare in childhood with an incidence throughout the world of less than 1 per million (1). Less than 6% of all colorectal cancers occur in patients under 30 years of age and in the first two decades of life account for less than 1% of all malignancies (59, 60). In childhood presentation is usually in the second decade (59, 61). Racial variation is noted in some reports that cite an increased incidence in non-White adolescents and young adults (60, 62). It is slightly more common in males (61). Presenting symptoms are similar in all age groups with abdominal pain, often vague, being the dominant childhood complaint.

There are however, major differences between paediatric and adult cases with regard to site, stage, histology, and outcome. Delay in diagnosis is a major problem in childhood cases and has been attributed to a low index of suspicion in doctors and patients (59, 62–64). In children carcinoma occurs throughout the colon, with 53% arising in the right and transverse colon compared to less than 33% in adults and under 10% in the rectum compared to a third of cases in adults (62, 65). Advanced stage at presentation is more common in paediatric cases. Most are Dukes Stage D (65%) and C (23%), with only 10% Stage B (59). In adults most are Stage B or C (64). Metastases occur to many sites, including omentum, ovary, liver, brain, and bone. Histologically the tumours are predominantly mucinous, moderately or poorly differentiated adenocarcinomas, often with signet ring cells (61, 65) (Fig. 16.3). In adults the situation is different as the mucinous subtype is infrequent, <5% compared to over 60% in childhood (60, 62).

A number of hereditary conditions predispose to colon cancer, most presenting in adulthood. In childhood cases a family history is rare and the majority, as in adults, appear to arise *de novo*. Synchronous tumours or polyps are rarely present. Ulcerative colitis, familial polyposis coli, and neurofibromatosis have been associated with a small number of paediatric cases (61, 63, 65). We have observed colonic mucinous adenocarcinoma in an adolescent with cystic fibrosis. An excess of gastrointestinal malignancy has been found in adult cystic fibrosis patients (66).

Familial polyposis syndromes are characterized by onset of multiple gastrointestinal polyps in childhood, close surveillance of these patients is necessary because of increased risk of gastrointestinal and other malignancies in these syndromes usually in later life (67, 68). These are autosomal dominant conditions and are characterized by adenomatous polyps in FAP and with hamartomatous polyps in the others. FAP is caused by germline mutation in the *APC* gene (5q21). The germline mutation is in the *SMAD-4* gene (18q21) in juvenile polyposis syndrome (JPS), and in the *LKBI* gene (19p15) in PJS (67, 68). The risk of gastrointestinal carcinoma developing is greatest in FAP (100%) followed by JPS (22–50%) and PJS (10%) (67). In Cowden's syndrome, which is caused by a germline mutation in the *PTEN* gene (10q25) the cancer risk is uncertain (67). The *PTEN* gene is also mutated in the Bannayan–Riley–Ruvalcaba syndrome but there is no associated cancer risk.

Hereditary non-polyposis colorectal cancer (HNPCC) accounts for approximately 3% of all colorectal cancer (69). It is a relatively common autosomal dominant disorder characterized by an increased incidence of cancers of the colon, endometrium, ovary, and stomach. Patients with HNPCC have a very high frequency of developing colorectal cancer (80%), and may present in early adulthood. HNPCC is due to germline mutations in one of the DNA mismatch repair genes (*hMSH2* (2p), *hMLH1* (3p), *hPMS2* (7p), *hPMS1* (2q)). The heterozygous phenotype is apparently normal. Expression of *hMSH2* gene is regulated throughout the cell cycle, with preferential expression in the proliferative portion of the colonic crypt. Somatic mutation causing inactivation of the wild-type allele results in complete loss of DNA mismatch repair activity. Aberrations of *hMSH2* and *hMLH1* genes appear to account for approximately 50% of all HNPCC families. There are no 'hotspots' in either of these genes that confer disease phenotype, however the occurrence of premature truncations makes *in vitro* transcription/translation assays useful for screening purposes (69). Fifteen to twenty percent of all colorectal cancers have microsatellite instability (MIS(+)) similar to that seen in HNPCC. Genes containing repetitive DNA sequences appear to be targets for inactivation by the MIS(+) phenotype in tumours. The type 2 tranforming growth factor beta (*TGF beta*) gene is the prototype gene mutated in these tumours.

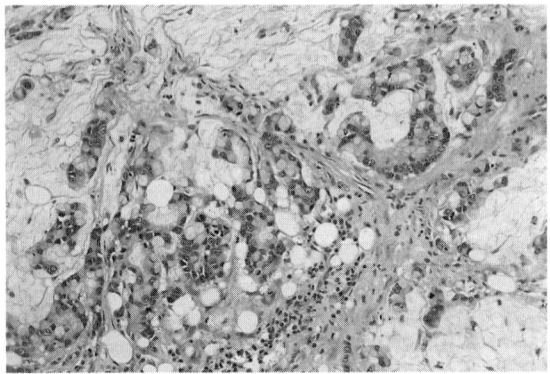

Fig. 16.3 In this poorly differentiated mucinous adenocarcinoma of the colon the malignant cells partly line mucin lakes separated by a fibrous stroma. Several cells show a signet ring appearance due to mucin distension of the cytoplasm with the nucleus pushed against the cell membrane. Detached clusters of cells are seen to 'float' in the mucin lakes (H&E).

The prognosis in children is very poor; most reports in the literature however have no 5-year survivors. Complete surgical resection, the main treatment for colon cancer, is possible in only 40% of children compared to 90% of adults (59). Partial resection is of value in obstruction relief and tumour debulking. Additional therapies such as chemotherapy or radiotherapy also have a palliative role. The poor prognosis in children is associated with the higher stage at diagnosis, incomplete resection, and mucinous morphology. Screening for CEA may be helpful in some cases in diagnostic workup and detecting recurrence (59, 62).

Carcinoma in the oesophagus is rarely encountered in children with Barrett's oesophagus due to gastro-oesophageal reflux (70). Gastric carcinoma is also rare and is usually signet ring type (71). The prognosis is also poor. Carcinoma of the liver is the most common epithelial malignancy of the digestive system in many parts of the world and is discussed in Chapter 15.

Adrenal carcinoma

Neuroblastoma is the most common tumour of the adrenal gland in children and is discussed in Chapter 8. Adrenal cortical tumours and phaeochromocytomas are rare accounting for less than 10–20% of adrenal neoplasms (72).

Adrenal cortical tumours in children and adults are usually benign adenomas. In contrast to adults however most paediatric tumours are hormone secreting. Adrenal cortical carcinoma (ACC) shows a bi-modal incidence with a peak in the first 5 years and a second peak in the 4th to 5th decade (73). ACC accounts for 0.2–0.3% of all malignancies in childhood and is predominantly a disease of White children (74). It is more common in girls in the 0–4-year age group, but no gender difference is found in 5–14-year olds (1). A high incidence is noted in Brazil where the annual rate is 4.7/1 million girls aged 0–4 years compared to 0.6 in the United States and 0.8 in the United Kingdom (1). Presentation can occur throughout childhood but the majority present in early childhood with a mean age at diagnosis of about 4 years (73–76). Rare congenital cases have been documented (74).

Virilization is the most common presentation, often combined with features of Cushing's syndrome (74, 75, 77). Signs of virilization include hirsutism, facial and pubic hair, increased muscle mass, rapid growth, and penile and clitoral enlargement. The children with Cushings syndrome exhibit moon face, obesity, hypertension, impaired glucose metabolism and growth arrest. Adrenocortical neoplasms account for 50–60% of childhood Cushing's syndrome (72). Feminization is the least common presentation. Girls exhibit precocious isosexual development while boys develop gynaecomastia. A mixture of feminizing and masculizing features is present in some patients. Serum and urine dehydroepiandrosterone, dehydroepiandrosterone sulphate, and testosterone are elevated in virilizing tumours, with raised 17 keto-steroids in Cushing's syndrome and oestrogen in feminizing tumours (75). Non-functional tumours are rare. The finding of virilization, Cushing's syndrome, or feminization in a child should raise clinical suspicion of an adrenal tumour.

Regional spread and metastases to liver, lung, and lymph nodes are definitive features of malignancy. Histological criteria for diagnosing malignancy have been difficult to establish. In adults a combination of histological features is associated with malignant behaviour (78). In children the situation is less clear-cut. Tumour weight has been cited as the only predictor of malignant behaviour in paediatric tumours in contrast to adults (79, 80). All tumours weighing more than 500 g were malignant and all weighing less than 100 g benign. Adrenocortical neoplasms consist of small polygonal cells with eosinophilic cytoplasm. Suggested criteria for the prospective diagnosis of ACC include presence of necrosis, multiple and atypical mitoses, nuclear pleomorphism, vascular invasion, broad fibrous bands, a diffuse growth pattern, and compact cell type, in addition to weight >300 g, local invasion, and features of virilization or feminization (Fig. 16.4) (72). Several features however, such as necrosis, mitoses, pleomorphism, and broad fibrous bands have been noted in benign paediatric tumours (79, 80). Tumour volume greater than 200 cm^3 has also been associated with malignant behaviour in children (76). In a review of small functioning adrenocortical tumours (<100 g, <200 cm^3) children had an excellent prognosis with surgery regardless of tumour morphology (81). Classification of tumours as adenoma, low-grade ACC, and high-grade ACC based on four of nine criteria used in adults showed that histological type and weight had statistical significance in outcome (82). The overall survival rate is 47–89% (83). Abdominal spread and metastases are poor prognostic features, with recurrence or death within 2 years in children with metastatic disease (75). Older age, delay of over 6 months in diagnosis, and increased urinary steroid levels are also associated with a poorer prognosis (76). The extent of

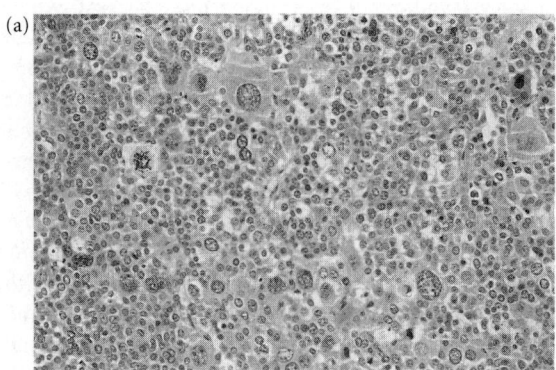 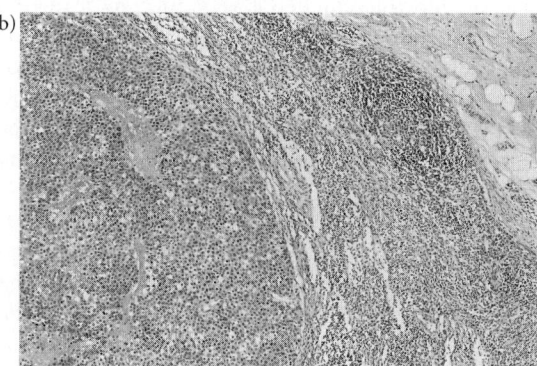

Fig. 16.4 (a) This virilizing adrenocortical carcinoma, weight 600 g, shows numerous large bizarre pleomorphic cells with atypical mitoses in a background of smaller, more compact cells (H&E). (b) Lymph node metastasis from the same adrenocortical carcinoma (H&E).

tumour resection is the most important factor for predicting patient outcome (83).

Adrenocortical neoplasms are associated with several syndromes (84). These include Li Fraumeni (germline mutation in *p53* on chromosome 17p), Beckwith Wiedemann (allelic loss of 11p15), and MEN 1 (germline mutation in the *menin* gene on 11q13). Childhood tumours are more strongly associated with *p53* germline mutations than those in adults (85). The occurrence of an ACC in a child may be the first indication of LiFraumeni syndrome in a family. The high incidence in Brazil is postulated to be related to agrotoxic agents (86). However in a recent study 35 of 36 patients had an identical germline point mutation of *p53*. There was no history of increased cancer incidence among family members and the mutation in *p53* was in codon 10, whereas in Li Fraumeni syndrome mutations are found in codons 5–8. This *p53* mutation appears to represent a low-penetrance *p53* allele that contributes in a tissue-specific manner to the development of paediatric ACC (87). The chromosomal regions in the syndromes associated with adrenocortical tumours have been more extensively investigated in adult tumours than in paediatric cases. Wilkin and colleagues studied four paediatric cases and demonstrated loss of structural abnormalities of 11p15, combined with mosaic LOH of 11p and increased insulin growth factor 2 (IGF 2) expression in all cases (88). In adults frequent genetic alterations of 11p and 17p, and high expression of IGF2 is more common in ACC (89, 90). This did not appear to be the case in the small number of childhood tumours in this report (88). The high IGF2 expression and steroidogenesis in these tumours supports origin from fetal adrenal cortex.

The majority of adrenocortical tumours are monoclonal (91). Cytogenetic analysis of short-term cultured cells from an 11-cm adrenocortical carcinoma in a 3.5-year-old girl revealed a complex karyotype (92). Recent comparative genomic hybridization studies suggest that the genetic events in paediatric adrenocortical neoplasia may be distinct from those in adults. In childhood cases gains in copy number of 9q, 12q, chromosomes 19, 5, and 20 are common (86, 93). Genetic losses are less common and are usually of 18q and 4q. In adult studies the results vary with gains of 4, 5, 7, 9q, 16q, 12q, 14q, 20q and losses of 2, 9p, 11q, 17p, 19p (84, 93).

Phaeochromocytoma is derived from chromaffin cells, which are of neural crest origin and secrete catecholamines. These cells are located in the adrenal medulla (phaeochromocytes), and in the paraganglia along the sympathetic chain and near the aorta (94). Twenty percent of all phaeochromocytomas occur in childhood, with an incidence of 2 per million (95, 96). In childhood studies there is an overall male preponderance, greater frequency of multifocality and extra-adrenal disease, and greater familial association than in adults (97). The mean age at diagnosis in childhood is 11 years (96, 97). The majority (95%) of paediatric phaeochromocytomas are intra-abdominal (97). Adrenal is the most common site. Fifty percent are extra-adrenal, usually upper abdominal para-aortic, followed by organs of Zuckerkandl and less commonly the bladder. Forty percent of cases are bilateral, 40% are multifocal, and about a third are familial (96–98). Recurrent tumours occur in 25–30% of cases up to 6 years post-operatively (96, 99). Multiple tumours may be synchronous or metachronous.

The majority of paediatric cases are sporadic. Familial cases are associated with several autosomal dominant syndromes: MEN 2 (usually MEN 2A, rarely MEN 2B); less frequently von Hippel–Lindau disease and rarely in type 1 neurofibromatosis (98, 100, 101). These diseases result from germline mutations in the *RET*, *VHL*, and *NF1* genes, respectively. Familial cases present at a younger age and are more often bilateral and multifocal than non-syndromic tumours (94). Mutations in *RET* and *VHL* genes may also be found in some sporadic tumours (102). Germline mutations in the *SDHB* gene at 11q23 have also been found in familial and sporadic phaeochromocytomas (103, 104). The gene encodes a subunit of succinate dehydrogenase, which is important in mitochondrial function. LOH at 1p, 3p, 17p, and 22q in both sporadic and familial phaeochromocytomas has also been reported (105).

The symptoms and signs are related to the catecholamine production by the tumour. The most common symptoms are sweating, visual blurring, nausea, vomiting, palpitations, flushing/pallor, with headache being infrequent (97, 106). Hypertension, usually sustained rather than paroxysmal, is the most common clinical finding but is absent in up to a quarter of cases (98, 106). Phaeochromocytoma is only responsible for about 1% of paediatric hypertension (107). The diagnosis is confirmed by the measurement of urinary catecholamine metabolites, vanillylmandelic acid (VMA), metanephrine, and normetanephrine, in urine; VMA is that most consistently elevated (106). Locating the tumour may necessitate use of a variety of radiological scanning techniques. The treatment is surgical excision of the tumour. Medical management of hypertension is critical before and during the operation (106, 108).

The majority of tumours are benign, 10% of cases are malignant (95, 97, 109). Malignancy is determined by tumour behaviour, that is, metastases and wide local invasion, rather than histology (96, 110). There appears to be a higher risk of malignancy in familial disease (97). Fifty percent of malignant tumours are extraadrenal, and in 45% of cases no metastases are present at diagnosis (109).

Most phaeochromocytomas weigh less than 100 g, are encapsulated, and solid with a fleshy cut surface (94). Microscopically they are composed of large polygonal tumour cells with abundant granular pink cytoplasm, a round or oval nucleus with coarse chromatin, and a single nucleolus. Immunohistochemically they react positively with chromogranin, neuron specific enolase (NSE), Leu 7, synaptophysin, and neurofilament antibodies as well as a variety of neuropeptides. The cells are grouped into solid nests (zellballen), cords, or ribbons in a rich capillary vascular framework. The nests are sometimes rimmed by spindle-shaped sustentacular cells, which are S100 and vimentin positive. Ultrastructurally they show neuronal differentiation with cell processes and neurosecretary dense core-granules. An uncommon variant, the composite phaeochromocytoma, consisting of a mixture of phaeochromocytoma with neuroblastoma, ganglioneuroblastoma, or ganglioneuroma is very rarely seen in childhood (94).

Adrenal medullary hyperplasia and the presence of sustentacular cells are features of familial tumours (111). Medullary hyperplasia may be diffuse or nodular and is determined by increased volume and extension into the tail and alar areas of the gland (94). There are no definite histological criteria to establish if a phaeochromocytoma is benign or malignant. Nuclear hyperchromasia and pleomorphism are common and are not indicative of malignancy, nor are mitoses or capsular invasion. Features considered suspicious of malignancy include large tumour size, small tumour cells, extensive necrosis, vascular invasion, and aneuploidy (112, 113). The only reliable criterion of malignancy is extensive local spread and the presence of metastases at sites normally devoid of chromaffin tissue.

Benign phaeochromocytoma has an excellent prognosis following complete excision. Unresectable and metastatic disease is treated by chemotherapy, usually according to a neuroblastoma protocol. Children with malignant disease have a mean 3-year survival of 75% (109). Genetic screening for the mutations in *RET* and *VHL* genes is advised in all patients with bilateral adrenal, recurrent, or multifocal phaeochromocytomas (108). Urinary screening for metabolites of catecholamine is mandatory not only in familial cases as these individuals have a life-long risk of developing further tumours but also in sporadic cases in order to detect recurrent or metachronous tumours.

Salivary gland carcinoma

Primary neoplasms of the salivary gland rarely present in childhood and account for <5% of tumours in all age groups (114, 115). The majority of salivary gland masses in childhood are non-neoplastic inflammatory/reactive conditions or vascular lesions (116). Capillary haemangioma is the most common cause of a parotid mass in childhood, especially in infancy, and shows a predilection for girls (117). Benign soft tissue tumours, sarcomas, lymphoma, and neuroblastoma may rarely present as a salivary gland mass (114, 117, 118). Sialoblastoma is a rare, congenital, epithelial tumour, unique to childhood (119). It presents usually in the perinatal period as a mass in the parotid gland, rarely in a minor salivary gland, and is generally benign. A small number show aggressive, malignant behaviour.

A parotid mass in a child is more likely to be malignant than in an adult. In their cumulative review of North American and European paediatric series of salivary gland tumours (vascular lesions excluded) Shikhani and colleagues found that almost 50% were malignant compared to adults where only 15–25% of neoplasms are malignant. A female predilection was noted, with a female to male ratio of 1.42 for all neoplasms, 1.57 for benign, and 1.28 for malignant tumours (114). The majority were epithelial tumours and usually presented in the second decade. Over 80% of epithelial neoplasms arise in the parotid gland; submandibular gland involvement is much less common and minor salivary gland involvement very infrequent. Although in adults minor salivary gland neoplasms are more likely malignant than benign, the reverse is true in children (114). As in adults the pleomorphic adenoma accounts for the vast majority of benign salivary gland tumours. Malignant epithelial salivary gland tumours show a morphological spectrum, with most types described in childhood. The most common malignant tumour in childhood, as in adulthood, is the mucoepidermoid carcinoma, followed by acinic cell carcinoma, adenoid cystic carcinoma, undifferentiated carcinoma, and adenocarcinoma (114, 117, 118).

Presentation is generally of a painless swelling in the parotid gland that usually has been present for some time. Facial nerve palsy and cervical lymph node involvement, although features of malignancy, are rarely observed. Rapid growth over a period of months is suspicious of malignancy. Lack of symptoms, even with malignant tumours, is common, making diagnosis on clinical grounds difficult.

Mucoepidermoid carcinoma is composed of a combination of mucus, epidermoid, and intermediate cells. Low-grade tumours have abundant cystic spaces lined mainly by these cells with mucus cells usually prominent. The nuclei are bland and mitoses rare (Fig. 16.5(a)). A solid pattern, nuclear pleomorphism, mitoses >4 per 10 high power fields, and necrosis are features of high-grade tumours (120).

Acinic cell carcinoma typically consists of sheets of polygonal cells resembling serous acinar cells that have well-defined cell borders with scanty intervening stroma. The nuclei are bland, small, round, and central (Fig. 16.5(b)). Cytoplasm is abundant and typically basophilic and granular due to the presence of zymogen granules. These are periodic acid stain (PAS) positive, diastase resistant, and mucicarmine negative. A prominent lymphocytic infiltrate is often present and helpful in diagnosis. Microcystic, papillary, and follicular variants can cause diagnostic concern. Mitoses, necrosis, and pleomorphism are worrying features but the behaviour if acinic cell carcinoma is generally not predictable on histology. Multiple recurrences and cervical node metastases are associated with a poor prognosis.

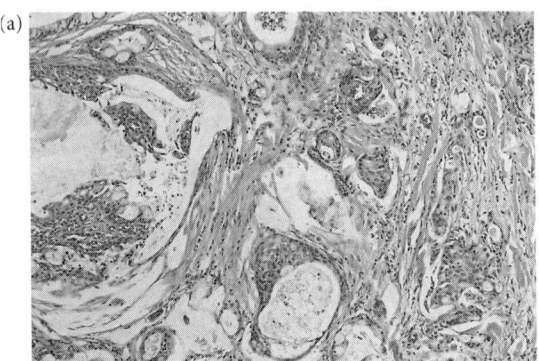 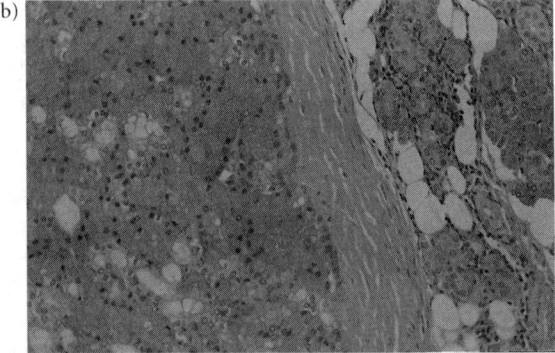

Fig. 16.5 (a) Mucoepidermoid carcinoma of the parotid gland with cystic spaces lined by bland intermediate cells and mucus cells (H&E). (b) The acinic cell tumour (*left*) has large cells with abundant granular cytoplasm and small bland central nuclei. A fibrous capsule separates it from the normal smaller serous cells of the normal parotid gland (*right*) (H&E).

Immunocytochemistry plays little role in the diagnosis of these tumours. Both are reactive for cytokeratins. Anti-amylase antibody may be useful in the diagnosis of problematic acinic cell carcinomas.

Little is known of the aetiology of salivary gland carcinoma. Radiation is a recognized risk factor for mucoepidermoid carcinoma. Presentation as a second malignancy is described in children (118, 121). Salivary gland neoplasms are not associated with heritable syndromes. Familial salivary gland carcinomas are rare (122). In adults chromosome 6q deletion is the most consistent abnormality and has been found in most types of salivary carcinoma, but is not unique to salivary gland neoplasms (123, 124). Loss of chromosomes 18, 21, Y and gain of chromosomes 2, 7, 8, 10, and X is described (125). Translocation t(11;19)(q14-21; p12-13) has been reported in several paediatric mucoepidermoid carcinomas and may be a diagnostic marker of this tumour (126–128).

The majority of mucoepidermoid and acinic cell carcinomas in children are low grade and have an excellent prognosis, as they are seldom fatal. Treatment is usually wide local excision. High-grade tumours, adenoid cystic carcinoma, undifferentiated carcinoma and adenocarcinoma have a poorer prognosis.

Melanoma

Malignant melanoma (MM) is very rare in children. Two percent of MM occurs in patients under the age of 20 years and it is seven times more common in the second decade of life than the first (129). It is more common in females than males and it is predominantly a disease of fair skinned races (130). The highest incidence in the world has been noted in Queensland, Australia. There the incidence rate is <1/million in children 0–4 years old but 30/million in 10–14-year olds (131). Worldwide an increasing incidence of melanomas in adults and children is well recognized. A doubling of melanoma cases over a 10-year period was found in a study of Swedish children aged 14–20 years (132). The incidence in younger children did not alter during this period.

The diagnosis of melanoma is difficult clinically and pathologically (133, 134). Problems arise with over-diagnosis because of misinterpretation of benign Spitz naevi and nodular, atypical proliferations in congenital giant naevi, as well as under-diagnosis because of reluctance to diagnose MM in a child. MM presents on the limbs, trunk, head, and neck (131, 135–137). In childhood melanoma may be congenital or acquired, arise *de novo* or in association with risk factors (134). As in adults the clinical features suspicious of malignant lesions are the classical ABCD criteria: Asymmetry, poorly defined Borders, change in Colour and large Diameter. Other features include bleeding, ulceration, itching, and pain (130, 138).

Risk factors for childhood MM include phenotype, number of common naevi, dysplastic naevus syndrome, congenital giant naevi, xeroderma pigmentosum, immunosuppression and family history (134, 137, 139). In an Australian study the risk factors were more than 10 naevi greater than 5 mm diameter, inability to tan on sun exposure and family history of melanoma (140).

The dysplastic naevus syndrome is either sporadic or familial and characterized by development of numerous large naevi on the trunk, limbs, and buttock with atypical features such as irregular margins and variation in colour (134, 137). The histological criteria include intraepidermal proliferation of naevomelanocytic cells with discontinuous arrangement of cells at the dermoepidermal junction, nuclear atypia, dermal fibrosis and inflammation, and fusion of rete ridges by nests of atypical cells (141). The lifetime risk of developing melanoma in familial dysplastic naevus syndrome and familial melanoma is high. If MM develops it is usually of superficial spreading type (142).

Xeroderma pigmentosum is a rare autosomal recessive disorder in which there is a defect DNA excision repair (142). The patient's skin is susceptible to damage by sun exposure. It affects all races and in those under 20 years old there is a 1000-fold greater prevalence than the general population for skin cancers. Skin tumours begin to appear in the first decade of life. MM occurs in up to 30% of individuals with xeroderma pigmentosa (134).

Giant congenital naevus is defined as a naevus present at birth comprising 5% of body surface in preadolescent children and >20 cm size in adolescents and adults (143). The cumulative 5-year risk of developing MM in a giant congenital naevus has been estimated to be 4.5–5.7% (143, 144). A number of nodular and atypical proliferations may arise in giant naevi and cause diagnostic concern (133, 143). Congenital melanoma is described in three circumstances—maternal MM, giant congenital naevus, and neurocutaneous melanosis (145). Transplacental spread of maternal melanoma with disseminated fetal disease is rare and has a poor prognosis (134, 137). Head and neck giant congenital naevus with leptomeningeal melanosis is associated with development of meningeal melanoma in

40% of cases and is usually fatal (134). Benign melanocytic proliferations may be present in the placenta in children with giant congenital naevi (146).

Histologically MM in children may be adult type superficial spreading MM, nodular MM, Spitz-like, and small cell type (136, 147). In children most melanomas are nodular type compared to adults where superficial spreading is more common (142). Lentigo maligna and acral lentiginous melanomas are quite uncommon in children. Histologically superficial spreading melanoma consists of epithelioid cells with large nuclei, prominent nucleoli, abundant cytoplasm with fine melanin pigment, arranged singly or in nests along the dermoepidermal junction in a lateral pattern. Single cells infiltrate upwards into the epidermis. Focal infiltration of papillary dermis is associated with a chronic inflammatory infiltrate (141). Nodular melanoma is characterized by vertical rather than lateral growth and expands down into the deep dermis and subcutaneous fat. The malignant melanocytes may be small, epithelioid, or spindle shaped with more numerous mitoses.

Distinguishing between Spitz naevus and MM remains challenging. Numerous morphological criteria have been assessed (138, 148, 149). Symmetry, maturation, presence of Kamino bodies, few mitoses, absence of atypical mitoses, and no mitoses in the deeper portion of the lesion favour the diagnosis of Spitz naevus. None is specific and diagnosis is made on a combination of features in each case. An atypical Spitz naevus is recognized and categorization into low- and high-risk groups based on morphological features has been proposed, although this has no predictive value (133). Atypical Spitz naevi with lymphnode metastases but no further progression is also described. The probability that atypical spitz tumour in a child under 12 years is malignant is very low (133). The small cell type of MM typically involves the scalp, is thick, and has a poor prognosis. It is the most common type of MM arising in giant congenital naevi (133). Immunohistochemically S100 is the most sensitive marker of melanocytic differentiation but is not specific. HMB-45 is helpful in diagnosis. Both stain benign and malignant melanocytic proliferations, as do more recently described antibodies Melan-A and peripherin (150). HMB-45 and peripherin have similar staining patterns. Benign, dysplastic, and Spitz naevi tend to show positive staining towards the skin surface, whereas positivity in the deeper portion of a lesion favours melanoma.

In familial MM germline mutations in several genes have been described. The first gene implicated was *CDKN2A* on chromosome 9p21 (151). Mutations are present in about 25% of large multicase families (152). This gene encodes p16, a negative growth regulator (cyclin dependent kinase inhibitor). Expression of p16 causes cell cycle arrest and forms part of a growth control pathway that involves cyclin-dependent kinases, cyclins and the retinoblastoma gene product pRb (153). Mutation of *CDKN2A* appears to be most important in early MM, with deletions of gene *PTEN/NMAC1* on 10q 23.3 and gene *AIM1* on 6q21, and mutations of *Ras* gene are associated with more advanced disease (154), mutation in the *CDK4* gene is also implicated and has been identified in three families (152). LOH for p16 has been noted in some sporadic dysplastic naevi (155). The application of molecular techniques may be helpful in the diagnosis of difficult melanocytic lesions. Comparative genomic hybridization of Spitz naevi showed the majority had a normal chromosomal content in contrast to melanoma in which there are frequent gains of chromosomes 8, 6p, and 1q and losses of 9p, 10q, 6q, and 8p (156). A small number of Spitz naevi had gains of 1p or 17q. A study of DNA content and proliferation markers in atypical nodules of giant congenital naevi showed a pattern intermediate between benign naevi and MM (157). Although only a small number of these studies are cited they support the view that melanocytic proliferations represent a disease continuum ranging from fully benign to fully malignant lesions (133).

Tumour thickness (Breslow depth of invasion) is the best predictor of melanoma prognosis (134, 137). Thin tumours (<0.76 mm), usually superficial spreading melanoma, have an excellent prognosis as in adults since the risk of metastases is low and surgery is usually curative (141, 142). However in children most melanomas are nodular type and thicker at diagnosis. The prognosis is poor as the risk of metastases increases with increasing Clark level, that is, depth of invasion (141). Overall 5-year survival in childhood MM is 40%, 100% in Stage 1 (localized) and 0% for Stages 2 (regional spread) and 3 (disseminated disease) (158). In another paediatric series the 5-year survival for localized disease was 78% and 30% in cases with regional metastases (130). The treatment of melanoma in children is similar to that in adults.

Pancreatic carcinoma

Primary malignant tumours of the pancreas are extremely uncommon in children. A 20-year review at one Canadian paediatric institution identified only six patients who were operated on for pancreatic neoplasms, five of which were malignant (159). Another 20-year review in the USA identified 4 cases of pancreatic carcinoma in children (160). Pseudocysts, insulinoma, cystadenomas, and infiltration by other small round cell childhood tumours must also be considered in the differential diagnosis of a pancreatic mass. The behaviour and morphology of childhood pancreatic carcinoma generally differs from that in the adult. The usual adult pancreatic ductular adenocarcinoma presents in the sixth decade and has a poor prognosis. Similar tumours very rarely occur in children, have a bimodal distribution with peaks in the first and second decades of life, and an equally poor outlook (161). Most pancreatic carcinomas in children are either pancreatoblastoma or solid-pseudopapillary tumour. These are indolent malignant tumours with an overall good prognosis.

Pancreatoblastoma is a tumour of young children with an average age at presentation of 6 years (162). A recent review of the literature identified 65 cases in children and 4 in adults since 1979 (163). It is twice as common in boys as girls and almost always presents as an abdominal mass. An association with Beckwith Wiedemann syndrome has been noted (162, 163). Raised serum alpha-fetoprotein is common and useful in diagnosis and follow-up (164). The tumour is usually large, encapsulated, predominantly solid, and arises in any part of the pancreas (164). Microscopically it shows lobules of cuboidal epithelial cells with a variable number of mitoses, clusters of acinar type cells with amphophilic cytoplasm containing PAS positive inclusions, small ducts, sometimes cystically dilated, and the characteristic squamous corpuscles, which are round whorls of elongated squamous cells. The lobules are separated by dense fibrous stroma. Necrosis and focal calcification may also be present. Rarely bone, cartilage and cellular spindle cell stroma have been noted (162). Immunohistochemically the tumour is usually strongly positive for alpha1 antitrypsin. In general neural and pancreatic enzyme markers are negative. Approximately 25% of cases have metastasises to liver and bone (163).

Pancreatoblastoma appears to be genetically distinct from adult ductular carcinoma. In the latter 90% harbour mutations of the *K-ras* oncogene. *p16* is inactivated in 80% of cases, *p53* in 50–75%, and *DPC4* in 50%. LOH of chromosomes 1p, 6p, 8p, 12q, 13q, 21q, and 22q has been described in greater than 40% of pancreatic tumours by Hruban *et al.* (165). The molecular pathogenesis of pancreatoblastomas is unknown. A tumour from a 4-year-old boy showed both near-diploid and near-teraploid cell populations with t(13;13)(q10;q10) and loss of one copy of chromosomes 1, 6, 13, and 22 in the near-tetraploid cells and t(13;22)(q10;q10) in the near-diploid cells (166). Trisomies of chromosomes 3, 10, 12, and 20 were found in a nodal metastasis (167). Their occasional occurrence in patients with Beckwith Wiedemann syndrome and occasionally with FAP suggests that they might bear a genetic similarity to other infantile embryonal tumours such as hepatoblastomas (168). In this recent study allelic loss on chromosome 11p was the most common genetic alteration in pancreatoblastomas, presenting in approximately 86% of cases. Molecular alterations in the *APC* gene/beta-catenin pathway were detected in 67% of tumours with activating mutations of the *beta-catenin* proto-oncogene. In contrast, loss of *DPC4* was infrequent and *K-ras* mutations and p53 expression not detected.

Surgical excision is the treatment of choice with chemotherapy and radiation therapy in certain cases (163). Complete surgical excision of a localized tumour is associated with an excellent prognosis. The presence of metastases however results in a poorer outlook although tumour progression is generally slow.

Solid-pseudopapillary tumour of the pancreas is a tumour of adolescent and young adult females. In a review of 292 reported cases 90% were female and mean age at diagnosis was 23 years (169). Presentation is usually related to the presence of an abdominal mass and the tumour is large, often encapsulated and may arise in any part of the pancreas (170). Over 90% are cystic. There are no known associations with heritable conditions and its histogenesis remains controversial. Extensive degenerative changes in the tumour are responsible for the cystic appearance. In solid areas the cells are polygonal and uniform with oval bland grooved nuclei (Fig. 16.6). Mitoses are usually rare. Hyaline globules are common, and are PAS positive but negative for mucin stains. Early degenerative changes lead to formation of pseudopapillae with central capillary and surface layer of attached cells (171). Immunohistochemically the cells are diffusely positive for vimentin and NSE and are focally positive for cytokeratin, alpha1 antitrypsin, and synaptophysin. Progesterone receptors are usually expressed but oestrogen receptors are generally negative. Pancreatic enzyme markers are also negative. Electron dense granules are the characteristic ultrastructural finding.

There is little information available about the molecular or genetic profile of this tumour. Of those studied most appear to be diploid (170, 172). Aneuploidy has been found in a few and may be a marker of tumours

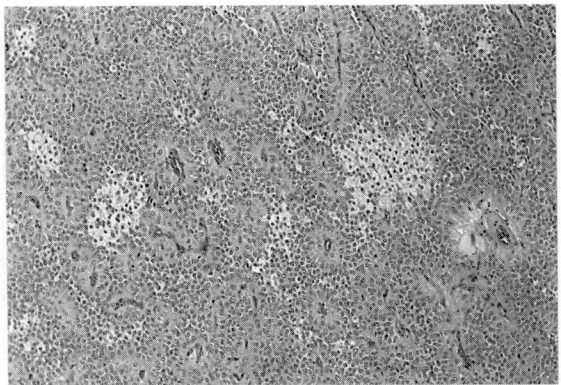

Fig. 16.6 The solid-pseudopapillary tumour of the pancreas shows solid areas of polygonal uniform cells as well as focal dissolution with early pseudopapilla formation characterized by a central capillary and radiating layers of attached cells (H&E).

with metastatic potential, but this requires further study (172, 173). An unbalanced translocation between chromosomes 13 and 17 has been reported in one case (der(17)t(13;17)(q14;p11)) (173). Another case showed double loss of the X chromosomes and trisomy of chromosome 3 (174). The molecular genetic features of adult ductular carcinoma (see above) have not been reported in this tumour.

The tumour is localized in 85% of cases with metastases in 15% usually in the liver (171). Histological determination of the behaviour of this tumour is difficult. Features such as high nuclear grade and mitotic rate, cellular pleomorphism, and venous invasion have been suggested as predictive of metastatic potential (172). However no correlation between any of these parameters and outcome has been established (171). Complete resection of localized tumours is curative and even with local extension and abdominal metastases the long-term survival is generally good.

References

1. Stiller CA. International variations in the incidence of childhood carcinomas. Cancer Epidemiol Biomarkers Prev 1994, 3, 305–10.
2. Pratt CB, George SL, Green AA, Fields LA, Dodge RK. Carcinomas in children. Clinical and demographic characteristics. Cancer 1988, 61, 1046–50.
3. McWhirter WR, Stiller CA, Lennox EL. Carcinomas in childhood—a registry based study of incidence and survival. Cancer 1989, 63(11), 2242–6.
4. al-Sheyyab M, Muir KR, Cameron AH, Raafat F, Pincott JR, Parkes SE, Mann JR. Malignant epithelial tumours in children: incidence and aetiology. Med Pediatr Oncol 1993, 21(6), 421–8.
5. Parkin DM, Stiller CA, Draper GJ, Bieber CA. The international incidence of childhood cancer. Int J Cancer 1988, 42(4), 511–20.
6. Lafferty AR, Batch JA. Thyroid nodules in childhood and adolescence—thirty years of experience. J Pediatr Endocrinol Metab 1997, 10, 479–86.
7. McHenry C, Smith M, Lawrence AM, Jarosz H, Paloyan E. Nodular thyroid disease in children and adolescents: a high incidence of carcinoma. Am Surg 1988, 54(7), 444–7.
8. Harach H, Williams ED. Childhood thyroid cancer in England and Wales. Br J Cancer 1995, 72, 777–83.
9. Goepfert H, Dichtel WJ, Samaan NA. Thyroid cancer in children and teenagers. Arch Otolaryngol 1984, 110(2), 72–5.
10. Ceccarelli C, Pacini F, Lippi F, Elisei R, Arganini M, Miccoli P, Pinchera A. Thyroid cancer in children and adolescents. Surgery 1988, 104(6), 1143–8.
11. Samuel AM, Sharma SM. Differentiated thyroid carcinomas in children and adolescents. Cancer 1991, 67, 2186–90.
12. Rosai J, Carcangiu ML, DeLellis R. Atlas of tumour pathology. Tumors of the thyroid gland, 3rd Series, Fascicle 5. Armed Forces Institute of Pathology, Washington, 1992.
13. Hallwirth U, Flores J, Kaserer K, Niederle B. Differentiated thyroid cancer in children and adolescents: the importance of adequate surgery and review of literature. Eur J Pediatr Surg 1999, 9(6), 359–63.
14. Schlumberger M, De Vathaire F, Travagli JP, Vassal G, Lemerle J, Parmentier C, Tubiana M. Differentiated thyroid carcinoma in childhood: long term follow up of 72 patients. J Clin Endocrinol Metab 1987, 65(6), 1088–94.
15. La Quaglia MP, Black T, Holcomb GW, Sklar C, Azizkhan RG, Haase GM, Newman KD. Differentiated thyroid cancer: clinical characteristics, treatment, and outcome in patients under 21 years of age who present with distant metastases. A report from the surgical Discipline Committee of the Children's Cancer Group. J Pediatr Surg 2000, 35(6), 955–60.
16. Zimmerman D, Hay ID, Gough IR, Goellner JR, Ryan JJ, Grant CS, McConahey WM. Papillary thyroid carcinoma in children and adults: long term follow up of 1039 patients conservatively treated at one institution during three decades. Surgery 1988, 104(6), 1157–66.
17. Fagin JA. Familial nonmedullary thyroid carcinoma—the case for genetic susceptibility. J Clin Endocrinol Metab 1997, 82(2), 342–4.
18. Scanlon EF, Sener SF. Head and neck neoplasia following irradiation for benign conditions. Head Neck Surg 1981, 4(20), 139–45.
19. Viswanathan K, Gierlowski TC, Schneider AB. Childhood thyroid cancer: characteristics and long-term outcome in children irradiated for benign conditions of the head and neck. Arch Pediatr Adolsc Med 1994, 148(3), 260–5.
20. de Vathaire F, Francois P, Schlumberger M, Schweisguth O, Hardiman C, Grimaud E, Oberlin O, Hill C, Lemerle J, Flamant R. Epidemiological evidence for a common mechanism for neuroblastoma and differentiated thyroid tumour. Br J Cancer 1992, 65, 425–8.

21. Kuefer MU, Moinuddin M, Heideman RL, Lustig RH, Rose SR, Burstein S, VanMiddlesworth L, Fleming I, Jenkins JJ, Shearer PD. Papillary thyroid carcinoma: demographics, treatment, and outcome in eleven pediatric patients treated at a single institution. Med Pediatr Oncol 1997, **28**(6), 433–40.

22. Thomas GA, Bunnell H, Cook A, Williams ED, Nerovnya A, Cherstvoy ED, Tronko ND, Bogdanova TI, Chiapetta G, Viglietto G, Pentimalli F, Salvatore G, Fusco A, Santoro M, Vecchio G. High prevalence of *RET/PTC* rearrangements in Ukrainian and Bellarussian post-Chernobyl thyroid papillary carcinomas: a strong correlation between RET/PTC3 and the solid-follicular variant. J Clin Endocrinol Metab 1999, **84**(11), 4232–8.

23. Nikiforov YE, Heffess CS, Korzenko AV, Fagin JA, Gnepp DR. Characteristics of follicular tumors and non-neoplastic thyroid lesions in children and adolescents exposed to radiation as a result of the Chernobyl disaster. Cancer 1995, **76**(5), 900–9.

24. Mizukami Y, Michigishi T, Nonomura A, Hashimoto T, Nogachi M, Matsubara F, Watanabe K. Carcinoma of the thyroid at a young age—a review of 23 patients. Histopathology 1992, **20**(1), 63–6.

25. Fenton CL, Lukes Y, Nicholson D, Dinauer CA, Francis GL, Tuttle RM. The *RET/PTC* mutations are common in sporadic papillary thyroid carcinoma of children and young adults. J Clin Endocrinol Metab 2000, **85**(3), 1170–5.

26. Nikiforov YE, Rowland JM, Bove KE, Monforte-Munoz H, Fagin JA. Distinct pattern of *ret* oncogene rearrangements in morphological variants of radiation-induced and sporadic thyroid papillary carcinomas in children. Cancer Res 1997, **57**(9); 1690–4.

27. Fenton C, Anderson J, Lukes Y, Dinauer CA, Tuttle RM, Francis GI. *Ras* mutations are uncommon in sporadic thyroid cancer in children and young adults. J Endocrinol Invest 1999, **22**(10), 781–9.

28. Zitzelsberger H, Lehmann L, Hieber L, Weier HU, Janish C, Fung J, Negele T, Spelsberg F, Lengfelder E, Demidchik EP, Salassidis K, Kellerer AM, Werner M, Bauchinger M. Cytogenetic changes in radiation-induced tumors of the thyroid. Cancer Res 1999, **59**(1), 135–40.

29. Millman B, Pellitteri PK. Thyroid carcinoma in children and adolescents. Arch Otolaryngol Head Neck Surg 1995, **121**(11), 1261–4.

30. Skinner MA, Wells SA. Medullary carcinoma of the thyroid gland and the MEN 2 syndromes. Semin Pediatr Surg 1997, **6**(3), 134–40.

31. Eng C, Mulligan LM. Mutations of the *RET* proto-oncogene in the multiple endocrine neoplasia type 2 syndromes, related sporadic tumours and Hirschsprung's disease. Hum Mutat 1997, **9**, 97–109.

32. Hansford JR, Mulligan LM. Multiple endocrine neoplasia type 2 and RET: from neoplasia to neurogenesis. J Med Genet 2000, **37**, 817–27.

33. Krueger JE, Maitra A, Albores-Saavedra J. Inherited medullary microcarcinoma of the thyroid: a study of 11 cases. Am J Surg Pathol 2000, **24**(6), 853–8.

34. Kebebew E, Ituarte PH, Siperstein AE, Duh QY, Clark OH. Medullary thyroid carcinoma: clinical characteristics, treatment, prognostic factors, and a comparison of staging systems. Cancer 2000, **88**, 1139–48.

35. O'Riordain DS, O'Brien T, Weaver AL, Gharib H, Hay ID, Grant CS, van Heerden JA. Medullary thyroid carcinoma in multiple endocrine neoplasia types 2A and 2B. Surgery 1994, **116**(6), 1017–23.

36. Kebebew E, Tresler PA, Siperstein AE, Duh QY, Clark OH. Normal thyroid pathology in patients undergoing thyroidectomy for finding a *RET* gene germline mutation: a report of three cases and review of the literature. Thyroid 1999, **9**(2), 127–31.

37. Alsanea O, Clark OH. Familial thyroid cancer. Mod Pathol 2001, **13**(1), 44–51.

38. Pratt CB, Douglass EC. Management of the less common cancers of childhood. In: Principle and practice of Paediatric Oncology (ed. PA Pizzo, Poplack). Lippincott, Philadelphia, 1993, 913–38.

39. Jereb B, Huvos AG, Steinherz P, Unal A. Nasopharyngeal carcinoma in children. Review of 16 cases. Radiat Oncol Biol Phys 1980, **6**(4), 487–91.

40. Jenkin RD, Anderson JR, Jereb B, Thompson JC, Pyesmany A, Wara WM, Hammond D. Nasopharyngeal carcinoma—a retrospective review of patients less than thirty years of age: a report of the Children's Cancer Study Group. Cancer 1981, **47**(2), 360–6.

41. Roper HP, Essex-Cater A, Marsden HB, Dixon PE, Campbell RHA. Nasopharyngeal carcinoma in children. Pediatr Hematol Oncol 1986, **3**, 143–52.

42. Hawkins EP, Krischer JP, Smith BE, Hawkins HK, Finegold MJ. Nasopharyngeal carcinoma in children—a retrospective review and demonstration of Epstein–Barr viral genomes in tumor cell cytoplasm: a report of the Paediatric Oncology Group. Hum Pathol 1990, **21**(8), 805–10.

43. Martin WD, Shah KJ. Carcinoma of the nasopharynx in young patients. Int J Oncology Biol Phys 1994, **28**(4), 991–9.

44. Shanmugaratum K, Sobin LH. The World Health Organization histological classification of tumors of the upper respiratory tract and ear. A commentary on the second edition. Cancer 1993, **71**(8), 2689–97.

45. Sham JS, Poon YF, Wei WI, Choy D. Nasopharyngeal carcinoma in young patients. Cancer 1990, **65**(11), 2606–10.

46. Huang TH. Cancer of the nasopharynx in childhood. Cancer 1990, **66**, 968–71.

47. Ayan I, Altun M. Nasopharyngeal carcinoma in children: retrospective review of 50 patients. Int J Radiat Oncol Biol Phys 1996, **35**(30), 485–92.

48. Marks JE, Phillips JL, Menck HR. The National Cancer Data Base report on the relationship of race and national origin to the histology of nasopharyngeal carcinoma. Cancer 1998, **83**(3), 583–8.

49. Liebowitz D. Nasopharyngeal carcinoma: the Epstein-Barr virus association. Semin Oncol 1994, **21**(3), 376–81.

50. Farrell PJ, Tidy J. Viruses and human cancer. Chapter 2. In: Recent advances in histopathology. Vol. 13 (ed. PP Anthony, NM MacSween). London, Churchill Livingstone, 1989.

51. Ning JP, Yu MC, Wang QS, Henderson BE. Consumption of salted fish and other risk factors for nasopharyngeal carcinoma (NPC) in Tianjin, a low risk region for NPC in the People's Republic of China. J Nat Cancer Inst 1990, **82**, 291–6.

52. Farrow DC, Vaughan TL, Berwick M, lynch CF, Swanson GM, Lyon JL. Diet and nasopharyngeal carcinoma in a low-risk population. Int J cancer 1998, **78**(6), 675–9.

53. Harn HJ, Fan HC, Chen CJ, Tsai NM, Yen CY, Huang SC. Microsatellite alteration at chromosome 11 in primary human nasopharyngeal carcinoma in Taiwan. Oral Oncol 2002, 38(1), 23–9.
54. Shao JY, Huang XM, Yu XJ, Huang LX, Wu QL, Xia JC, Wang HY, Feng QS, Ren ZF, Ernberg I, Hu LF, Zeng YX. Loss of heterozygosity and its correlation with clinical outcome and Epstein-Barr virus infection in nasopharyngeal carcinoma. Anticancer Res 2001, 21(4B), 3021–9.
55. Serin M, Erkal HS, Elhan AH, Cakmak AA. Nasopharyngeal carcinoma in childhood and adolescence. Med Pediatr Oncol 1998, 31(60), 498–505.
56. Tsai ST, Jin YT, Leung HW, Wang ST, Tsao CJ, Su IJ. Bcl-2 and proliferating nuclear antigen (PCNA) expression correlates with subsequent recurrence in nasopharyngeal carcinomas. Anticancer Res 1998, 18(4B), 2849–54.
57. Harn HJ, Hsieh HF, Ho LI, Yu CP, Chen JH, Chiu CC, Fan HC, Lee WH. Apoptosis in nasopharyngeal carcinoma as related to histopathological characteristics and clinical stage. Histopathology 1998, 33(2), 117–22.
58. Zaghloul MS, Dahaba, NW, Hussein MH, el-Kouthey M. Nasopharyngeal carcinoma in children and adolescents' successful role of retrieval therapy. Tumori 1993, 79(2), 123–7.
59. Rao BN, Pratt CB, Fleming ID, Dilawari RA, Green AA, Bradford AA. Colon carcinoma in children and adolescents. A review of 30 cases. Cancer 1985, 55, 1322–6.
60. Ibrahim NK, Abdul-Karim FW. Colorectal adenocarcinoma in young Lebanese adults. Cancer 1986, 58, 816–20.
61. Lamego CM, Tortloni H. Colorectal adenocarcinoma in childhood and adolescent. Report of 11 cases and review of the literature. Pediatr Radiol 1989, 19, 504–8.
62. Brown RA, Rode H, Millar AJ, Sinclair-Smith C, Cywes S. Colorectal carcinoma in children. J Pediatr Surg 1992, 27(7), 919–21.
63. Steinberg JB, Tuggle DW, Postier RG. Adenocarcinoma of the colon in adolescents. Am J Surg 1988, 156, 460–2.
64. Khan AM, Doig CM, Dickson AP. Advanced colonic carcinoma in children. Postgrad Med J 1997, 73(857), 169–70.
65. Pratt CB, Parham DM, Rao BN, Fleming, Dilawari R. Multiple colorectal carcinomas, polyposis coli, and neurofibromatosis. J Nat Cancer Inst 1988, 80(14), 1170–1.
66. Schoni MH, Maisonneuve P, Schoni-Affolter F, Lowenfels AB. Cancer risk in patients with cystic fibrosis: the European data. J Royal Soc Med 1996, 89(27), 38–43.
67. Corredor J, Wambach J, Barnard J. Gastrointestinal polyps in children: advances in molecular genetics, diagnosis, and management. J Pediatr 2001, 138(5), 621–8.
68. Wirtzfeld DA, Petrelli NJ, Rodriguez-Bigas. Hamartomatous polyposis syndromes: molecular genetics, neoplastic risk, and surveillance recommendations. Ann Surg Oncol 2001, 8, 319–27.
69. Boland CR. Hereditary non-polyposis colorectal cancer. In: The genetic basis of human cancer (ed. B Vogelstein, KW Kinzler). NY, USA, McGraw Hill, 1998.
70. Hoeffel JG, Nihoul-Fekete C, Schmitt M. Eosophageal adenocarcinoma after gastroeosophageal reflux in children. J Pediatr 1989, 115, 259–61.
71. Grabiec J, Owen DA. Carcinoma of the stomach in young persons. Cancer 1985, 56, 388–96.
72. Askin FB. Neoplasms of the thyroid and adrenal cortex. Chapter 6. In: Pathology of solid tumors in childhood (ed. JT Stocker, FB Askin). London, Chapman and Hall, 1998.
73. Sabbaga CC, Avilla SG, Schulz C, Garbers JC, Blucher D. Adrenocortical carcinoma in children: clinical aspects and prognosis. J Ped Surg 1993, 28(6), 841–3.
74. Lack EE, Mulvihill JJ, Travis WD, Kozakewich HPW. Adrenal and cortical neoplasms in the pediatric and adolescent age group. Clinicopathologic study of 30 cases with emphasis on epidemiological and prognostic factors. Pathol Ann 1992, 27(1), 1–53.
75. Neblett WW, Frexes-Steed M, Scott HW. Experience with adrenocortical neoplasms in childhood. Am Surg 1987, 53(3), 117–25.
76. Ribeiro RC, Neto RS, Schell MJ, Lacerda L, Sambaio GA, Cat I. Adrenocortical carcinoma in children: a study of 40 cases. J Clin Oncol 1990, 8, 67–74.
77. Lee PDK, Winter RJ, Green OC. Virilizing adrenocortical tumors in childhood: eight cases and a review of the literature. Pediatrics 1985, 76(3), 437–44.
78. Medeiros LJ, Weiss LM. New developments in the pathologic diagnosis of adrenal cortical neoplasms. A review. Am J Clin Pathol 1992, 97, 73–83.
79. Cagle PT, Hough AJ, Pysher J, Page DL, Johnson EH, Kirkland RT, Holcombe JH, Hawkins EP. Comparison of adrenal cortical tumors in children and adults. Cancer 1986, 57, 2235–7.
80. Hawkins EP, Cagle PT. Adrenal cortical neoplasms in children. Am J Clin Pathol 1992, 98(3), 382–3.
81. Michalkiewicz EL, Sandrini R, Bugg MF, Cristofani L, Caran E, Cardoso AM, de Lacerda L, Ribeiro RC. Clinical characteristics of small functioning adrenocortical tumors in children. Med Pediatr Oncol 1997, 28(3), 175–8.
82. Bugg MF, Ribeiro RC, Roberson PK, Lloyd RV, Sandrini R, Silva JB, Epelman S, Shapiro DN, Parham DM. Correlation of pathologic features with clinical outcome on pediatric adrenocortical neoplasia. Am J Clin Pathol 1994, 101, 625–9.
83. Wilkin F, Gagne N, Paquette, J, Oligny Ll, Deal C. Pediatric adrenocortical tumors: molecular events leading to insulin-like growth factor 11 gene expression. J Clin Endocrinol Metab 2000, 85(5), 2048–56.
84. Reincke M. Mutations in adrenocortical tumors. Horm Metab Res 1998, 30, 447–55.
85. Wagner J, Portwine C, Rabin K, Leclerc JM, Narod SA, Malkin D. High frequency of germline p53 mutations in childhood adrenocortical cancer. J Natl Cancer Inst 1994, 86(22), 1707–10.
86. Figueiredo BC, Stratakis CA, Sandrini R, DeLacerda L, Pianovsky MAD, Giatzakis C, Young HM, Haddad BR. Comparative genomic hybridization analysis of adrenocortical tumors of childhood. J Clin Endocrinol Metab 1999, 84(3), 1116–21.
87. Ribeiro RC, Sandrini F, Figueiredo B, Zambetti GP, Michalkiewicz E, Lafferty AR, DeLacerda L, Rabin M, Cadwell C, Sampaio G, Cat I, Stratakis CA, Sandrini R. An inherited p53 mutation that contributes in a tissue-specific manner to pediatric adrenal cortical carcinoma. Proc Natl Acad Sci USA 2001, 98(16), 9330–5.
88. Wilkin F, Gagne N, Paquette J, Oligny LL, Deal C. Pediatric adrenocortical tumors: molecular events leading to insulin-like growth factor 11 gene expression. J Clin Endocrinol Metab 2000, 85(5), 2048–56.

89. Gicquel C, Raffin-Sanson ML, Gaston V, Bertagna X, Plouin PF, Schlumberger M, Louvel A, Luton JP, Le Bouc Y. Structural and functional abnormalities at 11p15 are associated with the malignant phenotype in sporadic adrenocortical tumors: study of a series of 82 tumors. J Clin Endocrinol Metab 1997, **82**(8), 2559–65.
90. Borstein SR, Stratakis CA, Chrousos GP. Adrenocortical tumors: recent advances in basic concepts and clinical management. Ann Intern Med 1999, **130**(9), 759–71.
91. James LA, Kelsey AM, Birch JM, Varley JM. Highly consistent genetic alterations in childhood tumours detected by comparative genomic hybridisation. Br J Cancer 1999, **81**(2), 300–4.
92. Mertens F, Kullendorff CM, Moell C, Alumets J, Mandahl N. Complex karyotype in a childhood adrenocortical carcinoma. Cancer Genet Cytogenet 1998, **105**(2), 190–2.
93. Kjellman M, Kallioniemi OP, Karhu R, Hoog A, Farnebo LO, Auer G, Larsson C, Backdahl M. Genetic aberrations in adrenocortical tumors detected using comparative genomic hybridization correlate with tumor size and malignancy. Cancer Res 1996, **56**, 4219–23.
94. Kelly DR, Joshi VV. Neuroblastoma and related tumors. Chapter 6. In: Pediatric neoplasia. Morphology and biology (ed. DM Parham). USA Lippincott-Raven, 1996, 136–42.
95. Ein SH, Shandling B, Wesson D, Filler RM. Recurrent pheochromocytoma in children. J Pediatr Surg 1990, **25**(10), 1063–5.
96. Ciftci AO, Tanyel FC, Senocak ME, Buyukpamukcu N. Pheochromocytoma in children. J Pediatr Surg 2001, **36**(3), 447–52.
97. Ross JH. Pheochromocytoma. Special considerations in children. Paediatr Urol Oncol 2000, **27**(3), 393–402.
98. Caty MG, Coran AG, Geagen M, et al. Current diagnosis and treatment of pheochromocytoma in children. Arch Surg 1990, **125**, 978–81.
99. Ein SH, Weitzman S, Thorner P, Seagram CG, Filler RM. Pediatric malignant pheochromocytoma. J Pediatr Surg 1994, **29**(9), 1197–201.
100. Neumann HP, Berger DP, Sigmund G, et al. Pheochromocytomas, multiple endocrine neoplasia type2 and von Hippel Lindau disease. N Eng J Med 1993, **329**, 1531–8.
101. Walther MM, Herring J, Enquist E, Keiser HR, Linehan WM. von Recklinghausen's disease and pheochromocytomas. J Urol 1999, **162**, 1583–6.
102. Eng C, Crossey PA, Mulligan LM, Healey CS, et al. Mutations in the Ret proto-oncogene and von Hippel Lindau disease tumour suppressor gene in sporadic and syndromic pheochromocytomas. J Med Genet 1995, **32**, 934–7.
103. Astuti D, Douglas F, Ball S, Lennard L, Aliaganis I, Woodward ER, Evans DGR, Latif F, Maher. Germline SDHD mutation in familial pheochromocytoma. Lancet 2001, **357**, 1181–2.
104. Gimm O, Armanios M, Dziema H, Neumann HP, Eng C. Somatic and occult germline mutations mutations in *SDHD*, a mitochondrial complex 11 gene, in nonfamilial pheochromocytoma. Cancer Res 2000, **60**, 6822–5.
105. Khosla S, Patel VM, Hay ID, Schaid DJ, Grant CS, van Heerden JA, Thibodeau SN. Loss of heterozygosity suggests multiple genetic alterations in phaeochromocytoma and medullary thyroid carcinomas. J Clin Investig 1991, **87**, 1691–9.
106. Reddy VS, O'Neill JA, Holcomb GW, Neblett WW, Pietsch JB, Morgan WM, Goldstein RE. Twenty-five-year surgical experience with pheochromocytoma in children. Am Surg 2000, **66**(12), 1085–92.
107. Wyszynska T, Cichocka E, Wieteska-Klimezak A, Jobs K, Januszewicz P. A single pediatric center experience with 1025 hildren with hypertension. Acta Paediatr 1992, **81**, 244–6.
108. Karel P, Linehan WM, Eisenhofer G, Walther MM, Goldstein DS. Recent advances in genetics, diagnosis, localization, and treatment of pheochromocytoma. Ann Intern Med 2001, **134**(4), 315–19.
109. Coutant R, Pein F, Adamsbaum C, Oberlin O, Dubousset J, Guinebretiere JM, Teinturier C, Bougneres PF. Prognosis of children with malignant pheochromocytoma. Report of two cases and review of the literature. Haem Res 1999, **52**(3), 145–9.
110. Ein SH, Pullerits J, Creighton R, Balfe JW. Pediatric pheochromocytoma. A 36 year experience. Pediatr Surg Int 1997, **12**(8), 595–8.
111. Lloyd RV, Blaivas M, Wilson BS. Distribution of chromogranin and S100 in normal and abnormal adrenal medullary tissues. Arch Pathol Lab Med 1985, **109**, 633–5.
112. Medeiros LJ, Wolf BC, Balogh K, Federman M. Adrenal pheochromocytoma: a clinicopathologic review of 60 cases. Hum Pathol 1985, **16**(6), 580–9.
113. Werbel SS, Ober KP. Pheochromocytoma. Update on diagnosis, localization and management. Med Clin North Am 1995, **79**, 131–53.
114. Shikhani AH, Johns ME. Tumors of the major salivary glands in children. Head Neck Surg 1988, **10**, 257–63.
115. Luna MA, Batsakis JG, el Naggar AK. Salivary gland tumours in children. Ann Otol Rhinol Laryngol 1991, **100**(10), 869–71.
116. Orvidas LJ, Kasperbauer JL, Lewis JE, Olsen KD, Lesnick TG. Pediatric parotid masses. Arch Otol Head Neck Surg 2000, **126**, 177–84.
117. Lack EE, Upton MP. Histopathologic review of salivary gland tumors in childhood. Arch Otol Head Neck Surg 1988, **114**, 898–906.
118. Rogers DA, Rao BN, Bowman L, Marina N, Fleming ID, Schropp KP, Lobe TE. Primary malignancy of the salivary gland in children. J Pediatr Surg 1994, **29**(1), 44–7.
119. Luna MA. Sialoblastoma and epithelial tumors in children: their morphologic spectrum and distribution by age. Adv Anat Pathol 1999, **6**(5), 287–92.
120. Ellis GL, Auclair PL. Atlas of tumor pathology, tumors of the salivary glands, 3rd Series, Fascicle 17. Armed Forces Institute of Pathology, Washington, 1996.
121. Prasannan L, Pu A, Hoff P, Weatherly R, Castle V. Parotid carcinoma as a second malignancy after treatment of childhood acute lymphoblastic leukaemia. J Pediatr Hematol Oncol 1999, **21**(6), 535–8.
122. Depowski PL, Setzen G, Chui A, Koltai PJ, Dollar J, Ross JS. Familial occurrence of acinic cell carcinoma of the parotid gland. Arch Pathol Lab Med 1999, **123**(11), 1118–20.
123. Sandros J, Stenman G, Mark J. Cytogenetic and molecular observations in human and experimental salivary

124. Jin Y, Mertens F, Limon J, Mandahl N, Wennerberg J, Dictor M, Heim S, Mitelman F. Characteristic karyotypic features of lacrimal and salivary gland carcinomas. Br J Cancer 1994, **70**, 42–7.
125. Martins C, Fonseca I, Roque L, Pinto AE, Soares J. Malignant salivary gland neoplasms: a cytogenetic study of 19 cases. Eur J Cancer Oral Oncol 1996, **32B**(2) 128–32.
126. Dahlenfors R, Wedell B, Rundantz H, Mark J. Translocation (11; 19)(q14-21;p12) in a parotid mucoepidermoid carcinoma in a child. Cancer Genet Cytogenet 1995, **79**(2), 188.
127. El-Naggar AK, Lovell M, Killary AM, Clayman GL, Batsakis JG. A mucoepidermoid carcinoma of minor salivary gland with t(11;19)(q21;p13.1) as the only karyotypic abnormality. Cancer Genet Cytogenet 1996, **87**(1), 29–33.
128. Stenman G, Petursdottir V, Mellgren G, Mark J. A child with a t(11;19)(q14-21;p12) in a pulmonary mucoepidermoid carcinoma. Virchows Arch 1998, **433**(60), 579–81.
129. Bader JL, Li FP, Olmstead PM, Strickman NA, Green DM. Childhood malignant melanoma. Incidence and etiology. Am J Pediatr Hematol Oncol 1985, **7**(4), 341–5.
130. Saenz NC, Saenz-Badillos J, Busam K, LaQuaglia MP, Corbally M, Brady MS. Childhood melanoma survival. Cancer 1999, **85**(3), 750–4.
131. Whiteman D, Valery P, McWhirter W, Green A. Incidence of cutaneous childhood melanoma in Queensland, Australia. Int J Cancer 1995, **63**(6), 765–8.
132. Berg P, Lindelof B. Differences in malignant melanoma between children and adolescents. A 35-year epidemiological study. Arch Dermatol 1997, **133**(3), 295–7. Barnhill RL. Childhood melanoma. Semin Diagn Pathol 1998, **15**(3), 189–94.
133. Barnhill Rl. Childhood melanoma. Seminars in Diagnostic Pathology 1998, **15**(3), 189–94.
134. Spatz A, Avril MF. Melanoma in childhood: review and perspectives. Perspectives in pediatric pathology. Pediatr Dev Pathol 1998, **1**, 463–74.
135. Temple WJ, Mulloy RH, Alexander F, Marx LH, Jenkins M, Jerry LM. Childhood melanoma. J Pediatr Surg 1991, **26**(2), 135–37.
136. Barnhill RL, Flotte TJ, Fleischli M, Perez-Atayde A. Cutaneous melanoma and atypical Spitz tumors in childhood. Cancer 1995, **76**(10), 1833–45.
137. Ceballos PI, Ruiz-Maldonado R, Mihm MC. Melanoma in children. N Engl J Med 1995, **332**(10), 656–62.
138. Crotty KA, McCarthy SW, Palmer AA, Ng AB, Thompson JF, Gianoutsos MP, Shaw HM. Malignant melanoma in childhood: a clinicopathologic study of 13 cases and comparison with Spitz nevi. World J Surg 1992, **16**(2), 179–85.
139. Roth ME, Grant-Kels JM. Important melanocytic lesions in childhood and adolescence. Pediatr Clin N Am 1991, **38**(4), 791–809.
140. Whiteman DC, Valery P, McWhirter W, Green AC. Risk factors for childhood melanoma in Queensland, Australia. Int J Cancer 1997, **70**(1), 26–31.
141. Heasley DD, Toda T, Mihm MC. Pathology of malignant melanoma. In: Surg Clin N Am, Cutaneous malignant melanoma (ed. SPL Leong). 1996, **76**(6), 1223–55. WB Saunders Company, 1996.
142. Wyatt AJ, Hansen RC. Pediatric skin tumors. Pediatr Clin N Am 2000, **47**(4), 937–63.
143. Egan CL, Oliveria SA, Elenitsas R, Hanson J, Halpern AC. Cutaneous melanoma risk and phenotypic changes in large congenital nevi: a follow-up study of 46 patients. J Am Acad Dermatol 1998, **39**(6), 923–32.
144. Marghoob AA, Schoenbach SP, Kopf AW, Orlow SJ, Nossa R, Bart RS. Large congenital melanocytic nevi and the risk for the development of malignant melanoma. A prospective study. Arch Dermatol 1996, **132**(2), 170–5.
145. Mehregan AH, Mehregan DA. Malignant melanoma in childhood. Cancer 1993, **71**(12), 4096–103.
146. Ball RA, Genest D, Sander M, Schmidt B, Barnhill RL. Congenital melanocytic nevi with placental infiltration by melanocytes: a benign condition that mimics metastatic melanoma. Arch Dermatol 1998, **134**(6), 711–14.
147. Zhu N, Warr R, Cai R, Rigby HS, Burd DA. Cutaneous malignant melanoma in the young. Br J Plastic Surg 1997, **50**(1), 10–14.
148. Handfield-Jones SE, Smith NP. Malignant melanoma in childhood. Br J Dermatol 1996, **134**, 607–16.
149. Walsh N, Crotty K, Palmer A, McCarthy S. Spitz nevus versus spitzoid malignant melanoma: an evaluation of the current distinguishing histopathologic criteria. Hum Pathol 1998, **29**(10), 1105–12.
150. Shea CR, Prieto VG. Recent developments in the pathology of melanocytic neoplasia. Dermatol Clin 1999, **17**(1), 615–30.
151. Serrano M, Hannon GJ, Beach D. A new regulatory motif in cell-cycle control causing specific inhibition of cyclin/CDK4. Nature 1993, **366**, 704–7. 212 Pollock PM, Trent JM. The genetics of cutaneous melanoma. Clin Lab Med 2000, **20**(4), 667–90.
152. Pollock PM, Trent JM. The genetics of cutaneous melanoma. Clin Lab Med 2000, **20**(4), 667–90.
153. Kamb A, Herlyn M. Malignant melanoma. In: The genetic basis of human cancer (ed. B Vogelstein, KW Kinzler). NY, USA, McGraw Hill, 1998.
154. Saida T. Recent advances in melanoma research. J Dermatol Sci 2001, **26**(1), 1–13.
155. Park WS, Vortmeyer AO, Pack S, Duray PH, Boni R, Guerami AA, Emme Buck MR, Liotta LA, Zhuang Z. Allelic deletion at chromosome 9p21(p16) and 17p13(p53) in microdissected sporadic dysplastic nevus. Hum Pathol 1998, **29**(2), 127–30.
156. Bastian BC, Wesselmann U, Pinkel D, Leboit PE. Molecular cytogenetic analysis of Spitz nevi shows clear differences to melanoma. J Invest Dermatol 1999, **113**(60), 1065–9.
157. Fromont Hankard G, Fraitag S, Wolter M, Brousse N, Masood S. DNA content and cell proliferation in giant congenital melanocytic naevi (GCMN). An analysis by image cytometry. J Cutan Pathol 1998, **25**(8), 401–6.
158. Wu SJ, Lambert DR. Melanoma in children and adolescents. Pediatr Dermatol 1997, **14**(2), 87–92.
159. Jaksic T, Yaman M, Thorner P, Wesson DK, Filler RM, Shandling B. A 20-year review of pediatric pancreatic tumors. J Pediatr Surg 1992, **27**(10), 1315–17.

160. Grosfeld JL, Vane DW, Rescorla FJ, McGuire W, West KW. Pancreatic tumors in childhood: analysis of 13 cases. J Pediatr Surg 1990, **25**(10), 1057–62.
161. Jaffe R, Newman B. Pancreatic masses. In: Pathology of solid tumors in children (ed. JT Stocker, FB Askin). London, Chapman and Hall, 1998.
162. Kissane JM. Pancreatoblastoma and solid and cystic papillary tumor: two tumors related to pancreatic ontogeny. Semin Diagn Pathol 1994, **11**(2), 152–64.
163. Defachelles AS, de Lassalle EM, Boutard P, Nelken B, Schneider P, Patte C. Pancreatoblastoma in childhood: clinical course and therapeutic management of seven patients. Med Ped Oncol 2001, **37**, 47–52.
164. Murakami T, Ueki K, Kawakami H, Gondo T, Kuga T, Esato K, Furukawa S. Pancreatoblastoma: case report and review of treatment in the literature. Med Ped Oncol 1996, **27**, 193–7.
165. Hruban RH, Yeo CJ, Kern SE. Pancreatic cancer. In: The Genetic Basis of Human Cancer (ed. B Vogelstein, KW Kinzler). NY, USA, McGraw Hill, 1998.
166. Wiley J, Posekany K, Riley R, Hollbrook T, Silverman J, Joshi V, Bowyer S. Cytogenetic and flow cytometric analysis of a pancreatoblastoma. Cancer Genet Cytogenet 1995, **79**(2), 115–18.
167. Nagashima Y, Misugi K, Tanaka Y, Ijiri R, Nishihira H, Nishi T, Kigasawa H, Kato K. Pancreatoblastoma: a second report on cytogenetic findings. Cancer Genet Cytogenet 1999, **109**(2), 178–9.
168. Abraham SC, Wu TT, Klimstra DS, Finn LS, Lee JH, Yeo CJ, Cameron JL, Hruban RH. Distinctive molecular genetic alterations in sporadic and familial adenomatous polyposis-associated pancreatoblastomas: frequent alterations in the APC/beta-catenin pathway and chromosome 11p. Am J Pathol 2001, **159**(5), 1619–27.
169. Mao C, Guvendi M, Domenico DR, Kim K, Thomford NR, Howard JM. Papillary cystic and solid tumors of the pancreas: a pancreatic embryonic tumor? Studies of three cases and cumulative review of the world's literature. Surgery 1995, **118**(5), 821–8.
170. Pettinato G, Manivel JC, Ravetto C, Terracciano LM, Gould EW, Di Tuoro A, Jaszcz W, Albores-Saavedra J. Papillary cystic tumor of the pancreas. A clinicopathologic study of 20 cases with cytologic, immunohistochemical, ultrastructural and flow cytometric observations and a review of the literature. Am J Clin Pathol 1992, **98**, 478–88.
171. Klimstra DS, Wenig BM, Heffess CS. Solid-pseudopapillary tumor of the pancreas: a typically cystic carcinoma of low malignant potential. Semin Diagn Pathol 2000, **17**(1), 66–80.
172. Nishihara K, Nagoshi M, Tsuneyoshi M, Yamagichi K, Hayashi I. Papillary cystic tumors of the pancreas. Assessment of their malignant potential. Cancer 1993, **71**, 82–92.
173. Grant LD, Lauwers GY, Meloni AM, Stone JF, Betz JL, Vogel S, Sandberg AA. Unbalanced chromosomal translocation, der(17)t(13;17)(q14;p11) in a solid and cystic papillary epithelial neoplasm of the pancreas. Am J Surg Pathol 1996, **20**(3), 339–45.
174. Matsubara K, Nigami H, Harigaya H, Baba K. Chromosome abnormality in solid and cystic tumor of the pancreas. Am J Gastroenterol 1997, **92**(7), 1219–21.

Glossary of molecular terms

Anaphase	The separation of two sister chromatids at their centromeres.	Exon	The region of a gene that codes for a specific portion of the complete protein.
Bacterial artificial chromosome (BAC)	Large segments of DNA 100,000 to 200,000 bases from another species cloned into bacteria. Foreign DNA cloned into the host bacteria may be used to generate multiple copies.	Fluorescence *in situ* hybridization (FISH)	A process which paints chromosomes or portions of chromosomes with fluorescent markers, useful for identifying chromosomal abnormalities and gene mapping.
Chromosome	Packages of genes and other DNA in the nucleus of the cell. Humans have 23 pairs of chromosomes, 46 in total (44 autosomes and 2 sex chromosomes).	Gene	The functional unit of heredity passed from parent to offspring. Genes are pieces of DNA, most genes (coding genes) contain the information for making specific protein products.
Codon	Three bases in a DNA or RNA sequence which specify a single amino acid.	Gene amplification	An increase in the number of copies of any particular piece of DNA.
Deletion	A particular kind of mutation: loss of a piece of DNA from a chromosome. Deletion of a gene or part of a gene can lead to a disease or abnormality.	Gene expression	The process by which proteins are made from DNA.
		Gene mapping	Determining the relevant positions of genes on a chromosome and the distance between them.
Deoxyribo nucleic acid (DNA)	The chemical makeup of the nucleus within a cell that carries the genetic material instructing the production of living organisms.	Gene pool	The sum total of genes possessed by a particular species at any particular time.
DNA replication	The process by which DNA double helix unwinds and makes an exact copy of itself.	Genome	All the DNA contained in an organism or a cell, which includes both the chromosomes within the nucleus and the DNA in mitochondria.
Non-coding DNA	The strand of DNA that does not carry the information necessary to make a protein. The non-coding strand is the mirror image of the coding strand and is also known as the antisense strand.	Genetic code (ATCG)	The instructions in a gene that drive the production of specific proteins by cells. Adenine (A), Thymine (T),

	Cytosine (C), Guanine (G) are the letters of the DNA code. Each code combines the four chemicals (ATCG) in various ways to spell a three-letter "word" that specifies which amino acid is needed.	Microarray technology	Method to study large numbers of genes, their interaction and regulation by cell networks.
		Microsatellite	Repetitive stretches of short sequences of DNA used as genetic markers to follow inheritance in families.
Genetic screening	Testing a population group to identify a sub-set of individuals at high risk for having or transmitting a specific genetic disorder.	Mutation	A permanent, structural alteration in DNA: in most cases these mutations do not have an effect or cause harm, but sometimes the mutation can improve the survival chances of an organism which may be passed onto its descendants.
Heterozygous	Possessing two different forms of a particular gene, one inherited from each parent.		
Homozygous	Possessing two identical forms of a specific gene, one inherited from each parent.	Northern blot	A technique used to identify and locate mRNA sequences that are complementary to a DNA probe.
Human artificial chromosome (HAC)	A vector used to transfer or express large fragments of human DNA.		
Inherited	Transmitted through genes from parents to offspring.	Oncogene	A gene that is capable of transforming normal cells into cancer cells.
Intron	A non-coding sequence of DNA that is initially copied into RNA but is spliced out of the final RNA transcript. Often called junk DNA.	Polymerase chain reaction (PCR)	A rapid, inexpensive technique for making an unlimited number of DNA copies.
		Polymorphism	A common variant in the sequence of DNA
Linkage	The association of genes and/or markers that are close to each other on a chromosome. Linked genes and markers tend to be inherited together.	Proto-oncogene	A gene that if mutated or modified in some way to alter the normal regulation of the gene may become an oncogene.
Metaphase	The phase of cell division when chromosomes align along the centre of the cell. Metaphase chromosomes are highly condensed hence scientists use these chromosomes for gene mapping and identifying chromosomal aberrations.	Recessive	A genetic disorder that occurs only in patients with two copies of a mutant gene (one from each parent).
		Restriction fragment/length polymorphisms (RFLP)	Genetic variations at the site where a restriction enzyme cuts a piece of DNA. These sequences

Glossary of molecular terms

	can be used as markers on physical and linkage maps.	Southern blot	A technique used to identify and locate DNA sequences which are complementary to a second piece of DNA (probe).
Reverse transcriptase polymerase chain reaction (RT-PCR)	The conversion of RNA to cDNA using reverse transcriptase, allowing the amplification of cDNA by PCR. Used to amplify RNA sequences.	Spectral karyotype (SKY)	Visualization of the full complement of an organism's chromosomes together, each labelled with a different colour. This technique is useful for identifying chromosome abnormalities.
Ribonucleic acid (RNA)	A chemical similar to a single strand of DNA, that encodes the genetic message of the DNA to the cytoplasm of a cell where proteins are made. In RNA the letter U stands for uracil which substitutes T in the genetic code of DNA. Each set of three bases (codons) specifies a certain protein in the sequence of amino acids that comprise a protein. The strand of mRNA is based on the sequence of a complimentary strand of DNA.	Translocation	Breakage and removal of a large segment of DNA from one chromosome, followed by the segment's attachment to a different chromosome. May involve reciprocal exchange of DNA from one chromosome to another.
		Western blot	A technique used to identify proteins based on their size and ability to bind to specific antibodies.
Single nucleotide polymorphisms (SNP)	Common but minute variations that occur in human DNA at a frequency in 1 : 1000 bases. Can be used to track inheritance in families.	Yeast artificial chromosome (YAC)	Extremely large segments of DNA from another species spliced into DNA of yeast. Used to clone up to 1 million bases of foreign DNA into a host cell, where the DNA is propagated with the other chromosomes of the yeast cell.

Index

Page numbers in **bold** type refer to figures and page numbers in *italics* refer to tables

acetic acid fixatives 30
acinic cell carcinoma 308–9
adhesion molecules 132
adrenal carcinoma 305–7
adrenal medullary hyperplasia 307
adrenocortical carcinoma, cytogenetic analysis 306
adrenocortical tumours 305–**6**
Affymetrix GeneChips 49
aflatoxin 265, 283
AIDS 117
Alagille syndrome 280
 and liver tumors 266
alcohol fixatives 29, 32
aldehydes 28
allelic imbalance (AI)
 assay **60**
 study 61–2
 tumours associated with 62
alpha-fetoprotein 251, 253, 257
 liver tumor marker 278
 yolk sac tumour marker 278
alveolar soft part sarcoma 209–**10**
amplicon detection 65
anaesthetics, general 12
anaplasia 220–1, 223–4
androgen insensitivity syndrome 249
angiomyolipoma 270
angiosarcoma 211, 270
Ann Arbor staging system 118–19
anthracyclines 109
antibody
 binding specificity 21–2
 bound, detection 22
 in lymphoma characterization *127*
 therapy in leukaemias 110
antigen
 preservation 23
 retrieval methods *21*, 127
aponeuroses 210
arsenic trioxide 109
Askin tumour 171
astrocytoma 136–7
 cell kinetic analysis 141
 cell line **38**
 cerebellar 138
 fibrillary 140
 gemistiocytic 140
 molecular genetic analysis 141
 pilocytic 138, 140
 protoplasmic 140

 superficial cerebral 140
ataxia telangiectasia
 and familial thyroid cancer 301
 and liver tumors 266
ataxia-telangiectasia 76–7, 95, 117
Ataxia-Telangiectasia Society 76–7
Autoimmune Lymphoproliferative Syndrome 126

B-ALL gene 103
B-cell leukaemia *see* leukaemia
BCR-ABL fusion gene 102–3
Beckwith-Wiedemann syndrome 3, 81, 87–9, 186
 with adrenocortical tumours 306
 clinical features 88
 clinical genetics 89
 course 88
 hepatoblastoma risk 284
 and liver tumors 266
 molecular genetics 89
 screening policies 89
 and Wilms' tumour 219
beta-catenin proto-oncogene, mutations in pancreatoblastoma 311
bile duct adenomas 270
biotin 38, 72
Bloom's syndrome 74–5, 95
bone marrow transplant 112
bone tumors 238–46
 epidemiology 238
brain tumors
 cell kinetic studies 137–8
 classification 136
 molecular genetic studies 137–8
 sampling 136
British National Lymphoma Investigation 123
buffers
 concentration 34
 in fixation 29–30
Burkitt lymphoma 115, 117
 clinical presentation 116
 cytology **120**
 translocations 127–9
Byler syndrome 266

c-kit ligand 249
cancer
 5 year survival rates **4**
 aetiology 2–3
 diagnosis 4–5
 diagnostic evaluation 6–9

cancer (cont.)
  drugs causing 3
  environmental factors 3
  epidemiology 1–2
  incidence 2
  management stages 5
  outcome changes 3–4
  referral 5–6
  treatment 4–**5**
cancer predisposition syndromes
  autosomal dominant 81
  inherited 74–93
carcinoembryonic antigen 302
carcinoma 299–320
cell-cycle analysis 23–4
  DNA content 24
  strategies 24
central nervous system
  germ cell tumour 260–1
  tumours 85, 86, 140
cerebellum
  glioma 140
  pilocytic astrocytoma 140
Chaganti's hypothesis 248–9
chemoresistance associated genes in osteosarcoma 243
Children's Cancer Group 3, 97, 264, 267
  liver tumor chemotherapy 286
Children's Cancer Study Group 4, 247
chondrosarcoma, extraskeletal myxoid 210–11
choriocarcinoma 254, 255–6
choristoma 260
choroid plexus tumors **147–8**
chromic-acid formaldehyde 29
chromogenic detection 22–3
chromogranins 275, 302
chromosome
  analysis 23
  paints 44
  SKY visualization 44
  translocation breakpoints position 26
citrullinaemia 79
clear cell sarcoma
  kidney 217, 228, **229**–30
    genetics 229
    pathology 228–9
    prognosis 229–30
    treatment 229
  tendons 210
Coats' disease 151
Cockayne syndrome 78–81
colon, mucinous adenocarcinoma **304**
comparative genomic hybridization (CGH) 38, 47–8, 137–8
  DNA sequencing 69–71
  microarray 51–**2**
  neuroblastoma 163
core binding factor 102
Cowden's disease, and familial thyroid cancer 301
craniopharyngioma 136

cryopreservation 21
Cushing's syndrome 305
cyclin A 265
cytarabine 109
cytochemistry, ALL 98–9
cytogenetics
  7 and 5, abnormalities 109
  abnormalities, in hepatocarcinoma 277
  adrenocortical carcinoma 306
  analysis 8, 23, 25
    methods 37
  Ewing's sarcoma family of tumours (ESFT) 176–7
  germ cell tumours 250
  hepatoblastoma 280, 283–4
    abnormalities 276
  hepatocarcinoma 279–80, 283–5
  isochromosome 17q 144
  lymphoma 127–31
  neuroblastoma **162**–3
  rhabdomyosarcoma 191–2
  teratoma 250
  trisomy 18 and liver tumours 266–7
  trisomy 21 see Down's Syndrome 21
  tyrosinemia, hereditary, and liver tumours 266–7
  see also individual tumours and individual genes
cytology 17–**18**
cytosine arabinoside 111

data mining 50–1
de Sanctis-Cacchione variant, Cockayne syndrome 78
Denys-Drash syndrome 89–90
  intralobar nephrogenic rest with 221–2
  and Wilms' tumour 218
dermoid cyst 253
desmin 190, 233
desmoplastic cerebral astrocytoma 140
desmoplastic infantile ganglioglioma (DIG) 140–1
detergents, effect 31
dexamethasone 109
diabetes mellitus type 1, genome-wide study 61
diagnosis, routine 18–19
diagnostic process
  decision point 9–10
  flow diagram **16**
diagnostic samples 7–8
Diamond-Blackfan anaemia 96
digoxigenin 38
diktyoma 151
DNA
  amplification
    DOP PCR **70**
    Taq Man PCR 64–5
  array production 47–8
  chip 47
  complementary, microarray technology 71–2
  damage, DNA repair disorders 80

extraction techniques 25
finger-printing 63–4
measurements 24
probe 38
repair disorders 74–81
spacer 63
synthesis markers 23
template 59
DNA sequencing 66–9
chain termination 67, **68–9**
chemical 67
DNA-specific fluorescence 24
dot blot 57–8
Down's syndrome 90, 249
and AML 107
and germ cell tumour risk 248
and leukaemia 3
dysembryoplastic neuroepithelial tumor (DNET) 146
dysgerminoma **256**, 257, 259
dysplastic naevus syndrome 309

EBER RNAs 302
ectomesenchymoma, malignant 179–80
electron microscopy 23
embedding 19
embryonal carcinoma 254–5, **256**
and germ cell tumours 248
embryonal sarcoma
hepatic 267
renal *see* synovial sarcoma, renal
endodermal sinus tumour 255
ependymoma 144–5
epignathus 260
epithelial markers 139
epithelial membrane antigen (EMA) 123
epithelioid sarcoma **209**
Epstein-Barr virus
infection 125
nuclear antigen 302
risk for nasopharyngeal carcinoma 302
erythroleukaemia 106
esthesioneuroblastoma 180
Estren-Dameshek syndrome 77
Ewing's sarcoma 171
chromosomal G-banding **176**
family of tumours (ESFT) 171–2
clinical prognostic factors 177–8
cytogenetics 176–7
diagnosis 172–9
FISH **177**
genetic prognostic factors 179
immunohistochemistry 174, **175–6**
pathological prognostic factors 178–9
pathology 172–4
prognostic factors *178*
stains **175**
FISH analysis 39

EWS gene, fusion types in Ewing's sarcoma family of tumours (ESFT) *173*
EWS-FL11 fusion transcripts **176**
expression microarray analysis 49, 50–1

familial adenomatous polyposis
and familial thyroid cancer 301
hepatoblastoma risk 284
and liver tumours 266–7
familial cancer syndromes, and high penetrance genes 81
familial factors and germ cell tumours 248
familial medullary thyroid cancer 83
familial polyposis, hepatoblastoma in 265
familial polyposis syndromes, and nasopharyngeal carcima 304
familial predisposition 6
familial syndromes 74–93
Fanconi anaemia/anemia 77–8, 95, 266
fetal alcohol syndrome 186
fibrolamellar carcinoma 266, 267
immunocytochemistry 271, 273
prognostic factors 286
fibrosarcoma 201, 205–6
infantile 205–**6**
inflammatory 206
fine needle aspirate 261
FISH 23, 37–43, 128, 137–8
Ewing's sarcoma family of tumours (ESFT) **177**
multicolor (M-FISH) 43
neuroblastoma 163
signal evaluation and enumeration 42
FISH analysis
clinical samples 38, **39**–40
cytogenetic preparations 40–1
cytological specimens 41
hematologic malignancies *45*
interphase
analytical sensitivity 42–3
statistical consideration 43
paraffin-embedded specimens 41–2
results criteria 42
solid tumors *45*
FISH microscopy, cell selection 42–3
FISH probes
double fusion 112
suppliers 53
tumor assessment use 43
fixation
categories 27
cytochemical aspects 27–9
duration 34
non-tissue factors 29–30
rapid 18
secondary 31
time 31

fixatives 27–34
  chemical properties 32–4
  concentration importance 30
  solution osmolarity 30
  substance addition effect 30–1
fleurettes 149–50
Flexner Wintersteiner rosettes 149–50
flow cytometry 23–4
focal nodular hyperplasia 270
formaldehyde 28–9
  chemical properties 32
French/American/British (FAB) classification of ALL 98
frozen section 17
FWT1 gene 223

ganglioglioma 137, 146
ganglioneuroblastoma 156
  types 164–6
ganglioneuroma 156, 166–7
genes
  amplification, FISH analysis 44
  expression, hepatoblastoma *281–2*
  translocation detection, FISH analysis 44
genetic analysis, methods 37–55
genetics, DNA repair disorders 79–80
genome, human, maps *61*
genome analysis 60–1
  microarray-based 70–1
Genome Database 61
genomics, cancer 47
germ cell tumours/tumors 247–63
  aetiology and pathogenesis 248–9
  associated primary malignancies 248
  categories *250*
  cytogenetics 250
  environmental 248
  extragonadal
    pathogenesis 249
    sites 260
  gonadal 248, 258–9
  histopathological classification 252
  incidence 247
    ethnicity 247–8
  intratubular neoplasia (ITGCN) 249
  liver 267
  malignant 247, 254–5
    classification *252*
  mast cell proliferation post-mediastinal 248
  ovary 258–9
    pathogenesis 249
  pathology 253–6
  post-chemotherapy, histology 257
  sites *258*
    age and tumour type distribution 257–8
  staging 250, *251–2*
  testicular
    pathogenesis of adolescent and adult 249
    pathogenesis of infantile 249
  staging 259
  treatment 261–2
  WHO classification *252*
German Cooperative Soft Tissue Sarcoma Study *187*
German Hodgkin Disease study group 131
German Soft Tissue Tumor Study 192
germinoma 254, 256
  CNS 261
glial fibrillary acidic protein (GFAP) 138
  immunohistochemistry 140
gliofibroma 140
glioma
  brain stem 86–7
  cerebellar 140
  optic pathway 86
gliomatosis 258
glutaraldehyde 28–9, 30, 31
  chemical properties 32
glycogen storage disease, hepatocarcinoma in 265, 266–7
gonadal dysgenesis 249
gonadoblastoma 257, 259
Gorlin syndrome 85
growth factors in osteosarcoma 243
growth fraction 23

haemangioma, capillary 308
haematoxylin 19
Heifetz report 254
hemangioendothelioma 270, 275
hemangiopericytoma 201
hematologic malignancies, analysis 43
hemihypertrophy, and Wilms' tumour 219
hepatitis, neonatal giant cell 266
hepatitis B virus
  carrier rate 264
  core antigen **265**
hepatoblastoma
  with Beckwith-Wiedemann syndrome and hemihypertrophy **272**
  cholangioblastic 274
  classification 267
  "crowded fetal" 273–4
  cytogenetic abnormalities 276, 280, 283
  cytogenetics 280, 283
  gene expression *281–2*
  HBV in **265**
  histology 273–5
  incidence 264–5
  molecular genetics 284
  neuro-endocrine 275
  pretreatment evaluation of location 271
  prognostic factors 285
  small cell undifferentiated **273**, 275
  stage and histopathology *275*
  staging *270*
  teratoid **268**, 275

hepatocarcinoma
   chromosomal abnormalities 277
   of classical trabecular 272
   classification 267
   cytogenetics 280, 283
   etiology 264–7
   HBV in 264–5
   immunocytochemistry 271
   molecular genetics 279–80, 283–5
   prognostic factors 285–6
hereditary tyrosinemia, and liver tumors 266–7
high penetrance genes and familial cancer syndromes 81
Hirschprung's disease 84–5
histiocytoma, malignant fibrous 208
HLA linkage, risk for nasopharyngeal carcinoma 302
hereditary non-polyposis colon cancer (HNPCC)
   gene mutation in 80
   MSI in 62
   and nasopharyngeal carcinoma 304
Hodgkin lymphoma 115, 116
   classification 117, *118*
   cytology 123
   lymphocyte predominant 125
   mixed cellularity (MCHL), cytology 124–5
   nodular sclerosing (NSHL), cytology 123–4
Homer-Wright rosettes 156, 174
homovanillic acid 161
human chorionic gonadotrophin 251, 257
Human Genome Project 47
Hürthle cell carcinoma 300
hydantoin syndrome 186
hydroxyurea 111

imaging systems and optics, suppliers 53
immunochemistry, non-Hodgkin lymphoma 119–25
immunocytochemistry 8
   liver tumors 270–5
immunohistochemistry 19–23
   diagrammatical representation 22
   Ewing's sarcoma family of tumours (ESFT) 174, **175**–6
   evaluation 7
   germ cell tumour diagnosis 257
   germinoma 256
   glial fibrillary acidic protein 140
   markers 138–9
   neuroblastoma 156–7
   polyclonal and monoclonal antisera *21*
   pPNETs 173
   rhabdomyosarcoma 190–1
   tumor markers 127
immunophenotype
   ALL 99
   lymphoma cells 131
immunotherapy, in AML 110
immunotoxins 110
infants, testicular germ cell tumours, staging 259
insulin-like growth factor 1 (IGF-1) 243
insulin-like growth factor 2 (IGF-2) 223, 228

interferon 111
Intergroup Rhabdomyosarcoma Study, staging system *187*
International Agency for Research on Cancer 264
International Classification of Childhood Cancer 1
International Classification of Rhabdomyosarcomas *187*
International Germ Cell Cancer Collaborative Group 251
   protocol staging 259
International Neuroblastoma Pathology Committee (INPC) terminology 163–6
International Neuroblastoma Staging System 158
   conference 155
International Society of Paediatric Oncology (SIOP) 3
   clear cell sarcoma of kidney (CCSK) staging 229–30
   protocols 217
intestinal carcinoma 303–5
intraocular neoplasms 149–51
isochromosome 17q 144

Japanese Children's Cancer Registry 264

karyorrhexis 159
Klinefelter's syndrome and germ cell tumour risk 248
Knudson's two hit hypothesis 61, 149, 221, 241
Kostmann's disease 95

lactic dehydrogenase 251
laser capture microdissection 27, 70
latent membrane protein 302–3
Lennert's lymphoma 125
Leukaemia Working Group 3
leukaemia/leukemia 95–114
   acute lymphoblastic 95–6, 96–100
   age in 96
   B-lineage 99
   biologic factors 97
   chromosomal aberrations **101**
   chromosomal translocations 102
   chromosome number 101
   clinical risk factors 96–7
   gender 97
   genetic factors 100–1
   immunoglobulin and T-cell receptor rearrangements 100
   light microscopy 97–8
   MLL gene rearrangements 102
   peripheral blood smear **98**
   response to therapy 97
   risk groups *104*
   structural chromosomal abnormalities 101–2
   T-cell lineage translocations 103
   T-lineage 99–100
   trisomy 4 and 10 101
   acute megakaryoblastic 106

leukaemia/leukemia (cont.)
  acute monoblastic 106
  acute myeloblastic 103–9
    age at diagnosis 106
    classification 103–4
    clinical risk factors 106–7
    FAB classification 105
    genetics 107–9
    immunophenotypic analysis 107
    prognostic features 108
    recurrent chromosomal aberrations 108
    secondary 107
    therapy 109–10
    white cell counts 107
  acute myeloid 95, 104
  acute myelomonoblastic 106
  acute promyelocytic 104, 108, 109
  chronic myelocytic 95, 111–12
    clinical features 111
    G-banded analysis 100
    special features 111
    therapy 111–12
  CNS 97
  epidemiology 95–6
  FISH analysis 45
  infant 96
  juvenile chronic myelomonocytic 87
  megakaryoblastic 275
  minimal residual disease studies 110–11
  mixed-lineage 100, 102
  subtypes 7
leukocoria 149, 151
leukocyte count, in ALL 96–7
Li-Fraumeni syndrome 81–3, 95, 186, 242
  with adrenocortical tumours 306
  aetiology 2
  clinical aspects 82
  and germ cell tumours 248
  and liver tumors 266
  molecular genetics 82–3
  second cancer risk 82
  tumour spectrum 82
liposarcoma 208–9
  myxoid 208
Lisch nodules 85
liver
  adenoma 270
  carcinoids 267
  germ cell tumors 267
  nodular regeneration 275
  orthotopic transplantation 287
liver tumours/tumors 264–98
  age at presentation 269
  biochemical tests 278, 280
  blood tests for 278
  classification 267–70
  cytogenetic abnormalities 269
  epidemiology 264

immunocytochemistry 270–5
incidence 264, 278
multiple hepatocarcinomas 283
natural history and spread 270
staging 270–5
teratoid 267
treatment strategies 286–7
tumor markers 278, 280
loss of heterozygosity (LOH) 145
  liver tumors 283
  study 61–2
  tumours associated with 62
  Wilms' tumour 223
Louis-Bar syndrome 76–7
lymphoepithelioma 302
lymphoma 115–35
  see also Burkitt lymphoma; Hodgkin lymphoma;
    non-Hodgkin lymphoma
  anaplastic large cell 116
    chromosomal abnormalities 130
    cytology 122–3
  B cell 117, 122
    large 116, 117
  chromosomal abnormalities 128
  classification 117
  clinical presentation 116
  disorders mimicking 125–7
  epidemiology 115
  etiology 117
  immunophenotyping 127
  incidence 115
  large cell 115, 116
    chromosomal abnormalities 130
    cytology 121–2
  lymphoblastic 115, 116, 117
    chromosomal abnormalities 129–30
    cytology 121–2
  molecular factors 132
  natural history 116
  non-Hodgkin, classification 118
  peripheral T cell 117
    cytology 123
  prognosis 115–16
  staging 118–19
  T cell 117
    chromosomal abnormalities 130
  tumor markers 127
lymphoproliferative disease 126

magnetic resonance imaging 86
malignant peripheral nerve sheath tumour 87
marker chromosomes 44, 46
Maxam-Gilbert technique 67
medullary carcinoma thyroid 301–2
medulloblastoma 142–3
  cell kinetic analysis 144
  molecular genetic analysis 144
medulloepithelioma 151

melanoma 309–10
  congenital 309–10
  familial, germline mutations 310
  nodular 310
  tumour thickness 310
melanotic neuroectodermal tumour of infancy (MNETI) 180
menin gene 84
meningioma **148**
Menkes syndrome 79
mercuric chloride 28
  containing fixatives 33
mesenchymal hamartoma 269
methacran 32
microarray
  -based genomic analysis 70–**1**
  analysis methods 47–8
  cDNA technology 71–2
  comparative genomic hybridization (CGH) 51
  findings validation 51–2
  image processing and quantification 49–50
  manufacturing 49
  statistical analysis and data mining 50–1
  suppliers 53
  target preparation and hybridization 49
microsatellite
  analysis, chromosome 11 **60–1**
  associated with disease 62
  detection and scoring 59
  expansion in disease 62
  forensic and population study applications 63
  markers in human disease 62
  sequences 58
  uses in pathology 60–3
microsatellite instability (MSI)
  in human disease 62–3
  in nasopharyngeal carcinoma 303
microsatellite PCR 59–60
  analysis 58
  buffers 59
  dNTPs 59
  primers 59
microscopy
  FISH, cell selection 42–3
  light 17–18
microwave fixation 28
minisatellite sequences 58
minor groove binder probes 66
mitosis-karyorrhexis index (MKI) 159–61
MLL gene rearrangements in ALL 102, 109
mononucleosis syndrome 125
mucoepidermoid carcinoma 308–9
multiple endocrine neoplasia 83–5
  clinical implications 85
  genetic basis 84–5
  tumour spectrum 83
multiple endocrine neoplasia (MEN 1) 83–4
  clinical aspects 83–4

and familial thyroid cancer 301
multiple endocrine neoplasia (MEN 2) 83–4
  clinical aspects 84
  familial cancer syndromes 299
  familial medullary thyroid carcinoma 301–2
myelodysplasia 95
myofibroblastic tumors, inflammatory 206
myofibroblastoma, inflammatory 275
myofibrosarcoma 206
myogenin 26
myxofibrosarcoma 208

naevus
  giant congenital 309
  Spitz 309–10
    CGH 310
nasopharyngeal carcinoma 302–3
  genetic events 303
National Breast Screening Programme 77
National Institutes of Health 85
National Registry of Childhood Cancer 247
National Wilms' Tumor
  Pathology Center 211
  Study 217, 218
nephroblastoma *see* Wilms' tumour
nephroblastomatosis 221
nephrogenic rests 221–2
  intralobar 221–**2**
  perilobar 221–2
nephroma
  adult mesoblastic 228
  atypical mesoblastic 227
  congenital mesoblastic 225–8
    classical versus cellular 226
    genetics 227
    pathology 225, **226**–7
    prognosis 227
    treatment 227
  cystic 220
nerve sheath tumor, malignant peripheral (MPNST) 201, 202, **204**–5
neuroblastoma 155–69
  biochemical parameters 161
  biology 161–3
  clinical diagnosis 157–9
  cytogenetic abnormalities **162**–3
  diagnostic considerations 155
  differential diagnosis 156
  immunohistochemistry 156–7
  microscopy 156, 157
  MKI **160**
  morphological parameters 159–61
  olfactory 180
  prognostic parameters 157
  Schwannian stroma 156, 159, 165–6
  staging system *159*
  subtypes 164–**5**

neuroblastoma (cont.)
  terminology comparisons 164
  ultrastructure **158**
neurocytoma 145
neuroepithelioma *see* peripheral primitive neuroectodermal tumours and Ewing's sarcoma family of tumours (ESFT)
neurofibroma, plexiform 87
neurofibromatosis
  and liver tumors 266
  and rhabdomyosarcoma 186
neurofibromatosis-1 85
  aetiology 2
  associated malignancy 85–6
  leukaemia in 96
  pilocytic astrocytoma 138
  soft tissue sarcoma in 202, 204–5
neurofibromin 205
neurofilaments 138
neuron specific enolase 139
Nijmegen breakage syndrome 76
non-Hodgkin lymphoma 115
  histologic features 131–2
  histopathologic features 119, *120–5*
  international index 131
  molecular alterations 128
  prognostic factors 131
North American Oncologists, germ cell tumour categories 250
Northern blot 57
nucleic acids
  and formaldehyde 32
  interactions 28–9
  which fixative 33
nucleoproteins, which fixative 33

oligodendroglioma 145
omentalmesenteric myxoid hamartoma 206
optic nerve, pilocytic astrocytoma 139
osteosarcoma 238
  CGH microarray analysis 52
  classification 239–40
  clinical symptoms 238
  cytogenetic findings 240–1
  FISH analysis **39**
  histologic findings 239–40
  molecular and biochemical alterations **242**
  molecular findings 240–1
  oncogenes 242–3
  radiograph **238–40**
  radiologic findings 238–9
  and retinoblastoma 241–2
  treatment and prognosis 240
  variants *239*
ovary
  immature teratoma 253–4
  malignant tumours 258–9
  mature teratoma 258
overgrowth syndromes 87–9
oxidising agents 28

p53 immunohistochemistry 138
pancreas
  carcinoma 310–11
  solid-pseudopapillary tumour 311–12
pancreatoblastoma 311
pancytopaenia 77–8
papilloma, choroid plexus **147**
patient pathway 4, 5–14
Pediatric Oncology Group (POG) 96, 117, 199–*200*, 202, 210
  AML protocol 110
  hepatoblastoma 275
  hepatocarcinoma 278
  liver tumor chemotherapy 286
  soft tissue sarcoma grading scheme *200*
  staging system 270
pentagastrin stimulation test 84
peri-vascular rosettes 174
peripheral primitive neuroectodermal tumours (pPNETs) 171–85
  cytology **174**
  Ewing's sarcoma family of tumours (ESFT) 171–9
  immunohistochemistry 173
  nosology 142
  renal 232–3
Perlman syndrome 90
Peutz Jeghers syndrome, and familial thyroid cancer 301
pH
  concentration 34
  fixatives 29–30
phaeochromocytoma 84, 306–7
Philadelphia chromosome 7
picric acid fixatives 33
placental alkaline phosphatase 249, 257
plasma cell granuloma 206
Pollitt syndrome 79
polyacrylamide gel electrophoresis (PAGE) 59
polyembryoma **256**
polymerase chain reaction (PCR) 128, 137–8
  microsatellite *see* microsatellite
polymorphisms 63
predisposition syndromes 74–93
primitive neuroectodermal tumours (PNETs)
  cerebral 136, 137, **143**, 171–85
    cell kinetic analysis 144
    and cerebellar 142–3
    molecular genetic analysis 144
primordial germ cells 248, 249
probes
  cocktail 44–5
  DNA 38
  FISH, use 43
  minor groove binder 66
  Taq Man 64–6
  three color fusion, use 43
profiling techniques, future applications 52–3
progressive transformation of germinal centers (PTGC) 125, **126**
protein fixation 27–8

pseudolipoblasts 208
pseudopalisading necrosis 140
pseudorosettes 174
pseudotumor, inflammatory 206, 275

radiation
   and lymphomas 117
   risk factor for papillary thyroid cancer 300–1
RAR alpha rearrangements 108–9
recombinant DNA testing 63
Reed Sternberg cell 117, 122–3, 125, 127, 131
renal cell carcinoma 232
renal neoplasms 217–37
   classification 217
   primary *218*
   staging 217–18
      criteria *218*
restriction endonucleases 56
RET proto-oncogene 83–5
retinoblastoma 149, **150–1**
   and osteosarcoma 241
retinoids 288
reverse transcriptase polymerase chain reaction *see* RT-PCR
Revised European-American Lymphoma classification (REAL) 117
rhabdoid tumor 269–70
   extrarenal 211
   kidney 217, **230–1**
      genetics 231
      pathologic features 230–1
      treatment and prognosis 231
   malignant (MRT) 148–9
rhabdomyofibrosarcoma 205
rhabdomyosarcoma 186–98, 255, 270
   alveolar 189–**90**
   botryoid subtype of embryonal **188**
   classical embryonal 188–9
   classification *187*
   cytogenetics 191–2
   DNA ploidy 191
   electron microscopy 191
   embryonal **189**
   genetic predisposition 186
   immunohistochemistry 190–1
   molecular genetics 191–2
   prognostic factors 192
   spindle cell type of embryonal **188**
   staging *187*
   treatment strategies 192–3
RNA
   amplification, Taq Man PCR 64–6
   EBER 302
   extraction protocols 25
Roberts syndrome 186
rosettes 156, 174
Rothmund Thomson syndrome 90
round cell tumor
   desmoplastic small (DSRCT) 206–7
   G-band karyotype **207**
round cell tumor (RCT), small, of childhood 15
RT-PCR 158
   characterization, gene translocation 25
   tissue-specific mRNA identification 26
   tumour cells
      in bone marrow aspirates 27
      detection in blood **26–7**
   tumour-specific gene rearrangements 26
Rubinstein Taybi syndrome 90, 186

S101 protein 138
sacrococcygeal tumours 260
St Jude's lymphoma staging system *119*
salivary gland carcinoma 307, **308–9**
Sanger method, DNA sequencing 67, **68–9**
sarcoma amplified sequence (SAS) gene 243
satellite sequences 58
Schiller Duval bodies **255**
Schwachmann's syndrome 96
Schwannian stroma *see* neuroblastoma
schwannoma
   epithelioid malignant 204
   glandular malignant 204
seminoma 254
sertoli cell factor 249
severe combined immunodeficiency syndrome (SCID) 81, 117
sex steroids in hepatocellular neoplasms 265–6
short nucleotide polymorphisms 58
   uses in pathology 60–3
sialoblastoma 307
Simpson Golabi Behmel syndrome 87
slot blot 57–8
soft tissue tumors 199–216
   histologic category distribution *200*
Southern blot 63
   analysis 56–7, 128
spectral karyotyping (SKY) 38, 43–7
   assay 45, **46–7**
Spitz naevus *see* naevus
subependymal giant cell tumor (SEGT) **146–7**
supportive care 4–**5**, 11–12
sustentacular cells 307
synaptophysin 138–9
synovial sarcoma 199–202, **203**
   biphasic **202**
   cell types 200–1
   cytogenetic studies 202
   monophasic spindle cell 201, 205
   renal 233

T-cell leukaemia *see* leukaemia
T-cell receptor (TCR) gene 103
Taq Man
   PCR 64–6
      allelic discrimination **66**
      probe chemistry 64, **65**–6

TEL-AML 1 fusion gene t 102
telomerase activity 283–4
temperature in fixation 30
tendons, clear cell sarcoma 210
teratoma
　CNS 261
　cytogenetics 250
　immature (IT) 247, 253–4
　ovarian 258
　pathology 253–4
　and yolk sac tumour 260
testicular feminisation syndrome and germ cell tumour
　　risk 248
testis, germ cell tumours 259
thermocycling 59
thyroid carcinoma 299–302
　familial 301
　follicular 300–2
　medullary 301–2
　papillary 299–300
tissue
　cryopreservation 24–7
　fixative penetration 30
　handling 15–17
　preservation 23
　secondary changes 31
tissue arrays, suppliers 53
topotecan 8
transforming growth factor alpha 265
transforming growth factor *beta*, and nasopharyngeal
　　carcinoma 304
trichothiodystrophy 79
trisomy *see* cytogenetics
Triton tumor, malignant 204
tuberous sclerosis and liver tumors 266
tumour/tumor lysis syndrome 116
tumour/tumor markers 6
　serological 257
tyrosinemia, hereditary, and liver tumours *see*
　　cytogenetics

undifferentiated sarcoma 267–8
US National Cancer Institute Surveillance,
　　Epidemiology and End-Result (SEER)
　　program 264

vanillylmandelic acid 161, 307
variable number of tandem repeats (VNTRs) 61, **63**
vimentin 138, 175, 190, 233, 302
virilization 305
von Hippel Lindau syndrome 85

WAGR syndrome 89
　intralobar nephrogenic rest with 221–2
　and Wilms' tumour 218
West Midlands Regional Children's Tumor
　　Registry 264, 275
Western blot 57
WHO (World Health Organization)
　germ cell tumour classification 252
　lymphoma classification 117
　nasopharyngeal carcinoma classification 302
Wilms' tumour/tumor 89–90, 218–25
　anaplastic **220–1**
　cystic partially differentiated 220
　familial 223
　genetics 221–4
　malformations in 3
　pathology **219–20**
　prognosis 224–5
　teratoid 219
　therapy 224
Wiskott-Aldrich syndrome 117
WT-1 gene 222–3

xanthoastrocytoma, pleomorphic (PXA) 140–1
xeroderma pigmentosum 78, 309

yolk sac tumour 247, 254, **255**, 260
　hepatoid 248
　histology 255
　testicular 259